Endocrine Replacement Therapy

in Clinical Practice

CONTEMPORARY ENDOCRINOLOGY

P. Michael Conn, SERIES EDITOR

ENDOCRINE REPLACEMENT THERAPY IN CLINICAL PRACTICE

Edited by

A. WAYNE MEIKLE, MD

*University of Utah School of Medicine
and ARUP Laboratory
Salt Lake City, UT*

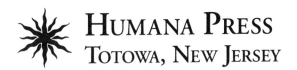

HUMANA PRESS
TOTOWA, NEW JERSEY

BS

Production Editor: Robin B. Weisberg.
Cover Design: Patricia F. Cleary.

Photocopy Authorization Policy:
Authorization to photocopy items for internal or personal use, or the internal or personal use of specific clients, is granted by Humana Press Inc., provided that the base fee of US $20.00 per copy is paid directly to the Copyright Clearance Center at 222 Rosewood Drive, Danvers, MA 01923. For those organizations that have been granted a photocopy license from the CCC, a separate system of payment has been arranged and is acceptable to Humana Press Inc. The fee code for users of the Transactional Reporting Service is: [1-58829-195-2/03 $20.00].

Printed in the United States of America. 10 9 8 7 6 5 4 3 2 1

Endocrine replacement therapy in clinical practice /edited by A. Wayne Meikle.
    p. cm.—(Contemporary endocrinology)
    Includes bibliographical references and index.
    ISBN 1-58829-195-2 (alk. paper); 1-59259-375-5 (e-ISBN)
    1. Hormone therapy. 2. Endocrine glands—Diseases—Hormone therapy. I. Meikle, A. Wayne. II. Contemporary endocrinology (Totowa, NJ).
RM286 .E53 2003
615'.36—dc21   2002032873

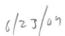
6/23/04

PREFACE

Endocrine Replacement Therapy in Clinical Practice, an update of *Hormone Replacement Therapy* published by Humana Press in 1999, aims to assist the endocrinologist, gynecologist, pediatrician, urologist, general surgeon, neurologist, neurosurgeon, psychiatrist, generalist, and trainee in management of their patients with hormonal deficiencies or altered hormonal synthesis or responses. Many new authors have added several new chapters, and all of the previous chapters have been updated. Endocrine testing used to diagnose endocrine disorders and monitor hormone replacement therapy is reviewed. However, detailed discussion of physiology and pathophysiology is not an aim of this book, and these topics are covered in other volumes on endocrinology. Although no one is considered an expert in all areas of endocrine replacement therapy, each of the authors here have extensive knowledge and experience in the management of patients with specific endocrine disorders requiring hormone replacement treatment.

Although some differences of opinion exist among experts in replacement therapy, each writer has attempted to give a balanced, unbiased recommendation. When comparable regimens exist, the authors have made this apparent to the reader who can then choose the best treatment for the individual patient. Cost, therapeutic effectiveness, and route of administration are all important considerations in making the final selection of replacement therapy.

Endocrine Replacement Therapy in Clinical Practice is divided into seven main sections covering hormone replacement therapy of the pituitary, parathyroid and vitamin D, thyroid, diabetes, adrenal, gonads of men, and gonads of women. In Part I, the management of diabetes insipidus and polydipsia in children is reviewed by Donald Zimmerman and Greg Uramoto and the treatment of diabetes insipidus in adults is covered by Gary Robertson and Andjela Drincic. Darrell Wilson covers growth hormone therapy with emphasis on growth disorders of children, and George Merriam focuses on growth hormone and growth hormone secretagogues in adults.

In Part II, issues related to treatment of disorders of calcium metabolism caused by diseases affecting parathyroid hormone and vitamin D are presented by Eric Orwoll. In Part III, Steven Sherman and Luis Lopez-Penabad's discussion on the use of thyroid-stimulating hormone in the diagnosis and management of thyroid diseases, including thyroid cancer, provides invaluable perspectives. David Cooper reviews current guidelines for thyroid hormone replacement therapy in patients with primary and secondary hypothyroidism. Special issues related to thyroid hormone replacement therapy in children with congenital and acquired hypothyroidism are reviewed by Stephen LaFranchi and thyroid hormone replacement during pregnancy is discussed by Amy Sullivan and T. Flint Porter.

Part IV includes six chapters discussing various aspects of hormone replacement therapy of diabetes. Dana Hardin focuses on the diagnosis and management of diabetes in children, while Donald McClain reviews insulin and oral agents in the treatment of type 2 diabetes. The special issues of management of diabetes during pregnancy are presented by Kay McFarland, Laura Irwin, and Janice Bacon. Raymond Plodkowski and Steven Edelman report on their expertise using insulin pump therapy. In her chapter, Susan Braithwaite develops an algorithm for diabetic therapy during glucocorticoid treatment of nonendocrine disease. The unique problems of treatment of the diabetic during exercise are summarized by Robert Jones.

Part V consists of three chapters. The first is by Lynnette Nieman and Kristina Rother and covers glucocorticoid therapy for prenatal and postnatal life. Robert Dluhy summarizes therapy of mineralocorticoid deficiency disorders; and Syed Tariq, Hosam Kamel, and John Morley carefully analyze the pros and cons for dehydroepiandrosterone and pregnenolone therapy.

Part VI has six chapters covering sex hormone replacement issues in men. A. Wayne Meikle details issues relating to androgen replacement therapy in children and men with androgen deficiency. The influence of androgen replacement therapy on sexual behavior, affect, and cognition is presented by Max Hirshkowitz, Claudia Orengo, and Glenn Cunningham. J. Lisa Tenover summarizes the merits and safety issues associated with testosterone therapy in older men. Shalender Bhasin, Atam Singh, Keith Beck, and Linda Woodhouse present the rationale and recommendations for androgen therapy in men with muscle-wasting disorders, particularly as related to AIDS. Christina Wang and Ronald S. Swerdloff discuss hormonal contraception, which is becoming more commonly used in men and requires hormonal therapy to suppress spermatogenesis while maintaining normal testosterone concentrations. Peter Liu and David Handelsman contribute an article on the status of hormonal therapy of the infertile man.

Part VII contains three chapters that focus on sex hormone replacement issues in women. Daren Watts, Howard Sharp, and C. Matthew Peterson make recommendations for hormone replacement therapy in women with primary and secondary hypogonadism. Androgen replacement therapy in women is still somewhat controversial, but is becoming more accepted. Susan Davis and Henry Burger present a rational basis for androgen therapy in women. Shahar Kol focuses on hormonal therapy of the infertile women.

Students, fellows, residents, generalists, and specialists in many disciplines will find *Endocrine Replacement Therapy in Clinical Practice* a highly practical reference for the management of patients. Patients will greatly benefit by receiving the best regimen for managing their hormonal deficits.

I express thanks to the distinguished, willing, and internationally recognized authors who accepted the invitation to share their expertise. Susan Brown provided invaluable assistance in correspondence and compilation of the manuscripts. My sincere thanks to Dr. P. Michael Conn for his trust and encouragement in making the project a reality and to the Editorial Director, Paul Dolgert, and to Craig Adams of Humana Press for their helpful suggestions.

A. Wayne Meikle, MD

CONTENTS

CONTRIBUTORS

JANICE BACON, MD, *Department of Obstetrics and Gynecology, University of South Carolina School of Medicine, Columbia, SC*

KEITH BECK, MD, *Division of Endocrinology, Metabolism, and Molecular Medicine, Charles R. Drew University of Medicine and Science, Los Angeles, CA*

SHALENDER BHASIN, MD, *Department of Medicine, Division of Endocrinology, Metabolism, and Molecular Medicine, Charles R. Drew University of Medicine and Science, Los Angeles, CA*

SUSAN S. BRAITHWAITE, MD, *UNC Diabetes Care Center, University of North Carolina, Durham, NC*

HENRY G. BURGER, MD, FRACP, *Prince Henry's Institute of Medical Research, Monash Medical Center, Clayton, Victoria, Australia*

DAVID S. COOPER, MD, *Division of Endocrinology, Sinai Hospital of Baltimore and Thyroid Clinic, Johns Hopkins Hospital, Johns Hopkins University School of Medicine, Baltimore, MD*

DAVID E. CUMMINGS, MD, *Division of Metabolism, Endocrinology, and Nutrition, Department of Medicine, University of Washington School of Medicine, Veterans Affairs Puget Sound Health Care System, Seattle, WA*

GLENN R. CUNNINGHAM, MD, *Department of Research and Development, Houston Veterans Affairs Medical Center and Departments of Medicine, Molecular and Cellular Biology, Baylor College of Medicine, Houston, TX*

SUSAN R. DAVIS, MBBS, FRACP, PhD, *The Jean Hailes Foundation, Clayton, Australia*

ROBERT G. DLUHY, MD, *Endocrine-Hypertension Division, Brigham and Women's Hospital, Harvard Medical School, Boston, MA*

ANDJELA T. DRINCIC, MD, *Division of Endocrinology, Department of Internal Medicine, VA Nebraska-Western Iowa Health Care System, Department of Veterans Affairs, Grand Island, NE*

STEVEN V. EDELMAN, MD, *Division of Endocrinology and Metabolism, University of California San Diego and VA San Diego Healthcare, San Diego, CA*

DAVID J. HANDELSMAN, MBBS, FRACP, PhD, *Department of Andrology, Concord Hospital and ANZAC Research Institute, University of Sydney, Sydney, Australia*

DANA S. HARDIN, MD, *Division of Endocrinology, Department of Pediatrics, University of Texas-Southwestern Medical School, Dallas, TX*

MAX HIRSHKOWITZ, PhD, *Sleep Disorder Center, Department of Medicine, Houston Veterans Affairs Medical Center and Departments of Psychiatry and Medicine, Baylor College of Medicine, Houston, TX*

LAURA S. IRWIN, MD, *Department of Obstetrics and Gynecology, Medical College of Georgia, Augusta, GA*

ROBERT E. JONES, MD, *Division of Endocrinology, Metabolism and Diabetes, Department of Internal Medicine, University of Utah School of Medicine, Salt Lake City, UT*

HOSAM KAMEL, MD, *Division of Geriatric Medicine, Medical College of Wisconsin and GRECC VA Medical Center, Milwaukee, WI*

SHAHAR KOL, MD, *Department of Obstetrics and Gynecology, Rambam Medical Center, Haifa, Israel*

STEPHEN LAFRANCHI, MD, *Division of Endocrinology, Department of Pediatrics, Oregon Health and Sciences University and School of Medicine, Portland, OR*

PETER Y. LIU, MBBS, FRACP, *Department of Andrology, Concord Hospital and ANZAC Research Institute, University of Sydney, Sydney, Australia*

LUIS LOPEZ-PENABAD, MD, *Department of Endocrine Neoplasia and Hormonal Disorders, University of Texas M.D. Anderson Cancer Center, Houston, TX*

DONALD A. MCCLAIN, MD, PhD, *Division of Endocrinology, Diabetes and Metabolism, Department of Internal Medicine, University of Utah School of Medicine, Salt Lake City, UT*

KAY F. MCFARLAND, MD, *Department of Medicine, University of South Carolina School of Medicine, Columbia, SC*

A. WAYNE MEIKLE, MD, *Division of Endocrinology, Diabetes and Metabolism, Departments of Medicine and Pathology, University of Utah School of Medicine and ARUP Laboratory, Salt Lake City, UT*

GEORGE R. MERRIAM, MD, *Division of Metabolism, Endocrinology, and Nutrition, Department of Medicine, University of Washington School of Medicine, Veterans Affairs Puget Sound Health Care System, Seattle, WA*

JOHN E. MORLEY, MB, BCh, *Division of Geriatric Medicine, Saint Louis University School of Medicine and GRECC VA Medical Center, St. Louis, MO*

LYNNETTE K. NIEMAN, MD, *Pediatric and Reproductive Endocrinology Branch, National Institute of Child Health and Human Development, NIH, Bethesda, MD*

CLAUDIA A. ORENGO, MD, PhD, *South Central Mental Illness Research, Education, and Clinical Center, Houston Veterans Affairs Medical Center and Department of Psychiatry and Behavioral Sciences, Baylor College of Medicine, Houston, TX*

ERIC S. ORWOLL, MD, *Department of Medicine, Oregon Health and Sciences University and Medical Service, Portland Veterans Affairs Medical Center, Portland, OR*

C. MATTHEW PETERSON, MD, FACOG, *Division of Reproductive Endocrinology and Infertility, Department of Obstetrics and Gynecology, University of Utah Medical Center, Salt Lake City, UT*

RAYMOND A. PLODKOWSKI, MD, *Division of Endocrinology, Diabetes, and Metabolism, University of Nevada School of Medicine, Reno and Sierra Nevada Veterans Affairs Medical Center, Reno NV*

T. FLINT PORTER, MD, *Division of Maternal-Fetal Medicine, Department of Obstetrics and Gynecology, University of Utah School of Medicine, Salt Lake City, UT*

GARY L. ROBERTSON, MD, *Division of Endocrinology and Metabolism, Northwestern University Medical School, Chicago, IL*

KRISTINA I. ROTHER, MD, *Transplant and Autoimmunity Branch, National Institute of Diabetes, Digestive and Kidney Diseases, NIH, Bethesda, MD*

HOWARD T. SHARP, MD, *Department of Obstetrics and Gynecology, University of Utah Medical Center, Salt Lake City, UT*

STEVEN I. SHERMAN, MD, *Department of Endocrine Neoplasia and Hormonal Disorders, University of Texas M.D. Anderson Cancer Center, Houston, TX*

ATAM B. SINGH, MD, *Division of Endocrinology, Metabolism, and Molecular Medicine, Charles R. Drew University of Medicine and Science, Los Angeles, CA*

AMY E. SULLIVAN, MD, *Division of Maternal-Fetal Medicine, Department of Obstetrics and Gynecology, University of Utah School of Medicine, Salt Lake City, UT*

RONALD S. SWERDLOFF, MD, *Division of Endocrinology, Department of Medicine, Harbor-UCLA Medical Center, UCLA School of Medicine, Torrance, CA*

SYED H. TARIQ, MD, *Division of Geriatric Medicine, Saint Louis University School of Medicine and GRECC VA Medical Center, St. Louis, MO*

J. LISA TENOVER, MD, PhD, *Division of Geriatric Medicine and Gerontology, Department of Medicine, Emory University School of Medicine, Atlanta, GA*

GREG URAMOTO, MD, *Department of Pediatrics, Mayo Clinic, Mayo Medical School, Rochester, MN*

CHRISTINA WANG, MD, *Department of Medicine and Clinical Research Center, Harbor-UCLA Medical Center, UCLA School of Medicine, Torrance, CA*

DAREN A. WATTS, MD, *Department of Obstetrics and Gynecology, University of Utah Medical Center, Salt Lake City, UT*

DARRELL M. WILSON, MD, *Department of Pediatric Endocrinology and Diabetes, Stanford University Medical Center, Stanford, CA*

LINDA WOODHOUSE, PhD, *Division of Endocrinology, Metabolism, and Molecular Medicine, Charles R. Drew University of Medicine and Science, Los Angeles, CA*

DONALD ZIMMERMAN, MD, *Department of Pediatrics, The Feinberg School of Medicine, Northwestern University, Chicago, IL*

I   PITUITARY

1

Diabetes Insipidus in Pediatrics

Donald Zimmerman, MD and Greg Uramoto, MD

CONTENTS

INTRODUCTION

Separate mechanisms supply and eliminate water to maintain fluid homeostasis. A variety of sensors modulate thirst to drive water-seeking behavior and water intake. The elimination of water is achieved via hormonal control of the kidney. To ensure that a healthy fluid balance is maintained, the mechanisms that accrue water can compensate for defects in the mechanisms that eliminate water and vice versa. Clinical problems arise when the capacity for this compensation is exceeded or when such compensation becomes unduly demanding.

When water losses increase for any reason, adults and children will drink more water in response to thirst if access to water is not limited. In this way, increased water intake can balance obligatory water outputs such as sweating or even mild diabetes. Infants, however, face unique problems with their inability to control their own water intake and with their reliance on fluids to meet both water and caloric needs. Compounding this problem, infants cannot differentially communicate thirst, hunger, pain, and other messages. Because of the inability of infants to precisely control their water intake, the mechanisms of water elimination primarily maintain their water balance. Problems with their elimination systems, therefore, rapidly lead to clinical problems. As infants mature into ambulatory and communicative children, their control over their water intake improves and problems with water balance resemble those found in adults.

In this chapter, we discuss the hormonal aspects of water balance and the problems that arise in this balance with emphasis on the pediatric population.

From: *Endocrine Replacement Therapy in Clinical Practice*
Edited by: A. Wayne Meikle © Humana Press Inc., Totowa, NJ

ANATOMY AND PHYSIOLOGY

Water Consumption

THIRST INDUCTION

The driving force behind water intake is the sensation of thirst. Consumed water replaces fluid losses to maintain the osmolality of body fluids and to increase the vascular volume. No receptors found to date directly sense the absolute volume of the vascular space. This critical parameter is inferred from several indicators, including the tonicity of the blood *(1)* and blood pressure *(2)*. Inputs that influence thirst include baroreceptors of the cardiovascular system, osmoreceptors of the hypothalamus, and, possibly, osmoreceptors of the viscera. The sensation of thirst is mediated, at least in part, by angiotensin II or a molecule that is similar to this peptide. Receptors that bind with angiotensin can be found in the lamina terminalis and other areas of the brain that are associated with fluid homeostasis and with hemodynamic control *(3)*. Stimulation of these receptors is associated with increased thirst. Closely tied to the sensation of thirst is the appetite for salt (sodium). This is the most active osmotic ion in the extracellular space and greatly influences the fluid shifts between the intracellular and extracellular spaces *(4)*.

Although only partially understood, several conditions contribute to the induction and suppression of this sensation. Increasing the serum osmolality by 1–2% or decreasing the plasma volume by 10% increases thirst. Plasma osmolalities above 290 mOsmol/kg have been strongly associated with the desire to drink *(5)*. The systemic infusion of solutes that do not easily traverse cell membranes like sodium chloride and sucrose will influence thirst more than permeable solutes like urea and glycerol. This probably reflects cellular fluid shifts between the intracellular and extracellular fluid spaces.

THIRST SUPPRESSION

Thirst is suppressed by decreasing plasma osmolality by 1–2% or by increasing plasma volume by 10%. Drinking water will suppress thirst before the serum osmolality decreases. Gastrointestinal (GI) stretch receptors convey a sense of fullness that inhibits thirst. In addition, temperature receptors in the oropharynx will inhibit thirst and vasopressin release when they are cooled *(6)*.

The stimuli for water-seeking behavior are related to the vascular fullness and to the osmolality of the plasma. Inhibitors of thirst, however, cannot be exclusively tied to these parameters because of the lag time between drinking water, absorbing water, and the desired effects on vascular volume and osmolality. If the drive to drink water was inhibited only when the vascular space was affected, a large amount of water may be consumed. To prevent this, other mechanisms, including oropharyngeal temperature receptors and GI stretch receptors, help to inhibit thirst more promptly. The subject of thirst and sodium hunger is complex. For a more thorough review, *see* refs. *3* and *4*.

Water Excretion

OVERVIEW

As organisms took to the land and as access to water became more restricted, opportunities to drink became more periodic. The intermittent acquisition of water necessitated a system that could dispose of water at controlled rates to keep the serum osmolality within a narrow window. The kidneys, under endocrine control, can excrete very dilute and very concentrated urine to accomplish this vital task. The hormone in large part responsible for this endocrine control is arginine vasopressin (AVP). To conserve water by concentrating the urine, AVP increases the permeability of the collecting duct and thus allows the osmotic gradient in the renal medulla to draw free water out of the filtrate flowing through these ducts. Drawing free water from these ducts concentrates the urine and saves this water for physiologic needs.

Under physiological conditions, AVP adjusts the water output of the kidney and helps to preserve both plasma osmolality and vascular volume. Conserving water in the vascular space by limiting the kidney excretion of water is important but not sufficient to maintain the vascular volume; osmotic pressure may draw free water out of the vascular space and into the tissues. The most important solute in maintaining the osmolarity of the serum, sodium, is conserved via the renin–angiotensin–aldosterone pathways. Working together, AVP and aldosterone help to maintain the serum volume and osmolality. The interaction between these pathways provides physiologic flexibility and allows for fine control of the system.

AVP PRODUCTION AND RELEASE

The gene for vasopressin has been localized to chromosome region 20p13 *(7,8)* (*see* Fig. 1). Expression of this 2.5-kb prepro-AVP-neuropressin (NP) II gene occurs in the magnocellular neurons of the hypothalamic and paraventricular nuclei in the hypothalamus. The gene consists of three exons and two introns that code for a macromolecular protein that contains vasopressin. This macromolecular protein is cleaved at dibasic amino acid sites by trypsin-like cleavage as the molecule travels down the pituitary stalk in secretory granules. Along with vasopressin, this macromolecular protein contains a signal peptide, neurophysin II-binding protein, and a glycoprotein of uncertain function called copeptin. Upon reaching the posterior pituitary, the AVP nonapeptide is ready for release (*see* Fig. 2).

Arginine vasopressin is comprised of a 6-amino-acid disulfide ring plus a 3-amino-acid tail that has an amide group attached to the carboxy terminus. This molecule is evolutionarily related to oxytocin, differing in two amino acids but retaining the disulfide ring. Vasopressin is bound to neurophysin II while stored in the neurohypophysis. The function of this combination is still under investigation, but it has been hypothesized that the binding of neurophysin to vasopressin conveys some protection against degradation.

Vasopressin release is mediated by a stimulus-release coupling mechanism commonly found in many types of neurons. The action potential stimulus for the release of vasopressin permits the influx of extracellular calcium. This influx, in turn, stimulates the movement of the stored granules to the cell membrane and subsequent exocytosis.

STIMULI OF AVP RELEASE

Argine vasopressin allows for the reabsorption of water at the level of the kidney. The blood tonicity, the blood pressure, and the blood volume estimate the need for more or less water reabsorption. These parameters, then, logically influence AVP release.

The tonicity of the blood is sensed by osmoreceptors of the anterolateral hypothalamus near the supraoptic nuclei in the anterolateral hypothalamus *(9)* (*see* Fig. 3). These osmoreceptors are functionally outside of the blood-brain barrier as evidenced by the measurement of similar serum levels of AVP in response to changing the serum tonicity

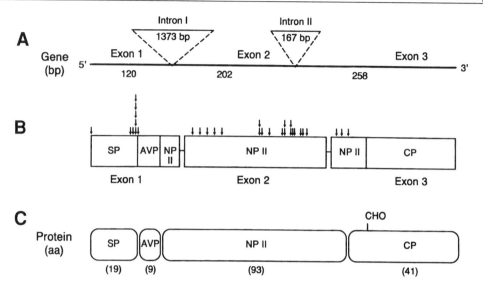

Fig. 1. Arginine vasopressin–neurophysin II–copeptin gene on chromosome 20. (**A**) Introns and exons. Exon 1 codes for a signal peptide (SP), arginine vasopressin (AVP), and the N-terminus of neurophysin II (NPII). Exon 2 codes for most of NPII. Exon 3 codes for the C-terminus of NPII and copeptin (CP). (**B**) The positions of known mutations in the gene. (**C**) Gene product. The signal peptide, AVP, neurophysin, and the glycopeptide (copeptin) are cleaved from this precurser.

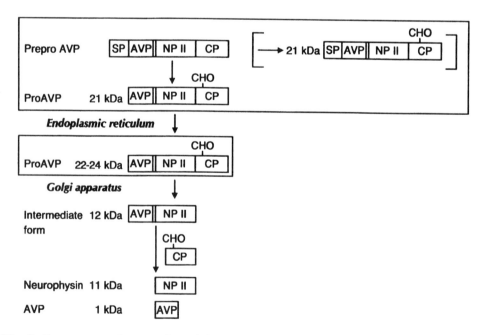

Fig. 2. Compartmental processing of the prepo-AVP–NPII–CP gene product. Prepo-AVP is converted to pro-AVP by removal of the signal peptide and the addition of carbohydrate side chains in the endoplasmic reticulum. Pro-AVP that is partially glycosylated in the endoplasmic reticulum is further glycosylated in the Golgi apparatus. The glycosylated portion, copeptin, is cleaved in the process of axonal transport in secretory vesicles. Upon reaching the posterior pituitary, vasopressin is available for release into the bloodstream.

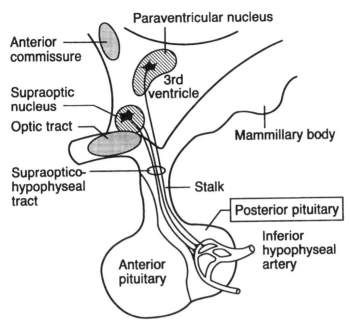

Fig. 3. Anatomy of the hypothalamus and the pituitary. Magnocellular neurons of the supraoptic and paraventricular nuclei extend down the supraopticohypophyseal tract and synapse with capillaries of the posterior pituitary.

with urea versus sodium. These receptors synapse with both the paraventricular (PVN) and supraoptic (SON) nuclei to influence the release of AVP from the magnocellular neurons in these nuclei. The amount of AVP released in response to the osmolality of the serum is precisely controlled. Under physiologic conditions, vasopressin blood levels rise linearly in response to rising serum osmolalities after a minimum set point of serum osmolality is reached. This set point of AVP release has been shown to be approx 275 mOsm/kg (10). Studies have shown that AVP rises approx 1 pg/mL for every 3 mOsm/kg above this threshold for vasopressin release. The levels of vasopressin are also influenced by diurnal variations in older children with nighttime vasopressin levels that are approximately two to three times higher than daytime levels (11). Released in response to increasing serum tonicity, AVP will induce more water conservation through the kidney and, thus, counteract the rising serum tonicity.

Blood pressure changes contribute to the release of AVP via the high-pressure barore-ceptors of the aortic arch and the carotid sinuses. The baroreceptors of the aortic arch and the carotid sinuses send projections to the SON and the PVN via cranial nerves IX and X (12). Signals from these pressure receptors are first routed through the nucleus tractus solitarious in the brainstem. Neurons from this nucleus then synapse with the supraoptic and paraventricular nuclei and tonically inhibit vasopressin release. Under normal physiologic conditions, these neurons tonically inhibit AVP release. Blood pressure decreases of 5–15% will lead to an exponential increase in vasopressin levels as a result of barore-ceptor stimulation (13). This is unlike the linear increase in vasopressin levels in response changes in osmolality described earlier (see Fig. 4). The levels of AVP found in hypotensive states will far exceed the 5 pg/mL needed for maximal antidiuresis. AVP concentrations in this range will induce vasoconstriction via the V1 receptor on the vascular smooth muscle and will help to support the falling blood pressure. The true physiologic importance of this effect is not yet clear (14).

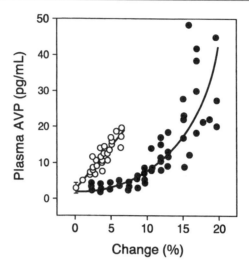

Fig. 4. Relationship between osmotic and nonosmotic stimuli for vasopressin release. Relationship of plasma AVP concentration to the percent increase in blood osmolality (open circles) or decrease in blood volume (closed circles).

Stretch receptors of the left atrium respond to changes in atrial blood volume. Like the baroreceptors of the aortic arch and the carotid sinuses, these stretch receptors induce vasopressin release during hypovolemic states. The influence of these neurons, however, is thought to be less important than the baroreceptors of the carotid sinuses and the aortic arch.

Nausea increases vasopressin levels above those needed for maximum antidiuresis. Nausea resulting from motion sickness, drugs, or illness can increase vasopressin levels 100-fold. The mechanism for this vasopressin release in these settings seems to be unrelated to the mechanisms that mediate vasopressin release as a result of changes in blood pressure and blood osmolality. Blockade of nausea with antiemetics will not suppress the vasopressin response to hypovolemia and hypernatremia.

Vasopressin release is inhibited by glucocorticoids. Patients illustrate this modulating effect with glucocorticoid deficiency when vasopressin is "inappropriately" released *(15)*. The mechanism for this tonic inhibition of vasopressin by glucocorticoids remains elusive. Studies in transgenic mice implicate the involvement of a proximal cis-acting element that is suppressed by glucocorticoid action *(16)*.

RESPONSE TO AVP

The kidneys respond to serum vasopressin via the V_2 receptor. The binding of vasopressin to this receptor induces an incorporation of aquaporin-2 molecules into the luminal membrane of the collecting ducts. This incorporation creates water channels through the walls of the collecting duct that allow water to flow down the concentration gradient in the renal medulla *(17,18)* *(see* Fig. 5). This flow draws free water out of the filtrate in the collecting ducts and thus concentrates the urine. These aquaporin-2 molecules are a part of a family of membrane proteins that are responsible for channel-mediated water transport. They are stored in the membranes of intracytoplasmic vesicles until these vesicles are incorporated into the cellular membranes via an exocytotic process. Without the stimulation of AVP, membrane endocytosis pulls these transmem-

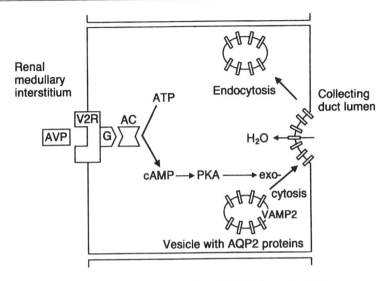

Fig. 5. Action of AVP in the collecting duct cell. AVP binds to the V2 receptor, causing the G-protein to activate adenylate cyclase (AC), resulting in an increase in cAMP and activation of protein kinase A (PKA). The catalytic subunit of PKA, via an undetermined phosphorylation step, causes fusion of membrane bodies bearing aquaporin-2 (AQP2) water channel and VAMP2 with the collecting duct luminal membrane, resulting in an increase in water flow from the urine into the renal medullary interstium. Demeclocycline, lithium, high calcium, and low potassium interfere with these processes, possibly at the level of cAMP generation and AQP2 synthesis or action.

brane proteins back into intracytoplasmic vesicles. The incorporation and removal of aquaporins from the luminal surface via exocytosis and endocytosis comprises a membrane shuttle mechanism.

DIABETES INSIPIDUS

The term *diabetes insipidus* (DI) is applied to conditions in which patients produce high volumes of dilute and glucose-free urine. DI may arise from different underlying causes. A lack of AVP secretion is usually called neurogenic, cranial, central or hypothalamic DI. A failure to respond to circulating AVP is called nephrogenic DI. Excessive water intake resulting from a lesion in the thirst centers is called dipsogenic DI. Excessive water intake as a result of psychosis or other mental illnesses is called psychogenic DI. Finally, symptoms of DI associated with pregnancy and a physiologically higher metabolism of AVP is called gestational DI. Moreover, patients may have only a partial defect in either their production or response to AVP. Each of the categories just listed can be further subdivided:

Neurogenic:
　Idiopathic
　Hypothalamic or pituitary lesion
　　Head trauma/surgical trauma
　　Central Nervous System (CNS) infection
　　Lymphocytic infundibulohypophysitis
　　Ischemia

    Mass lesion
       Germinoma
       Craniopharyngioma
       Hematoma
    Infiltrative lesion
       Langerhans cell histiocytosis
       Neurosarcoidosis
  Familial
    Autosomal dominant
    X-linked recessive
    Part of other syndrome
       Diabetes insipidus, diabetes mellitus, optic atropy, and neurosensory deafness
       (DIDMOAD)
Nephrogenic:
  Idiopathic
  Kidney lesion
    Nephrocalcinosis
    Obstructive uropathy
    Medullary cystic disease
    Sickle cell disease
  Drugs
    Lithium
    Rifampin
    Aminoglycosides
    Acetohexamide
    Vinblastine
    Cisplatin
    Methoxyflurane
  Electrolyte abnormalities
    Hypokalemia
    Hypercalcemia
  Familial
    X-linked recessive: V_2 receptor
    Autosomal recessive: aquaporin II
    Autosomal recessive and mitochondrial DIDMOAD
Dipsogenic:
  Idiopathic
  Hypothalamic lesion
    Head trauma
    Drugs
       Lithium
       Carbamazepine
    Infection
       Tuberculosis
    Mass lesion
       Germinoma
    Infiltrative lesion
       Neurosarcoid
       Langerhans cell histiocytosis

Psychogenic:
    Compulsive water drinking
    Schizophrenia

Pathology of DI

Problems with either vasopressin production or vasopressin response can lead to DI. The pathologies are divided at an anatomic level according to the site of the defect.

Neurogenic Diabetes Insipidus

The pathologies involved in neurogenic DI are quite varied. Any lesion that damages the neurons that produce and release vasopressin will lead to DI. In broad cateories, these lesions include trauma, surgical damage, mass lesions, and infiltrative lesions. Of particular interest are the genetically transmitted forms of the disease. In patients with this pathology, vasopressin-producing neurons selectively degenerate, leaving the rest of the brain intact *(19)*. The genetic defects are in the AVP-NPII gene on chromosome 20. The mutations isolated to date mainly cluster within the coding sequences of either the signal peptide of the precursor or within the coding sequence for neurophysin II *(20,21)*. At the time of this writing, only one mutation in the vasopressin sequence has been described. Accumulation of the improperly cleaved molecule most likely leads to the destruction of the cells. Wolfram syndrome consists of DIDMOAD. Genetic defects have been found in the WFSI/Wolframin gene on chromosome 4p16.1, which encodes an endoglycosidase H-sensitive membrane glycoprotein, which is primarily found in endoplasmic reticulum *(22,23)*. Other genes may produce a similar phenotype. One is located on chromosome 4q22-q24 and another may be on the mitochondrial chromosome *(24,25)*. Idiopathic DI is usually sporadic, although autosomal-dominant and X-linked recessive forms have been described. The prevalence in the two sexes is approximately equal. Antibodies may be found against AVP-secreting cells in approx 30% of cases *(26)*.

Nephrogenic Diabetes Insipidus

In nephrogenic diabetes insipidus, the kidneys fail to respond to AVP. This failure can result from an inability to establish and maintain a hyperosmotic medullary interstitium or from an inability to sense the AVP signal. The osmotic gradient in the kidney is necessary to pull water from the collecting ducts in order to concentrate the urine. The collecting ducts must also be able to allow this gradient to draw water from the collecting ducts. The permeability of the collecting duct membrane is under vasopressin control.

The concentration gradient in the kidneys is generated by sodium–potassium pumps in the ascending loops of Henle. In renal failure, the kidneys may not be able to generate an effective concentration gradient. Several primary kidney diseases, including obstructive pathologies, medullary cystic disease, and infarctions may impair the kidney's ability to establish a concentration gradient. Similarly, systemic diseases such as sarcoidosis, amyloidosis, and Sjogren syndrome lead at times to DI. The loops of Henle, and the concentration gradients that they produce, are also affected in hypercalcemia and hypokalemia *(27)*. Studies in animals have shown that hypokalemia interferes with sodium transport in the thick ascending limb of the loop of Henle *(28,29)*. Recent work has suggested that a particular calcium receptor, the Ca^{2+}-sensing receptor, may play a role in water metabolism and may explain hypercalcemia-mediated DI *(30)*. In addition to influencing the concentration gradient in the kidney, hypercalcemia may also play a role in the response of the kidney to AVP *(31,32)*.

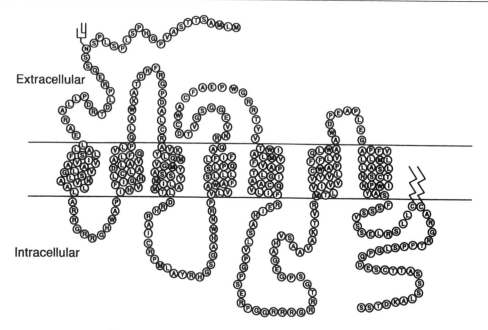

Fig. 6. Schematic representation of the V2 receptor.

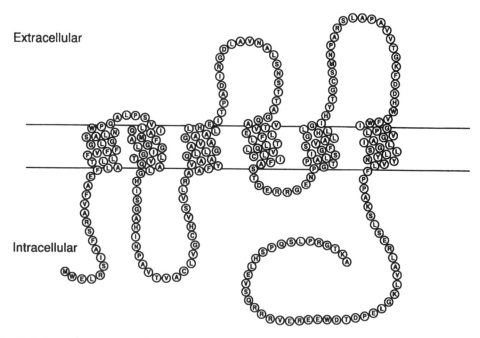

Fig. 7. Schematic representation of aquaporin-2 protein, based on the proposed topology of the rat homolog and of aquaporin-1.

A defect in the receptor for AVP can also lead to an inability to respond to AVP *(33,34)*. Familial transmission of the disorder has been reported and it most commonly manifests an X-linked dominant pattern of inheritance *(35,36)*. The females in these families manifest some degree of DI but do not have as many clinical problems as do the males. The gene involved has been localized using linkage analysis to the long arm of the X chromosome at band *(34,37,38)*. It codes for the V_2 receptor, which activates the membrane shuttle mechanism via cyclic AMP in response to arginine vasopressin.

Specific mutations in the V_2 receptor have been elucidated in patients with nephrogenic DI *(39,40)*. These can be classified into at least three distinct phenotypes *(41)* (*see* Fig. 6). In the first phenotype, the mutant receptor can be transported to the surface of the cell but is unable to combine with vasopressin. In the second phenotype, the mutant receptor may accumulate in intracellular compartments but is unable to reach the cell surface. In the third phenotype, the mutant gene is ineffectively translated or the protein is rapidly degraded.

Mutations in the gene for aquaporin-2 can also lead to nephrogenic DI (*see* Fig. 7). The family history is consistent with an autosomal recessive inheritance *(42)*. Defects in the aquaporin-2 gene have included a missense mutation *(43)* that probably result in an inability to properly transport the protein to the plasma membrane and a nonsense mutation *(44)* that results in an early stop codon for the aquaporin-2 molecule.

Evaluation of Children

The most common presenting symptoms of postinfancy DI include polyuria and polydipsia, with a preference for consuming ice-cold water. In a patient with this history, the differential diagnosis includes diabetes insipidus, diabetes mellitus, hypercalcemia, hypokalemia, renal failure, and psychogenic polydipsia. An initial screen for serum osmolality, serum electrolytes, BUN, serum glucose, and urine osmolality will aid in establishing the diagnosis of the patient. The hallmark of DI is a urine osmolality that is inappropriately low compared to the serum osmolality. In normal subjects, serum osmolalities above 295 mOsm/L will induce urine concentrations above 700 mOsm/L. In patients with partial DI, serum sodium levels greater than 143 mmol/L and serum osmolality of above 295 mOsm/L induce urine concentrations of approx 500–700 mOsm/L. Patients with complete DI will concentrate their urine to approx 250 mOsm/L or less under these conditions. To definitively establish an inability to concentrate the urine resulting from a defect in the release of vasopressin or the response to vasopressin, a water-deprivation test can be used.

WATER-DEPRIVATION TEST IN CHILDREN

The purpose of this test is to evaluate the urine osmolality in response to a slightly hyperosmolal and volume-contracted state. Under these conditions, the urine concentration should rise as free water is conserved. Before starting the test, children should be taken off of any desmopressin acetate or diuretics for at least 1 d. Children should be endocrinologically normal except for to the suspected deficit in vasopressin or should be well replaced before starting the test.

The test would optimally begin with the child's first void in the morning after awakening. Serum should be drawn at this time and both the serum and the urine should be analyzed for osmolality. The initial blood pressure and weight should be recorded. From this time to the end of the study, the child must be prevented from consuming any food or fluids and watched carefully for compliance. The volume and timing of all urine samples should be recorded. With each void, serum is collected and the osmolality of both the serum and the urine should be determined. Weights should be determined every 1–2 h and an early termination of the test should be considered if the weight falls by >3%. Patients with psychogenic polydipsia may be overhydrated by >3% of the body weight.

Thus, if this diagnosis is strongly suspected, body weight may be allowed to fall more markedly. If symptoms of hypoglycemia develop, serum glucose should be obtained.

If the urine osmolalities exceed 1000 mOsm/L at any time, a diagnosis of DI can be ruled out. If the urine osmolality is <250 mOsm/L with a concurrent serum osmolality of >295 mOsm/L, a diagnosis of DI is confirmed. If neither of these conditions is met, the test could continue for 12 h in children and 9 h in toddlers.

When a diagnosis of DI is confirmed, a distinction between nephrogenic and neurogenic DI can be made by injecting aqueous vasopressin subcutaneously at a dose of 1 U/m^2 (45). Patients with neurogenic DI will respond by doubling the concentration of their urine within approx 3 h. If available, measuring the AVP levels at time of maximal dehydration is also helpful in differentiating between nephrogenic and neurogenic DI.

In psychogenic DI, the initial polyuric state is an appropriate response to the increased water intake. The urine concentrating ability as demonstrated by a water deprivation test is therefore usually normal. With a long-standing problem, the high turnover of water may compromise the kidney's ability to concentrate urine. Under these circumstances, they may be resistant to AVP and may transiently resemble other forms of nephrogenic DI.

RADIOLOGY

Patients with DI often have characteristic magnetic resonance imaging (MRI) findings of the posterior pituitary. In normal subjects, the T_1 weighted MR image shows a distinctly bright signal that is thought to represent intracellular storage granules of processed vasopressin and neurophysin (46,47). This bright signal is lost in patients with DI because of a wide range of pathologies associated with injury to the magnocellular neurons, including trauma, mass lesions, and infiltrative lesions. In patients with nephrogenic DI, the magnocellular neurons are intact, but much of the stored vasopressin has been released, giving a similar loss of the bright signal. In some instances, the development of this MRI finding may lag behind clinical signs of DI (48). For this reason, the initial MRI may be normal in patients with polyuria and polydipsia who eventually are found to have a CNS lesion. Because MRI findings will change over time, serial scans may be useful (49).

FUTURE DIAGNOSTIC APPROACHES

Given the time and cost needed to establish a diagnosis of neurogenic diabetes insipidus in some patients, new ways to test for the condition are being sought. One promising avenue of exploration is the measurement of urinary aquaporins. Saito et al found that patients with neurogenic DI secrete much less aquaporin-2 per milligram of creatinine in the urine compared to normal patients under ad libitum water intake (50).

Evaluation of Infants

In the infant age range, the most common clinical presentation of DI is failure to thrive. The differential diagnosis, then, is very broad and includes both organic and nonorganic pathologies. The major endocrine disorders that could present as failure to thrive include hypothyroidism, adrenal insufficiency, hyperparathyroidism, diabetes mellitus, and diabetes insipidus. Infants with DI may not be satisfied with feedings but are quieted by water. Vomiting and constipation may be present. Parents may report that the infant's diaper is always wet. In decompensated states, the infant will lose enough water to develop dehydration, hypernatremia, and hyperthermia. Repeated episodes of hypernatremia and seizures may lead to brain damage and mental impairment.

WATER-DEPRIVATION TEST IN INFANTS

In infants with frank polyuria, a dilute urine, and a classic serum profile, a diagnosis of DI may be made without a water-deprivation test. In cases when the diagnosis is not clear, a water-deprivation test may be helpful. The purpose of this test is still to evaluate the ability of the kidney to concentrate urine appropriately. Serum samples should be obtained with each void after starting the test in the morning. Both of these samples should be sent to the laboratory for determinations of osmolality. This test should be a done in a hospital setting, especially as infants may easily develop hypoglycemia with prolonged fasting. For this reason, testing should include a serum glucose with the serum osmolalities and should stop after 6–7 h if no definitive results are obtained. The period of time between determinations of the serum glucose should not exceed 1 h during the test. If the infant does not void for over 1 h, a glucose level should be obtained without waiting for the void. Interpreting the results of the serum and urine osmolalities resembles that for children.

THERAPEUTIC COMPOUNDS AND TREATMENT STRATEGIES

Desmopressin Acetate

Desmopressin acetate is a clinically valuable tool for treating DI (*see* Fig. 8). In children with neurogenic diabetes insipdus who have free access to water, desmopressin acetate is used widely. Treatment with desmopressin acetate in infants and any other patient who cannot directly control their own fluid intake can be difficult and requires close monitoring.

Desmopressin acetate (1-deamino-8-D-arginine vasopressin) is an arginine vasopressin analog that has approximately twice the antidiuretic potency of the parent molecule in addition to a greatly decreased pressor effect (51,52). Tablets, nasal solutions, and injectable forms are available. Orally administered desmopressin acetate doses are 20-fold larger than the usual nasal doses. For the oral route, antidiuretic effects may be seen approx 1 h after administration of the medication with a peak effect seen approx 4–7 h after administration. The peak effects of nasally administered desmopressin acetate can be seen at approx 1–5 h with a duration of 5–20 h. The exact mechanism of the metabolism of the drug is unknown, but the duration of the effect has been shown clincally to depend on the size of the dose. Resulting probably from more predictable absorption, the clinical effects following nasal administration of desmopressin acetate usually varies less than that following the oral route. The timing, duration, and magnitude of the antidiuresis of a single dose can be quite variable between different patients.

The optimum route of administration and the dosage will be influenced most strongly by the patient's ability to swallow pills, the absorption rate of desmopressin acetate from the GI track and the nasal mucosa in the individual patient, and the presence of nasal congestion. The convenience of the tablet forms of desmopressin acetate, which do not have to be refrigerated, may be preferred by teenagers.

A low starting dose and titration of this dose for effect is recommended. A nasal dose of desmopressin acetate at 1 μg/kg daily divided into two doses has been used successfully in premature infants (53). Term infants can be started on 1 μg nasally every 12 h. In children less than 12 yr old, a reasonable initial dose of nasally administered desmopressin acetate is approx 5 μg/d divided qd or bid. In children able to swallow tablets, the initial dosage can be 0.1–0.2 μg/d divided qd or bid. The dosages of both of

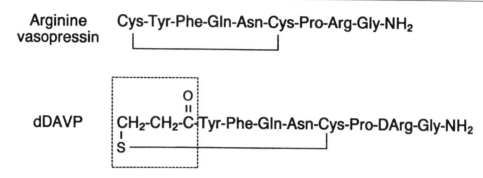

Fig. 8. Structural sequence of arginine vasopressin and desmopressin acetate (dDAVP).

these routes should be adjusted to allow for periods of diuresis between doses. Controlling nocturia is usually a priority for toilet-trained patients and may be the only goal of treatment. In patients with only mild symptoms, a single dose at night without a morning dose can be enough to sufficiently control their problem.

Care must be taken to avoid water intoxication. Such a complication is particularly likely if patients are given intravenous fluid and therefore are not regulating intake strictly by thirst. Patients treated with carbamazepine and patients with cortisol deficiency are at increased risk of water intoxication *(54)*.

Diuretics

This pharmacologic strategy is used in patients with nephrogenic DI, in infants, and as an adjunct to desmopressin acetate therapy. Thiazide and furosemide diuretics have been found to help conserve water by inducing a mildly hypovolemic state. By doing this, these diuretics promote better sodium resorption in the proximal tubules of the kidney with a resulting reabsorption of more water at this level of the nephron. Thus, the volume of the filtrate that reaches the collecting ducts, the site of AVP action, will be modestly reduced. A failure to concentrate the urine at the level of the collecting ducts will then have a smaller clinical impact.

Treatment with hydrochlorothiazide in combination with mild salt depletion would be a reasonable first choice in the management of DI in infants. Doses can range from 1 to 3 mg/kg/d divided into three doses. If this treatment is unsuccessful in ameliorating the infant's failure to thrive, then treatment with vasopressin or a vasopressin analog can be considered. The use of desmopressin acetate in an infant is difficult because fluid intake is regulated by hunger and thirst. With this dual control of fluid intake, infants may drink when they are already fluid overloaded.

In children, a reasonable starting dose of hydrochlorothiazide is 1–3 mg/kg/d divided bid or tid. The addition of ameloride at 0.2–0.7 mg/kg/d may improve the potassium status in patients receiving diuretic therapy *(55)*. A salt-restricted diet is usually necessary to induce the slight degree of hypovolemia and to prevent hypokalemia.

Inhibitors of Prostaglandin Synthesis

When used alone, these drugs have little effect on water conservation. When used with a thiazide diuretic, however, water conservation improves markedly in patients with nephrogenic DI *(55)*. This property has been attributed to the elimination of the prostaglandin inhibition of sodium absorption at the tubules. As a result, sodium reabsorption improves and the osmolality of the renal interstitium is more efficiently increased. Following the solute reabsorption, water reabsorption is also augmented. This effect has been shown with indomethacin, tolmetin, and acetylsalicylic acid (56–58).

SPECIAL CONDITIONS

Primary Polydipsia and Psychogenic Polydipsia

Mimicking DI, these disorders can present with polydipsia and polyuria. In primary polydipsia, the patient has an increased desire to drink. With our incomplete knowledge of mechanisms behind thirst, the exact etiology of this disorder remains unexplained. Patients with this disorder may consume excessive amounts of water in the belief of specific health benefits or other reasons. Excessive water intake leads to chronic volume expansion and impairment of AVP release (59). The differentiation of primary polydipsia and DI can be aided by the use of MRI. A hyperintense signal in the neurohypophysis on a T_1-weighted scan has been demonstrated in one series of patients with primary polydipsia but not in patients with diabetes insipidus (60).

Hypodipsia

Lesions as a result of trauma, hydrocephalus, granulomatous disease, tumor, histiocytosis, surgery, or congenital malformation can involve the thirst centers of the brain and can lead to hypodipsic states. Patients who lack thirst to control water intake rely heavily on varying urine concentrations to maintain water homeostasis. In patients with DI in addition to hypodipsia, the mechanisms that control both fluid intake and fluid conservation are lost. The combination of DI and hypodipsia, then, is very clinically challenging. In children with this combination of problems, the treatment regimen must be tailored to meet the needs of the patient and the family. A careful account of the water intake is necessary. Weights should be obtained once or twice each day and should be checked more often with illnesses. Desmopressin acetate may be used to reduce urine output. Serum sodium levels should be monitored frequently when starting or changing regimens. In growing children, target weights must be changed to take appropriate weight gain into account.

Chemotherapy

Children receiving chemotherapy need adequate fluid management for optimal care. Saline diuresis is often employed to reduce the renal toxicity of the chemotherapy agents. Children with DI in addition to their oncologic problem require special attention. Longer-acting preparations of AVP such as desmopressin acetate are difficult to use in this setting because the effects are difficult to turn off quickly. Aqueous vasopressin is available and has been used successfully to manage DI in patients receiving chemotherapy (61). This agent has a short half-life and can be administered intravenously via a drip. By adjusting the drip rate, the patient's urine output can be varied to achieve the goals of the chemotherapy protocol. As an initial dose, a continuous infusion of aqueous AVP at a rate of between 0.08 and 0.1 mU/kg/h during the hydration phase is recommended. This rate is much lower than the 1.0–3.0 mU/kg/h necessary to maintain homeostasis in a patient receiving maintenance fluids (62). Frequent monitoring of urine output, urine specific gravity, weight, and serum sodium levels are needed to allow appropriate hydration. Blood pressure and pulse must also be monitored closely as well in view of the presser effects of AVP.

Surgery

Fluid management during surgery of DI patients may follow one of two general strategies. The first strategy comprises administration of the long-acting vasopressin analog desmopressin acetate. Fluids should be given to replace insensible fluid losses and urine output. Alternatively, an intravenous infusion of aqueous vasopressin may be given and titrated to allow for fine control of the urine output. Aqueous vasopressin doses of 1–3 mU/kg/h have been used in this setting. Monitoring the urine output, urine specific gravity, and the serum sodium levels are necessary during and after the procedure. Fluids should be administered to replace insensible fluid losses in addition to urine output. This method allows minute-to-minute control of both the intake and output of fluids. The first strategy allows close regulation of fluid intake; output is changeable only when the activities of medications used to treat the DI begin to wane.

SUMMARY

Diabetes insipidus may arise from abnormalities of vasopressin secretion or from aberations of renal responsiveness to vasopressin. Although it presents with polyuria and polydipsia in childhood, it may present as failure to thrive in infancy. Treatment is predicated on adequate understanding of the etiology.

Chronic treatment of children with desmopressin is usually straightforward. Other strategies may be needed for special circumstances. Infants may be effectively treated with thiazide diuretics. Adipsic patients may be treated with desmopressin acetate but must be given maintenance fluids with appropriate supplements as directed by frequent body weight determinations and by less frequent measurements of serum sodium. Intravenous fluid administration should comprise insensible losses in addition to urine output. Urine output may be controlled with desmopressin or with aqueous vasopressin.

REFERENCES

1. Robertson GL. Physiology of ADH release. Kidney Int 1987;31:S20.
2. McKinley MJ. Common aspects of the cerebral regulation of thirst and renal sodium excretion. Kidney Int 1992;37:S102.
3. Denton DA, McKinley MJ, Weisinger RS. Hypothalmic integration of body fluid regulation. Proc Natl Acad Sci USA 1996;93:7397–7404.
4. Johnson AK, Thunhorst RL. The neuroendocrinology of thirst and salt appetite: visceral sensory signals and mechanisms of central integration. Front Neuroendocrinol 1997;18:292–353.
5. Coggins CH, Leaf A. Diabetes insipidus. Am J Med 1967;42:807–813.
6. Salata RA, Verbalis JG, Robinson AG. Cold water stimulation of oropharyngeal receptors in man inhibit release of vasopressin J Clin Endocrinol Metab 1987;65:561.
7. Gopal Rao VVN, Loffler C, Battey J, Hansmann I. The human gene for oxytocin-neurophysin I OXT is physically mapped to chromosome 20p13 by in situ hybridization. Cell Genet 1992;61:271
8. Riddell DC, Mallonnee R, Phillips JA. Chromosomal assignment of human sequences encoding arginine vasopressin-neurophysin II and growth hormone releasing factor. Somat Cell Mol Genet 1985;11:189.
9. Robertson GL, Shelton RL, Athar S. The osmoregulation of the vasopressin. Kidney Int 1976;10:25.
10. Zerbe, RL, Miller JZ, Robertson GL. Osmoregulation of thirst and vasopressin secretion in human subjects: effects of various solutes. Am J Physiol 1983;224:E607.

11. Rittig S, Knudsen VB, Norgaard JP. Abnormal diurnal rhythm of plasma vasopressin and urinary output in patients with enuresis Am J Physiol 1989;256:F664.
12. Robertson GL. Thirst and vasopressin function in normal and disordered states of water balance. J Lab Clin Med 1983;101:351.
13. Wiggins RC, Basar I, Slater JD, et al. Vasovagal hypotension and vasopressin release. Clin Endocrinol 1977;6:387.
14. Hirsch AT, Majzoub JA, Ren CJ, et al. Contribution of vasopressin to blood pressure regulation during hypovolemic hypotension in humans. J Appl Physiol 1993;95:721.
15. Green HH, Harrington AR, Valtin H. On the role of antidiuretic hormone in the inhibition of acute water diuresis in adrenal insufficiency and the effects of gluco- and mineralocorticoids in reversing the inhibition. J Clin Invest 1970;49:1724.
16. Burke ZD, Ho MY, Morgan H, et al. Repression of vasopressin gene expression by glucocorticoids in transgenic mice: evidence of a direct mechanism mediated by proximal 5' flanking sequence. Neuroscience 1997;78:1177–1185.
17. Deen PMT, Verdijk MAJ, van Oost BA, et al. Requirement of human renal water channel aquaporin-2 for vasopressin-dependent concentration of urine. Science 1994;264:92.
18. Saito T, Ishikawa SE, Saito T, et al. Urinary excretion of aquaporin-2 in the diagnosis of central diabetes insipidus. J Clin Endocrinol Metab 1997;82:1823.
19. Ito M, Oiso Y, Murase T, et al. Possible involvement of inefficient cleavage of preprovasopressin by signal peptidase as a cause for familial central diabetes insipidus. J Clin Invest 1993;91:2565.
20. Rittig S, Robertson GL, Siggard C. Identification of 13 new mutations in the vasopressin-neurophysin II gene in 17 kindreds with familial autosomal dominant neurohypophyseal diabetes insipidus. Am J Hum Genet 1996;58:107–117.
21. Rauch F, Lenzner C, Nurnberg P, Frommel C, Vetter U. A novel mutation in the coding region for neurophysin-II is associated with autosomal dominant neurohypophyseal diabetes insipidus. Clin Endocrinol (Oxf.) 1996 Jan;44(1):45–51.
22. Inove H, Tanizawa Y, Wasson J, et al. A gene encoding α transmembrane protein is mutated in patients with diabetes mellitus and optic atrophy (Wolfram syndrome). Nat Genet 1998;20:143–148.
23. Takeda K, Inove K, Tanizawa Y, et al. WFSI (Wolfram syndrome I) gene product: predominant subcellular localization to endoplasmic reticulum in cultured cells and neuronal expression in rat brain. Hum Mol Genet 2001;10:477–484.
24. El-Shanti H, Lidral AC, Jarrah N, et al. Homozygosity mapping identifies an additional locus for Wolfram syndrome on chromosome 4q. Am J Hum Genet 2000;66:129–136.
25. Bundey S, Poulton K, Whitwell H, et al. Mitochondrial abnormalities in DIDMOAD syndrome. J Inherit Metab Dis 1992;15:316–319
26. Scherbaum WA, Wass IA, Besser GM, et al. Autoimmune cranial diabetes insipidus: its association with other endocrine diseases and with histiocytosis X. Clin Endocrinol 1986;25:411–420.
27. Schwartz WB, Relman, AS. Effects of electrolyte disorders on renal structure and function. N Engl J Med 1967;276:452–458.
28. Bennett CM. Urine concentration and dilution in hypokalemic and hypercalcemic dogs. J Clin Invest 1970;49:1447–1457.
29. Galla IH, Booker BB, Luke RG. Role of loop segment in the concentrating defect of hypercalcemia. Kidney Int 1986;29:977–982.
30. Hebert SC, Brown EM, Harris HW. Role of the Ca(2+)-sensing receptor in divalent mineral ion homeo- stasis. J Exp Biol 1997;200:295–302.
31. Berl T. The cAMP system in vasopressin-sensitive nephron segments of the vitamin D-treated rat. Kidney Int 1987;31:1065–1071.
32. Beck N, Singh H Reed SW, et al. Pathogenic role of cyclic AMP in the impairment of urinary concentrating ability in acute hypercalcemia. J Clin Invest 1974;54:1049–1055.
33. Bichet DG, Razi M, Lonergan M, et al. Hemodynanic and coagulation responses to 1-desamino (8-D-arginine) vasopressin in patients with congenital nephrogenic diabetes insipidus. N Engl J Med 1988;318:881–887.
34. Moses AM, Miller IL, Levine MA. Two distinct pathophysiological mechanisms in congenital nephrogenic diabetes insipidus. J Clin Endocrinol Metab 1988;66:1259–1264.
35. Knoers N, van der Heyden H, van Oost BA, et al. Three-point linkage analysis using multiple DNA polymorphic markers in families with X-Iinked nephrogenic diabetes insipidus. Genomics 1989;4:434–437.

36. Oksche A, Schulein R, Rutz C, et al. Vasopressin V2 receptor mutants that cause X-linked nephrogenic diabetes insipidus: analysis of expression, processing, and function. Mol Pharmacol 1996;50:820–828.
37. Kambouris M, Dlouhy SR, Trofatter IA, et al. Localization of the gene for X-Iinked nephrogenic diabetes insipidus to Xq28. Am K Med Genet 1988;29:239–246.
38. Rosenthal W, Seibold A, Antaramian A, et al. Molecular identification of the gene responsible for congenital nephrogenic diabetes insipidus. Nature 1992;359:233–235.
39. Merendino JJ Jr, Speigel AM, Crawford, et al. Brief Report: A mutation in the vasopressin V2-receptor gene in a kindred with X-linked nephrogenic diabetes insipidus. N Engl J Med 1993:328:1538.
40. Holtzman EI, Harris HW Ir, Kolakowski LF, et al. Brief report: a molecular defect in the vasopressin V2-receptor gene causing nephrogenic diabetes insipidus. N Engl J Med 1993;328:1562,1563.
41. Tsukaguchi H, Matsubara H, Taketani S, et al. Binding-, intracellular transport-, and biosynthesis-defective mutations of vasopressin type-2 receptor in patients with X-linked nephrogenic diabetes insipidus. J Clin Invest 1995;96:2043–2050.
42. Langley IM, Balfel W, Selander T, et al. Autosomal recessive inheritance of vasopressin-resistant diabetes insipidus. Am J Med Genet 1991;38:90–94.
43. Deen PMT, Croes H, van Aubel RA, et al. Water channels encoded by mutant aquaporin-2 genes in nephrogenic diabetes insipidus are impaired in their cellular routing. J Clin Invest 1995;95:2291–2296.
44. Hochberg Z, Van Lieburg A, Even L, et al. Autosomal recessive nephrogenic diabetes insipidus caused by an aquaporin-2 mutation. J Clin Endocrinol Metab 1997;82:686–689.
45. Muglia LI, Majzoub IA. Pediatric endocrinology. In: Sperling MA, ed. Disorders of the Posterior Pituitary. WB Saunders Co, Philadelphia, 1996, p. 206.
46. Abernethy LI, Qunibi MA, Smith CS. Nonnal MR appearances of the posterior pituitary in central diabetes insipidus associated with septo-optic dysplasia. Pediatr Radiol 1997;27:45–47 .
47. Colombo N, Berry I, Kucharczyk I, et al. Posterior pituitary gland: appearance on MR images in nonnal and pathologic states. Radiology 1987;165:481–485.
48. Weimann E, Molenkemp G, Bohles HJ. Diabetes insipidus due to hypophysis. Horm Res 1997;47:81–84.
49. Mootha SL, Barkovich AI, Grumbach MM, et al. Idio-pathic hypothalamic diabetes insipidus, pituitary stalk thickening, and the occult intracranial genninoma in children and adolescents. J Clin Endocrinol Metab 1997;82:1362–1367.
50. Saito T, Ishikawa S, Sasaki S, et al. Urinary excretion of aquaporin-2 in the diagnosis of central diabetes insipidus. J Clin Endocrinol Metab 1997;82:1823–1827.
51. Kimbrough RD, Cash WD, Branden LA, et al. Synthesis and biologic properties of 1-desamino-8-lysine vasopressin. J Biol Chem 1963;238:1411.
52. Sawyer WH, Grzonka Z, Manning M. Neurohypophysialpeptides: design of tissue specific agonists and antagonists. Mol Cell Endocrinol 1981;22:117–134.
53. Giacoia GP, Watson S, Karathanos A. Treatment of neonatal diabetes insipidus with desmopressin. Southern Med 1984;77:75–77.
54. Rizzo V, Albanese A, Stanhope R. Morbidity and Mortality associated with vasopressin replacement therapy in children. J Pediat Endocrinol 2001;14:861–867.
55. Knoers N, Monnens LA. Amiloride-hydrochlorothiazide versus indomethacin-hydrochlorothiazide in the treatment of nephrogenic diabetes insipidus. J Pediatr 1990;117:499–502.
56. Fichman MP, Speckhart P, Zia P, Lee A. Antidiuretic response to prostaglandin inhibition by indomethacin in nephrogenic diabetes insipidus. Clin Res 1976;24:161A.
57. Chevalier RL, Rogol AD. Tolmetin sodium in the management of nephrogenic diabetes insipidus. J Pediatr 1982;101:787–789.
58. Monn E. Prostaglandin synthetase inhibitors in the treatment of nephrogenic diabetes insipidus. Acta Pediatr Scand 1981;70:39–42.
59. Moses AM, Clayton B. Impairment of osmotically stimulated A VP release in patients with primary polydipsia. Am J Physiol 1993;265:RI247–RI252.
60. Moses AM, Clayton B, Hochhauser L. The use of Tl-weighted MR imaging to differentiate between primary polydipsia and central diabetes insipidus. Am J Neuroradiol 1992;13:1273–1277.
61. Bryant WP, O'Marcaigh AS, Ledger GA, Zimmerman D. Aqueous vasopressin infusion during chemotherapy in patients with Dl. Cancer 1994;74:2589–2592.
62. McDonald IA, Martha PM, Kerrigan I, et al. Treatment of the young child with postoperative central diabetes insipidus. Am J Dis Child 1989;143:201–204.

2

Treatment of Diabetes Insipidus in Adults

Andjela T. Drincic, MD
and Gary L. Robertson, MD

CONTENTS

INTRODUCTION

Diabetes insipidus (DI) is a syndrome characterized by the excretion of abnormally large volumes of dilute urine. The polyuria causes symptoms of urinary frequency and nocturia and sometimes, incontinence and enuresis. It is also associated with thirst and/or a commensurate increase in fluid intake (polydipsia).

Diabetes insipidus is divisible into three types, each of which has a different pathogenesis and must be managed in a different way *(1)*. The most common type of DI is that caused by a deficiency of the antidiuretic hormone, arginine vasopressin (AVP). It is usually, if not always, caused by destruction of the neurohypophysis and is variously referred to as pituitary, neurohypophysial, cranial, or central DI. This destruction can be caused by various acquired *(1)* or genetic disorders *(2)*. It can also be caused or uncovered by the increased metabolism of AVP that occurs during pregnancy, in which case it is known as gestational DI *(3)*. A second type of DI is the result of renal insensitivity to the antidiuretic effect of AVP. It is caused by defects in the AVP receptor or postreceptor elements that mediate antidiuresis and is usually referred to as nephrogenic DI. It, too, can be caused by various acquired *(1)* or genetic disorders *(4)*. The third type of DI is caused by excessive intake of water. It is generally referred to as primary

From: *Endocrine Replacement Therapy in Clinical Practice*
Edited by: A. Wayne Meikle © Humana Press Inc., Totowa, NJ

polydipsia and is divisible into three forms based on the patient's explanation for the polydipsia. One is thirst, which appears to be due to an abnormality in osmoregulation (5). It is referred to as dipsogenic DI and is nearly impossible to distinguish from partial pituitary or nephrogenic DI without special tests (see below). The second form of primary polydipsia results from a more generalized cognitive defect and is usually called psychogenic polydipsia (6,7). It is not attributed to thirst but to other, irrational motives. The third form is motivated by therapeutic advice of physicians, nurses or the popular media and may be designated as iatrogenic polydipsia. Because it is important, but not always easy, to distinguish among the three major types of DI, a brief review of the basic anatomy, biochemistry, physiology, and diagnostic methodology of antidiuretic function is in order before discussing management.

VASOPRESSIN

Arginine vasopressin is a nonapeptide hormone (see Fig. 1) synthesized and secreted by magnocellular neurohypophysial neurons that originate in the supraoptic and paraventricular nuclei and terminate on capillaries in the median eminence and posterior lobe of the pituitary gland (8). The gene encoding AVP is located on chromosome 20 near the gene for a closely related neurosecretory hormone, oxytocin (9). It has three exons and directs the production of a preprohormone that contains 166 amino acids and comprises a signal peptide, AVP, an AVP binding protein known as neurophysin (NP) II and a glycosylated peptide known as copeptin (CP). Like other preprohormones, the AVP precursor is formed by cleavage of signal peptide in the endoplasmatic reticulum, transported through the Golgi to neurosecretory vesicles, where it is further processed to AVP, NPII, and CP and stored until released into the systemic circulation.

The main if not the only important physiological action of AVP in humans is to regulate urinary concentration and flow by altering the hydro-osmotic reabsorption of solute-free water in the distal and collecting tubules of the kidney. This effect is mediated by special receptors (V2) that activate adenyl cyclase and cause preformed water channels composed of a protein known as aquaporin-2 to be inserted in the luminal membrane of tubular cells (10,11). The insertion of these water channels permits solute-free water to be reabsorbed osmotically down the gradient that exists between the hypertonic medulla and the hypotonic tubular fluid. This results in a reduction in urine output to as little as 0.5 mL/min and a rise in urine concentration (osmolality) to levels as high as 1200–1500 mOsm/kg. When AVP is low or absent, relatively little solute-free water is reabsorbed in the collecting tubules and the urine that issues from them is not only much greater in volume (10–15 mL/min) but is also unconcentrated and may reach osmolality levels as low as 40–50 mOsm/kg. This condition is known as a maximum water diuresis.

Supraphysiologic amounts of AVP or a synthetic analog desmopressin (1-deamino-8-D-arginine vasopressin DDAVP) also act via V_2 receptors to stimulate the release of Factor VIII and von Willebrand factor from endothelium (12). This effect is probably of no physiologic importance but has important implications for treatment of certain bleeding disorders (see below, DDAVP). AVP can also act via a different type of receptor (V_1) to stimulate contraction of vascular and gastrointestinal smooth muscle, urinary excretion of potassium, and prostaglandin production by the kidney. However, it is not yet clear if these effects are of any physiologic or pharmacologic importance.

The secretion of AVP and, presumably, NPII and CP are regulated primarily by the effective osmotic pressure of extracellular fluid (13). This effect is mediated via

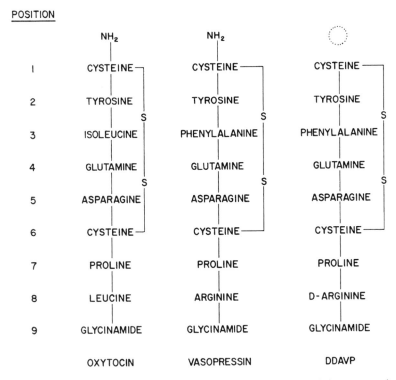

POSITION

Fig. 1. The amino acid sequence of oxytocin, vasopressin, and desmopressin.

osmoreceptors that are located in the anterior hypothalamus near the supraoptic nucleus. These osmoreceptors appear to operate like a discontinuous or "set-point" receptor and are extremely sensitive to changes in the plasma concentration of sodium and certain other solutes. Among healthy adults, the "set" and sensitivity of the osmoregulatory system shows relatively large, genetically determined differences. On average, however, plasma AVP begins to rise at a plasma osmolality or sodium concentration around 280 mOsm/kg or 135 meq/L and it reaches levels sufficient to produce maximum antidiuresis at a plasma osmolality and sodium of only about 295 mOsm/kg and 143 meq/L. AVP secretion can also be stimulated by hypotension, hypovolemia, nausea, and certain other nonosmotic factors, but these influences probably are important only under certain pathological conditions.

DIFFERENTIAL DIAGNOSIS OF DI

In a patient with symptoms or a voiding diary suggestive of DI, the diagnosis should always be verified by collecting a 24-h urine to confirm that the volume is abnormally high (>50 mL/kg body wt), the osmolality is abnormally low (<300 mOsm/kg), and glucosuria or other types of solute diuresis are absent (>20 mOsm/kg body wt). Measurement of osmolality or specific gravity of a random urine sample should not be relied upon because they can give false-negative or false-positive results. Physical or routine laboratory indicators of hydration status are rarely of value since they are almost always within normal limits in DI.

Once the diagnosis of DI is established, it is necessary to determine the type *(14)*. The history and physical or clinical setting may be helpful, but it can also be ambiguous or even misleading. Therefore, it is usually necessary or prudent to rely on laboratory criteria. Measurements of plasma osmolality and/or sodium under basal conditions of ad libitum fluid intake are usually of no value because they vary widely and overlap extensively in the three major types of DI; that is because the excessive water loss in patients with pituitary or nephrogenic DI is usually offset by thirst and a commensurate increase in fluid intake, whereas the excessive intake in primary polydipsia is offset by suppression of AVP and a commensurate increase in water excretion. These compensatory responses occur at slightly different levels of plasma osmolality and sodium in different patients because of genetic differences in the "set" of the osmoregulatory mechanisms. However, they are always within the reference range for plasma osmolality and sodium unless the patient also has a defect in thirst (hypodispia) or urinary dilution (e.g., SIADH). Therefore, a fluid deprivation test is usually needed to determine if dehydration elicits an appropriate increase in urine concentration and decrease in urine flow. If a rise in plasma osmolality and sodium above the normal range does not result in a rise in urine osmolality above 300 mOsm/kg, primary polydipsia is largely excluded and an injection of AVP (1 IU Pitressin®) or its synthetic analog, desmopressin (4 μg DDAVP) will suffice to differentiate between severe pituitary and nephrogenic DI. However, if dehydration results in concentration of the urine, partial pituitary or partial nephrogenic DI are not excluded and the subsequent urinary response to AVP or DDAVP is of no diagnostic value. In this case, another approach to the differential diagnosis is required.

There are several different ways to differentiate reliably among primary polydipsia, partial pituitary, and partial nephrogenic DI. One is to measure basal plasma AVP. If it is clearly elevated (>2 pg/mL), the patient has nephrogenic DI and further investigation should be focused on finding the cause. On the other hand, if basal plasma AVP is low or not clearly elevated, nephrogenic DI is unlikely and further evaluation should be directed toward determining if the patient has partial pituitary DI or some form of primary polydipsia. One way to do this is to perform a combined fluid deprivation/ hypertonic saline infusion test (3% saline iv at 0.1 mL/kg/min for 1–2 h) and repeat the measurements of plasma AVP when plasma osmolality and/or sodium exceed the normal range (usually approx 300 mOsm/kg or 150 meq/L).

In a patient with partial pituitary DI, plasma AVP may rise slightly, but its relationship to plasma osmolality or sodium always falls below the normal range. In dipsogenic DI, however, the rise in plasma AVP is normal for the concurrent rise in plasma osmolality or sodium. Another way to differentiate primary polydipsia from partial pituitary DI is to perform a magnetic resonance imaging (MRI) of the brain to determine if the hyperintense signal ("bright spot") normally emitted by the posterior pituitary on T_1-weighted images is present *(15)*. If it is present, the patient almost certainly has some form of primary polydipsia rather than partial pituitary DI. However, if the bright spot is absent, the patient probably has partial pituitary DI, although it is also absent about 5% of the time in primary polydipsia.

A third way to differentiate among the three types of DI is to give a short (24–48 h) closely monitored therapeutic trial of DDAVP (2–4 μg subcutaneously [sc] every 12 h or 20 μg intranasally [in] every 8 h). If DDAVP promptly abolishes thirst and polydipsia as well as polyuria without excessive retention of water (i.e., plasma sodium concentration remains within the normal limits), the patient probably has pituitary DI. If DDAVP has no effect, the most likely diagnosis is nephrogenic DI. If DDAVP abolishes the poly-uria but causes smaller reductions in thirst and polydipsia and/or results in development of water intoxication (i.e., plasma sodium concentration below the normal limits) the odds are about 20 to 1 that the patient has primary polydipsia (probably the dipsogenic form).

During pregnancy, the measurement of plasma AVP is not recommended for the differential diagnosis of DI because special protease inhibitors must be used during collection of the sample to prevent rapid degradation of AVP in vitro. The other approaches, including fluid deprivation or therapeutic trial of DDAVP, may be used, although with particularly close monitoring because of the possible risk to the fetus of severe maternal dehydration or overhydration. In this regard, it should also be remembered that the normal range for serum sodium in pregnancy is about 5 meq/L lower in the gravid than in the nongravid state.

TREATMENT OF DI

In general, the goal of DI treatment is to improve the patients' quality of life by restoring urinary volume to normal or, at least, reducing urinary frequency to minimize interference with daytime activities or sleep at night. Because DI *per se* usually does not cause significant morbidity (if the patient has intact thirst mechanism and unrestricted access to water), the modality of treatment chosen should not only be effective but also safe.

TREATMENT OF PITUITARY DI

Because pituitary DI is the result of a primary deficiency of AVP that is rarely if ever reversible, it can be and should be treated by replacing the hormone or giving other drugs that mimic its antidiuretic effect. Agents currently available are as follows:

1. Arginine vasopressin (Pitressin®) is a synthetic form of the natural hormone. When given as a subcutaneous injection in a dose of 1–5 U, aqueous Pitressin has a very short half-life with onset of action within 30 min and duration of action of 3–6 h. Given intravenously, it has an equally rapid onset of action and a duration that persists for 1–2 h after stopping the infusion. Therefore, its principal use is for acute, short-term treatment of DI. Aqueous Pitressin comes as a buffered solution of L-arginine vasopressin in 1 mL snap-top vials at a concentration of 20 U/mL. Because it is so highly concentrated, it must be diluted several-thousand-fold to achieve the desired concentration in the infusate. We recommend that it be prepared in 5% dextrose and water at a concentration of 1–2 mU/mL and infused at a rate of 0.5 mL/kg/h. Side effects of Pitressin occur only at very high doses and are primarily nausea, vomiting, and abdominal cramps.

2. Vasopressin tannate in oil (Pitressin Tannate®) is an extract of bovine posterior pituitary in depot preparation. When given in a dose of 5–10 U sc or im, it has an antidiuretic effect that lasts up to 72 h. The duration of action varies markedly because of variable bioavailability. For many years it was a standard of treatment for pituitary DI. However, it is no longer available in the United States.

3. Lysine vasopressin (Lypressin, Diapid®) is a synthetic vasopressin that has a lysine in place of arginine at position 8. When given intranasally, Diapid has a very short half-life, with rapid onset of action (30 min) and short duration of action (4–6 h). The recommended dose is one to two sprays intranasally (providing 2–4 U of vasopressin) four to six times a day. Side effects are essentially the same as those encountered with AVP. Diapid is currently available on a compassionate basis through Novartis Pharmaceutical.

4. Desmopressin: 1-deamino-8-D-arginine vasopressine (DDAVP®) *(16)* is a synthetic analog of L-arginine vasopressin in which the amino group at position 1 has been removed and the naturally occurring levo-isomer of arginine at position 8 has been replaced by its dextro-isomer *(see* Fig. 1). DDAVP has no significant side effects except for a slight reduction in blood pressure and rise in pulse rate when given iv or sc at supraphysiologic doses. Because it is less susceptible to degradation by N-terminal peptidases, it can be given by the oral as well as parenteral and intranasal routes.

a. Oral DDAVP is provided as tablets of 0.1 or 0.2 mg *(17,18)*. It is easy to use, does not require refrigeration, and is the treatment of choice in situations where poor absorption from intranasal mucosa is expected *(see* item 4b, intranasal DDAVVP). It may also be preferred in children. The usual dose is 100–200 µg po two or three times daily. In some patients, its effects can be erratic because of, presumably, variable absorption of the peptide from the gastrointestinal (GI) tract.

b. Intranasal DDAVP is supplied as a 2.5-mL bottle containing 100 µg/mL of desmopressin. It is available for two different modes of administration: a calibrated rhinal tube applicator that can be used to deliver volumes of 50–200 µL containing 5–20 µg of DDAVP or a nasal spray pump that delivers a fixed 100-µL containing 10 µg of desmopressin. The main advantage of the rhinal tube is the ability to give small, graded doses of medication. However, the technical skills required for proper use render it impractical for many patients. The nasal spray is easier to use, but provides a higher minimal dose and larger graduations of 10 µg that may be more than is necessary for some patients. The usual dose by either route is 10–20 µg intranasally two or three times a day but individual requirements vary widely. Poor or erratic responses usually result from incomplete absorption owing to inflammation of the nasal mucosa secondary to upper respiratory infections, allergic rhinitis, or sinusitis. Poor vision and severe arthritis also make intranasal DDAVP difficult to use. Allergy to DDAVP, with or without resistance to its biologic effects, is rare.

c. Parenteral DDAVP is supplied as a 10-mL vial containing 4 µg/mL of desmopressin and is available for intravenous and subcutaneous use. It is the treatment of choice for patients who, because of their age or intercurrent illness, are unable to take or absorb the drug by the intranasal or oral route. The usual dose in adults is 1–4 µg once or twice daily.

After more than 20 yr of clinical experience, desmopressin has become the drug of choice for the treatment of pituitary DI. In uncomplicated patients, administration of the drug completely eliminates the polyuria and polydipsia *(see* Fig. 2) both acutely and during long-term therapy. Desmopressin is equally effective in all patients with pituitary DI, irrespective of the severity or cause of their vasopressin deficiency. Because of individual differences in absorption and metabolism, the dose required to achieve complete, around-the-clock control varies from patient to patient. Increasing the dose size generally increases the duration of action rather than magnitude of antidiuresis. Thus, once-a-day dosing is possible, but it is more expensive because a higher total dose must be used. Desmopressin therapy is also safe for patients with uncomplicated pituitary DI. At doses that are 5–10 times higher than those conventionally used to treat pituitary DI, DDAVP does stimulate the release of Factor VIII and Von Willebrand factor (which is the basis of its hemostatic applications). However hypercoagulability is not a risk with the usual antidiuretic doses.

A major misconception in DDAVP therapy is the fear that the drug will induce hyponatremia unless the patient is allowed to "escape" frequently from the antidiuretic effect. However, even high doses of DDAVP do not induce hyponatremia in patients with

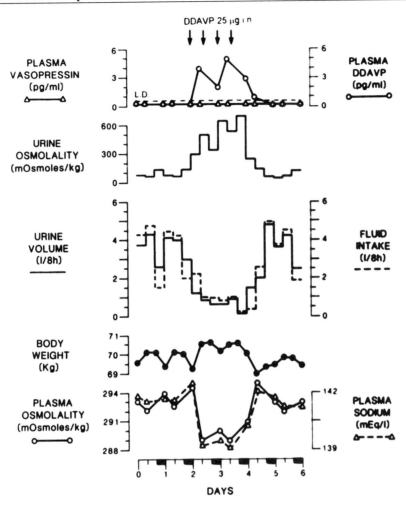

Fig. 2. The effect of DDAVP on water balance in pituitary DI. DDAVP was given intranasally in dose of 25 μg every 8 h. The urinary values are for successive 8-h collections. Note that the treatment produced a commensurate, contemporaneous decrease in fluid intake and urinary output with minimal retention of water as indicated by slight increase in body weight and decrease in plasma osmolality/sodium, both of which remain within normal range.

uncomplicated pituitary DI because the drug induces slight retention of water, which reduces plasma osmolality/sodium and promptly suppresses thirst and fluid intake. Hyponatremia develops only if the patient has an associated abnormality in thirst or drinks excessively for other reasons. Therefore, when initiating therapy, patients always should be instructed to drink only enough fluid to satisfy their thirst. They should avoid drinking for any other reason (such as to avoid dehydration or treat a cold or the flu) and should be warned that excessive fluid intake can result in life-threatening water intoxication. When hospitalized for other medical or surgical care, even routine maintenance or "keep open" rates of iv fluids may induce water intoxication if given while the patient is taking DDAVP. Therefore, the patient should carry a bracelet or card indicating that he or she has pituitary DI, is taking DDAVP, and will require very close monitoring and management of fluid balance and serum sodium if unconscious or otherwise unable to

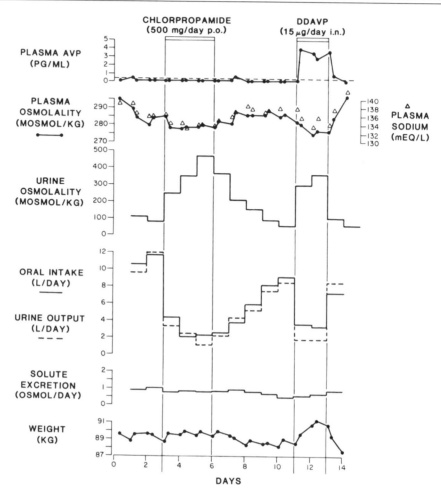

Fig. 3. The effects of chloropropamide and DDAVP on water balance in pituitary DI. Note that the urinary volumes are for 24-h urinary collections. Given separately, both chlorpropamide and DDAVP produced a significant rise in urine osmality and a decrease in fluid intake and urinary output with minimal water retention as indicated by the slight increase in body weight and decrease in plasma osmolality/sodium, both of which remain within the normal range. Note that the magnitude of antidiuretic effect is similar in both drugs.

regulate intake via the thirst mechanism (also, *see* below, Special Considerations, Post-operative and Posttraumatic DI).

5. Chlorpropamide also increases urine concentration and reduces urine volume in patients with pituitary DI (*see* Fig. 3) *(19,20)*. Its mechanism of action is uncertain, but may involve enhancing the secretion as well as the antidiuretic action of residual AVP *(21)*. It may also act via some independent mechanism *(20)*, because it is often most effective in patients with severe if not complete deficiencies of vasopressin (*see* below; this section) and its antidiuretic action begins sooner in patients with a prolonged deficiency of antidiuretic hormone (often in 24–48 h) than in patients recently exposed to AVP or DDAVP (in which case, the maximum effect may not occur for 7–10 d). This fact as well as the lack of antidiuretic effect of chlorpropamide in normal subjects or patients with primary polydipsia suggests that the mechanism requires some change in antidiuretic function that results from prolonged deficiency of the hormone.

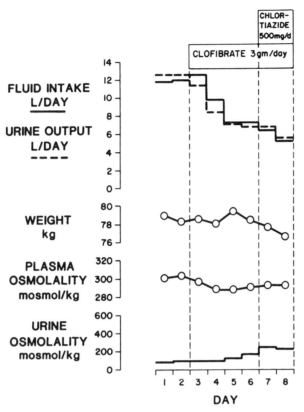

Fig. 4. The effect of clofibrate and hydrochlorothiazide (HCTZ) on water balance in pituitary DI. Note that both clofibrate given alone or with HCTZ produce an increase in urine osmolality as well as fall in fluid intake and urine output with minimal water retention, as evidenced by the slight fall in plasma osmolality and increase in body weight that remains within normal limits.

Contrary to widespread views, chlorpropamide is equally effective in patients with severe or partial pituitary DI. Its antidiuretic effect seems to diminish with water loading, making it a safer alternative to DDAVP in the management of patients with abnormal thirst as well as a deficiency of AVP. Efficacy also varies widely from patient to patient. Some can be completely controlled on a dose as low as 100 mg/d, whereas others will achieve only a 50% reduction in urine output at doses as high as 500 mg/d. In these patients, the addition of chlorothiazide (250–500 mg bid) or hydrochlorothiazide (25–50 mg bid) potentiates the antidiuretic effect of chlorpropamide and usually reduces urine output to the normal range. Chlorpropamide should not be given with DDAVP, because this combination is no more effective than DDAVP alone. The most serious side effect of chlorpropamide is hypoglycemia, but this is uncommon unless the patient has associated adrenal insufficiency, engages in strenuous, prolonged physical activity, or severely restricts food intake. Nevertheless, because of this risk, the drug should be used with caution (if at all) in children, the elderly, and patients with chronic renal failure or concurrent hypopituitarism or hypoadrenalism, even if treated. Chlorpropamide can also produce an antabuse-like reaction to alcohol in about 30% of patients, but this effect is well tolerated if the patient is forewarned and usually attenuates or stops with repeated exposure.

6. Clofibrate in divided doses of 1–3 g/d also increases urine concentration and decreases urine volume in patients with pituitary DI (*see* Fig. 4). Like chlorpropamide, its mecha-

nism of action is uncertain and may involve potentiation of AVP action, enhanced secretion or an AVP-independent effect *(22)*. Its antidiuretic effect is usually but not always less than that of chlorpropamide *(23)*. It is not widely used because of limited efficacy and related side effects, the most important being induction of gallstone formation and subsequent increase in risk for gallbladder cancer.

7. Carbamazepine in doses of 200–600 mg/d has a pronounced antidiuretic effect in patients with pituitary DI. Its mechanism of action is unknown *(24–26)*. Its most serious potential side effect is agranulocytosis, which necessitates periodic hematologic monitoring.

8. Thiazide diuretics also reduce urine volume and increase urine concentration in patients with pituitary DI *(see Fig. 4)*. They act via two vasopressin-independent mechanisms related to their natriuretic effect. One is interference with sodium absorption in the ascending limb of Henle's loop, which impairs urine dilution, and the other is mild volume depletion, which increases reabsorption of glomerular filtrate in proximal tubule, thereby decreasing distal delivery *(27–29)*. When combined with dietary sodium restriction, the thiazides reduce urine volume by an average of 50%. This effect is usually inadequate for sole therapy of pituitary DI, but it is very useful as an adjunct to the other oral agents. The usual recommended dose of hydrochlorothiazide is 25–50 mg once or twice daily. Side effects are mainly related to consequences of electrolyte and metabolic disturbances, namely hypokalemia, hypercalcemia, and, rarely, hyperglycemia with glycosuria.

Special Considerations in the Therapy of Pituitary DI

POSTOPERATIVE AND POSTTRAUMATIC DI

Postsurgical and posttraumatic DI occur secondary to trauma to the median eminence, pituitary stalk, or posterior pituitary *(30)*. Incidence of postsurgical DI varies from 5 to 25% following transsphenoidal surgery to almost 75% after suprasellar operations for craniopharyngioma *(31)*. Posttraumatic DI usually occurs in a setting of a head trauma in a motor vehicle accident and is thought to be caused by a shearing force on a pituitary stalk or hemorrhagic ischemia of the hypothalamus or posterior pituitary. In either case, more than 80% of supraoptic nuclei need to be destroyed in order for clinically overt DI to occur. There are several special problems associated with the diagnosis and treatment of DI in this clinical setting:

1. The first question is whether the polyuria is the result of a solute diuresis or a water diuresis. This can usually be answered by testing for glucosuria, checking on the administration of mannitol or a radiocontrast dye and determining if the solute excretion rate (urine volume × urine osmolality) exceeds 15 μmol/kg/min. If these investigations are negative, the polyuria probably is the result of a water diuresis.

2. The next question is whether a water diuresis is caused by excessive administration of fluid or to pituitary or nephrogenic DI. Usually, this can be answered by slowing or stopping iv fluids while closely monitoring urine output, urine osmolality, and serum sodium. If the patient does not concentrate his or her urine before plasma sodium reaches 145 meq/L, excessive fluid intake can be eliminated as a cause and AVP or DDAVP can be injected to determine if the patient has pituitary or nephrogenic DI.

3. If the patient has pituitary DI, the next question is how best to treat it. A depressed sensorium and/or edema and inflammation of nasal mucosa after transsphenoidal surgery usually preclude the administration of DDAVP by the oral or intranasal route. Therefore, the parenteral formulation of the drug should be injected in a dose of 1–2 μg im, sc, or iv once or twice daily. The intravenous route is sometimes preferable to im or sc admin-

istration because it provides a quicker "on–off" time. The aim should be to maintain a relatively constant level of antidiuresis and regulate water balance solely by varying the rate of fluid administration.

4. The next question is how to manage fluid replacement during treatment with parenteral DDAVP. If the patient has normal thirst and is able to drink, it is best to allow him or her to self-regulate intake and completely avoid the use of iv fluids. If the patient lacks thirst or cannot drink or requires iv fluids for other reasons, the latter cannot be given indiscriminately but should be carefully and constantly matched to total urinary and insensible losses to prevent overhydration or underhydration. The effectiveness of the regimen should be monitored by measuring plasma osmolality or sodium at least twice a day. A rise in either variable indicates dehydration and should be treated by administering supplemental fluid and increasing the dose of DDAVP if the DI is not adequately controlled. A decrease in plasma osmolality or sodium to subnormal levels indicates overhydration and should be treated by reducing fluid intake or, as a last resort, stopping the DDAVP therapy. Attempting to regulate water balance by titrating the dose of DDAVP is not recommended, because the resultant changes in urinary flow are impossible to control precisely and often lead to large and rapid fluctuations in salt and water balance. In some patients, massive head trauma and/or radical surgeries may be associated with damage to hypothalamic osmoreceptors for thirst and vasopressin secretion. Therefore, DDAVP treatment in such patient poses a risk for water intoxication when the patient attempts to regulate his or her own fluid intake. We will deal with management of this challenging clinical scenario in a separate section.

5. Another problem unique to the management of postsurgical and posttraumatic DI is possible fluctuations in the natural course of the DI during the first 4–6 wk. This is often referred to as the triple-phase response, which is characterized by initial DI followed by SIADH with or without return of permanent DI (32,33). For this reason, it is advisable to stop treatment periodically during the first month to determine if DI recurs. It should be remembered that the development of associated adrenal insufficiency may mask signs of DI. Therefore, spontaneous resolution of signs or symptoms should always prompt evaluation of adrenal function.

THIRST DISORDERS WITH DI

Hyperdipsia. As previously mentioned, water intoxication is an uncommon side effect of desmopressin therapy in uncomplicated pituitary DI. However, it may arise in patients who also have hyperdipsia resulting from associated damage to the inhibitory component of the thirst mechanism (34). The treatment of this combined defect is problematic because no method has been devised for abolishing abnormal thirst. Therefore, standard doses of DDAVP cannot be given to these patients, because they will invariably result in water intoxication. However, the nocturia and sleep disturbances can be prevented by a small dose of desmopressin at bedtime. This regimen will not result in water intoxication if the dose of desmopressin is titrated to permit recurrence of polyuria during the day, when most of the abnormal water intake occurs. Chlorpropamide may also be useful in treating patients with a combined defect because it allows more modulation of urine output in accordance with changes in hydration.

Hypodipsia. Patients with pituitary DI can also develop hypernatremic dehydration if they have hypodipsia resulting from associated damage to the stimulatory component of the thirst mechanism. This condition has been observed with head trauma, tumors such as craniopharyngioma, histiocytosis, neurosarcoidosis, and congenital developmental defects. It can also occur with aging (35). The dehydration results presumably from failure to sense and replenish excessive free water loss caused by untreated DI or insensible loss. However, in some cases, it is also aggravated by a secondary carbohydrate intolerance that results in hyperglycemia, glucosuria, and a solute diuresis. The carbohydrate intolerance is usually a temporary phenomenon caused by the dehydration, but the basic mechanism is unclear. Hypokalemia may also be present as a result of hypovolemia and secondary hyperaldosteronism.

The acute treatment of hypernatremic dehydration entails, first, the elimination of excessive urinary water losses and, second, replacement of the free water deficit (FWD) as well as ongoing urinary or insensible losses. If DI is present, AVP or DDAVP should be given parenterally as described in the previous section. If glucosuria is present, the patient should also be given regular insulin in doses sufficient to control blood sugar until the dehydration is corrected when the carbohydrate intolerance usually subsides. Parenteral potassium supplementation should also be given as needed to correct the hypokalemia. If hypotension and/or hyperglycemia are present, the free water deficit should be replaced initially with normal (0.9%) saline, because it is slightly hypotonic relative to body fluids, does not aggravate the hyperglycemia, and restores extracellular volume more rapidly with less effect on osmolality than comparable volumes of free water (i.e., 5% dextrose). Once the blood pressure or blood sugar are normalized, fluid can be given iv as half-normal saline and 5% dextrose in water or 5% dextrose in water alone.

The amount required to replenish the free water deficit (FWD) can be estimated from the formula:

$$FWD = 0.55 \times BW \times (pNa^* - 140)/140$$

where BW is body weight and pNa* is effective plasma sodium. The latter should be corrected for any hyperglycemia that may be present by the formula:

$$pNa^* = pNa\text{-}m + 0.5 (BS - 100)/18$$

where BS is the measured blood sugar (in mg/dl) and pNa-m is the measured plasma sodium. This volume should be supplemented by amounts equal to ongoing urinary and estimated insensible losses and administered over a 24- to 48-h period. Progress should be monitored continuously by repeat measurements of plasma sodium and glucose and the rate of fluid administration adjusted accordingly.

Once the acute dehydration has been corrected, the patient should be placed on an individually tailored regimen of weight-controlled water intake in conjunction with DDAVP *(36,37)*. In some patients, chlorpropamide may be more effective than DDAVP because it allows more modulation of urine output in accordance with changes in hydration and may also stimulate thirst *(38)*.

Vasopressin Antibodies

Antibodies to vasopressin do not occur spontaneously in untreated DI *(39)*. However, they occasionally develop during treatment with antidiuretic hormone, usually lysine vasopressin, and when they do, they almost always result in secondary resistance to its antidiuretic effect. Antibodies to vasopressin do not impair the response to other forms of therapy such as chlorpropamide. They may interfere with the diagnosis of DI by falsely suggesting partial nephrogenic DI, probably because the hormone that is extracted and assayed is biologically inactive as a result of antibody binding.

PREGNANCY

Women who develop DI during pregnancy usually have a deficiency of AVP caused by the combination of a preexisting subclinical impairment in secretion and a marked increase in metabolic clearance by a vasopressinase produced by placenta *(40–42)*. DDAVP is ideal treatment for such a condition because it is not degraded by vasopressinase and because it is free of any uterotonic effect. Use of DDAVP during pregnancy does not constitute a significant risk for the fetus *(43)*. Nursing while using DDAVP is also safe because the baby is not exposed to the clinically significant amounts of hormone and is not at risk for water intoxication.

Women with preexisting pituitary DI who are on a stable dose of DDAVP usually do not need any dose adjustment during pregnancy. The occasional reports of a need to increase the dose may reflect the misinterpretation of symptoms associated with physiological decrease in the threshold for thirst that normally occurs during pregnancy *(43)*. AVP and lysine vasopressin are much less effective for treating DI during pregnancy because they are quickly degraded by vasopressinase. Chlorpropamide and clofibrate are contraindicated because of possible teratogenic effects.

WOLFRAM SYNDROME

Wolfram syndrome is a rare disorder characterized by diabetes insipidus, diabetes mellitus, optic atrophy, and deafness (DIDMOAD syndrome) *(44,45)*. Dilatation of the urinary tract and gonadal dysfunction have also been noted. Many cases appear to be inherited in an autosomal recessive manner because of a mutation in a gene on chromosome 4 *(46)*.

The DI in DIDMOAD syndrome appears to be secondary to an AVP deficiency *(47)*. It ranges in severity from partial to complete and the vast majority of patients respond to treatment with DDAVP. The reason for poor response to DDAVP that is occasionally noted is unclear but may represent a partial nephrogenic component to the DI resulting from chronic dilatation of the collecting system.

Diabetes mellitus (DM) in DIDMOAD varies from impaired glucose tolerance to diabetic ketoacidosis. Chlorpropamide can be used to treat both DI and DM, but one should be alert to a progressive decline in insulin secretory capacity and institute insulin treatment when needed.

TREATMENT OF NEPHROGENIC DI

Because nephrogenic DI is caused by renal resistance to AVP, it cannot be treated with standard therapeutic doses of desmopressin or any of the other agents effective in pituitary DI (except thiazide diuretics). Some patients with partial nephrogenic DI do respond to high doses of DDAVP, but the great expense of this approach currently makes it impractical for long-term treatment. Therefore, treatment is currently limited to sodium restriction in combination with a few drugs that reduce urine output by vasopressin-independent mechanisms. They are as follows:

1. Thiazide diuretics are the mainstay of therapy for nephrogenic DI. Their pharmacology has been described earlier in the section on pituitary DI. One should remember that thiazide-induced hypokalemia may impair glucose tolerance and urinary concentrating ability, either of which could exaggerate polyuria and polydipsia in patients with nephrogenic DI.

2. Amiloride reduces polyuria in nephrogenic DI. In most forms, it tends to be less effective than chlorothiazide because it is a weaker natriuretic. However, it can be used to augment the effect of the thiazides *(48)*. Moreover, it is the drug of choice for treatment of lithium-induced nephrogenic DI *(49)* because it acts, at least in part, by blocking aldosterone-sensitive sodium channels that are the site of lithium entry into the collecting tubule cell. Thus, it reduces lithium toxicity by minimizing lithium accumulation in the distal nephron. At the usual recommended dose of 5–10 mg bid, urinary volume is reduced by 35%, but the onset of action may require several weeks *(49)*. Because the blockade of sodium sensitive aldosterone channel also impairs secretion of potassium and hydrogen ions, amiloride may cause hyperkalemia and metabolic acidosis.

3. Nonsteroidal antiinflammatory agents (NSAIDs) also have an antidiuretic effect in patients with nephrogenic diabetes insipidus. They appear to act by inhibiting the synthesis of prostaglandins, which impair urinary concentration by increasing medullary blood flow and solute washout, thereby decreasing osmolar gradient and water reabsorption *(50–52)*. When given in recommended dose of 1.5–3 mg/kg/d or 50 mg bid or tid, indomethacin can decrease urinary volume 30–52% both acutely (within hours of administration) and during chronic use *(52,53)*. It should be remembered that chronic use of nonsteroidal agents is associated with gastrointestinal, hematopoietic, central nervous system, and renal toxicity. Combining NSAIDs with hydrochlorothiazide diuretics may or may not give additive effects on urine output *(51,54)*.

Special Considerations in the Therapy of Nephrogenic DI (NDI)

1. Lithium is the most common cause of acquired nephrogenic DI (NDI). The impairment in urinary concentrating ability correlates with duration of therapy, average serum lithium ion level, and total lithium carbonate dose *(55)*. Because lithium-induced NDI may be fully reversible if the drug is discontinued in the first year or two of treatment, the necessity of prolonged lithium use should be discussed with the prescribing physician before alternatives are considered. If discontinuation of lithium is not possible or effective, lithium-induced polyuria can be reduced by administration of thiazide diuretics *(56)*, nonsteroidal agents *(53)*, or amiloride *(49)*. Thiazide diuretics cause volume contraction, which increases renal reabsorption of lithium and increases the risk of lithium toxicity. Therefore, it is important to closely monitor serum lithium levels after starting the treatment. Nonsteroidal agents appear to be efficacious but have not been extensively studied. Amiloride is currently considered to be the drug of choice for treatment of this form of nephrogenic DI. The major drawback is slow onset of action and relatively modest antidiuretic effect. The limited efficacy probably can be explained by the presence of lithium-induced structural tubulointerstitial damage *(55)*.

2. Demeclocycline, usually used for acne therapy, often causes a dose- and duration-dependent, reversible form of NDI. Complete restoration of renal concentration capacity usually occurs several weeks after treatment is stopped.

3. Because electrolyte imbalances such as hypokalemia (with potassium deficit greater than 200 meq) and hypercalcemia (Ca > 11 mg/dL) cause a reversible form of NDI, the mainstay of therapy in these forms remains the treatment of underlying cause.

TREATMENT OF PRIMARY POLYDIPSIA

Because patients with primary polydipsia have a physiological or psychological compulsion to drink excessive amounts of fluid, treatment with standard doses of AVP, DDAVP, thiazides, or any other drugs that reduce free water excretion is contraindicated

DDAVP
25 µg i.n.

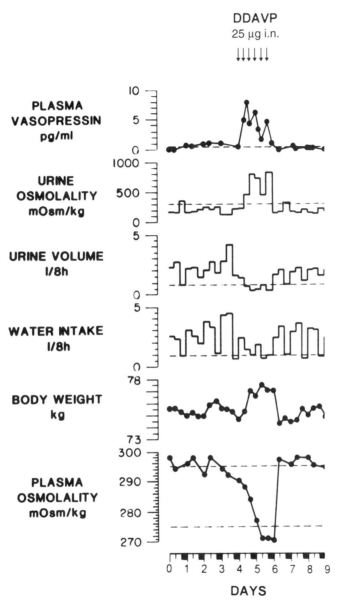

Fig. 5. The effect of DDAVP on water balance in a patient with dipsogenic DI. DDAVP was administered intranasally in a dose of 25 µg every 8 h. Note that the treatment produced an increase in urine osmolality and a decrease in fluid intake but only after excessive water retention, as evidenced by an abnormally large gain in weight and a fall in plasma osmolality and sodium to well below normal limits.

because they invariably cause symptomatic water intoxication (*see* Fig. 5). The only safe and effective way to treat this type of DI is to eliminate the excessive fluid intake. Unfortunately, there is currently no way to do this in either the psychogenic or the dipsogenic form of primary polydipsia. Therefore, the only treatment possible at present is to ameliorate some of the more annoying symptoms of nocturia and to educate the patient to prevent, recognize, and rapidly treat potentially serious complication of water intoxication.

1. The symptoms of nocturia can be relieved by small bedtime doses of DDAVP or lysine vasopressin. This treatment generally should be limited to patients with dipsogenic DI because the potential for misuse is much greater in patients with psychogenic polydipsia. To minimize the risk of water intoxication, the dose and/or form of treatment should be selected to permit recurrence of polyuria the following morning. Because of its shorter duration of action (only 4–6 h), Diapid (LVP) may offer an advantage over DDAVP, whose effect can last 12 h or longer. Regardless of the medication used, patients should have plasma osmolality and/or sodium measured periodically to rule out dilutional hyponatremia.
2. The risk of water intoxication in patients with either form of primary polydipsia can be minimized by instructing them to avoid the use of nicotine or drugs such as thiazide diuretics, which can impair water excretion *(27,57,58)*. In addition, they should be warned about the possibility of developing acute water intoxication during influenza or other febrile illnesses that often cause SIADH. Specifically, they should be advised to avoid any and all advice to increase fluid intake, should be educated as to the symptoms of water intoxication, and should advised to obtain measurements of plasma sodium at the first suggestion of these symptoms such as headaches, nausea, and anorexia.

CONCLUSIONS

Optimal treatment of DI requires an adequate diagnostic evaluation to determine the cause and the type of DI. A search for possible collateral damage to other organ systems is also needed. In pituitary or dipsogenic DI, the search should include computed tomography and/or magnetic resonance imaging of the brain and tests of anterior pituitary function. In nephrogenic DI, the search should include screening for potentially reversible metabolic causes such as hypercalcemia, as well as drugs. In both forms, a search for genetic causes *(2,4)* may also be indicated, particularly if there is a family history or presence of the disorder during early childhood.

ACKNOWLEDGMENTS

The authors thank the staff of Northwestern University's General Clinical Research Center for assistance in caring for the many patients who have greatly contributed to the understanding of this topic. The authors also express their appreciation to Mary Beth Gaskill for help with figure preparation and to James Macchione and Marie Avery for technical assistance in the preparation of this manuscript.

REFERENCES

1. Robertson GL. Diabetes insipidus. Endocrinol Metab Clin North Am 1995;24:549–572.
2. Hansen LK, Rittig S, Robertson GL. Genetic basis of familial neurohypophysial diabetes insipidus. TEM 1997;8:363–372.
3. Durr JA. Diabetes insipidus in pregnancy. Am J Kidney Dis 1987;9:276–283.
4. Bichet DG. Nephrogenic diabetes insipidus. Am J Med 1998;105:431–442.
5. Robertson GL. Dipsogenic Diabetes insipidus: a newly recognized syndrome caused by a selective defect in the osmoregulation of thirst. Trans Assoc Physician 1987;100:241–249.
6. Illowsky BP, Kirch DG. Polydipsia and hyponatremia in psychiatric patients. Am J Psychiatry 1988;145:675–683.
7. Goldman MB, Luchins DJ, Robertson GL. Mechanisms of altered water metabolism in psychotic patients with polydipsia and hyponatremia. N Engl J Med 1988;318:397–403.

8. Zimmerman EA, Ma LY, Nilaver G. Anatomical basis of thirst and vasopressin secretion. Kidney Int 1987;32:S14–S19.
9. Schmale H, Fehr S, Richter D. Vasopressin biosynthesis-from gene to peptide hormone. Kidney Int 1987;32:S8–S13.
10. Knepper MA, Wade JB, Terris J, et al. Renal aquaporins. Kidney Int 1996;49:1712–1717.
11. Nielsen S, Marples D, Frokiaer J, et al. The aquaporin family of water channels in kidney: an update on physiology and pathophysiology of aquaporin-2. Kidney Int 1996;49:1718–1723.
12. Mannucci PM. Desmopressin: a nontransfusional form of treatment for congenital and acquired bleeding disorders. Blood 1988;72:1449–1455.
13. Zerbe RL, Robertson GL. Osmotic and nonosmotic regulation of thirst and vasopressin secretion. In: Narins RG, ed. Clinical Disorders of Fluid and Electrolyte Metabolism. McGraw Hill, New York, NY, 1994, pp. 81–100.
14. Robertson GL. Differential diagnosis of polyuria. Ann Rev Med 1988;39:425–442.
15. Elster AD. Modern imaging of the pituitary. Radiology 1993;187:1–14.
16. Richardson DW, Robinson AG. Desmopressin. Annu Intern Med 1985;103:228–239.
17. Fjellstad-Paulsen A, Paulsen O, d'Agay-Abensour L, Lundin S, Czernichow P. Central diabetes insipidus: oral treatment with dDAVP. Reg Pep 1993;45:303–307.
18. Lam KS, Wat MS, Choi KL, Ip TP, Pang RWC, Kumana CR. Pharmacokinetics, pharmacodynamics, long-term efficacy and safety of oral 1-deamino-8-D-arginie vasopressin in adult patients with central diabetes insipidus. Br J Clin Pharm 1996;42:379–385.
19. Robertson GL. Posterior pituitary. In: Felig P, Baxter JD, Frohman LA, eds. Endocrinology and Metabolism, 3rd ed. McGraw Hill, New York, 1995, pp. 385–432.
20. Byun KY, Gaskill MB, Robertson GL. The mechanism of chlorpropamide antidiuresis in diabetes insipidus. Clin Res 1984;32:483A.
21. Moses AM, Numann P, Miller M. Mechanism of chlorpropamide-induced antidiuresis in man: evidence for release of ADH and enhancement of peripheral action. Metabolism 1973;22:59–66.
22. Moses AM, Howanitz J, van Gemert M, Miller M. Clofibrate-induced antidiuresis. J Clin Invest 1973;52:535–542.
23. Thompson P Jr, Earl JM, Schaaf M. Comparison of clofibrate and chlorpropamide in vasopressin-responsive diabetes insipidus. Metabolism 1977;26:749–762.
24. Van Amelsvoort T, Bakshi R, Devaux CB, Schwabe S. Hyponatremia associated with carbamazepine and oxacarbazepine therapy: a review. Epilepsia 1994;35:181–188.
25. Stephens WP, Coe JY, Baylis PH. Plasma arginine vasopressin concentration and antidiuretic action of carbamazepine. Br Med J 1978;1:1445–1447.
26. Gold PW, Robertson GL, Ballenger JC, et al. Carbamazepine diminishes the sensitivity of the plasma arginine vasopressin response to osmotic stimulation. J Clin Endocrinol Metab 1983;57:952–957.
27. Friedman E, Shadel M, Halkin H, Farfel Z. Thiazide-induced hyponatremia: reproducibility by single dose rechallenge and an analysis of pathogenesis. Ann Intern Med 1989;110:24–30.
28. Walter SJ, Skinner J, Laycock JF, et al. The antidiuretic effect of chronic hydrochlorothiazide treatment in rats with diabetes insipidus: water and electrolyte balance. Clin Sci 1982;63:525–532.
29. Shirley DG, Walter SJ, Laycock JF. The antidiuretic effect of chronic hydrochlorothiazide treatment in rats with diabetes insipidus: renal mechanisms. Clin Sci 1982;63:533–538.
30. Seckl JR, Dunger DB. Postoperative DI. Br Med J 1989;298:2,3.
31. Ciric I, Ragin A, Baumgartner C, Pierce D. Complications of transsphenoidal surgery: results of a national survey, review of the literature and personal experience. Neurosurgery 1997;40:225–236.
32. Seckl JR, Dunger DB. Neurohypophysial peptide function during early postoperative diabetes insipidus. Brain 1987;110:737–746.
33. Lindsay RS, Seckl JR, Padfield PL. The triple phase response-problems of water balance after pituitary surgery. Postgrad Med J 1995;71:439–441.
34. Robertson GL. Disorders of thirst in man. In: Ramsay DJ, Booth DA, eds. Thirst: Physiological and Psychological Aspects. Springer-Verlag, New York, 1991, pp. 453–475.
35. Phillips PA, Phil D, Rolls BJ, Ledingahm JGG, Forsling ML, Morton JJ, Crowe MJ, Wollner L. Reduced thirst after water deprivation in healthy elderly men. N Engl J Med 1984;311:753–759.
36. Robertson GL. Abnormalities of thirst regulation. Kidney Int 1984;25:460–469.
37. Perez GO, Ostre JR, Robertson GL. Severe hypernatremia with impaired thirst. Am J Nephrol 1989;9:421–434.
38. Nandi M, Harrington AR. Successful treatment of hypernatremic thirst deficiency with chlorpropamide. Clin Nephrol 1978;10:90–95.

39. Vokes TJ, Gaskill MB, Robertson GL. Antibodies to vasopressin in patients with diabetes insipidus. Ann Inter Med 1988;108:190–195.
40. Iwasacki Y, Oiso Y, Kondo K, et al. Aggravation of subclinical diabetes insipidus during pregnancy. N Engl J Med 1991;324:522–526.
41. Durr JA, Hoggard JG, Hunt JM, Schrier RW. Diabetes insipidus in pregnancy associated with abnormally high circulating vasopressinase activity. N Engl J Med 1987;316:1070–1074.
42. Lindheimer MD, Davison JM. Osmoregulation, the secretion of arginine vasopressin and its metabolism during pregnancy. Eur J Endocrinol 1995;132:133–143.
43. Kallen BAJ, Carlsson SS, Bengtsson BKA. Diabetes insipidus and use of desmopressin (Minirin) during pregnancy. Eur J Endocrinol 1995;132:144–146.
44. Kinsley BT, Swift M, Dumont RH, Swift RG. Morbidity and mortality in the Wolfram syndrome. Diabetes Care 1995;18:1566–1570.
45. Barett TG, Bundey SE. Wolfram (DIDMOAD) syndrome. J Med Genet 1997;34:838–841.
46. Karasik A, O'Hara C, Sriknata S, et al. Genetically Programmed Selective Islet b-cell loss in diabetic subjects with Wolfram's syndrome. Diabetes Care 1989;12:135–138.
47. Thompson CJ, Charlton SW, Walford S, et al. Vasopressin secretion in the DIDMOAD (Wolfram) syndrome. QJM 1989;71:333–345.
48. Alon U, Chan JCM. Hydrochlorothiazide-amiloride in the treatment of congenital nephrogenic diabetes insipidus. Am J Nephrol 1985;5:9–13.
49. Battle DC, von Riotte AB, Gaviria M, Grupp M. Amelioration of polyuria by amiloride in patients receiving long-term lithium therapy. N Engl J Med 1985;312:408–414.
50. Libber S, Harrison H, Spector D. Treatment of nephrogenic diabetes insipidus with prostaglandin synthesis inhibitors. J Pediatr 1986;108:305–311.
51. Jakobsson B, Berg U. Effect of hydrochlorothiazide and indomethacin treatment on renal function in nephrogenic diabetes insipidus. Acta Pediatr 1994;83:522–525.
52. Monn E. Prostaglandin synthetase inhibitors in the treatment of nephrogenic diabetes insipidus. Acta Pediatr Scand 1981;70:39–42.
53. Allen HM, Jackson RL, Winchester MD, Deck LV, Allon M. Indomethacin in the treatment of lithium-induced nephrogenic diabetes insipidus. Arch Intern Med 1989;149:1123–1126.
54. Monnens L, Jonkman A, Thomas C. Response to indomethacin and hydrochlorothiazide in nephrogenic diabetes insipidus. Clin Sci 1984;66:709–715.
55. Boton R, Gaviria M, Battle DC. Prevalence, pathogenesis and treatment of renal dysfunction associated with chronic lithium therapy. Am J Kidney Dis 1987;10:329–345.
56. Himmelhoch JM, Forrest J, Neil JF, Detre TP. Thiazide-lithium synergy in refractory mood swings. Am J Psychiatry 1977;134:149–152.
57. Hariprasad MK, Eisinger RP, et al. Hyponatremia in psychogenic polydipsia. Arch Intern Med 1980;140:1639–1642.
58. Siegler El, Tamres D, Berlin JA, et al. Risk factors for the development of hyponatremia in psychiatric inpatients. Arch Intern Med 1995;155:953–957.

3

Growth Hormone Therapy in Children and Adults

Darrell M. Wilson, MD

INTRODUCTION

The first documented therapeutic use of growth hormone occurred in 1958 in an effort to treat a growth-hormone-deficient adolescent *(1)*. Further studies confirmed that human growth hormone improved the growth of children with severe growth hormone deficiency (GHD). However, because of the limited supply of pituitary-derived growth hormone (GH), treatment was limited to only a few thousand patients and therapy was often sporadic. The use of the pituitary-derived human GH continued until 1985. At that time, a link between the pituitary-derived hormone and Jakob–Creutzfeldt disease was reported, resulting in the cessation of the therapeutic use of this medication *(2,3)* in the United States. Fortunately, biosynthetic forms of GH quickly became available. With improved safety and essentially limitless supplies, the therapeutic use of GH has increased dramatically.

From: *Endocrine Replacement Therapy in Clinical Practice*
Edited by: A. Wayne Meikle © Humana Press Inc., Totowa, NJ

Growth hormone therapy remains extremely expensive and quite cumbersome. Despite decades of use, substantial debate regarding who are appropriate candidates for therapy remains. The role of GH stimulation tests, the traditional tests of the GH axis, in selecting patients who will benefit from GH therapy is increasingly controversial. Although GH is approved for use in GHD adults, questions about the long-term benefits of this therapy remain. There are many potential uses for GH therapy, but because it can induce serious adverse reactions, the efficacy and benefits must be thoroughly studied in each clinical condition before it should be accepted as an appropriate therapy.

GROWTH IN CHILDREN

The primary goal of GH therapy in children and adolescents with growth abnormalities is to increase linear growth and final adult height. Essential to this process is the identification of abnormal growth patterns. The initial evaluation of growth involves accurate measurement and recording of height. Height is most consistently and accurately measured by using a calibrated, wall-mounted stadiometer for those children who can stand unassisted. The flexible-arm type of measuring devices, as often attached to scales, give misleading measurements. If the child is too young or unable to stand, then a lying height, using fixed measurement devices is the next best option. Although not necessary for screening purposes, triplicate height measurements ensure accuracy in children receiving GH therapy. Wherever possible, height should be measured by a single experienced person.

Once an accurate height is obtained, it should be recorded on a standard growth curve. There are two families of growth curve available—cross-sectional curves and longitudinal curves. The most common cross-sectional curve is based on height and weight data of normal US children that are available electronically from the Center for Disease Control (4). These curves list the height values from the 3rd to 97th percentile of normal children. Although these curves are useful for screening children, the limited percentile ranges make it difficult to quantify the deviation from normal of the very short or very tall child. Furthermore, these curves reflect heights for children going through puberty at various ages and can be misleading for the evaluation of growth of adolescents. The longitudinal curves, based on the expected growth during puberty, may be more helpful for an adolescent patient (5). When compared to the cross-sectional curve, the longitudinal curve better reflects the transient increase in growth velocity at the time of puberty (*see* Fig. 1).

In addition to noting the impact of pubertal development on growth, it is also important to assess other factors that influence growth. Chronic diseases, malnutrition, genetic abnormalities, and a history of intrauterine growth retardation can all play a significant role in affecting growth and final height. The genetic potential, based on parental heights, is also a strong determinant of adult height. It is helpful to adjust population-derived growth curves for genetic growth potential of the patient. Formulas can be used to calculate patient specific 5th to 95th percentile target range, based on parental heights (*see* Table 1).

In addition to assessing stature, it is important to assess the growth velocity. The growth velocity should be at a reasonable rate, when compared to normal standards. In the United States, the minimum growth rate is approx 4–5 cm/yr in the prepubertal ages, and 8–9 cm/yr during puberty. The growth rate is calculated by reassessing growth every 4–6 mo.

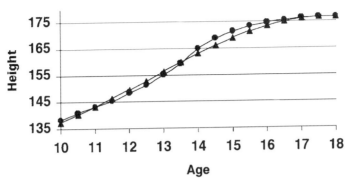

Fig. 1. Cross-section vs longitudinal growth curves. (Circles represent the median height on longitudinal curves; triangles represent cross-sectional data.)

Table 1
Calculating a Target Height Range Based on Parental Heights

1. Calculate parental mid-height (cm) accounting for the mean difference between adult men and women of 13 cm.
   For a boy: (Father's height + Mother's height + 13)/2
   For a girl: (Father's height – 13 + Mother's height)/2
2. Adjust the parental mid-height for the tendency of children's height to regress to the mean. The difference between the calculated midparental height and average adult height (177 cm for men, 164 cm for women) should be reduced to 80% of original difference.
3. Calculated the 95% confidence interval for the target range by adding and subtracting 10 cm for boys and 9 cm for girls.
   Example:
   For a boy:
     Father's height = 165 cm
     Mother's height = 154 cm
        Parental mid-height: (165 + 154 + 13)/2 = 166 cm
        Regression to the mean: 177 – 166 = 11
           11 × 0.8 = 8.8
        Corrected parental mid-height: 177 – 8.8 = 168.2 cm
        Target range: 158.2–178.2 cm
   For a girl:
     Father's height = 165 cm
     Mother's height = 154 cm
        Parental mid-height: (165 – 13 + 154)/2 = 153 cm
        Regression to the mean: 164 – 153 = 11
           11 x 0.8 = 8.8
        Corrected parental mid-height:- 164 – 8.8 = 155.2 cm
        Target range: 146.2–164.2 cm

EVALUATION OF ABNORMAL GROWTH IN CHILDREN

The initial growth assessment entails a thorough history *(6)*. Birth history, including birth weight, past medical history of chronic illness, and use of chronic medications should be detailed. The pregnancy history and birth weight are especially important as approximately one-third of patients with intrauterine growth retardation (IUGR) will continue to have poor growth velocity beyond infancy and will have a subnormal adult height *(7)*, despite normal pituitary function. Family history should include parental heights, any endocrine abnormalities, and age of onset of puberty of the parents as an indication of a family history of constitutional delay.

A complete physical exam should include height, measured with a stadiometer, and complete pubertal staging. It is important to assess the weight and weight gain in relation to the height and growth velocity. If the weight gain has been inadequate, then malnutrition, which negatively impacts growth velocity, must be initially addressed. Follow-up measurements, using the same equipment, should be performed at 4- to 6-mo intervals to assess the growth velocity.

Many factors, both endocrine and nonendocrine, play important roles in growth. Hypothyroidism is one of the more common endocrine disorders to cause growth failure in children. Thyroid-stimulating hormone (TSH) and thyroxine levels are essential to determine if hypothyroidism is present. Other endocrine disorders that can present as poor growth velocity include cortisol excess, delayed puberty, and poorly controlled diabetes mellitus. These endocrine maladies can be assessed with a thorough history, physical exam, and specific blood tests.

If the growth rate is subnormal, based on historical data or follow-up data, and there are no confounding factors, GHD should be considered. However, as discussed below, the interpretation of GH testing has become increasingly controversial.

GROWTH HORMONE SECRETION

Growth hormone is one of the primary hormones influencing linear growth. Produced by the anterior pituitary gland, GH is regulated by the hypothalamic hormones GH-releasing hormone and somatostatin, as well the recently described ghrelin *(8,9)*. GH secretion is pulsatile, with peak secretion occurring during sleep in the early morning hours *(10)*. GH values are initially high in the newborn and decline by 1 mo of age toward the prepuberty GH levels *(11)*. Growth hormone values increase in puberty with an increase primarily in the amplitude of the GH pulses. The mean GH secretion peaks during early puberty in girls and late puberty in boys *(12,13)*. The daily GH secretion plateaus in adulthood, followed by a decline by the fourth decade of life. By the eighth decade of life in men, the mean GH values are less than one-third of the values found in men in their 20s to 30s *(14)*.

Severe stress, exercise, and hypoglycemia also increase the secretion of GH. Severe psychosocial deprivation reduces the GH secretion, and obesity is associated with a decrease in the frequency and intensity of the peaks of GH secretion, primarily during the day *(15)*.

Growth hormone mediates its growth effects primarily through insulinlike growth factor-1 (IGF-1). The production of IGF-I, stimulated by GH, occurs mainly in the liver, but also takes place in many other tissues in the body *(16)*. IGF-1 stimulates tissue proliferation and thus directly affects growth. Recent data from mouse models where liver, but not local, IGF-1 production is knocked out suggest that the circulating IGF-1 is not as important as previous thought *(17)*. Most of the circulating IGF-1 is bound to specific binding proteins, with the majority bound to IGF-1-binding protein-3 (IGFBP-3). Both IGF-1 and IGFBP-3 concentrations are stable in the serum and lack the pulsatile variation as observed in serum GH measurements. Similar to GH, IGF-1, and IGFBP-3 vary with age, gender, and the degree of pubertal development. Serum IGF-1 levels increase from infancy to puberty, with pubertal IGF-1 peaks occurring later in boys than girls (14.4 yr of age form males, compared to 12.6 yr for females) *(18)*. The IGF-1 levels tend to decrease after the 30th yr of life and by the 7th decade of life, the values are approx 60% of the young adult level, and by the 90th yr at 30% of the 20- to 30-yr-old level. These two proteins also correlate with the peak stimulated GH levels *(19,20)* and may be good indicators of GH production.

EVALUATION OF GROWTH HORMONE AXIS

Clinical Signs in Children

Growth hormone deficiency in children should be suspected when a patient's height is less than three standard deviations below the mean or when the growth velocity declines with the growth curve crossing percentile lines *(21)*. Traditionally, children have been considered GHD if they have a peak GH response of less than 10 µg/L following two stimulation tests (e.g., using clonidine, insulin-induced hypoglycemia, exercise, etc.) *(22)*. In the past, the insulin-induced hypoglycemia test is considered to be the best method to assess GHD, however these tests have inherent risks. Many children experience side effects from the tests, including vomiting, abdominal pain, and hypoglycemic symptoms *(23)*. More serious complications (hypotension, bradycardia, seizures, and death) have also been reported *(24,25)*.

GH Testing Problems

Serum GH has a short half-life in blood and is normally secreted in a pulsatile manner. As such, random sampling to measure GH directly rarely yields useful information. GH can be measured following a large variety of physiological and metabolic/hormonal stimuli. Most clinicians have used the peak GH concentration obtained during a combination of GH stimulation tests as the "golden standard" of diagnosing GHD. The data regarding these GH stimulation tests (GHSTs) make this a questionable practice.

Golden Standard

Rather than validating various tests for GHD by comparing them to GHST, the utility of any diagnostic test (including GHSTs) should be determined in a population in which the diagnosis of GHD has been made using other criteria, often referred as a "golden standard." Investigators comparing diagnostic tests frequently fall prey to circular logic, concluding that the test under consideration is better because it agrees with itself more than it agrees with another test. When the results of IGF-1 or IGFBP-3 are discordant, as an example, it is impossible to select the better test without an independent method of determining if the patient has GHD. Patients who have had their pituitaries surgically removed demonstrate this point. Adan et al. *(26)* used clinical criteria (pituitary stalk interruption, familial GHD, and/or microphallus and hypoglycemia) as the golden standard for GHD in children. Stimulated GH, 24-h GH profiles, IGF-1, or IGFBP-3 are all dramatically low. For children and adolescents with classical GHD, all of the procedures discussed in the following section are quite consistent with the clinical impression. Except for these classically GHD patients, meeting all these criteria is quite difficult. Without growth as a clinical sign, the diagnosis of GHD in adults is potentially more difficult. Moreover, many investigators report that impaired IGF-1 and IGFBP-3 concentrations are not found as consistently among adults with GHD.

Reproducibility

Growth hormone stimulation tests have poor reproducibility. Carel et al. *(27)* reviewed paired GHSTs in more than 3200 children and adolescents and concluded reliability of the estimate of the GH peak value was poor. The 95% confidence limit for the difference in peak GH concentrations on two GHSTs was huge, −5 to +5 μg/L. These data confirm those of Tassoni et al. *(28)*, who performed various growth hormone stimulation tests twice in a group of 49 short children. Repeated arginine GHSTs were discordant in 40% of the patients (using a GH concentration cutoff of 7 μg/L).

In severe GHD, with peak stimulated GH values less than 4 μg/L, the stimulation tests are generally reliable. However, peak GHSTs are notoriously unreliable for the majority of patients with GH responses between 5 and 9.9 μg/L *(29)*. Many of the studies involving GHD adults are using lower GH cutoffs to confirm the diagnosis of GHD. This seems to improve the reliability of GHSTs. GHST results are generally unnecessary in the evaluation of GHD, at least among children and adolescents.

Repeat GHSTs *(30,31)* in early adulthood frequently fail to confirm the childhood diagnosis of GHD, particularly when no hypothalamic or pituitary anatomical abnormality is detected by head magnetic resonance imaging (MRI).

Physiological Factors

A number of factors alter both the endogenous production of GH and the GH response to various stimuli. Patients in puberty have a more robust response to GHST. Many investigators advocate "priming" prepubertal children with sex steroids immediately prior to GH-stimulation testing. Marin et al. *(32)* perform arginine–insulin and exercise GH-stimulation tests in 84 children and adolescents with heights in the expected normal range. They demonstrated a dramatic effect of the stage of puberty on the GH response in adolescents. The mean peak GH concentration of 6.9 μg/L among normal prepubertal subjects was four times lower than that found among adolescents with stage 5 puberty. In fact, only 4 out of 18 (22%) of stage 1 subjects had unprimed peak GH concentrations greater than 10 μg/L on any of the three tests. Eleven prepubertal subjects had a second set of tests following 2 d of pretreatment with estrogen. The lower limit of the 95% confidence interval for stimulated GH concentrations increased from 1.7 to 7.2 μg/L. Of note, this value is still substantially below the commonly accepted pediatric cutoff of 10 μg/L. Likewise, Mauras et al. *(33)* have shown that about 50% of normal children have peak concentration less than 7 μg/L and 30% below 5 μg/L. Guyda has recently review this controversial area *(34)*.

As discussed earlier, both GH and IGF-1 concentrations rise with puberty and decrease with aging *(35)*, implying that age-specific normal ranges be used to develop criteria for diagnosing GHD. Finally, obese patients have reduced endogenous GH production *(36)* and decreased GH hormone response to GH-stimulation tests.

GH Assays

Growth hormone assays are quite variable. Celniker et al. *(37)* compared two different radioimmunoassays (RIAs) and two immunoradiometric assays for GH and found a threefold difference in GH concentrations. Granada et al. *(38)* compared 11 commercially available GH assays and found 3.3-fold variation in mean GH concentration done on the same samples. Many investigators have found that polyclonal RIAs generally gave higher serum GH values than two-site immunoradiometric assays employing monoclonal antibodies. Factors found to contribute to these discrepancies included variable standards, different buffers, and the ability of the different antibodies to recognize the 20K GH variant. The variable nature of these assays makes the common practice of using a fixed cutoff value untenable.

24-H GH Profiles

The most consistent period of GH secretion occurs approx 1 h after the onset of deep sleep. Spontaneous GH secretory patterns are generally obtained by obtaining serum at 20- to 30-min intervals. However, GH secretion can be affected by many factors, and it is not clear what GH secretory patterns reflect. The reproducibility of such patterns is poor (39), and the test is quite cumbersome.

Spiliotis et al. (40) measured serum GH levels in samples obtained at 20-min intervals from indwelling catheters and found minimal overlap between GHD children and controls. The correlation of pharmacological provocative tests and measures of physiological GH secretion (measured at 30-min intervals) in short children was assessed by Plotnick et al. (41). They found a significant correlation between the 24-h integrated serum GH concentration and the peak stimulatory GH levels ($r = 0.67$). Despite this correlation, 25% of the children who were considered GHD (peak GH of less than 10 µg/L following a stimulation test) had 24-h GH concentrations that were within the normal range. Furthermore, Bercu et al. (42) and Rose et al. (43) have reported that measurements of spontaneous GH secretion correlated poorly with provocative testing or with any "golden standard" for the diagnosis of GHD.

IGF-1 and IGFBP-3

The diagnostic significance of low serum levels of radioimmunoassayable IGF-1 was first reported in the mid-1970s. It was quickly discovered that normal concentrations are influenced by chronological age, degree of sexual maturation, and nutritional status. Thus, clinical information is essential to properly interpret IGF-1 or IGFBP-3 concentrations.

Rosenfeld et al. (44) subsequently measured plasma IGF-1 levels in 197 patients with normal heights, compared with 68 children with GHD (provocative GH levels <7 µg/L) and 44 normal short children (provocative GH levels >7 µg/L). Eighteen percent of the GHD children had IGF-I levels within the normal range for age. Furthermore, 32% of normal short children had low IGF-1 levels, although all children in this group had provocative GH levels >7 µg/L. Many other investigators have shown similar overlaps. Measurement of IGF-2 levels provided limited discrimination between GH-deficient and GH-replete patients. Among children, the general lack of good concordance between measurements of GH secretion (either provocative or spontaneous) and plasma IGF-1 or IGFBP-3 levels appears to primarily reflect the failure of standard GH tests to adequately measure GH secretion (45). Additionally, see the discussion in this section regarding a serious lack of diagnostic concordance in young adults initially diagnosed with GHD in childhood during follow-up GHSTs.

Among adult patients, a different picture may be emerging. Hoffman et al. (46) compared 23 subjects with organic pituitary disease (age range: 17–77 yr) with 35 normal subjects. The subjects were defined as having GHD if they had a structural lesion of the pituitary or hypothalamus that was treated with surgery and/or radiotherapy ($n = 20$) or if they required replacement therapy of at least two other pituitary hormones ($n = 3$). The investigators found complete separation of the two groups when they used insulin-induced hypoglycemia as a GH stimulus and a GH cutoff of 4 µg/L. However, integrated 24-h GH, IGF-1, and IGFBP-3 concentrations all showed substantial overlap between the two groups. Despite the dangers and inconvenience of insulin-induced hypoglycemia, these authors conclude that it is the test of choice. This area has recently reviewed by Ghigo et al. *(47)*.

In contrast, Baum et al. *(48)* compared the GH secretion of 23 adult men (aged 32–62 yr) with adult onset GHD with 17 normal adult men. All of the GHD subjects had undetectable GH concentrations (less than 0.5 µg/L) following two GHSTs. Of note, these investigators did not use insulin-induced hypoglycemia in any subjects older than 50 yr because of concerns of cardiovascular complications of hypoglycemia. Each GHD subject had additional pituitary hormone deficiencies. Because the diagnosis of GHD was based on GHSTs, these data cannot be used to evaluate the role of stimulation tests in the diagnosing GHD among adults. These subjects, however, met clinically reasonable criteria for GHD and can be used to evaluate other biochemical measures that might be useful to diagnose GHD. Of note, the mean peak GH response following arginine stimulation among the normal subjects was only 5.8 µg/L (range: 0.8–16.6). Thirty-five percent of the normal subjects had no GH response at all to clonidine (0.15 mg). Twenty-four-hour GH sampling revealed mean GH concentrations that were clearly lower in the GHD group. The overlap seen with the normal subjects resulted from the very low GH concentrations seen in about 30% of normal subjects, a phenomenon also seen among children.

The IGF-1 concentrations demonstrated good separation between the groups, with only three of the GHD subjects overlapping with the concentrations seen in normal subject. Unfortunately, the investigators did not normalize the IGF-1 concentrations for age. As noted earlier, the mean IGF-1 concentration falls by approx 30% over the age range of the GHD subjects. IGFBP-3 fared less well, with substantial overlap between the two groups.

As part of the baseline evaluation for a trial of GH therapy, Attanasio et al. *(49)* reported on 173 subjects with GHD as diagnosed by a peak GH follow a single GHST of less than 5 µg/L. Seventy-four of these subjects had the onset of their GHD in childhood and 99 had adult onset. Of note, the mean concentrations of both IGF-I and IGFBP-3 among those with adult-onset GHD were nearly twice as high as the mean concentrations among the child onset group.

Among adults, IGF-1 remains an effective indicator of GH secretion. IGFBP-3, a useful indicator of GHD in children, however, is frequently normal among adults with GHD. Paradoxically, one possible explanation for this may be the generally lower IGF-1 concentrations seen in older adults. The molar concentration of serum IGFBP-3 approximates the sum of IGF-1 and IGF-2 in most clinical settings. Among pediatric subjects, normal IGF-1 concentrations are high and fall with GHD, whereas IGF-2 concentrations remain more constant. The lower normal IGF-1 concentrations found in adults implies that IGFBP-3 concentration mainly reflect serum IGF-2, a hormone that is not as GH dependent as IGF-1.

AUXOLOGIC ASSESSMENT

Among children, poor growth is the most important sign of GHD. Thus, auxologic data are essential in the diagnosis of GHD. In Australia, auxologic data and close clinical follow-up alone (rather than biochemical testing) have been utilized to select patients for growth hormone therapy and dictate the duration of treatment (50). Although concerns exist about over prescribing GH by using auxologic data alone, the preliminary study indicates that the percentage of children treated with growth hormone in Australia is comparable to many other countries, and less than the United States, Sweden, and Japan (50). The rate of adverse side effects is low and the authors assert that this method is effective in selecting appropriate candidates for growth hormone therapy. However, final height data are not yet available on children selected by auxologic criteria alone.

APPROVED USES OF RECOMBINANT GROWTH HORMONE

Currently, growth hormone has been approved by the US Food and Drug Administration (FDA) for children and adults with GHD, girls with Turner syndrome, Prader–Willi syndrome, small-for-gestational-age toddlers who have not had catch-up growth, children with chronic renal insufficiency, and the treatment of acute immune deficiency syndrome (AIDS)-associated wasting syndrome (see Table 2). Growth hormone therapy has been effectively utilized clinically for other problems such as hypoglycemia in infants and children resulting from panhypopituitarism.

Of note, GH therapy is dangerous in some settings. Although GH therapy for severely malnourished patients has shown short-term improvement in the nitrogen balance (51), subsequent controlled trials of GH in adults in intensive care settings demonstrate a significantly increased mortality rate (52,53).

GROWTH HORMONE THERAPY

Historically, patients were treated with GH purified from human pituitaries obtained at autopsy. Following the reports of Jakob–Creutzfeldt disease in 1985 (2), the use of human-derived GH stopped in the United States. Since that time, all US GH preparations have been biosynthetically produced.

GH Preparations

Growth hormone is supplied as either as a powder requiring reconstitution, a liquid premixed solution, or a recently approved depot preparation. The premixed solution is dispensed in vials or cartridges, for which can be used in a number of different pen injection systems. The pen device, where one can "dial" the appropriate volume, is beneficial to those patients who have difficulties in drawing up medication and for some children who seek independence when administering their GH. Fidotti (54) has reviewed different injection systems. The recently developed depot formulation of GH (55) is given by subcutaneous injection either every 2 or 4 wk. Although this preparation has not been directly compared with daily injections of GH, estimates are that the growth response is somewhat less. Moreover, the injections are generally considered more painful.

GH Dose for Children

In most children, GH therapy, given as subcutaneous injection, is most effective if given daily or six times per week (56). Dosing is usually in the range of 25–50 µg/kg-d, with most children receiving approx 50 µg/kg-d.

Table 2
Uses for Recombinant Human Growth Hormone

FDA approved uses:
   Growth failure as a result of lack of adequate endogenous growth hormone secretion
   Short stature associated with Turner syndrome
   Growth failure associated with chronic renal insufficiency (up to time of renal transplantation)
   Replacement therapy in adults with somatotropin deficiency syndrome
   AIDS wasting (cachexia)
   Turner syndrome
   Prader–Willi syndrome
   Short stature because of intrauterine growth retardation in children
Speculative uses:
   Idiopathic short stature (ISS) in children

Children are generally followed every 3–4 mo in the first year, then at a minimum of every 6 mo thereafter, to assess the growth rate and to monitor for complications. Most children, regardless of their diagnosis, have an increase in their growth velocity in the first 1–3 yr of treatment. Whenever the growth velocity on GH is lower than expected, the patient should be re-evaluated, with particular attention to compliance. Thyroid function should be checked at least annually. Although not yet universal, many advocate monitoring the insulin-like growth factor axis as well. Using the paradigm, the dose of GH is adjusted based on the physiological response, most commonly IGF-1 concentrations, rather than using weight or body surface area. Patients in puberty (57) require more GH to "normalize" IGF-1 concentrations. Drake et al. (58) has recently reviewed many of the issues involved in GH therapy.

GH Dose for Adults

Early studies of GH therapy among adults generally used dosing regimens similar to those used in pediatric patients. These doses of GH resulted in a high incidence of complications. De Boer et al. (59) compared three doses of GH (approx 5, 10, and 15 µg/kg/d) in 46 GHD adult males. The dose of GH was reduced in 67% of the subjects receiving the highest dose because of side effects. Dose reductions were required in 35 and 18% of subjects in the middle- and lowest-dose groups, respectively. Using normalization of IGF-I concentrations as a goal, these authors recommend a maintenance dose of about 7 µg/kg/d, roughly sevenfold lower than the pediatric dose. The current suggested starting dose in the FDA approved package insert is 6 µg/kg/d, rising to a maximum of 12.5 µg/kg/d and many clinicians suggest even lower doses to initiate therapy. Men appear to be more responsive to GH than women (60–62), implying that women will likely require higher doses than men.

Psychosocial Aspects of GH Therapy

Effective GH therapy in children requires intense parental involvement and commitment. If there is concern about poor compliance with therapy, this can be assessed through the pharmacy records and biochemically. If GH is not requested in a timely fashion or if a given supply lasts for an inappropriately long time, then noncompliance is very likely. IGF-1 and IGF-BP3 levels increase with GH therapy so these tests can be used to monitor compliance. Not all children will have an improved growth velocity in

Table 3
Complications Associated with Growth Hormone Therapy

Complications in children	Complications in adults
• Injection-site hypertrophy	• Injection-site hypertrophy
• Pain/bruising at injection site	• Pain/bruising at injection site
• Glucose intolerance/hyperglycemia	• Glucose intolerance/hyperglycemia
• Benign idiopathic intracranial hypertension/pseudotumor cerebri	• Benign idiopathic intracranial hypertension/pseudotumor cerebri
• GH Antibody production	• GH Antibody production
• Slipped capital femoral epiphysis (SCFE)	• Fluid retention/edema
• Leukemia	• Carpel tunnel syndrome
• Gynecomastia	• Arthralgia
• Worsening of scoliosis	• Psychological effects/depression
• Allergic reaction	• Decreased survival in intensive care settings
• Testicle atrophy and decreased function	

response to GH, despite good compliance. If the growth response is poor, continuation of GH therapy must be re-evaluated.

Complications of GH Therapy in Children and Adults

Therapy with GH is not only costly but is also associated with some significant side effects (63) (see Table 3). Growth hormone is a parenteral drug and small bruises or pain can occur at the injection sites. Furthermore, hypertrophy at injection sites can occur if the injection sites are not rotated. This hypertrophy may interfere with GH drug absorption.

Development of antibodies to the GH preparation occurs in some patients. Antibody production was more notable in the patients receiving earlier human-derived GH preparations and methionyl-recombinant human growth hormone (64). A high percentage of patients (65–95%) who received methionyl-GH developed antibodies, although the titers were low and there was no effect in the growth velocity in these patients (65,66). A more recent study (67) showed that the GH preparations derived from *Eschericha coli* DNA-recombinant techniques induced very little immunogenicity (1.4–2.8%) and the GH produced by mammalian cell lines resulted in a 8.5% antibody rate. The antibody presence was transitory, and at low titers, and it did not influence the growth velocity.

Benign increased intracranial hypertension (pseudotumor cerebri) is a rare complication. Twenty-three cases (22 children and 1 adult) were reported between 1986 and 1993 (68). It usually occurs within the first 8 wk of therapy; however, some patients reported symptoms up to 5 yr after the initiation of therapy. More than one-third of the reported cases involved children with chronic renal insufficiency. Symptoms include headache, nausea, vomiting, and vision changes. Signs include papilledema, which may only be evident with a thorough ophthalmology examination. If pseudotumor cerebri is suspected, GH treatment should be suspended and an ophthalmology referral and brain imaging study considered. Of the reported cases, all patients had papilledema, the majority had increased cerebral spinal fluid pressure, and most had normal brain imaging studies. The increased pressure and associated symptoms resolves after discontinuation of GH therapy.

Hyperglycemia and glucose intolerance can also occur with GH therapy in children and adults, although it is rare. Furthermore, most of these cases occurred among individuals who had an increased risk of glucose intolerance, such as patients with Turner syndrome or children with other syndromes with a known increased risk for glucose intolerance. In the majority of the reported cases, the hyperglycemia resolved once GH therapy was discontinued. However, any signs of hyperglycemia, such as polyuria, polydypsia, polyphagia, must be immediately investigated. Long-term studies do not indicate any increased risk for the future development of diabetes among GH-treated patients *(51)*.

A slight increased risk of SCFE has also been reported among children receiving GH. The incidence of SCFE among treated children is 21/7719 *(51)*, whereas the incidence of SCFE observed in adolescents is 1–8/100,000. Furthermore, animal models suggest that GH may weaken growth plates *(45)*, which may play a role in the development of SCFE. Any complaints of knee or hip pain while on GH therapy should be assessed with a complete examination and radiological studies, as indicated.

Fifty to seventy-five percent of normal boys experience some transient increase in the breast glandular tissue during puberty, and spontaneous resolution occurs in the majority of these males. The occurrence of prepubertal gynecosmastia is much less frequent, although incidence rates are unknown. Among boys treated with GH therapy through 1995, there were 28 reported cases of gynecomastia, with more than half of them occurring in pubertal boys. Of the prepubertal boys, about half had some resolution of the gynecomastia while continuing GH therapy and the remaining had resolution with GH therapy cessation *(69)*. Malozowski *(70)* also discussed the problem. The etiology of the breast enlargement among these patients is not clear. Whether it was a normal physiologic occurrence or related to the GH therapy is unknown and why only a limited number of treated boys experienced it remains a mystery. Growth hormone may have played a causal role in the development of gynecomastia in some of these males. Although Bertelloni et al. *(71)* reported that GH might be related to decreased testicular function, a more recent randomized controlled trial *(72)* detected no adverse effect on testes.

Scoliosis is also a fairly prevalent complaint in the general pediatric population, with mild scoliosis (10–20° curvature) occurring in up to 3% of the population. It is more commonly seen in girls and tends to progress during childhood and worsen during peak growth periods. Among children treated with GH and followed by the National Cooperative Growth Study, less than 1% of the patients reported a new diagnosis of scoliosis *(69)*. Therefore, there does not seem to be an increased risk of the development of scoliosis among GH-treated individuals. However, because GH therapy does result in increased growth velocity, it is important to monitor existing cases of scoliosis for progression so appropriate intervention can be provided.

There was initial concern that GH therapy increased a child's risk for malignancy, however recent data casts doubt on that assertion. Watanabe et al. *(73)* reported an increase risk of leukemia in pediatric GHD patients following GH therapy. To date, these results have not been duplicated *(74)*. Among more than 24,000 children followed by the National Cooperative Growth Study, no increased risk of leukemia was detected. Eleven cases of new leukemia among 24,417 GH-treated individuals were noted; however, eight of these children had known risk factors for leukemia, such as previous central nervous system tumor or aplastic anemia. Therefore, when compared to the incidence rate of leukemia in the general pediatric population (approx 1/2,000 persons under 15 yr of age), there was not an apparent increased cancer risk among GH-treated children. On the other hand, the confidence limits for these studies remain large *(75)*.

However, reports imply a greater risk of cancer among children who have risk factors, such as previous cancer or radiation therapy or certain syndromes, such as Bloom or Down syndrome. Therefore, caution should be taken when treating recovered cancer patients with GH. Although most of the clinical evidence suggests that GH therapy does not increase the risk of cancer, increased IGF-1 have been associated with certain malignancies *(76)*, leading to the suggestion that IGF-1 and IGF-BP3 be monitored during GH therapy.

Among adults, GH therapy has been associated with increased fluid retention and edema. In a small study, 18% of the adult patients experienced edema with therapy, although the majority had resolution of symptoms when the GH dose was decreased *(77)*. Other reported side effects include carpel tunnel syndrome and arthralgias, which also resolve when dosing is reduced *(78)*.

GROWTH HORMONE DEFICIENCY

GHD in Children

Growth hormone deficieny can be congenital or acquired (*see* Table 4). The genetic causes of the GHD have been nicely reviewed by Procter et al. *(79)*. Patients with structural brain defects, such as with septo-optic dysplasia, or genetic defects may present in the neonatal period with hypoglycemia. Poor growth issues tend to present later in life, frequently around 6 mo of age.

The acquired forms of GHD can present at any age and are clinically detected by an acute decline in the growth velocity with the growth rate at less than that expected for age. The reported incidence of GHD varies widely from 1/1500 to 1/30,000. A recent US survey of school children reported GHD in 1/3500 children, with a slight male:female predominance of 2.7:1 *(80)*.

If GHD is suspected, an MRI of the brain, with specific attention to the hypothalamus and pituitary, should be considered to detect tumors or other structural abnormalities. Furthermore, other pituitary hormone deficiencies, such as TSH, adrenocorticotropic hormone (ACTH), and, in pubertal aged children, gonadotropins, should be sought.

Most studies indicate that children with classic GHD dramatically improve their growth rate in the first few years of GH therapy. Growth velocity in one study increased from a mean of 4 to 10 cm/yr *(21)*. One can expect at least a doubling in the pretreatment growth velocity in the first year of treatment *(81)*. Children also experience an improvement in their final adult height, however, many children did not reach their predicted genetic height, based on their parental heights *(81)*. This long-term deficit in adult height may be the result of the late diagnoses or the limited supply of GH at the time of these earlier studies.

A study *(82)* evaluated GH therapy in children with growth hormone deficiency and suggested that the normal genetic growth pattern was not restored, despite therapy. This study initially enrolled more than 3000 patients, however, approx 35% did not complete the study because of insufficient response or "tiredness." The mean age at the start of treatment was 10.5 yr and most were diagnosed with GHD, based on stimulation tests, with a mean peak GH level of 6.7 µg/L. The treatment ended when the growth velocity was less than 2 cm in 6 mo and the bone age was greater or equal to 13 yr for girls and 14.5 yr for boys.

Table 4
Etiology of Growth Hormone Deficiency
in Children

Congenital
    Pituitary dysplasia or absence
        Septo-optic dysplasia, midline defects
    Hypothalamus dysplasia
    Neurosecretory disorders
    Biochemically inactive growth hormone
Acquired
    Chemotherapy/irradiation
    Trauma
    Infection/inflammation
    Hypoxia
    Central nervous system tumor/mass
        Hamartoma, craniopharyngioma
    Histiocytosis
    Vascular lesion or infarction
    Idiopathic

The average treatment time was 4.3 yr and most children did have a gain in their growth velocity in the first year of treatment. The pubertal children in the study had an increase in their height standard deviation (SD) score from 0.5 to 0.8. Among the pre-pubertal children, their mean final height was at −1.9 SD and lower than the genetic target, but their height SD score increased by 1.2 SD over the treatment years. This study reports smaller gains in height SD scores compared to previous studies; however, many of these children were pubertal and the injection doses and frequencies were 30–50% lower than doses recommended and routinely used in other countries (13 µg/kg/wk vs 35 µg/kg/wk). The diagnosis of GHD was based on stimulation tests that are difficult to interpret, especially the range in which most of the study children were detected. It is quite possible that many of these children were not truly GH deficient. These children were also treated for only a relatively short period, and it is unclear from this study if the final height may have improved if the children began treatment earlier. It is generally believed that the earlier that GH therapy is started, the better the final height outcome. Furthermore, the study only reports near-final adult height. Therefore, this study does not provide definitive information about treatment of GHD. More recently, Coutant et al. (83) reported the final height data in a large series of patients receiving GH. Height improvement was substantially greater among the subset of 15 patients with documented anatomical abnormalities in the hypothalamus or pituitary compared with those who only had GHSTs indicating GHD. Among this subset, the final height SD was higher (−1.1 vs −1.7 SD) even though they were shorter at the onset of treatment.

GHD in Adults

An ever increasing number of studies (for reviews, see ref. 84) are examining the hypothesis that GH replacement in GHD adults can significantly improve their lives. Most of the published studies demonstrate some clinically significant improvement. Many questions about risk vs benefit, ideal doses, and appropriate duration of therapy remain incompletely answered at this time. A pair of articles (85,86) frame the debate

Table 5
Possible Benefits of GH Therapy in GHD Adults

Body composition
    Increased muscle mass
    Improved muscle strength and exercise capacity
    Decreased fat mass
Increase bone mineral density
Increased cardiac output
Improved sleep patterns
Improved perceived health status

regarding various aspects of GH therapy in adults. Possible benefits of GH therapy for adults are list in Table 5. A few of the larger, controlled trials are reviewed next.

Growth hormone deficiency in adults can be of childhood or adult onset. Attanasio et al. *(49)* found significant baseline differences when comparing 74 childhood-onset GHD subjects (mean age 28.8 yr) with 99 adult-onset GHD (mean age 43.5 yr). Men with childhood-onset GHD were 12 cm shorter (~50% shorter than –2 SD) and 22 kg lighter. Similar differences were seen among the women. Of note, the IGF-1 and IGFBP-3 concentrations were nearly twice as high among the subjects with adult-onset GHD. Clearly, there are substantial differences in the baseline characteristics between these two groups, and it is reasonable to expect differences in the response to GH therapy.

GHD: CHILDHOOD ONSET

The primary outcome of GH treatment during childhood and adolescence is increased adult height. As such, most clinicians stopped GH therapy as linear growth waned. As the supply of GH increased, many investigators suggested that GH therapy be continued because of GH's other salutary metabolic effects. Nicolson et al. *(87)* repeated GHSTs in 88 adults who had been treated with GH for GHD as children. Originally, these children were diagnosed as GHD if they failed to achieve a peak GH 20 mU/L (approx 7–10 μg/L) following one (29 subjects) or two (59 subjects) tests. Re-evaluating the initial data, the proposed peak GH cutoff for adult GHD of <9 mU/L resulted in only 65% being classified as GHD. The 88 subjects were retested as adults with either one (33 subjects) or two (55 subjects) GHSTs. Sixty percent had peak GH concentrations of <9 mU/L as adults. Of note, 26 of the 55 of the adults (47%) undergoing two GHSTs had discordant results using this more conservative cutoff. Fifteen of the 55 subjects who had two GHSTs with a GH concentration of <9 mU/L (approx 4 μg/L) had additional pituitary hormone deficiencies.

Clearly, not all children who receive GH during adolescence should continue to receive it as adults. On the other hand, repeat GHSTs are not necessary in the setting of clear GHD (e.g., surgical removal of the pituitary, multiple pituitary hormone deficiencies). Which GH-treated adolescents should continue GH as adults remains unclear.

In a randomized, placebo-controlled trial of 74 subjects with childhood-onset GHD, Attanasio et al. *(49)* studied GH therapy at a dose of 12.5 μg/kg/d (half this dose for the first month) for 6 mo. The GH-treated subjects had an 8.5% increase in lean body mass and a 17% decrease in body fat (measured by bioelectrical impedance). IGF-1 concentrations tripled and IGFBP-3 concentrations increased by 70%. No treatment effect was seen on quality-of-life measures (Nottingham Health Profile). Of note, these subjects reported substantially fewer adverse effects than those subjects with adult-onset GHD.

GHD: ADULT ONSET

In a randomized, placebo controlled trial of 99 subjects with adult-onset GHD, Attanasio et al. *(49)* studied GH therapy at a dose of 12.5 µg/kg/d (half this dose for the first month) for 6 mo. The GH-treated subjects had an 6% increase in lean body mass and a 17% decrease in body fat. As with subjects with childhood-onset GHD, IGF-1 concentrations tripled. IGFBP-3 concentrations, however, increased only by 40%. Only the social isolation and physical mobility subscales of the Nottingham Health Profile were improved ($p < 0.01$).

Nass et al. *(88)* examined the effect of GH on exercise performance in 20 adults with adult-onset GHD. Those randomly assigned to receive 12.5 µg/kg/d of GH for 6 mo increased their IGF-1 concentrations nearly fivefold to a mean of 303 µg/L. Their maximum oxygen consumption increased by 37% in the GH-treated group. Multiple measures of exercise performance increased in the treated group, but remained constant in the placebo group.

NON-GROWTH-HORMONE-DEFICIENCY IDIOPATHIC SHORT STATURE

Most short children do not have any endocrinologic abnormality. The short stature most often is explained by constitutional delay, genetic components (based on predicted parental mid-heights) or a combination of both. Some children with severe short stature and a height below the –2 SD curve or a growth velocity that is slightly decreased are not GHD by standard stimulation tests. This may be a reflection of the unreliability of the provocative GH tests or, alternatively, these children may have a neurosecretory defect in GH production and delivery. The issue of whether GH therapy is effective in this group of children is controversial as the data are inconclusive.

Studies on the final height achieved among these children with non-GHD ISS, have had varied results. Most reports indicate that these children have an initial increase in growth velocity in the first few years of treatment *(89)*, although the response is not as great as that seen in GHD patients. There were no reported side effects with treatment, and puberty was initiated at a comparable time, compared to controls. However, there is an indication that the bone age advances at a slightly greater rate during puberty among GH-treated individuals *(90)*. Guyda *(91)* has recently reviewed 10 studies comparing final height or near-final height to the pretreatment predicted adult height in 413 GH-treated non-GHD children. The mean increase was 2.7 cm, with an approximate average duration of treatment of 5 yr. When the GH-treated groups were compared to untreated non-GHD controls, the results varied from no difference in height change, to improved height change, and to decreased height change. The varied results in final-height comparisons likely reflect the age of diagnosis and length of treatment in the different studies. However, all of the final heights were less than the predicted target heights, based on parental heights. The final height data from a randomized, blinded, controlled trial *(72)* have not yet been published.

The data to date regarding final adult height are generally disappointing, showing only minor increases in final height. These facts plus the cost and potential side effects of GH, make therapy in this group generally inappropriate. If the child's height is below the –2 SD curve, but he or she is growing with a normal growth velocity, then close observation, instead of medical therapy, is warranted.

TURNER SYNDROME

Turner syndrome (TS) is classically associated with significant short stature. If untreated, US women with TS are expected to reach a mean adult height of 142 cm. Although the etiology of the short stature is unknown, it is suspected that both skeletal dysplasia and GH neurosecretory defects both play roles. Often, girls with TS tend to have normal GH responses to stimulation tests and normal IGF-1 levels *(92)*, although the IGF-I levels tend to decrease after 10 yr of age *(93)*. Whether the decrease in IGF-1 levels is related to the delayed puberty, as a result of gonadal dysgenesis, is unknown. However, clinically, the growth velocity tends to dramatically decrease at this time.

One study indicated that girls with TS with isochromosomes had a greater incidence of an abnormal GH response to a stimulation test, compared to the TS girls with an XO or mosaic karyotype *(94)*. However, the short- and long-term responses to GH therapy could not be predicted by the results of the GHSTs. The short-term response to GH therapy was significantly better among the girls with amosaic karyotype, although the final height was significantly greater among the girls with isochromosomes. As discussed by Schmitt et al., this greater adult height could be explained by the greater delay in bone age at the start of GH therapy among this subgroup.

Growth hormone therapy is approved by the FDA for girls with TS. The degree of improved final height depends on treatment duration, although the exact increase in final height varies according to different studies. European studies indicate a mean increase in final height of 5–8 cm among TS girls treated with GH-treated compared to untreated TS girls *(95)*, Japanese TS subjects had a mean improvement of final height of 4–6 cm among GH-treated TS girls, with a mean treatment period of 10 yr, compared to untreated Japanese TS girls *(96)*. The US study showed that treatment with GH improved TS adult height by approx 8–9 cm, after an average of 6 yr of therapy *(97)*. In a large review of these and other studies, Guyda *(91)* reports on the results of 16 articles following 2217 GH-treated girls with TS. Among the girls the mean difference between final and predicted heights was 5.7 cm.

The optimal time to start GH therapy in TS is unknown, but earlier treatment results in further improvement of adult height. Growth hormone therapy is often initiated when the height is less than the 5th percentile on the normal female curve, which usually occurs at 4–5 yr of age. Because the classic GH stimulation testing yields little diagnostic information, GH testing should not be routinely performed in girls diagnosed with TS.

The optimal duration of GH therapy is unknown. Many physicians continue GH therapy until the growth velocity slows to less than 2.5 cm/yr and the bone age is greater than 14 yr. Although the complications with GH therapy do not differ with TS girls, TS itself is associated with glucose intolerance so one must be vigilant about assessing possible signs of hyperglycemia while treating these patients.

CHRONIC RENAL INSUFFICIENCY

Severe short stature and impaired growth velocity are common complications of chronic renal insufficiency (CRI). Many children with CRI prior to puberty will have adult heights less than 2.0 SDs below the mean *(98)*. GH therapy is FDA approved for children with short stature and CRI, prior to transplant. In order to optimize the response to GH therapy, these patients should be managed by an experienced pediatric nephrologist and should have good metabolic and nutritional status, with minimal renal osteodystrophy.

Placebo-controlled studies indicate that GH therapy will significantly improve growth velocity *(99)* in patients with CRI and does not interfere with subsequent transplant success. In a study of long-term treatment (5 yr) *(100)* of children with CRI, the mean increase in height was 40 cm with a 1.9-SD height improvement. Furthermore, these children did not have excessive increase in their bone age or any adverse effects and did not experience any significant worsening of renal function. Although the potential impact on adult height has been reviewed *(101)*, it is as yet unclear if what the ultimate impact will be.

Criteria for initiation of GH in CRI do not require GHST *(98)*. GH responses to GHST, IGF-1, and IGFBP-3 levels can be variable among CRI patients and are of little diagnostic value. Patients should be followed on a quarterly basis in order to assess the responsiveness to therapy and possible complications. Growth hormone therapy is discontinued in most CRI patients at the time of renal transplant.

Growth hormone therapy following renal transplant has been shown to be effective for children with short stature. In one study *(102)*, GH therapy improved growth velocity following transplant. Furthermore, there was no relationship between therapy and rejection or graft survival. Although the study duration was only for 3 yr, further studies may indicate whether GH therapy will ultimately improve adult height among these patients without any change in renal function.

Growth hormone therapy has not been indicated in adults with CRI, although other growth factors have been studied to determine if they will improve renal function in acute renal failure.

SMALL FOR GESTATIONAL AGE

Newborns with birth weights less than the 10th percentile for their gestation age (2.5 kg for term infants) have intrauterine growth retardation, also referred to as small for gestational age (SGA). Although most of these infants exhibit catch-up growth, approx 10% remain short into adulthood *(103)*. Both Sas et al. *(104)* and de Zegher et al. *(105)* report on long-term study of GH in children born SGA who were still short at 2 yr of age. De Zegher et al. *(106)* recently conducted an epianalysis of four randomized, multicenter trials of GH therapy in children born SGA. Across the four studies, 188 children with a mean age of 5.2 yr were randomized. Forty-nine were untreated and 139 received GH in varying regimes with GH doses ranging from 33 to 100 µg/kg/d. Of note, in all four studies, control subjects were only followed for 2 yr before being offered GH therapy. During these first 2 yr, the treated subjects had a clear increase in their height SDS. Those receiving 0.24 mg/kg/wk had a 1.2 (SDs) increase in their mean height, whereas those receiving 0.88 mg/kg/wk increased by 1.7 SDs (compared with 0.1 in the control group). Height continued to improve, although more slowly for as long as four additional years. Although these height gains are impressive, the increase in bone ages was greater in the treated groups as well. The impact on final height remains unknown. Based on these data, the FDA recently approved the use of GH for the long-term treatment of growth failure in children born SGA who fail to manifest catch-up growth by age 2.

PRADER–WILLI SYNDROME

As patients with Prader–Willi syndrome (PWS) have poor linear growth, earlier experiments with GH examined primarily the growth response *(107)*. Subsequent studies revealed a substantial impact on body composition *(108–112)* with a reduction of body fat mass and an increase in lean body mass. Patients with PWS have a high incidence of glucose intolerance *(113)* and this should be monitored during GH therapy. The rationale for GH therapy in PWS have recently been reviewed in a consensus statement *(114)*.

SUMMARY

The therapeutic use of GH for short stature has greatly expanded since the emergence of a biosynthetic product in 1985. In the United States, recombinant GH is currently approved for children with GHD, TS, PWS, short children who were SGA without catch-up growth or CRI, and adults with GHD or AIDS-associated wasting syndrome. There continues to be speculative uses for GH in children for other causes of short stature, such as genetic syndromes.

There continues to be controversy regarding GH testing issues, identification of appropriate patients for GH, and efficacy of therapy among children and adults. As the patient population for GH therapy expands, the benefits of therapy for each group need to be thoroughly explored to yield the best outcome with the least risks.

REFERENCES

1. Raben M. Treatment of pituitary dwarf with human growth hormone. J Clin Endocrinol Metab 1958;18:901–903.
2. Hintz RL. The prismatic case of Creutzfeldt-Jakob disease associated with pituitary growth hormone treatment. J Clin Endocrinol Metab 1995;80(8):2298–2301.
3. Fradkin JE, Schonberger LB, Mills JL, et al. Creutzfeldt-Jakob disease in pituitary growth hormone recipients in the United States. JAMA 1991;265(7):880–884.
4. CDC. Clinical growth charts. Centers for Disease Control, Atlanta, GA, 2001.
5. Tanner JM, Davies PS. Clinical longitudinal standards for height and height velocity for North American children. J Pediatr 1985;107(3):317–229.
6. Tanner JM. Auxology. In: Kappy MS, Blizzard RM, Migeon CJ, eds. Wilkins: The Diagnosis and Treatment of Endocrine Disorders in Childhood and Adolescence. Charles C. Thomas Publisher, Illinois, 1994, pp. 137–192.
7. Fitzhardinge PM, Inwood S. Long-term growth in small-for-date children. Acta Paediatr Scand 1989;349:27–33; discussion 34.
8. Horvath TL, et al. Minireview: ghrelin and the regulation of energy balance—a hypothalamic perspective. Endocrinology 2001;142(10):4163–4169.
9. Pombo M, et al. Hormonal control of growth hormone secretion. Horm Res 2001;55:11–16.
10. Van Cauter E, Plat L. Physiology of growth hormone secretion during sleep. J Pediatr 1996;128(5 Pt 2):S32–37.
11. Radetti G, Bozzola M, Pagamini C, et al. Growth hormone bioactivity and levels of growth hormone, growth hormone-binding protein, insulinlike growth factor I, and insulinlike growth factor-binding proteins in premature and full-term newborns during the first month of life. Arch Pediatr Adolesc Med 1997;151(2):170–175.
12. Rose SR, Municchi G, Barnes KM, et al. Spontaneous growth hormone secretion increases during puberty in normal girls and boys. J Clin Endocrinol Metab 1991;73(2):428–435.
13. Costin G, Kaufman FR. Growth hormone secretory patterns in children with short stature. J Pediatr 1987;110(3):362–368.
14. van Coevorden A, Mockel J, Laurent E, et al. Neuroendocrine rhythms and sleep in aging men. Am J Physiol 1991;260(4 Pt 1):E651–661.
15. Martin-Hernandez T, Galvaz MD, Cuadro AT, et al. Growth hormone secretion in normal prepubertal children: importance of relations between endogenous secretion, pulsatility and body mass. Clin Endocrinol (Oxf) 1996;44(3):327–334.
16. Humbel RE. Insulin-like growth factors I and II. Eur J Biochem 1990;190(3):445–462.
17. Le Roith D, Scavo L, ButlerA. What is the role of circulating IGF-I? Trends Endocrinol Metab 2001;12(2):48–52.

18. Hesse V, Jahreis G, Schambach H, et al. Insulin-like growth factor I correlations to changes of the hormonal status in puberty and age. Exp Clin Endocrinol 1994;102(4):289–298.

19. Attie KM, Julius JR, Stoppani C, et al. National Cooperative Growth Study substudy VI: the clinical utility of growth-hormone-binding protein, insulin-like growth factor I, and insulin-like growth factor-binding protein 3 measurements. J Pediatr 1997;131(1 Pt 2):S56–60.

20. Nunez SB, Municchi G, Barnes KM, et al. Insulin-like growth factor I (IGF-I) and IGF-binding protein-3 concentrations compared to stimulated and night growth hormone in the evaluation of short children—a clinical research center study. J Clin Endocrinol Metab 1996;81(5):1927–1932.

21. Neely EK, Rosenfeld RG. Use and abuse of human growth hormone. Annu Rev Med 1994;45:407–420.

22. Frasier SD. A review of growth hormone stimulation tests in children. Pediatrics 1974;53(6):929–937.

23. Ghigo E, Bellone J, Aimaretti G, et al. Reliability of provocative tests to assess growth hormone secretory status. Study in 472 normally growing children. J Clin Endocrinol Metab 1996;81(9):3323–3327.

24. Shah A, Stanhope R, Matthew D. Hazards of pharmacological tests of growth hormone secretion in childhood. Br Med J 1992;304(6820):173,174.

25. Rowe DW, Sare Z, Kelley VC. Possible complications of the levodopa-propranolol test. Pediatrics 1977;60(1):132,133.

26. Adan L, Souberbielle JC, Brauner R. Diagnostic markers of permanent idiopathic growth hormone deficiency. J Clin Endocrinol Metab 1994;78(2):353–358.

27. Carel JC, Tresca JP, Letrait M, et al. Growth hormone testing for the diagnosis of growth hormone deficiency in childhood: a population register-based study. J Clin Endocrinol Metab 1997;82(7):2117–2121.

28. Tassoni P, Cacciari E, Cau M, et al. Variability of growth hormone response to pharmacological and sleep tests performed twice in short children. J Clin Endocrinol Metab 1990;71(1):230–234.

29. Rosenfeld RG, Albertsson–Wikand K, Cassorla F, et al. Diagnostic controversy: the diagnosis of childhood growth hormone deficiency revisited. J Clin Endocrinol Metab 1995;80(5):1532–1540.

30. Van den Broeck J, et al. Interpretative difficulties with growth hormone provocative retesting in childhood-onset growth hormone deficiency. Horm Res 1999;51(1):1–9.

31. Maghnie M, et al. Growth hormone (GH) deficiency (GHD) of childhood onset: reassessment of GH status and evaluation of the predictive criteria for permanent GHD in young adults. J Clin Endocrinol Metab 1999;84(4):1324–1328.

32. Marin G, Domene HM, Barnes KM, et al. The effects of estrogen priming and puberty on the growth hormone response to standardized treadmill exercise and arginine-insulin in normal girls and boys. J Clin Endocrinol Metab 1994;79(2):537–541.

33. Mauras N, et al, Growth hormone stimulation testing in both short and normal statured children: use of an immunofunctional assay. Pediatr Res,2000;48(5):614–618.

34. Guyda HJ. Growth hormone testing and the short child. Pediatr Res 2000;48(5):579,580.

35. Florini JR, Prinz PN, Vitello MV, et al. Somatomedin-C levels in healthy young and old men: relationship to peak and 24-hour integrated levels of growth hormone. J Gerontol 1985;40(1):2–7.

36. Veldhuis JD, Iranmanesh A. Physiological regulation of the human growth hormone (GH)-insulin-like growth factor type I (IGF-I) axis: predominant impact of age, obesity, gonadal function, and sleep. Sleep 1996;19(Suppl 10):S221–224.

37. Celniker AC, Chen AB, Wert RM Jr, et al. Variability in the quantitation of circulating growth hormone using commercial immunoassays. J Clin Endocrinol Metab 1989;68(2):469–476.

38. Granada ML, Sanmarti A, Lucas A, et al. Assay-dependent results of immunoassayable spontaneous 24-hour growth hormone secretion in short children. Acta Paediatr Scand 1990;370:63–70; discussion 71.

39. Donaldson DL, Hallowell JG, Pan F, et al. Growth hormone secretory profiles: variation on consecutive nights. J Pediatr 1989;115(1):51–56.

40. Spiliotis BE, August GP, Hung W, et al. Growth hormone neurosecretory dysfunction. A treatable cause of short stature. JAMA 1984;251(17):2223–2230.

41. Plotnick LP, Lee PA, Migeon CJ, et al. Comparison of physiological and pharmacological tests of growth hormone function in children with short stature. J Clin Endocrinol Metab 1979;48(5):811–815.

42. Bercu BB, Shulman D, Root AW, et al. Growth hormone (GH) provocative testing frequently does not reflect endogenous GH secretion. J Clin Endocrinol Metab 1986;63(3):709–716.

43. Rose SR, Ross JL, Uriarte M, et al. The advantage of measuring stimulated as compared with spontaneous growth hormone levels in the diagnosis of growth hormone deficiency. N Engl J Med 1988;319(4):201–207.

44. Rosenfeld RG, Wilson DM, Lee PK, et al. Insulin-like growth factors I and II in evaluation of growth retardation. J Pediatr 1986;109(3):428–433.

45. Rosenfeld RG. Is growth hormone deficiency a viable diagnosis? J Clin Endocrinol Metab 1997;82(2):349–351.
46. Hoffman DM, O'Sullivan AJ, Baxter RC, et al. Diagnosis of growth-hormone deficiency in adults. Lancet 1994;343(8905):1064–1068.
47. Ghigo E, et al. Diagnosis of GH deficiency in adults. Growth Horm IGF Res 1998;8:55–58.
48. Baum HB, Biller BMK, Katznelson L, et al. Assessment of growth hormone (GH) secretion in men with adult-onset GH deficiency compared with that in normal men—a clinical research center study. J Clin Endocrinol Metab 1996;81(1):84–92.
49. Attanasio AF, Lamberts SWJ, Matranga AMC, et al. Adult growth hormone (GH)-deficient patients demonstrate heterogeneity between childhood onset and adult onset before and during human GH treatment. Adult Growth Hormone Deficiency Study Group. J Clin Endocrinol Metab 1997;82(1):82–88.
50. Werther GA. Growth hormone measurements versus auxology in treatment decisions: the Australian experience. J Pediatr 1996;128(5 Pt 2):S47–51.
51. Wilson DM. Clinical actions of growth hormone. Endocrinol Metab Clin N Am 1992;21(3):519–537.
52. Ruokonen E, Takala J. Dangers of growth hormone therapy in critically ill patients. Ann Med 2000;32(5):317–322.
53. Takala J, et al. Increased mortality associated with growth hormone treatment in critically ill adults. N Engl J Med 1999;341(11):785–792.
54. Fidotti E. A history of growth hormone injection devices. J Pediatr Endocrinol Metab 2001;14(5):497–501.
55. Reiter EO, et al. A multicenter study of the efficacy and safety of sustained release GH in the treatment of naive pediatric patients with GH deficiency. J Clin Endocrinol Metab 2001;86(10):4700–4706.
56. MacGillivray MH, Baptista J, Johanson A. Outcome of a four-year randomized study of daily versus three times weekly somatropin treatment in prepubertal naive growth hormone-deficient children. Genentech Study Group. J Clin Endocrinol Metab 1996;81(5):1806–1809.
57. Mauras N, et al. High dose recombinant human growth hormone (GH) treatment of GH-deficient patients in puberty increases near-final height: a randomized, multicenter trial. Genentech, Inc., Cooperative Study Group. J Clin Endocrinol Metab 2000;85(10):3653–3660.
58. Drake WM, et al. Optimizing gh therapy in adults and children. Endocr Rev 2001;22(4):425–450.
59. de Boer H, Blok GJ, Popp-Snijders C, et al. Monitoring of growth hormone replacement therapy in adults, based on measurement of serum markers. J Clin Endocrinol Metab 1996;81(4):1371–1377.
60. Johansson AG. Gender difference in growth hormone response in adults. J Endocrinol Invest 1999;22(Suppl 5):58–60.
61. Span JP, et al. Gender differences in rhGH-induced changes in body composition in GH-deficient adults. J Clin Endocrinol Metab 2001;86(9):4161–4165.
62. Hayes FJ, Fiad TM, McKenna TJ. Gender difference in the response of growth hormone (GH)-deficient adults to GH therapy. Metabolism 1999;48(3):308–313.
63. Maneatis T, et al. Growth hormone safety update from the National Cooperative Growth Study. J Pediatr Endocrinol Metab 2000;13(Suppl 2):1035–1044.
64. Massa G, Vanderschueren-Lodeweyckx M, Bouillon R. Five-year follow-up of growth hormone antibodies in growth hormone deficient children treated with recombinant human growth hormone. Clin Endocrinol (Oxf) 1993;38(2):137–142.
65. Kaplan SL, August GP, Blethen SL, et al. Clinical studies with recombinant-DNA-derived methionyl human growth hormone in growth hormone deficient children. Lancet 1986;1(8483):697–700.
66. Milner RD, Barnes ND, Buckler JMH, et al. United Kingdom multicentre clinical trial of somatrem. Arch Dis Child 1987;62(8):776–779.
67. Pirazzoli P, Cacciari E, Mandini M, et al. Follow-up of antibodies to growth hormone in 210 growth hormone-deficient children treated with different commercial preparations. Acta Paediatr 1995;84(11):1233–1236.
68. Malozowski S, Tanner LA, Wysowski D, et al. Growth hormone, insulin-like growth factor I, and benign intracranial hypertension. N Engl J Med 1993;329(9):665,666.
69. Allen DB. Safety of human growth hormone therapy: current topics. J Pediatr 1996;128(5 Pt 2):S8–13.
70. Malozowski S, Stadel BV. Prepubertal gynecomastia during growth hormone therapy. J Pediatr 1995;126(4):659–661.
71. Bertelloni S, et al. Can growth hormone treatment in boys without growth hormone deficiency impair testicular function? J Pediatr 1999;135(3):367–370.
72. Leschek EW, et al. Effect of growth hormone treatment on testicular function, puberty, and adrenarche in boys with non-growth hormone-deficient short stature: a randomized, double-blind, placebo-controlled trial. J Pediatr 2001;138(3):406–410.

73. Wantanabee S, Tsunematsu Y, Fujimoto J, et al. Leukaemia in patients treated with growth hormone. Lancet 1988;1(8595):1159,1160.
74. Allen DB, et al. Risk of leukemia in children treated with human growth hormone: review and reanalysis. J Pediatr 1997;131(1 Pt 2):S32–36.
75. Shalet SM, Brennan BM, Reddingius RE. Growth hormone therapy and malignancy. Horm Res 1997;48(Suppl 4):29–32.
76. Cohen P, Clemmons DR, Rosenfeld RG. Does the GH-IGF axis play a role in cancer pathogenesis? Growth Horm IGF Res 2000;10(6):297–305.
77. Beshyah SA, Freemantle C, Shah M, et al. Replacement treatment with biosynthetic human growth hormone in growth hormone-deficient hypopituitary adults. Clin Endocrinol (Oxf) 1995;42(1):73–84.
78. Baum HB, Biller BMK, Finklestein S, et al. Effects of physiologic growth hormone therapy on bone density and body composition in patients with adult-onset growth hormone deficiency. A randomized, placebo-controlled trial. Ann Intern Med 1996;125(11):883–890.
79. Procter AM, Phillips JA 3rd, Cooper DA. The molecular genetics of growth hormone deficiency. Hum Genet 1998;103(3):255–272.
80. Lindsay R, et al. Utah Growth Study: growth standards and the prevalence of growth hormone deficiency. J Pediatr 1994;125(1):29–35.
81. Drug and Therapeutics Committee of the Lawson Wilkins Pediatric Endocrine Society. Guidelines for the use of growth hormone in children with short stature. J Pediatr 1995;127(6):857–867.
82. Coste J, Letrait M, Carel JC, et al. Long-term results of growth hormone treatment in France in children of short stature: population, register based study. Br Med J 1997;315(7110):708–713.
83. Coutant R, et al. Growth and adult height in GH-treated children with nonacquired GH deficiency and idiopathic short stature: the influence of pituitary magnetic resonance imaging findings. J Clin Endocrinol Metab 2001;86(10):4649–4654.
84. Bengtsson BA, et al. Treatment of growth hormone deficiency in adults. J Clin Endocrinol Metab 2000;85(3):933–942.
85. Barkan AL, et al. Growth hormone therapy for hypopituitary adults: time for re-appraisal. Trends Endocrinol Metab 2000;11(6):238–245.
86. Carroll PV, Christ ER, Sonksen PH. Growth hormone replacement in adults with growth hormone deficiency: assessment of current knowledge. Trends Endocrinol Metab 2000;11(6):231–238.
87. Nicolson A, et al. The prevalence of severe growth hormone deficiency in adults who received growth hormone replacement in childhood (see comment). Clin Endocrinol (Oxf) 1996;44(3):311–316.
88. Nass R, Huber RM, Klauss V, et al. Effect of growth hormone (hGH) replacement therapy on physical work capacity and cardiac and pulmonary function in patients with hGH deficiency acquired in adulthood. J Clin Endocrinol Metab 1995;80(2):552–557.
89. Allen DB, Brook CGD, Bridges NA, et al. Therapeutic controversies: growth hormone (GH) treatment of non-GH deficient subjects. J Clin Endocrinol Metab 1994;79(5):1239–1248.
90. Loche S, Cambiaso P, Setzu S, et al. Final height after growth hormone therapy in non-growth-hormone-deficient children with short stature. J Pediatr 1994;125(2):196–200.
91. Guyda HJ. Four decades of growth hormone therapy for short children: what have we achieved? J Clin Endocrinol Metab 1999;84(12):4307–4316.
92. Wit JM, Massarano AA, Kamp GA, et al. Growth hormone secretion in patients with Turner's syndrome as determined by time series analysis. Acta Endocrinol (Copenh) 1992;127(1):7–12.
93. Ranke MB, Blum WF, Haug F, et al. Growth hormone, somatomedin levels and growth regulation in Turner's syndrome. Acta Endocrinol (Copenh) 1987;116(3):305–313.
94. Schmitt K, Haeusler G, Blumel P, et al. Short- and long-term (final height) growth responses to growth hormone (GH) therapy in patients with Turner syndrome: correlation of growth response to stimulated GH levels, spontaneous GH secretion, and karyotype. Horm Res 1997;47(2):67–72.
95. Pasquino AM, Passeri F, Municchi G, et al. Final height in Turner syndrome patients treated with growth hormone. Horm Res 1996;46(6):269–272.
96. Takano K, Ogawa M, Tanaka T, et al. Clinical trials of GH treatment in patients with Turner's syndrome in Japan—a consideration of final height. The Committee for the Treatment of Turner's Syndrome. Eur J Endocrinol 1997;137(2):138–145.
97. Rosenfeld RG, et al. Growth hormone therapy of Turner's syndrome: beneficial effect on adult height. J Pediatr 1998;132(2):319–324.

98. Kohaut EC, Fine RN. Testing for growth hormone release is not necessary prior to treatment of children with chronic renal insufficiency with recombinant human growth hormone. Kidney Int 1996;53:S119–122.

99. Fine RN, et al. The impact of recombinant human growth hormone treatment during chronic renal insufficiency on renal transplant recipients. J Pediatr 2000;136(3):376–382.

100. Fine RN, Kohaut E, Brown D, et al. Long-term treatment of growth retarded children with chronic renal insufficiency, with recombinant human growth hormone. Kidney Int 1996;49(3):781–785.

101. Haffner D, Schaefer F. Does recombinant growth hormone improve adult height in children with chronic renal failure? Semin Nephrol,2001;21(5):490–497.

102. Mentser M, Breen TJ, Sullivan D, et al. Growth-hormone treatment of renal transplant recipients: the National Cooperative Growth Study experience—a report of the National Cooperative Growth Study and the North American Pediatric Renal Transplant Cooperative Study. J Pediatr 1997;131(1 Pt 2):S20–24.

103. Luo ZC, Albertsson-Wikland K, Karlberg J. Length and body mass index at birth and target height influences on patterns of postnatal growth in children born small for gestational age. Pediatrics 1998;102(6):E72.

104. Sas T, et al. Growth hormone treatment in children with short stature born small for gestational age: 5-year results of a randomized, double-blind, dose- response trial. J Clin Endocrinol Metab 1999;84(9):3064–3070.

105. de Zegher F, et al. Early, discontinuous, high dose growth hormone treatment to normalize height and weight of short children born small for gestational age: results over 6 years. J Clin Endocrinol Metab 1999;84(5):1558–1561.

106. de Zegher F, et al. Growth hormone treatment of short children born small for gestational age: growth responses with continuous and discontinuous regimens over 6 years. J Clin Endocrinol Metab 2000;85(8):2816–2821.

107. Lee PD, et al. Linear growth response to exogenous growth hormone in Prader-Willi syndrome. Am J Med Genet 1987;28(4):865–871.

108. Lindgren AC, et al. Effects of growth hormone treatment on growth and body composition in Prader-Willi syndrome: a preliminary report. The Swedish National Growth Hormone Advisory Group. Acta Paediatr Suppl, 1997;423:60–62.

109. Carrel AL, et al. Sustained benefits of growth hormone on body composition, fat utilization, physical strength and agility, and growth in Prader-Willi syndrome are dose-dependent. J Pediatr Endocrinol Metab 2001;14(8):1097–1105.

110. Myers SE, et al. Sustained benefit after 2 years of growth hormone on body composition, fat utilization, physical strength and agility, and growth in Prader-Willi syndrome. J Pediatr 2000;137(1):42–49.

111. Eiholzer U, et al. Body composition abnormalities in children with Prader-Willi syndrome and long-term effects of growth hormone therapy. Horm Res 2000;53(4):200–206.

112. Lee PD. Effects of growth hormone treatment in children with Prader-Willi syndrome. Growth Horm IGF Res 2000;10(Suppl B):S75–79.

113. Zipf WB. Glucose homeostasis in Prader-Willi syndrome and potential implications of growth hormone therapy. Acta Paediatr 1999;88(433):115–117.

114. Lee P, et al. Consensus statement Prader-Willi syndrome: growth hormone (GH)/insulin-like growth factor axis deficiency and GH treatment. Endocrinol 2000;10:S71–73.

4

Growth Hormone and Growth Hormone Secretagogues in Adults

George R. Merriam, MD
and David E. Cummings, MD

Contents

INTRODUCTION

The association of growth hormone (GH) with the promotion of linear growth in childhood has focused attention away from its role in adults, but GH continues to play an important metabolic role in adult life, as a partitioning hormone regulating body composition and function. Patients who aquire GH deficiency (GHD) in adult life lack the obvious failure of linear growth that brings GHD children to medical attention, but they have an increase in cardiovascular and cerebrovascular mortality and well-documented, clinically significant abnormalities in hormone profiles, body composition, and physical and mental functions that are largely reversed by treatment, with some studies now reporting durable benefits over as long as 10 yr of treatment. This has led to a consensus that in most GHD patients, GH replacement should be continued indefinitely even after final adult stature is attained. Although adults are often more sensitive to the side effects of GH and there are still no data directly demonstrating improved functional performance, GH treatment of GHD adults has been approved by drug-regulatory agencies in the United States, Europe, and other regions.

Growth hormone secretion continues throughout life, reaching a maximum in late adolescence and then declining progressively with age. Many age-related changes resemble those of patients with classical GHD, including a reduction in muscle and bone mass, an increase in body fat, diminished exercise capacity, and adverse changes in lipoprotein profiles *(1)*. Successful experience with treating GHD in adults has led to speculation that GH could also be used as an anabolic agent in other conditions in patients

From: *Endocrine Replacement Therapy in Clinical Practice*
Edited by: A. Wayne Meikle © Humana Press Inc., Totowa, NJ

without GHD or to prevent or reverse some of the age-associated changes that resemble those of GHD. Short-term studies of GH treatment of normal older men date to the early 1990s, and a number of clinics have been organized specifically to promote off-label GH treatment.

However, interest in aging as a partial phenocopy of GHD has also highlighted the differences between normal aging and GHD syndrome in adults of similar ages. At any given age, the decrement in GH secretion remains more severe in patients with documented GHD than in healthy age-matched controls *(2)*. An indication for treatment in one group is not necessarily an indication in the other, and it remains an important goal to improve the ability to diagnose GHD specifically in adult life, especially in older patients. Nor is it clear that open-ended chronic replacement therapy is necessarily the optimum approach in so large and heterogeneous a group as aging: Short-term treatment focused on recovery from disease or injury might better balance benefits, costs, and risks.

And these risks are not trivial. The high prevalence of side effects such as edema and carpal tunnel syndrome in studies both of GHD and normal aging has forced major dose reductions below those that are well tolerated in childhood, and a study of high-dose GH treatment in critically ill patients found a marked *increase* in mortality in the GH-treated group *(3)*. Thus, GH treatment in aging should be approached with caution and, should be based on appropriately focused studies of clinically relevant outcomes, not just hormonal or body composition measurements.

Except for patients with hypopituitarism, pituitary somatotrophs are intrinsically normal in most cases of childhood-onset GHD and in normal aging. Stimulating the pituitary with GH-releasing hormone (GHRH) with GH-releasing peptides (GHRPs) or with other mimetics of the recently characterized gastric GH secretagogue (GHS) ghrelin (*see* the following section) can evoke an acute GH response, and repeated administration of these agents can chronically increase GH secretion and circulating levels of IGF-I.

GH AND IGF-I: A NOTE ON UNITS

Measurements of GH and of IGF-I concentrations and the preparation of pituitary-derived GH for therapy began before their chemical identity and structure were determined. To calibrate assays and doses, reference was made to standard preparations and expressed in somewhat arbitrary units. With their structures now known, concentrations are now generally expressed in mass units (ng/mL or µg/L for assays, and µg for GH dosing). However, much of the earlier literature used units, and many clinicians are still familiar with dosing in IU.

Conversion of units to mass is fairly straightforward for GH and more complex for IGF-I. Therefore, this chapter approaches the two sets of units differently.

GH: GH levels and dosing are expressed in mass units (µg/L or ng/mL). Doses are sometimes also listed in International Units, using the conversion 1 mg = 3 IU.

IGF-I: Early studies of IGF-I reported values in U/mL. These were calibrated with reference to a standard in which the mean value for young adults was set as 1 U/mL, with a normal range of approx 0.5–1.5 U/mL. Given the heterogeneity of antisera, there is no singel conversion factor that would accurately report these values in ng/mL; therefore, we retain the original units in discussing articles that used this system. More recent studies are reported in ng/mL, but readers should be aware that the normal range varies from study to study depending on the antisera and reference preparations used.

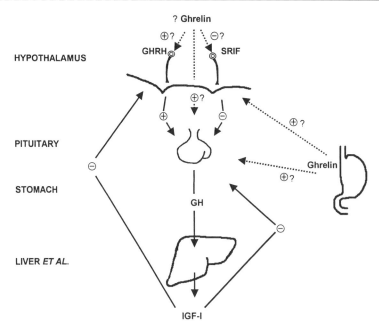

Fig. 1. Neuroendocrine regulation of GH secretion. Only the most proximal hypothalamic factors and feedback regulators are shown. A large number of converging neurotransmitter and neuromodulator pathways, in turn, regulate the loops illustrated here to provide the pattern of episodic GH secretion and the responses to factors such as sleep, stress, exercise, and meals. GHRH, GH-releasing hormone; SRIF, somatostatin; IGF-1, insulinlike growth factor-1. Whether ghrelin directly contributes to the pattern of episodic GH secretion is still uncertain. (From ref. 5).

These agents could therefore also potentially be used as treatments for GHD and normal aging, and there are both physiologic and practical reasons why their use might be attractive. Because of ongoing variability in secretion of somatostatin and perhaps other factors, GH secretion remains pulsatile even during continuous administration of GHRH or GHRPs, and there is evidence that the pattern as well as the amount of GH secreted may modulate its responses. Feedback regulation at the pituitary level is preserved during GHRH or GHRP administration, perhaps buffering somewhat against over-treatment. Of great practical importance, some GHS, particularly the GHRPs and nonpeptidyl ghrelin agonists, are active when administered orally, avoiding the need for GH injections. Several preliminary studies have explored the short-term effects of GHRH and ghrelin mimetics in adult GHD and aging, but their use is still investigational.

This chapter reviews replacement therapy with GH and the GHS in adult GHD and aging. Of these uses, only GH for adult GHD syndrome has received full regulatory approval, but we summarize the results of clinical trials that may possibly lead to other treatment indications in the future.

MECHANISMS OF REDUCED GH SECRETION

Physiologic Regulation of GH Secretion

Growth hormone is regulated by several hypothalamic factors. Without these signals, GH synthesis and secretion fall to low levels, and pituitary somatotrophs atrophy. GHRH, a 44-amino acid peptide, is the principal hypothalamic stimulator of GH synthesis and secretion. Somatostatin (SRIF), a family of 14- and 28-amino-acid peptides, is a noncompetitive inhibitor of GH secretion. After these two peptides were characterized, the prevailing consensus has until recently been that the pattern of episodic GH secretion derives from the interplay of hypothalamic GHRH and SRIF acting on the pituitary (*see* Fig. 1) (for review, *see* ref. *4*).

In the early 1980s, a group of enkephalin derivatives were found to have GH-releasing activity that appeared to act by a different mechanism from GHRH. Successive modification of these small peptides has led to the development of GHRPs, rendered devoid of opioidergic activity but with potent GHS activity *(6)*. High-affinity GHS binding sites distinct from the receptors for GHRH were demonstrated in both pituitary and hypothalamus, and recently cloned *(7)*, pointing to the existence of an endogenous ligand and a separate physiologic mechanism of GH release. In 1999, Kojima and colleagues identified a 28-amino-acid peptide from the oxyntic glands of the stomach that showed high-affinity binding for these GHS receptors and stimulated GH release in a manner similar to the GHRPs, and these authors called it *ghrelin*, from an Indo-European word meaning "to grow" *(8)*. Its structure is novel in having an octanoyl side chain, which is obligatory for biological activity, and its actions extend well beyond GH release; indeed, its major physiological role may be as an endogenous appetite stimulant *(9,10)*. Although ghrelin/GHS receptors are clearly present in hypothalamus and pituitary, whether there are also hypophysiotropic ghrelin-secreting neurons in the hypothalamus or whether instead the hypothalamus is only a target for peripherally secreted ghrelin is still a matter of controversy: Some recent abstracts claim to demonstrate small but discrete populations of ghrelin-containing neurons *(11)* and others can find no such neuronal ghrelin *(12)*. The former, positive findings seem very credible, but further independent studies will be needed to lay the issue to rest. Although ghrelin/GHS's can act directly and independently on the pituitary to release GH, their full GHS effect in vivo appears to involve a secondary release of endogenous GHRH and synergism with the pituitary effects of GHRH. Thus, there is a potent synergism when GHRH and GHRP or ghrelin are given together, and administration of a GHRH antagonist markedly reduces the effect of administered GHRP *(13,14)*.

GHD and Aging

Childhood-onset GHD is a heterogeneous disorder, but most often results from reduced hypothalamic secretion of GHRH. Thus, the pituitary is usually intrinsically normal, and GHD is often the only hormonal deficiency. Immune tolerance to GH typically develops, so that GH replacement generally does not evoke a clinically significant immune response, and the pituitary can respond to exogenous GHRH or GHRP *(15)*. Among adults with GHD, however, the majority of patients—approx 85% of the total—acquire GHD as adults, and for most of these, the deficiency results from a pituitary tumor or its treatment with radiation or surgery. In this setting, patients frequently have multiple pituitary hormone deficiencies; GHS would not be expected to be effective because the pituitary itself has been damaged.

Although normal aging mimics many of the features of GHD, the causes are likely to be different and the deficiency less severe. There are at least four possible mechanisms that could underlie the age-related decline in GH secretion: loss of pituitary responsivity to secretagogues, increased sensitivity to negative feedback by insulinlike growth factor -I (IGF-I), declining hypothalamic stimulation, and increased somatostatin inhibition.

Although both spontaneous and stimulated GH secretion is reduced in aging, the pituitary remains responsive to secretagogues, and when some of the other factors that blunt GH responses are removed, GH responses to GHRH can remain vigorous *(16)*. Thus a primary loss of somatotroph responsivity is unlikely to underlie the age-related decline in GH secretion. Chapman and colleagues examined dose-response curves for the suppression of GH secretion by infusions of IGF-I, and found no age-related shift in sensitivity to IGF-I negative feedback *(17)*.

Growth hormone responses to both GHRH and to GHRPs and ghrelin are reduced in aging, but can be increased by agents such as arginine, which are believed to suppress somatostatin secretion. The arginine effect is enhanced in older vs younger subjects *(18)*, suggesting that aging is associated with an increase in endogenous somatostatin tone, perhaps secondary to increased abdominal visceral fat. Although increases in GH secretion and IGF-I in response to administered GHRH suggest a relative deficiency of GHRH secretion in aging, it has been suggested that secretion of ghrelin may also decline. Reduced GH responses to GHRP or ghrelin, which cannot be fully restored by antagonism of somatostatin have led, Bowers to postulate an age-related decline in a hypothesized intermediate for GHRP action, the so-called "U factor" *(6)*.

At this stage, it is reasonable to conclude that the decline in GH secretion with aging is multifactorial and arises above the level of the pituitary.

Differential Diagnosis: GHD vs Aging

Because the causes, severity, and consequences of adult GHD and aging may differ, it is important to make the diagnosis of *bona fide* GHD in adults. With linear growth no longer a clue, the symptoms of GHD in adults can be nonspecific (*see* section on Adult GHD Syndrome) and available biochemical tests are imperfect. Therefore the most important indicator of the likelihood of GHD is the clinical context. The presence of a pituitary macroadenoma, a history of surgical or radiation treatment, and deficiencies of other pituitary-dependent hormones should all suggest GHD. Conversely, the absence of any factors pointing toward damage to the hypothalamic–pituitary system makes GHD unlikely and, given the imperfections of available stimulation tests (see below), testing may yield a false-positive diagnosis of GHD and so may not be prudent.

There is less information available on the best biochemical tests for GHD in adults than in children. Hoffman and colleagues compared several potential measures in hypopituitary patients with presumed GHD vs age-matched controls *(2)*. GH stimulation with insulin-induced hypoglycemia (ITT) provided the clearest distinction between patients and controls, whereas simpler integrated measures such as levels of IGF-I and IGF-binding protein-3 (IGFBP-3) showed substantial overlap and, thus, were poor discriminants. The ITT was the only provocative test examined in this study, but because this test has significant side effects and contraindications, it is important to assess whether other better-tolerated tests can provide comparable discrimination. Ghigo and colleagues reported data suggesting that the combination of GHRH with arginine (to eliminate the variable effects of somatostatin) also discriminates well between GHD and normal aging, with fewer side effects than the ITT *(18)*. This test combines the standard arginine infusion test with a bolus dose of GHRH. L-Arginine (e.g., Argine®, Pharmacia), 0.5 g/kg to a maximum dose of 30 g, is infused iv over 30 min into a free-flowing iv line, followed by GHRH (e.g., Geref Diagnostic®, Serono), 1 µg/kg iv as a bolus, 15 min into the arginine infusion, with sampling for GH at 0, 30, 60, 90, 120, and 180 min. A recently published multicenter study compared the sensitivity and specificity of six GH provocative tests *(19)*. Although ITT remained the "best" test, the combination of GHRH and arginine was a close second. Arginine by itself was a weak stimulus that failed to provoke a rise in GH in many normal subjects. Thus, although there is still not a large literature, it would appear that ITT or GHRH/arginine would be the best test choices in patients in whom the diagnosis of GHD is an open question. The ITT is more thoroughly documented, but is contraindicated in patients with a history of seizures or ischemic disease. Even in healthy subjects, it requires close direct supervision and access to appropriate medical backup test, and so may not be practical in office practice settings. In this context, the GHRH/arginine provides an effective alternative, and its use is likely to become more widespread. When there are no other pituitary deficiencies or an antecedent history of pediatric GHD, prudence often dictates performing two tests, as some normal subjects fail to respond even to the ITT.

Although most insurers still require a GH stimulation test to cover the (substantial) cost of GH therapy, it has been argued that in some patients one can legitimately presume GHD without such testing—e.g., in patients with multiple other pituitary deficiencies or panhypopituitarism, or in patients without other illness and very low levels of IGF-I (below 84 ng/mL in one reference laboratory assay) *(20)*. If it should be administratively necessary to perform a GH stimulation test to satisfy insurance coverage requirements, then one should appropriately choose a test as free as possible of side effects. This may assure at least a temporary ongoing utility for the arginine stimulation test.

Food and Drug Administration (FDA)-approved guidelines for treatment with GH in adults in the United States recommend using a peak GH response to provocative testing of <5 µg/L (tests using polyclonal GH antibody) or <2.5 µg/L (monoclonal GH antibody) as a cutoff. Although Ghigo's original study of the GHRH– arginine test suggested that a higher cutoff (ca. 9 µg/L) should be used as the dividing line between GHD and normal in this test *(18)*, the more recent multicenter study found that the same cutoffs could be used for this test as for the traditional ones *(19)*. The prudent clinician will weigh the results of one or two provocative tests together with the clinical context in forming a diagnostic impression. In the gray zone of possible "partial" or "mild" GHD, a definitive biochemical diagnosis may not be possible, and one may choose to undertake a trial of 6–12 mo of GH therapy to determine whether there is a beneficial subjective or objective response.

GHD vs GH Resistance

The somatic response to GH involves several intermediate steps, most visibly the generation of IGF-I; and inhibition of IGF-I can create a syndrome of relative GH resistance in which GH effects are reduced while GH secretion remains high. For example, fasting, malnutrition, or high-dose estrogen therapy causes a rapid fall in IGF-I levels, often with a compenstory increase in GH secretion. In prolonged severe systemic illness, however, GH secretion (and that of other pituitary hormones) can also fail. Several studies of critically ill hospitalized patients have shown reduced spontaneous GH secretion and profoundly decreased levels of IGF-I *(21,22)*. These patients most likely have both GHD and GH resistance. It has been suggested that in some catabolic states, such as burns and fractures, high-dose GH administration might overcome GH resistance, promote an anabolic response, and hasten recovery. This is pharmacologic rather than replacement therapy. The indications, doses, and side effects—some of which may be severe—are different in the two contexts, and the clinician should keep clearly in mind whether the intent of therapy is physiologic replacement or supraphysiologic therapy. This context also provides a caution in the anabolic use of pharmacologic doses of GH. In a large international multicenter study, Takala and colleagues reported the effects of high-dose (100 µg/kg/d) GH given to critically ill intensive care patients. The investigators had hoped to see a beneficial anabolic effect, but instead high-dose GH was associated with a near doubling of the already high mortality, from 20 to 38% *(3)*. Although the relatively large sample size makes it unlikely that this is a statistical artifact, there does not appear to be a single or simple explanation for this adverse effect. This cautionary report is reminiscent of earlier studies of the use of tri-iodothyronine (T_3) in critical illness, which also showed an adverse effect. Such an increase in mortality has not been seen in the use of high-dose GH in more chronic catabolic illnesses but indicates that each indication must be evaluated independently, and cautiously.

GH TREATMENT OF ADULT GHD SYNDROME

Adult GHD is commonly categorized in terms of whether the defect arose in childhood or in adult life. The former condition is usually congenital and idiopathic and may be characterized by an isolated GH deficit, but it accounts for only a minority (approx 20%) of patients presenting for treatment as adults. Adult-onset GHD, which is far more prevalent (approx 85% of patients), is most often iatrogenic, resulting from the treatment of pituitary or peripituitary tumors. Less common causes include trauma, pituitary apoplexy, Sheehan's syndrome, autoimmune or infiltrative diseases, infections, and metastases. Adult-onset GHD is generally accompanied by deficits in other anterior pituitary hormones. This is because treatment of pituitary tumors usually causes panhypopituitarism, and GH is often the first hormone to be lost from most noniatrogenic causes of hypopituitarism. Consequently, GHD is almost always a component of adult hypopituitarism, regardless of the cause. Yet, traditionally reduced GH has not been treated in adults who have completed linear bone growth, whereas inadequate thyroid, adrenal, and reproductive hormonal axes are almost always restored.

Adult GHD Syndrome

In recent years, it has become widely accepted that GH and its effector IGF-I subserve numerous important functions throughout adult life. GHD adults are physically and emotionally less healthy than age-matched peers, and suffer from a distinct clinical syndrome with widespread manifestations that are evident even when other pituitary hormone deficits are adequately corrected (*see* Table 1) (reviewed in refs. *23–29*).

This syndrome includes several adverse changes in body composition. GH has been shown to promote lipolysis and inhibit lipogenesis, as well as to redistribute fat from an android to a gynoid pattern. Accordingly, fat mass in GHD adults is increased by 7–10%. The excess fat is located preferentially in the visceral compartment of the abdomen, a pattern that in other contexts is associated with increased risk of cardiovascular disease and diabetes. The similarity between this preferentially central distribution of fat and that seen in Cushing's syndrome has been noted, although the severe catabolic changes of Cushing's patients are not present. GH inhibits the conversion of cortisone to cortisol through 11β-hydroxysteroid reductase type I, and it has been suggested that in GHD or GH resistance, a relative enhancement in the ratio of hormonally active cortisol to inactive cortisone may underlie this phenotypic similarity *(29)*.

Conversely, lean body mass is decreased 7–8% in GHD adults, and skeletal muscle volume at various sites has been shown to be diminished by up to 15%. GH exerts antinatriuretic effects, both directly by stimulating renal tubular sodium–potassium pumps and indirectly by facilitating the renin/aldosterone system. The net effect is that GH increases total-body water. Consequently, at least some of the loss of lean body mass seen in GHD adults arises from deficits in total-body sodium and fluid, especially in the

Table 1
Clinical Features of the Adult GHD Syndrome

↑ Fat mass (especially abdominal fat)
↓ Lean body mass
↓ Muscle strength
↓ Cardiac capacity
↓ RBC volume
↓ Exercise performance
↓ Bone mineral density
Atherogenic lipid profile
Thin, dry skin; poor venous access
Impaired sweating
Psychosocial problems
    Low self-esteem
    Depression
    Anxiety
    Fatigue/listlessness
    Sleep disturbances
    Emotional lability and impaired self-control
    Social isolation
    Poor marital and socioeconomic performance

extracellular compartment. However, GH is also anabolic toward muscle. It has been shown to increase the proliferation of muscle satellite cells, which can become myofibers. In mature muscle cells, GH stimulates glucose and amino acid uptake, as well as amino acid and protein synthesis. This suggests that the reduced lean body mass found in GHD adults probably does not result solely from decreased total-body water, but also from muscular atrophy.

Growth-hormone-deficient adults lose cardiac muscle in addition to skeletal muscle. Most notably, diminished left ventricular (LV) wall thickness has been demonstrated. This is associated with impaired ventricular function and cardiac capacity, as revealed by decreases in LV ejection fraction, stroke volume, and cardiac index. Furthermore, GHD generates an atherogenic lipid profile characterized by increased total cholesterol (by 20%), low-density lipoprotein cholesterol (LDL-C) (34%), and triglycerides (76%), and decreased high-density lipoprotein cholesterol (HDL-C) (34%). Thrombogenic blood components such as fibrinogen and plasminogen activator inhibitor-1 are also elevated, and hypertension may be more common. These changes combine to cause premature atherosclerosis (30). Hypopituitary patients suffer a twofold increase in cardiovascular mortality, a 3.4-fold increase in cerebrovascular mortality, and decreased life expectancy overall compared with normals (31,32). Because thyroid, adrenal, and gonadal hormones are replaced in these individuals, the untreated GHD has been implicated as the cause of increased mortality (33). It remains possible, however, that other factors such as the sequelae of pituitary radiotherapy are also involved, especially in the increase in cerebrovascular disease.

Exercise capacity is markedly compromised in GHD adults. Maximal oxygen intake (VO$_2$ max), an indicator of overall aerobic fitness, is decreased by 20–30%. This can be explained in part, by a 10–15% loss of strength that accompanies the reduced muscle mass. However, exercise performance is impaired out of proportion to muscular defects alone and is undoubtedly exacerbated by diminished cardiac capacity, as well as reduced red blood cell (RBC) volume.

Growth hormone exerts important influences on bone physiology even after linear bone growth has ceased, and its absence in postpubertal adults is unequivocally associated with osseous pathology. In general GH is anabolic with regard to bone, as it is with muscle. It enhances all of the following: intestinal absorption of Ca^{2+} and $PO4^{2-}$, 25-hydroxy-vitamin D-1α-hydroxylase activity, renal tubular $PO4^{2-}$ reabsorption, osteoblast proliferation, and synthesis of DNA and procollagen mRNA in bone. The overall effect is a stimulation of both bone formation and resorption. Bone mineral density at various skeletal sites is decreased in GHD adults by at least one standard deviation compared with age-matched controls. Consequently, these individuals have an increased incidence of osteoporotic fractures.

The skin of GHD adults is cool, dry, and thin. Patients have poor venous access and are often cold intolerant. These changes are partially the result of compromised cardiac capacity. However, the fact that acromegalics develop abnormally thick skin suggests that GH also stimulates skin growth directly. In addition, eccrine sweat glands express GH receptors, and acromegalics suffer from excessive sweating. Conversely, GHD leads to impaired sweat formation, probably contributing to exercise intolerance.

Growth-hormone-deficient adults suffer numerous psychological and social difficulties. Using a variety of questionnaires, investigators have described these as including diminished self-esteem, depressed mood, low energy and vitality, listlessness, fatigue, disturbed sleep, social isolation, anxiety, emotional lability, and impaired self-control. Objectively, patients demonstrate poor marital and socioeconomic performance. In the studies conducted to establish these findings, controls are typically matched for age, gender, socioeconomic status, and sometimes height. Nevertheless, it is difficult to determine to what degree the impaired well-being and quality of life arises directly from effects of insufficient GH vs from self-consciousness regarding a body habitus that is likely to be abnormally fatty, and possibly short if the disease originated in childhood.

Benefits of GH Replacement in GHD Adults

In view of the symptoms and signs suffered by GHD adults, it is reasonable to query whether some or all of these problems would be alleviated by GH replacement. Historically, GH treatment has been reserved for children. It was first proposed in 1921 that pituitary extracts might have growth-promoting effects (34). Beginning in the 1950s such extracts were administered to GHD children, and it quickly became axiomatic that GH increases linear bone growth in these patients. The severely limited availability of pituitary extracts prohibited serious research into the impact of exogenous GH on adults for another three decades. However, a case study was reported in 1962 describing improved vigor, ambition, and well-being in a 35-yr-old hypopituitary adult who received pituitary-derived GH, suggesting that the hormone might perform meaningful functions in adults (35). Purified recombinant human GH (rhGH) became available in 1984, and 1 yr later, pituitary-derived GH was removed from the market because of concerns over the transmission of Creutzfeldt–Jakob disease (36). The first placebo-controlled trials of GH replacement in GHD adults were reported in 1989 (37,38). Numerous related human trials have ensued since that time, each seeking to determine whether specific facets of the adult GHD syndrome are ameliorated by GH replacement (reviewed in ref. 39) (25–28,40–45). The results of these studies (detailed below) were sufficient to justify approval by the FDA in late 1996 for the use of rhGH in GHD adults and in individuals with Turner's syndrome.

Bona fide primary GHD arising in adulthood is rare (roughly 10 cases/million people/ yr) *(46)*. However, GH levels fall progressively in the course of normal aging *(47)*, and there is considerable overlap between the geriatric and GHD phenotypes, as detailed earlier. Furthermore, it has been proposed that the anabolic actions of GH on muscle and bone might also benefit patients with diverse catabolic conditions such as acquired immunodeficiency syndrome (AIDS), severe burns, extensive surgery, and malnutrition, despite the fact that GH levels are generally normal in these situations. GH has been approved by the FDA for use in AIDS-related wasting under the auspices of an expanded access program, despite a relative paucity of convincing evidence of its clinical benefits in this setting. Thus, there is a potentially vast target population for GH therapy. However, before exploring these uses, it was first necessary to prove that GH replacement is worthwhile in genuine nonaging-related GHD, which is the most logical paradigm for its use.

Several thousand GHD adults have now been administered rhGH in controlled trials. In order to recruit adequate study cohorts, investigators have typically combined patients with childhood-onset and adult-onset GHD. In most cases where these groups were analyzed separately, the findings were qualitatively similar, although a recent direct comparison of the two suggested that there may be some important differences in the response to GH therapy. Table 2 summarizes the major effects of GH replacement in GHD adults for which there is a general consensus among published reports.

Among the reported trials that examined body composition as a principal end point, it is uncontested that GH replacement causes a loss of fat and gain of lean body mass. Such consensus is impressive in view of the diverse methods of measurement employed, including bioelectrical impedance, dual-energy X-ray absorptiometry (DEXA), ^{40}K-counting, D_2O dilution, computed tomography (CT), MRI, skin-fold thickness, and waist-to-hip ratios. GH therapy decreases fat mass and volume by 7–15%, with the greatest reductions seen in abdominal visceral adipose tissue. In contrast, both lean body mass and skeletal muscle volume increase by 5–10%. Total-body water increases, especially that in the extracellular compartment. Although this explains at least some of the increase in lean body mass, total-body K^+ is also elevated, suggesting that GH promotes genuine muscular growth as well. Most studies showed no major changes in overall body weight, but rather a shift from fat to lean mass. Body composition changes in response to GH treatment are greatest in men (compared with women) and in young patients with low GH-binding protein levels at baseline.

There is also no controversy regarding the finding that GH replacement improves cardiac performance in GHD, as judged by increases in LV ejection fraction, stroke volume, and cardiac output, as well as decreased peripheral vascular resistance. These favorable changes are sustained for at least 3 yr on therapy. As the GH-induced expansion of extracellular volume includes increases in plasma volume (seen at 3 wk) and total blood volume (seen at 3 mo), at least some of the enhanced cardiac capacity may be the result of preload augmentation. Studies to date are fairly evenly divided between those that report minor (approx 5%) increases in LV muscle mass and those that deny this. The long-term impact of GH replacement on cardiac function is unknown, but warrants caution. Acromegalics develop hypertension, LV hypertrophy, and ultimately cardiac failure, which explains their increased incidence of cardiovascular mortality. It is likely that these problems can be avoided by restoring GH only to physiological levels, which may need to be adjusted for age.

Table 2
Effects of GH Replacement in GHD Adults

↓ Fat mass (especially abdominal fat)
↑ Lean body mass
↑ Total-body water and plasma volume
↑ Muscle mass and strength
Improved cardiac capacity
↑ Red blood cell volume
↑ Skin thickness
↑ Sweating
↑ Exercise capacity
↑ Resting energy expenditure
↑ Bone mineral density (after 1 yr of treatment)
Altered lipid profile
    Decreased total cholesterol
    Decreased LDL-C
    Decreased Apo B
    Decreased triglycerides (if initially elevated)
    Increased HDL-C (not seen in all studies)
    Increased Lp(a)
↓↑ Insulin sensitivity (↓ acutely, ↑ after changes in body composition)
Common side effects
    Fluid retention; edema
    Arthralgias
    Carpal tunnel syndrome
    Decreased insulin sensitivity (acutely); hyperglycemia

Another universal finding is that GH restoration significantly improves exercise performance and aerobic capacity. Usually assessed on treadmill or bicycle ergometers, subjects show increases in VO_2 max to nearly normal levels. Isometric and isokinetic muscle strength have been tested in various muscle groups. Although muscle volume increases shortly after initiating GH therapy (resulting, in part, from fluid retention), at least 6 mo treatment is required to generate appreciable changes in strength. One study showed no differences in skeletal muscle fiber areas and the proportions of type I vs II fibers after 6 mo of therapy (although these parameters were also normal in GHD patients at baseline), whereas a more recent report did see effects on these proportions (48). Limb girdle strength appears to respond to therapy by approx 6 mo, whereas quadriceps strength may take up to 1 yr to improve. Muscle strength continues to recover for as many as 3 yr of continued GH administration. The impressive improvement in exercise capacity is presumably the result of a combination of enhanced cardiac performance, increased muscle mass and strength, and a shift in body composition from fat to lean mass. In addition, GH replacement in this setting expands RBC volume (and hence oxygen-carrying capacity), via an IGF-I-mediated stimulation of erythropoiesis. Finally, GH replacement augments the capacity to sweat (as measured by response to pilocarpine iontophoresis) and, thus, dissipate heat during exercise.

Numerous studies have examined the effects of GH replacement on bone metabolism. All have shown GH treatment to increase markers of both bone formation (osteocalcin, bone alkaline phosphatase, procollagen I and III, and bone Gla) as well as bone resorption (urinary pyridinoline and deoxypyridinoline, cross-linked telopeptides of type I collagen, and urinary hydroxyproline and Ca^{2+}). The conclusion is that GH replacement stimulates bone turnover and remodeling in general. Of the studies that have examined bone mineral density (BMD), there is a roughly even split between those that lasted less than 1 yr and reported no change in this parameter vs those that lasted more than 1 yr and reported increases in BMD of 4–10%. Interestingly, the response of bone to GH restoration is biphasic. Initially, bone resorption is predominantly stimulated, and BMD may fall within the first year on therapy. Later, this change is counterbalanced by a delayed induction of bone formation, increasing BMD (up to at least 2 yr). Effects are maximal in patients with low initial BMD and least impressive in the elderly, where unrelated causes of osteopenia may be at work. The GH-induced increase in bone mass occurs fastest in trabecular bone and is, thus, manifest in vertebrae before the appendicular (cortical) skeleton. Investigators have reported no effects of GH on parathyroid hormone (PTH) or 25-hydroxy-vitamin D, whereas there are conflicting reports of either increased or unchanged 1,25-hydroxy-vitamin D.

Growth hormone regulates hepatic lipoprotein metabolism in a complex fashion, and its absence in adults is associated with an atherogenic lipid profile. Several placebo-controlled trials, typically lasting 6 mo, have examined the impact of GH replacement on lipids in GHD adults. Most reported decreases in total cholesterol, LDL-C, and Apo B, although these changes were not significant in all cases. Triglycerides tended to fall in patients who had elevated baseline values. Most investigators reported GH-mediated increases in HDL-C, although this change was not always statistically significant. Longer-term studies demonstrated that these lipoprotein changes were sustained for up to 4 yr on GH therapy. All of the above lipid alterations are favorable with respect to cardiovascular risk. However, most studies have also found that GH replacement increased Lp(a), a lipoprotein that poses an independent risk for premature atherogenesis and myocardial infarction. Given GH's opposing actions to decrease LDL-C and increase Lp(a), it is unclear what the net effect of GH replacement would be on cardiovascular risk.

Growth-hormone-deficient adults tend to be centrally obese and, consequently, demonstrate insulin resistance and elevated basal insulin levels. The effect of GH replacement on these parameters is complex and multiphasic. GH directly antagonizes insulin action, which should worsen insulin resistance; yet it also decreases central obesity, which should ameliorate the problem. In fact, trials that have specifically addressed this question using hyperinsulinemic euglycemic clamps or intravenous glucose tolerance tests have shown that both effects occur in sequence over time. GH replacement worsens insulin resistance during the first several weeks of therapy, presumably becuase of its direct counterregulatory actions. However, these changes begin to reverse after 3–6 mo of therapy. Although resting hyperinsulinemia persists, carbohydrate metabolism returns to baseline, presumably because of lost visceral fat. Several studies in which glycemic parameters were not primary end points reported mild elevations in basal insulin and/or glucose levels at some point during GH therapy, although these values generally remained within normal ranges and were never associated with significant elevations of $HgbA_{1C}$. Thus, GH treatment is not specifically contraindicated in GHD patients with diabetes, although one may need to titrate the dose more gradually than in nondiabetics (*see* section on Recommended Dosing Strategies).

Growth hormone replacement in GHD results in a rapid 12–18% elevation in resting energy expenditure (REE). Although much of this effect can be accounted for by increased lean body mass (LBM), some studies show increases in REE even when it is corrected for LBM, suggesting an actual increase in metabolic rate. GH has been shown to facilitate T_4 to T_3 conversion as well as to increase both protein synthesis and fat oxidation. All of these effects could contribute to its calorigenic potency.

Skin thickness and total skin collagen are reduced in adults with GHD, as well as in normal aging. Although trials of GH replacement in GHD adults have not examined this end point, GH supplementation was shown to increase skin thickness in one study of normal elderly men who had been selected on the basis of low IGF-I levels.

Despite the plethora of trials examining GH replacement in GHD adults, there is a dearth of data regarding clinically germane final outcomes, as opposed to surrogate or intermediate outcomes. For example, there is a great deal of data regarding effects on BMD but none on fractures, on muscle strength and exercise capacity but not functional status, and on body composition and lipids but little on morbidity or mortality. Data do exist about parameters that are overtly manifest (i.e., things that patients notice directly) in the psychosocial arena. In all controlled trials to date, subjects receiving GH replacement reported improvements in mood, energy, subjective well-being, emotional reaction, sleep, pain perception, behavior, and overall quality of life. Several questionnaires have been developed (e.g., AGHDA, QLS) which focus on the most salient symptoms in GHD (49,50). Not all of these parameters were significantly altered in every study in which they were examined, and the changes that were seen were often subtle and mutable over time. Furthermore, maintaining blindedness in these studies is difficult, because of GH-related symptoms such as fluid retention and arthralgias. Nevertheless, there has been remarkable concordance among numerous diverse studies suggesting that GH replacement improves overall well-being in GHD adults, although the mechanism by which this occurs is not known.

Adverse Effects of GH Replacement

Because rhGH is identical to the endogenous hormone, undesired consequences of GH administration should arise solely from the hormonal effects of overreplacement. By far the most common untoward effects of GH therapy in GHD adults are consequences of fluid retention arising from the antinatriuretic actions of GH. Roughly 40% of patients studied in experimental trials developed clinically apparent edema. About 20% complained of joint swelling (especially in the hands) and/or noninflammatory arthralgias, and approx 16% developed myalgias. Joint symptoms may be caused by excessive fluid in the joint space, as neither joint inflammation nor X-ray changes are detected, although the exact mechanism is unknown. These problems are generally mild and resolve after a few weeks on therapy. However, approx 10% of subjects develop symptoms of carpal tunnel syndrome. Although increased blood pressure has occasionally been reported, most studies do not demonstrate this, even after as many as 3 yr of therapy.

As discussed earlier, GH replacement may mildly impair glucose tolerance, at least transiently. Thus, patients should have glycemic markers checked periodically, especially when initiating therapy. In addition, GH influences the metabolism of certain medications, which may thus require dose adjustment after GH therapy is begun. In particular, panhypopituitary patients may require increases in thyroid, glucocorticoid, and vasopressin replacement (see subsection, Recommended Dosing Strategies).

Some concern has been expressed over potentially mitogenic properties of GH, based on highly controversial in vitro data using cells of many lineages (51), as well as the observation that acromegalics have an increased incidence of colon cancer compared with matched controls (52–55). It may be inappropriate to extrapolate conclusions from acromegalics, who have greatly excessive GH levels, to GHD patients in whom only physiological restitution is sought. Some epidemiological studies have reported a cor-relation between circulating IGF-I levels and subsequent risk for breast *(56)* or prostate cancer *(57)* in otherwise normal individuals, although there are methodologic limitations to these studies and other investigators have not uniformly concurred. Reassuringly, however, GH replacement has been practiced for four decades in children, at higher doses per kilogram than those intended for adults, with systematic surveillance studies; and there are few data to suggest either an increased incidence of *de novo* cancer as a result of GH therapy in these patients, nor is there an increased likelihood of recurrence of preexisting malignancies, although rates of both are higher in GHD children than in the general pediatric population (e.g., in children who are GHD because of cranial radiotherapy for leukemia). One recent study, however, does report increased risks of colorectal cancer and Hodgkin's disease when these children were followed into adult life *(57a)*. The risk of cancer is generally higher in adults than children, especially in AIDS patients and the elderly—two populations currently being considered for GH therapy. Nevertheless, at this time, adults receiving GH therapy are not recommended to require additional cancer surveillance beyond standard age- and gender-appropriate practices for prevention and early detection, and the only absolute cancer-related con-traindication to GH treatment is the presence of active malignancy.

There have been isolated case reports associating GH therapy with cerebral side effects such as headaches, tinnitus, encephalocele, and benign intracranial hypertension (typically with papilledema). Most of these were in children receiving high-dose GH and were reversible with cessation of therapy. Atrial fibrillation and gynecomastia have been rarely reported in association with GH treatment in elderly adults *(58)*.

Grwoth hormone administration is thus contraindicated in the setting of active malig-nancy, benign intracranial hypertension, and proliferative or preproliferative diabetic retinopathy. Although early pregnancy is not a contraindication, GH therapy may be discontinued in the second trimester, as a GH variant is secreted by the placenta. GH is a full lactogen (bovine GH is marketed to increase milk production in dairy cows), and in humans, this effect may either be an undesirable side effect or a beneficial support to lactation in postpartum hypopituitary patients, although formal trials are lacking.

Several manufacturers of GH sponsor postmarketing (phase IV) surveillance studies of adult GHD patients. Although they are not randomized controlled trials and so are less able to document efficacy outcomes, the largest of these each follow several thousand patients over an extended period and are already publishing useful information on the actual rates of complications of GH therapy as it is practiced. Physicians prescribing GH may wish to inform their patients about the possibility of enrolling in one of these studies, which can be conducted in practice as well as academic settings.

Recommended Dosing Strategies

Because all GH-related side effects are dose dependent, they may be avoided by titrating GH injections to the minimum effective dose. Serum IGF-I levels can be a useful indicator of GH treatment because IGF-I has virtually no diurnal variation, whereas serum GH levels fluctuate widely as a result of pulsatile release, diurnal variation, and sensitivity to numer-ous environmental stimuli. Early studies employed GH doses extrapolated from those used in GHD children (approx 15–50 μg/kg/d). These proved to be too high for adults, as judged by the supraphysiological IGF-I levels and high incidence of side effects that they gener-ated, both of which improved at lower doses. More recent trials have typically used lower doses and have still demonstrated salutary effects. It has been noted that patients who developed adverse side effects tend to have supraphysiologic IGF-I levels, whereas those whose IGF-I levels were maintained around the 50th percentile of the normal range had the greatest level of desired responses with few or no adverse effects (58).

The GH Research Society Workshop on Adult GH Deficiency published consensus guidelines for the diagnosis and treatment of adult GHD in 1998 (59). They recommend initiating GH at a low dosage not specifically pegged to body weight (150–300 µg/d; 0.45–0.90 IU/d), lower in older or frailer patients, administered subcutaneously in the evening (because approximately two-thirds of GH release usually occurs during sleep (60,61). The dose should be gradually titrated upward, at approximately monthly intervals, monitoring clinical and biochemical responses until a maintenance level is achieved. This can be defined as the minimal dose that normalizes serum IGF-I values without causing unacceptable side effects; we use the 50th percentile for age and sex as a general target (see Table 3). IGFBP-3 and urine GH have proven to be less helpful indicators. The considerable interindividual variation in GH sensitivity dictates equally variable final doses among different patients, although these should seldom exceed 1 mg/d (3 IU/d). The groups most sensitive to GH are elderly people, men, and women not taking oral estrogen replacement (see section on GH Secretagogues). Variability in both subcutaneous absorption and individual sensitivity preclude using body weight or surface area to predict dosage. Pulsatile administration of GH enjoys the theoretical advantage of being more physiological, but it is much more cumbersome and has not yet been proven to have clinical advantages that would justify the use of pump therapy. GHS (see below) may offer a more practical future way to reconsitute pulsatile GH secretion.

Several reports have suggested that women are less sensitive to the effects of GH than men and may require higher GH doses to achieve similar biological responses. Burman and colleagues gave similar doses (adjusted for body surface area) to 21 men and 15 women for 9 mo and found greater increases in IGF-I levels and greater effects on bone markers, lipoproteins, and body fat in the men (63). Using a dose-titration strategy similar to that of the GH Research Society, Drake and co-workers found that women required significantly higher mean GH doses than did men to achieve similar results (64). When titrated to similar IGF-I responses, Cook and colleagues found that women taking oral estrogens required nearly twice the GH dose as men—950 vs 550 µg/d, and that switching these patients to transdermal estrogen markedly reduced GH requirements or enhanced the response to a constant GH dose (62). Although circulating IGF-I largely derives from the liver, evidence suggests that estrogen may also blunt GH responses in many other target tissues.

A recently completed multicenter trial directly compared conventional weight-based dosing with an individualized dose titration regimen similar to that recommended by the GH Research Society (65). A total of 387 GH deficient adults were randomized to one of the two strategies, and a subset of 29 also had a detailed study of aerobic capacity (66). The individualized dosing (ID) regimen achieved similar increases in IGF-I with lower GH doses (540 vs 700 µg/d) and fewer reports of edema than fixed weight-based dosing (FD). Given the differences in final doses, treatment effects on some end points did differ (e.g., FD produced a greater reduction in total body fat in men [–13 vs –9%] but not in women, whereas ID resulted in a greater reduction in systolic blood pressure) but most measures of clinical efficacy, including the increase in aerobic capacity, were similar between the two dosing regimens. Thus, it appears that an individualized dose titration strategy yields generally similar treatment effects at a lower GH dose, with fewer of the most common side effects. As shown by the differences in effects on body fat, however,

Table 3
Summary of Recommendations for Adult GH Replacement Therapy

- Begin treatment at a dose of 150–300 µg/d in the evening. (This dose approximates 2–4 µg/kg/d.) Older patients should begin at the low end of this range.
- Titrate the dose at monthly or longer intervals based on clinical response, IGF-1 levels, side effects, and individual considerations such as glucose tolerance.
- In general, aim for an IGF-1 level near the 50th percentile for age and gender unless side effects are significant. Final doses average 400–500 µg/d in men, 500–600 µg/d in nonestrogenized women, and 900 µg/d in women taking oral estrogens, but there is wide interindividual variability.
- Growth hormone should not be used in the presence of active malignancy. Glucose intolerance is not an absolute contraindication to GH therapy: Although insulin resistance may be acutely worsened, changes in body composition often improve insulin sensitivity over time. However, these patients require close monitoring, as do patients with preexisting carpal tunnel syndrome.
- Adults given chronic GH therapy should receive age- and gender-appropriate periodic cancer screening such as colonoscopy, PSA levels, and mammography. There is currently no consensus on whether enhanced cancer surveillance is appropriate unless a patient has individual risk factors.

Source: Adapted from refs. 59 and 62 and other sources.

normalizing IGF-I levels alone may not guarantee maximal clinical benefits, and physicians may need to follow specific end points of interest to assure that the desired result has been achieved.

As the dose of GH is titrated upward, it is important to monitor its effects on other medications, including hydrocortisone, thyroid hormone, and desmopressin (DDAVP). A dose increase of approx 10% may be necessary to maintain free-T_4 levels constant, and symptoms of mild adrenal insufficiency or changes in DDAVP dosing frequency may suggest the need for adjustments of similar magnitude in hydrocortisone and DDAVP. The inhibition of 11β-hydroxysteroid type I by GH, shifting the equilibrium between cortisol and cortisone toward the latter, probably underlies part of this need for increased glucocorticoid replacement (29). GH accelerates the conversion of T_4 to T_3 and, therefore, it is not clear whether the decrease in free T_4 (which is usually accompanied by an increase in free T_3) reflects a true reduction in thyroid hormone effect; unfortunately, because the hypothyroidism is central, thyroid-stimulating hormone (TSH) levels are not helpful and one must base dose adjustments on the clinical impression. Once a maintenance GH dosage is achieved, follow-up visits every 6–12 mo are sufficient, at which times free-T_4 and IGF-I levels and an inventory of effects and side effects should be used for dose adjustments. Measurements to monitor efficacy objectively might include simple anthropometric determinations such as waist:hip ratio or skin-fold thickness, possibly supplemented by DEXA. The latter is also helpful in following BMD. Lipids should be assessed when indicated.

The cost of GH therapy is significant. At a current wholesale price of approx $35–40/mg, the annual cost of drug for a man receiving a typical dose of 500 µg/d would be about $7000, and twice that for a woman taking oral estrogen replacement. Given that cost, some insurers and health plans still question the medical necessity for GH replacement in adults, although policies and requirements vary widely. The savings in reducing the GH dose when patients are switched from oral to transdermal estrogen more than offsets the cost of estrogen patches.

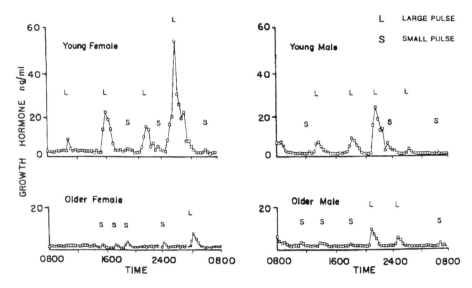

Fig. 2. Patterns of episodic GH secretion in younger and older women and men, sampled at 20 min intervals over 24 h. With aging, there is a decrease in the mean amplitude of the pulses, especially during sleep, but no overall change in pulse frequency. Young women have higher GH pulse amplitude than young men and higher 24-h integrated GH secretion. This difference is currently believed to reflect the relative GH resistance induced by estrogen and the consequent increase in GH secretion needed to maintain normal IGF-1 levels. With aging, estrogen levels fall and the gender difference in pulse amplitude is lost. In addition, there is an overall sex-hormone independent decrease in GH secretion and a loss of diurnal GH rhythms in both men and women. (From ref. *61*).

GH THERAPY IN AGING

In the course of normal aging, there is a gradual decrease in GH secretion *(1,5,67,68)* mediated, at least in part, by an age-related diminishment of endogenous GHRH release *(69,70)*. This is reflected in a progressive decrement in the amplitude of GH pulses, particularly at night, so that the sleep-related rise in GH secretion is lost *(61)* (*see* Fig. 2). Consequently, serum IGF-I levels in elderly people are less than half as high as those in younger adults. Hyposomatomedinemia is especially marked in the frail elderly *(47)*. Many of the untoward changes associated with aging mimic those seen in the GHD syndrome, including muscle atrophy, osteopenia, obesity, cardiovascular deterioration, exercise intolerance, decreased metabolic rate, dyslipidemia, thinning of the skin, mild anemia, and depression. Aging is thus a partial phenocopy of adult GHD. This has led to the speculation that pituitary somatotrope activity may be a pacemaker of aging *(44)*, and raised the possibility that GH supplementation might reverse or slow some features of geriatric deterioration *(71)*.

GH Treatment Studies in Aging

The first major trial examining the impact of GH replacement in the elderly was reported to wide public interest by Rudman, et al. in 1990 *(72)*. Twenty-one healthy elderly men aged 61–81 yr with physiologically low serum IGF-I levels[1] (<0.35 U/mL)

---

[1]See note on units at beginning of this chapter.

were randomized to receive 30 µg/kg of GH three times per week vs placebo for 6 mo. IGF-I levels in the GH group rose to a range that would be normal for men in the third decade of life (0.5–1.5 U/mL). These subjects enjoyed an 8.8% increase in LBM, a 14.4% decrease in adipose tissue mass, and a 7.1% increase in skin thickness. LBM was assessed by ^{40}K counting, which should not be spuriously elevated as a result of fluid retention. There was a slight (1.6%) increase in lumbar vertebral BMD in the GH group, but no change in BMD in the radius or proximal femur in either group. In a larger follow-up study using a similar cohort of healthy, GH-insufficient elderly men and the same GH dose, Rudman and colleagues demonstrated that increases in LBM, muscle cross-sectional area, and skin thickness persisted for as long as 1 yr in GH-treated individuals (73).

Since Rudman's landmark studies, there have been surprisingly few published investigations of GH treatment for the "somatopause" associated with normal aging. Among these, there is a consensus that GH causes advantageous changes in body composition among the elderly similar to those seen when it is replaced in younger GHD adults. For example, Thompson et al. demonstrated significant increases in LBM and decreases in fat mass among older women (72 ± 1 yr) administered either GH or IGF-I for just 4 wk (74). The treatments promoted whole-body and skeletal muscle protein synthesis and nitrogen retention. Similarly Cohn et al. reported a 6% increase in LBM and a 16% decrease in adipose tissue mass among elderly men (69 ± 2 yr) treated with GH for 1 yr (58). All of the studies of GH usage in the elderly that are described in this subsection noted changes similar to these among GH-treated subjects.

Although these alterations in body composition are favorable, it would be more meaningful to demonstrate improvement in strength and functional status with GH treatment, especially because at least some of the augmentation in LBM arises from GH-mediated fluid retention rather than from actual muscle growth. Taaffe et al. reported that there was no increase in muscular response to strength training among elderly men treated with GH for 10 wk, and concluded that deficits in GH do not underlie the time-dependent leveling off of muscle strength seen with aging (75).

In a larger study, Papadakis et al. assessed whether restoration of GH to youthful physiological levels improved functional ability in older men (76). Fifty-two healthy elderly men (70–85 yr) with well-preserved functional ability but low serum IGF-I levels were randomized to receive 30 µg/kg of GH three times per week vs placebo for 6 mo in a double-blinded fashion. Once again, LBM increased by 4.3% and fat mass decreased by 13.1% in the treatment group, whereas there were no significant changes in body composition seen with placebo. However, there was no difference between GH and placebo with regard to grip strength at the hand or knee, nor in systemic endurance. Several tests were employed to assess cognitive function and mood. Mean score in the Trails B Test, which measures visual and motor tracking and attention, improved by 8.5 s in the GH group and deteriorated by 5 s in the placebo group ($p = 0.01$). However, on the Mini-Mental State Examination, which assess orientation, attention, calculation, language, and memory, scores deteriorated by 0.4 in the GH group and improved by 0.2 in the placebo group ($p = 0.11$). Neither group showed changes in results on the Digital Symbol Substitution test, which measures cognitive ability, or in the Geriatric Depression Scale. The authors concluded that GH supplementation in healthy older men for 6 mo improves body composition but not functional status.

A small number of trials examined the effects of GH administration on bone physiology in healthy, postmenopausal women. They both showed that GH increases bone turnover, but reported somewhat conflicting results regarding GH effects on BMD. Holloway et al. randomized 27 elderly women (67 ± 3 yr) to receive either placebo or GH at an initial dose of 43 µg/kg/d for 6 mo *(77)*. At this starting dose, half of the subjects receiving GH required dose reduction within the first few weeks because of adverse side effects, most commonly related to fluid retention and carpal tunnel syndrome. GH treatment was associated with 20–80% increases in markers of both bone formation (osteocalcin) and bone resorption (urinary hydroxyproline and pyridinoline). These changes were especially marked in women not taking supplemental estrogens, and they persisted for as long as 12 mo in a subset of subjects who remained on therapy after the formal trial was completed. There was no change in BMD at the lumbar spine or hip in the GH group, whereas the placebo group showed a 1.7% decrease in BMD at the femoral trochanter and a 3% decrease at Ward's triangle. The authors concluded that although GH is a powerful initiator of bone remodeling in elderly women, it exerts, at best, a protective, not enhancing, effect on BMD. Similar increases in markers of both bone formation and resorption have been reported using GH in a mixed group of elderly men and women *(78)*.

Because GH stimulates both bone formation and resorption, it seems logical to administer it in conjunction with a resorption inhibitor such as a bisphosphonate, in order to treat osteoporosis. Accordingly, Erdtsieck et al. examined the effects of supplemental GH on bone turnover and mass among healthy, postmenopausal women in the presence of pamidronate *(79)*. Twenty-one women received pamidronate for 1 yr, either with or without concomitant GH therapy (22 µg/kg, three times per week) for the first 6 mo. GH blocked the pamidronate-induced decrease in biochemical markers of bone turnover. Furthermore, although subjects receiving only pamidronate showed a 5% increase in bone mineral mass at the lumbar spine and distal forearm, these changes were not seen in individuals receiving GH as well. Thus, somewhat surprisingly, GH blocked the pamidronate-induced decrease in bone turnover and the accumulation of bone mineral mass.

Several groups have examined the use of GH to enhance body weight in malnourished elderly people *(80–82)*. In one study, subjects over 60 yr of age selected on the basis of low body weight, recent weight loss, low serum albumin, and low IGF-I levels were administered GH for 3 wk. IGF-I levels were restored to the high end of the youthful range. This was associated with significant nitrogen retention, accompanied by a 2.2- to 2.3-kg weight gain and increased mid-arm muscle circumference. No increase in albumin was achieved, although the duration of therapy may have been too short for this. Although these findings show that GH supplementation bolsters body weight in the malnourished elderly, the results can be attributed, at least in part, to fluid retention. Further studies are required to determine whether GH improves strength or functional ability in this setting.

Given the relative dearth of well-controlled studies of GH effects in normal aging, the National Institute on Aging issued a request for applications in the early 1990s and ultimately supported several studies of GH, IGF-I, or GH secretagogues, alone or in combination with exercise or sex-hormone replacement therapy. These studies are now completed and are beginning to be published, although many are still only available as presented abstracts. Broadly summarizing the results currently available, these more recent reports all confirm the positive effects of GH and GHS on body composition, but they do not fully concur on physical or psychological function. Thus, all protocols reported a decrease in body fat and an increase in lean body mass *(83)*, with one study reporting an increase in the proportion of type 2 muscle fibers on biopsy *(48)*. There is an increase in markers of bone turnover, leading to an effect on BMD *(84)*. As with the treatment of adult GHD, the effects of GH or GHRH are more pronounced in men than in women, with a particular blunting of responses in women receiving estrogen replacement therapy *(83,85)*.

There is less agreement on functional measures. Hennessey and colleagues assigned moderately frail older subjects to receive GH, resistance exercise conditioning, or both, for 6 mo *(48)*. Muscle strength was increased by exercise but not by GH alone; the effect was marginally but not significantly greater in the combined GH/exercise group (which showed a 56% increase) than with exercise alone (48%). Weltman and colleagues studied healthy older subjects in a similar GH/exercise protocol over 1 yr of treatment and also reported no ehancement by GH of the effects of exercise conditioning *(86)*. In studies using treatment with GHRH or placebo in combination with exercise conditioning, we examined effects on both strength and physical functional performance, using tests which replicate activities of daily living in a standardized fashion. A preliminary analysis of these measurements shows improvement with exercise but not with GHRH alone, although there was a decrease in functional performance scores in nonexercising placebo-treated subjects that appeared to be mitigated by the drug *(87)*. A study using GH in higher effective doses, however, has reported a small but significant 3.2% increase in aerobic capacity after 6 mo of treatment *(88)*. Given the wide variety of types of tests used, it is difficult to compare these disparate results directly. Thus in contrast to treatment of GHD, there is no current consensus as to whether the increase in LBM produced by GH or GHS in normal aging is accompanied by improvements in strength, endurance, or physical functional performance.

Few of the recent studies since the 1996 report of Papadakis have reported effects on sleep, cognition, or affect. Since GH secretion is associated with slow-wave sleep (SWS) in younger subjects, and GH secretion and SWS decline in parallel with aging, several groups have inquired whether GH might affect sleep as well as the other way around (*see* refs. *89* and *90* for reviews). In short-term studies, GHS have variously been reported to have an acute effect boosting SWS, but in a more chronic 5-mo intervention with GHRH, deep sleep was not enhanced, possibly the result of the short duration of action of the GHRH formulation *(90)*. Unexpectedly, however, the same treatment showed improvement in several measures of cognitive performance, particularly those sensitive to changes in psychomotor and perceptual processing speed, including digit symbol substitution, finding-A's, and the single–dual tasks *(91)*. This finding is consistent with earlier observational studies showing a correlation between circulating levels of IGF-I and similar cognitive measures, but still requires confirmation.

Patient Selection, GH Dosage, and Adverse Effects in the Elderly

Two important questions must be addressed if GH supplementation is to be considered in the non-GHD elderly. Who should be classified as functionally GH deficient and to what level should IGF-I values be normalized? The answer to both questions depends on which healthy reference group is chosen as a standard: young adults or elderly people. The normal IGF-I range, as defined by 95% confidence intervals, for healthy men in their 20s is 240–460 ng/mL in this assay *(92)*. Values less 240 ng/mL are below the 2.5 percentile and are classified as abnormally low if this reference group is used. More recent studies define a wider population normal range, but by this standard, 80% of men over 60 yr of age would be deemed hyposomatomedinemic. Clearly, the definition of GH deficiency and, thus, the prevalence of the condition, are critically dependent on the reference range employed. The situation is similar to that encountered with the use of T vs Z scores to characterize bone density.

At present, there is insufficient evidence to clarify which reference group makes the most sense to use for the geriatric population, either in defining abnormal GHD or in establishing target IGF-I values to dictate GH dosage. Essentially, we do not yet know whether the age-related decline in GH secretion is a pathological or an adaptive condition, or whether it confers some still unknown benefits in the elderly. The experimental trials cited above have generally used young adults as the standard, and corrected IGF-I levels to a range that would be normal for that population. Additional studies are required to determine whether the risk–benefit ratio for GH treatment in the elderly is optimized by this strategy or by the more conservative approach of normalizing IGF-I levels only to the middle or high end of the age-appropriate geriatric reference range.

Adverse effects of GH therapy are unequivocally dose related, and several studies have shown that elderly people are considerably more susceptible to these untoward consequences than are the young. Indeed, nearly all of the above discussed trials reported high incidences of GH-related side effects in the geriatric population, especially fluid retention, carpal tunnel syndrome, gynecomastia, and insulin resistance. Some investigators noted that when IGF-I levels in elderly people were restored to the youthful normal range, side effects were far more prevalent among those individuals brought to the high end of that range (45,58,74). Subjects with levels in the lower half of the normal range generally enjoyed the benefits of GH therapy with far fewer adverse consequences.

As discussed earlier, GH has mitogenic properties on a number of cell lineages in vitro (51), and epidemiological evidence suggests that untreated acromegalics have an increased risk of neoplasia (52–54). Although these findings do not necessarily mean that people given physiological replacement doses of GH would suffer any increased cancer risk, it will be very difficult to prove or disprove definitively whether this is the case in humans. Theoretical concerns about carcinogenic properties of GH are likely to be greatest in the elderly, where there is an increased cancer risk in general.

In summary, if GH therapy ever becomes accepted for use in aging, physicians should seek to restore IGF-I levels to no more than the low normal range for young adults because of the enhanced sensitivity of elderly people for the adverse effects of supplemental GH. These levels can often be achieved with doses much lower than those reported in the earlier studies (93). It would be reasonable to adopt a strategy similar to that developed by the GH Research Society for use in adult GHD, beginning with a low dose and raising it gradually. Thus, one might initiate GH therapy at 100 μg sc at bedtime (approx 2 μg/kg), and increase as necessary until the desired IGF-I level is achieved (59,94) or until limiting side effects develop. Active malignancy is considered an absolute contraindication. In principle, complications of therapy could also be minimized by excluding patients with conditions that might be exacerbated by exogenous GH, such as carpal tunnel syndrome, diabetes, arthritis, congestive heart failure, and hypertension. However, as this list would exclude a large fraction of those who might benefit and sensitivity to GH side effects varies widely among individuals, these conditions are flags for caution and conservative dosing regimens rather than absolute contraindications. The effects of GH on body composition may improve glucose tolerance despite its acute insulin antagonism, and its effects on cardiac contractility may override its acute effects on fluid retention.

Both long- and short-term GH replacement strategies can be envisaged in the elderly. As discussed earlier, long-term therapy could theoretically reverse or slow many of the catabolic features of aging such as muscle and bone atrophy, although convincing evidence to prove this is lacking. In addition, short-term GH treatment might be indicated to maintain LBM when impaired nutrition and/or catabolic states develop, such as major surgeries, trauma such as hip fracture, or illnesses. Although the results of Takala et al. in critically ill patients raise an appropriate caution (3), it is still plausible that short-term GH therapy could facilitate the recovery of acutely debilitated elderly patients.

Summary of GH Therapy for Aging

Very little evidence exists to judge whether GH supplementation can ameliorate the physical and cognitive deterioration of aging. Although there is considerable public excitement about this possibility, most of the optimistic contentions are speculations derived from the treatment of GHD young adults. It is true that the handful of studies examining GH usage in healthy elderly people have all demonstrated beneficial changes in body composition: notably increased LBM and decreased adiposity. In their original article, Rudman et al. stated that these alterations were "equivalent in magnitude to the changes incurred during 10 to 20 yr of aging" (72)—a statement that was (mis)construed by the news media to suggest that GH reverses the effects of aging. However, it has still not been shown that these changes correlate with any meaningful clinical improvements. In contrast to the situation with nonelderly GHD adults, investigators have not yet documented among healthy elderly people any improvement from GH treatment in functional status, cognitive ability, or overall physical or emotional well-being. Thus, scientific evidence is lacking to support the popular perception of GH as an ergogenic aid in the elderly. Although GH may exert a maintenance effect on BMD in the hip among postmenopausal women, a variety of antiresorptive agents currently perform at least as well in this regard; and it would be difficult to justify the use of GH over such agents in view of its cost and inconvenient delivery. No studies have yet been reported to assess the impact of GH in the elderly with regard to such clinically germane outcomes as fracture risk, cardiac capacity, cardiovascular risk, cost-effectiveness, recovery, overall morbidity, or mortality.

In view of the fact that GH has not been clearly shown to confer important lasting benefits in the elderly, that this population is especially susceptible to GH-related side effects, and that GH therapy remains remarkably expensive, the use of GH in otherwise healthy aging people is not yet warranted. Nevertheless, GH replacement in the elderly has theoretical appeal, and longer studies may someday show it to have rejuvenating properties in this population. If so, it is likely that GH will be used first in frail and debilitated patients, in whom the risk/benefit ratio of treatment may be most favorable (95).

OTHER CONDITIONS: CATABOLISM, HIV, AND CRITICAL ILLNESS

Growth hormone has also been recommended as treatment for a variety of conditions in which the relationship of symptoms to reduced GH secretion is less clear (e.g., fibromyalgia and chronic fatigue syndrome and Crohn's disease [96], where it has been suggested that GH may reduce mucosal inflammation as well as promote general anabolism). Most of these suggested indications still rest on a very small number of studies. It has been suggested, for example, that GH secretion may be reduced in some fibromyalgia patients. A placebo-controlled trial of GH in 50 patients with fibromyalgia and low levels of IGF-I reported a reduction in symptoms over 9 mo of treatment, with most improvement occurring after 6 mo (97). At this time there are no confirmatory studies, and the FDA has not approved the use of GH for this indication.

Well-controlled data supporting the use of GH are even sparser for most other non-traditional indications, except for those associated with protein catabolism or wasting, such as chronic illnesses including AIDS, renal failure, burns, fractures, or malnutrition. In these settings GH secretion is normal or even elevated, but partial GH resistance may be present. Since the GH resistance in these conditions is relative rather than absolute, it has been suggested that pharmacologic doses of GH might overcome it and promote anabolism, often in conjunction with nutritional supplementation. For example, Horber and Haymond demonstrated that very high-dose GH treatment (100 µg/kg/d) counter-acted prednisone-induced leucine and nitrogen catabolism over 1 wk of treatment (98). Similar effects were shown in burn patients using even higher doses of GH (200 µg/kg/d) (99), and the use of GH has been suggested for patients with renal failure, based on some success in promoting growth in children (100). Because high-dose GH produces insulin resistance and often hyperglycemia, the combination of GH with recombinant IGF-I, which shares anabolic effects but reduces insulin resistance, has been advocated and evaluated in a few studies.

Early studies such as these were of brief duration and so have reported only metabolic end points, but a few more recent trials have reported favorable effects on clinically relevant end points such as decreased hospital stays and mortality in burn patients (see ref. 101 for review). The adverse experience in critical illness (3), however, has damp-ened the recent pursuit of these studies.

Of these catabolic states, the only one that has received FDA approval for GH treat-ment is AIDS-associated wasting. Published studies of GH in human immunodeficiency virus (HIV) illness are still relatively few. Mulligan and colleagues showed increased nitrogen retention and decreased protein oxidation in six men with HIV-associated wasting during 7 d of treatment with 100 µg/kg/d GH (102), and then 3 mo treatment with the same high GH dose (103). There was an increase in LBM, a decrease in body fat, and an increase in treadmill work output in patients receiving GH vs placebo. Lee and colleagues administered a lower GH dose (approx 12 µg/kg/d) together with IGF-I (5 mg bid) for 3 mo, but they found no significant anabolic effects with this regimen (104). There are still no data available showing an effect of GH on meaningful functional status, quality of life, or survival in HIV; further studies are needed to define its indica-tions. Current studies explore the effects of GH on the pseudo-Cushingoid lipodystrophy seen in AIDS patients treated with protease inhibitors (105).

Hospitalized patients with critical illness appear to have a dual GH disorder. They suffer marked protein catabolism and appear to share a relative GH resistance with other catabolic states; however, in severe illness, GH secretion is also markedly reduced (21,22). These patients would thus seem to be appropriate candidates for high-dose GH treatment, but the experience of Takala et al. also highlights the potential hazards of its use (3).

Doses of GH proposed for use in most wasting syndromes are high and it is not clear that GH resistance is uniform in all tissues, carrying the possibility of greater dose related side effects in fragile patients. Although protein catabolism is a serious clinical problem, the reductions in GH secretion or action may be adaptive in other ways that we override at our peril. Less acutely or seriously ill patients with catabolism report the usual gamut of GH side effects, including edema and compression neuropathies but have not shown serious morbidities or the excess mortality seen in critical illness. We recommend that clinicians wishing to use GH in catabolism, even for FDA-approved indications such as AIDS, obtain informed consent after thorough discussion with their patients, use graduated doses, and monitor side effects very closely.

GH SECRETAGOGUES

Growth hormone secretagogues—GHRH, ghrelin, and their mimetics—stimulate GH secretion, and in patients in whom the pituitary is intact, administered GHS can replace GH by boosting endogenous secretion. GHS have several potential and practical advantages over administered GH. Even when infused continuously, GHRH and GHRPs stimulate an episodic pattern of GH pulses that resembles physiologic secretion, presumably because of the effects of intermittent endogenous somatostatin. The GH response is modulated by IGF-I negative feedback at the pituitary level, which offers a relative (but not absolute) protection against overtreatment. Also, because secretagogues are much smaller molecules than GH, some can be administered orally or even transdermally. GHRH can be administered transnasally in high doses, and both the peptide and nonpeptide GHRPs are resistant to proteolysis and can be given orally.

At this writing, the only GHS approved for use as replacement therapy is GHRH(1-29)NH$_2$ (Geref®, Serono), which has been licensed for the treatment of idiopathic GHD in children (106). Single nightly subcutaneous injections have been given to GHD children in doses of 15–30 µg/kg/d, with restoration of normal growth velocity (107). In principle, this treatment could be continued in adult patients with hypothalamic GHD as well, and a few studies have examined the effects of short-term administration of GHRH in GHD adults (108). However, because the majority of adults with GHD have pituitary disorders and would be unlikely to respond, there are no published studies of long-term GHRH treatment of adult GHD.

Most adult studies have focused instead on the effects of GHRH in normal aging. Acute administration of GHRH continues to elicit an acute GH response in aging (16), although the magnitude of the rise may be less than in young adults. Corpas and colleagues found that twice-daily subcutaneous administration of 1 mg GHRH (approx 15 µg/kg) for 2 wk to healthy older men could elevate plasma IGF-I levels to the young adult normal range (109). Vittone et al. reported the effects of the same total daily GHRH given as a single 2-mg nightly injection for 6 wk (110). Two measures of muscle strength improved, but IGF-I and IGFBP-3 levels did not rise, and the authors concluded that divided doses of GHRH might be more effective than single higher doses. Khorram and colleagues described a study of 16-wk treatment with single nightly injections of a GHRH analog in healthy older men and women (111). IGF-I levels rose in both men and women, but there was a gender difference in effects on body composition, with an increase in LBM in men but not in women. These published studies have been of relatively brief duration, long enough to assess hormonal effects but not effects on body composition or function.

We recently completed two studies of a 5- to 6-mo intervention with single nightly sc doses of 1–2 mg GHRH(1-29)NH$_2$. In the study examining men and estrogenized women, there, was an approx 35% rise in IGF-2 levels (112), a reduction in body fat, and an increase in LBM. As noted earlier (see section GH Therapy in Aging), GHRH by itself did not increase physical functional performance, but appeared to block the decline seen in the placebo-treated group *(87)*.

A small number of studies have examined the effects of GHRH on sleep and cognition, some of which may possibly be mediated by GH secretagogues themselves and not by GH. Sleep promotes GH secretion, but the reverse may also be true. Steiger and colleagues *(113)* and Kerkhofs et al. *(114)* have reported that GHRH acutely stimulates slow-wave sleep in healthy young adults and that somatostatin inhibits this effect. In our studies of GHRH treatment, however, there was no beneficial effect on deep sleep *(90)*. This lack of effect may be the result of the very short duration of action of the currently available GHRH formulation, which, when given at bedtime, does not support and may even inhibit GH secretion later in the night. Several firms are attempting to develop longer-acting GHRH preparations, which may have a different, more positive effect.

Despite its short duration of action, GHRH treatment for 5 mo was associated with improvement in certain cognitive measures responsive to changes in processing speed *(91)*. This noteworthy finding currently stands alone and requires confirmation.

Short-term studies of the effects of the GHRPs and the nonpeptide GHRP mimetics in older subjects have also been conducted. Even brief 24-h infusions significantly elevated IGF-I levels. Daily oral administration of the nonpeptide ghrelin mimetic MK677 in two different doses (10 and 25 mg) for 14–28 d in healthy older men and women markedly elevated 24-h pulsatile GH and plasma IGF-I levels *(115)*. Effects of longer-term treatment with ghrelin agonists in adults have not yet been formally published, although there have been press reports of only modest effects on body composition in one study of 6 mo oral administration of the nonpeptide ghrelin mimetic CP-424,391 *(116)*. In GHD children treated with GHRP for 6 mo, there was a restoration of normal growth velocity *(117)*. Although that might lead one to speculate that GHRPs or other ghrelin mimetics will have effects similar to those of GHRH in adults as well, the orexigenic effect of ghrelin on appetite may oppose the loss of body fat induced by GHRH. Indeed, in the same study of GHD children treated with GHRP-2, 7 of 10 patients reported marked increases in appetite *(118)*.

A few studies of the effects of GHRH or ghrelin mimetics in catabolic conditions have been conducted but are not yet published. One study of treatment of children with chronic renal failure and growth retardation using GHRH(1-29)NH$_2$ (Geref®) twice daily for 3–6 mo reported an acceleration of growth *(119)*, and this encourages further study of the use of GHS in adult catabolic states. If ghrelin proves to be a potent orexigen in humans, this effect could also boost anabolism in catabolic or anorectic disorders. The reverse is also true and potentially affects a much greater target population: Ghrelin receptor antagonists might be effective treatments for obesity or primary hyperphagic disorders such as Prader-Willi Syndrome.

In contrast to GH administration, the effects of the GHS are affected by the same factors which modulate endogenous GHRH secretion. Increased somatostatin tone, in particular, can markedly reduce the GHRH response to GHRH or the GHRPs. Because obesity appears to suppress GH secretion, at least in part, through increased somatostatin, this inhibition can blunt the therapeutic response to repeated administration of GHRH, GHRPs, or their mimetics *(120)*. This effect has led investigators to examine the potential utility of adjuvants that could enhance the response to secretagogue treatment. Ghigo and colleagues have shown that arginine markedly potentiates the acute GH response to GHRH in aging *(18)*. β-Adrenergic antagonists such as propranolol and atenolol also boost the acute GH response to GHRH, probably through inhibition of somatostatin secretion, and are active by oral administration. We examined the effect of atenolol cotreatment in a group of GHD children treated with subcutaneous GHRH. In doses commonly used to treat hypertension, atenolol significantly increased the growth velocity acceleration during the first year of treatment, as compared to treatment with GHRH and placebo *(121)*.

Because GHRH and GHRP exert synergistic effects on GH release, in principle the combination of agents of these two categories would be more potent than either given alone. Our study of the treatment of GH children with GHRP included a final 2-mo treatment period with GHRP and GHRH given together *(122)*. Combination therapy produced a greater rise in peak nighttime GH than GHRP alone. The growth response was no greater, but the brief 2-mo treatment period limits the conclusions that can be reached from growth data. There are no comparable published studies of enhancing adjuvants to GH secretagogue therapy in adults.

In theory, the moderating effects of feedback regulation should make the GHS freer from side effects than is GH. This has generally been the case in published series, but occasional patients have reported typical GH side effects such as edema and carpal tunnel syndrome, and a small number of patients have had erythema or urticarial responses consistent with allergic reactions. At this date, it is not clear whether the apparently lower incidence of side effects reflects a qualitative advantage of GHS or simply the lower potency of the doses that have been employed.

Current formulations of the GHS are quite short acting and do not fully realize their potential for restoring physiologic pulsatile GH secretion. A preparation that provides secretagogue effect for at least 8–12 h is needed to attempt to restore the nighttime GH profile. The existing formulation of GHRH(1-29)NH$_2$ and the research formulations of the GHRPs and their mimetics appear to stimulate an acute rise in GH after administration but do not support GH secretion for the rest of the night *(121,122)*. Thus, the role for GHS in GH replacement for adults is likely to remain very limited until longer-acting drugs or formulations become available.

SUMMARY AND FUTURE PROSPECTS

Growth hormone has been available for adult replacement therapy for less than 15 yr. Although there is still some skepticism about whether all GHD adults need GH replacement, there is wide consensus about its beneficial effects in most patients, and lifelong GH replacement has become the standard of practice. However, we still have much to learn about its use, effects, and side effects; and we can expect treatment practices to continue to change as the published experience from investigational trials is supplemented by surveillance of clinical experience in a much larger number of subjects. The recommended dosage has been reduced progressively since the first studies of GH in adult GHD, and practice is shifting rapidly toward an individualized dose titration as recommended by the GH Research Society and currently practiced by many endocrinologists. It is already clear that appropriate replacement doses and sensitivity to the side effects of GH vary widely among individuals, especially in aging.

Although experience regarding long-term risks of cancer or other disorders has so far been reassuring, it is not yet clear whether patients receiving GH require periodic screening over and above population-based recommendations for colon, prostate, or other malignancies, or for other conditions.

The majority of GHD adults also have deficiencies of other pituitary hormones, and aging reduces levels of sex steroids, melatonin, and other hormones as well as growth hormone. Thus many patients are candidates for hormone replacement with more than one agent, but the interactions among these trophic factors have not been well defined. Subjects given growth hormone may also receive thyroid hormone, glucocorticoids, estrogen, testosterone, or DDAVP treatment. Their several effects may oppose, add to, or synergize with each other, and these interactions can arise from effects both on the secretion or metabolism of other hormones as well as on mutual target organs *(123–125)*. It is already clear that estrogen administration causes relative GH resistance, especially when administered by the oral route, and that GH treatment can increase dose requirements for patients receiving glucocorticoid, thyroid, and possibly antidiuretic hormone replacement; however, most other potential interactions are still largely undefined.

In addition to other hormones and drugs, GH may be used in conjunction with lifestyle interventions such as exercise conditioning. Exercise is also trophic, producing some of the same changes in fat, muscle, and bone as GH, while improving glucose tolerance. Although exercise acutely stimulates GH, most of these consequences are probably mediated through different effectors, suggesting the possibilities that the effects of GH and of exercise could be additive and that exercise might reduce some of the glucose intolerance initially induced by GH treatment. Results of recent studies of GH or GHRH treatment suggest that GH clearly improves physical performance in GHD, but its functional effects in normal aging are less clear. Studies of combined interventions have reaffirmed the benefits of exercise in normal aging but not demonstrated additional benefit from adding GH or GHRH, and parallel studies of exercise and GH in GHD have not been reported.

Thus with new GH formulations and secretagogues under development and new information about its beneficial and adverse effects as well as interactions with other treatment regimens, the practice of adult GH replacement therapy remains in a state of rapid development. Consensus opinions on strategies for making the diagnosis of adult GHD, and on other indications and contraindications for GH treatment in adult patients are likely to continue to evolve significantly in the coming years.

REFERENCES

1. Cummings DE, Merriam GR. Age-related changes in growth hormone secretion: should the somatopause be treated? Semin Reprod Endocrinol 1999;17:311–325.
2. Hoffman DM, O'Sullivan AJ, Baxter RC, Ho KKY. Diagnosis of growth-hormone deficiency in adults. Lancet 1994;343:1064–1068.
3. Takala J, Ruokonen E, Webster NR. Increased mortality associated with growth hormone treatment in critically ill adults. N Engl J Med 1999;341:785–792.
4. Gelato MC, Merriam GR. Growth hormone-releasing hormone. Ann Rev Physiol 1986;48:569–591.
5. Anawalt BD, Merriam GR. Neuroendocrine aging in men: andropause and somatopause. Endocrinol Metab Clin N Am 2001;30:647–669.
6. Bowers CY. Growth hormone-releasing peptide (GHRP). Cell Mol Life Sci 1998;54:1316–1329.
7. Patchett AA, Nargund RP, Tata JR, et al. Design and biological activites of L-163,191 (MK- 0677): a potent, orally active growth hormone secretagogue. Proc Natl Acad Sci USA 1995;92:7001–7005.
8. Kojima M, Hosoda H, Date Y, Nakazato M, Matsuo H, Kangawa K. Ghrelin is a growth- hormone-releasing acylated peptide from stomach. Nature 1999;402:656–660.
9. Muccioli G, Tschöp M, Papotti M, Deghenghi R, Heiman M, Ghigo E. Neuroendocrine and peripheral activities of ghrelin: implications to metabolism and obesity. Eur J Endocrinol 2002;440:235–254.

10. Cummings DE, Schwartz MW. Genetics and pathophysiology of human obesity. Ann Rev Med 2002;54:in press.

11. Tschöp MH, Horvath TL, Cowley ML, et al. Integration of hypothalamic ghrelin in central circuits regulating energy homeostasis, Endocrine Society 84th Annual Meeting, 2002, abstract OR44–42.

12. Katakami H, Hashida S, Usui T, Matsukara S. Role of endogenous ghrelin in the control of GH secretion in conscious rats, Endocrine Society 84th Annual Meeting, 2002, abstract P2–110.

13. Mericq V, Cassorla F, Garcia H, Avila A, Bowers CY, Merriam GR. Growth hormone (GH) responses to GH-releasing peptide and to GH-releasing hormone in GH-deficient children. J Clin Endocrinol Metab 1995;80:1681–1684.

14. Pandya N, DeMott-Friberg R, Bowers CY, Barkan AL, Jaffe CA. Growth hormone-releasing peptide-6 requires endogenous hypothalamic GH-releasing hormone for maximal GH stimulation. J Clin Endocrinol Metab 1998;83:1186–1189.

15. Gelato MC, Malozowski S, Caruso-Nicoletti M, et al. Growth hormone (GH) responses to GH-releasing hormone during pubertal development in normal boys and girls: comparison to idiopathic short stature and GH deficiency. J Clin Endocrinol Metab 1986;63:174–179.

16. Pavlov EP, Harman SM, Merriam GR, Gelato MC, Blackman MR. Responses of growth hormone (GH) and somatomedin-C to GH-releasing hormone in healthy aging men. J Clin Endocrinol Metab 1986;62:595–600.

17. Chapman IM, Hartman ML, Pezzoli SS, et al. Effect of aging on the sensitivity of growth hormone secretion to insulin-like growth factor-I negative feedback. J Clin Endocrinol Metab 1997;82:2996–3004.

18. Ghigo E, Goffi S, Nicolosi M, et al. Growth hormone (GH) responsiveness to combined administration of arginine and GH-releasing hormone does not vary with age in man. J Clin Endocrinol Metab 1990;71:1481–1485.

19. Biller BMK, Samuels MH, Zagar A, et al. Sensitivity and specificity of six tests for the diagnosis of adult growth hormone deficiency. J Clin Endocrinol Metab 2002;87:2067–2079.

20. Hartman ML, Crowe BJ, Biller BMK, Ho KY, Clemmons DR, Chipman JJ. Which patients do not require a growth hormone (GH) stimulation test for the diagnosis of adult GH deficiency? J. Clin Endocrinol Metab 2002;87:477–485.

21. van den Berghe G, de Zegher F, Veldhuis JD, et al. The somatotrophic axis in critical illness: effect of continuous growth hormone (GH)-releasing hormone and GH-releasing peptide-2 infusion. J Clin Endocrinol Metab 1997;82:590–599.

22. Van den Berghe G. Is severe illness also an endocrine disorder? In: Bouillon R, ed. Targets for Growth Hormone and IGF-I Action. Vol. 5. Bioscientifica, Bristol, UK, 2001, pp. 293–304.

23. Cuneo RC, Salomon F, McGauley GA, Sonksen PH. The growth hormone deficiency syndrome in adults. Clin Endocrinol Oxf 1992;37:387–397.

24. Jorgensen JO, Muller J, Moller J, et al. Adult growth hormone deficiency. Horm Res 1994;42:235–241.

25. Labram EK, Wilkin TJ. Growth hormone deficiency in adults and its response to growth hormone replacement. Quart J Med 1995;88:391–399.

26. Rosén T, Johannsson G, Johansson JO, Bengtsson B-Å. Consequences of growth hormone deficiency in adults and the benefits and risks of recombinant human growth hormone treatment. Horm Res 1995;43:93–99.

27. Lieberman SA, Hoffman AR. Growth hormone deficiency in adults: characteristics and response to growth hormone replacement. J Pediatr 1996;128:S58–60.

28. Christ ER, Carroll PV, Russell JDL, Sonksen PH. The consequences of growth hormone deficiency in adulthood, and the effects of growth hormone replacement. Schweiz Med Wochenschr 1997;127:1440–1449.

29. Stewart P, Toogood A, Tomlinson J. Growth hormone, insulin-like growth factor, and the cortisol-cortisone shuttle. Horm Res 2001;56:1–6.

30. Markussis V, Beshyah SA, Fisher C, Sharp P, Nicolaides AN, Johnston DG. Detection of premature atherosclerosis by high-resolution ultrasonography in symptom-free hypopituitary adults. Lancet 1992;340:1188–1192.

31. Rosén T, Bengtsson B-Å. Premature mortality due to cardiovascular disease in hypopituitarism. Lancet 1990;336:285–288.

32. Bates AS, Van't Hoff W, Jones PJ, Clayton RN. The effect of hypopituitarism on life expectancy. J Clin Endocrinol Metab 1996;81:1169–1172.

33. Shahi M, Beshyah SA, Hackett D, Sharp PS, Johnston DG, Foale RA. Myocardial dysfunction in treated adult hypopituitarism: a possible explanation for increased cardiovascular mortality. Br Heart J 1992;67:92–96.

34. Evans HM, Long JA. The effect of the anterior lobe administered intraperitoneally upon growth, maturity and oestrous cycles of the rat. Anat Rec 1921;21:62,63.

35. Raben MS. Clinical use of human growth hormone. N Engl J Med 1962;266:82-86.

36. Buchanan CR, Preece MA, Milner RD. Mortality, neoplasia, and Creutzfeldt-Jakob disease in patients treated with human pituitary growth hormone in the United Kingdom. Br Med J 1991;302:824–828.

37. Salomon F, Cuneo RC, Hesp R, Sonksen PH. The effects of treatment with recombinant human growth hormone on body composition and metabolism in adults with growth hormone deficiency. N Engl J Med 1989;321:1797–803.

38. Jorgensen JO, Pedersen SA, Thuesen L, et al. Beneficial effects of growth hormone treatment in GH-deficient adults. Lancet 1989;1:1221–1225.

39. Carroll PV, Christ ER, Bengtsson B-Å, et al. Growth hormone deficiency in adulthood and the effects of growth hormone replacement: a review. Growth Hormone Research Society Scientific Committee. J Clin Endocrinol Metab 1998;83:382–3-95.

40. Clark W, Kendall MJ. Growth hormone treatment for growth hormone deficient adults. J Clin Pharm Ther 1996;21:367–372.

41. Meling TR, Nylen ES. Growth hormone deficiency in adults: a review. Am J Med Sci 1996;311:153–166.

42. Mantzoros CS, Moses AC. Whither recombinant human growth hormone? Ann Intern Med 1996;125:932–934.

43. Powrie J, Weissberger A, Sonksen P. Growth hormone replacement therapy for growth hormone-deficient adults. Drugs 1995;49:656–663.

44. Lamberts SW, Valk NK, Binnerts A. The use of growth hormone in adults: a changing scene. Clin Endocrinol Oxf 1992;37:111–115.

45. Jorgensen JO. Human growth hormone replacement therapy: pharmacological and clinical aspects. Endocr Rev 1991;12:189–207.

46. Bengtsson B-Å. The consequences of growth hormone deficiency in adults. Acta Endocrinol Copenh 1993;2:2–5.

47. Abbasi AA, Drinka PJ, Mattson DE, Rudman D. Low circulating levels of insulin-like growth factors and testosterone in chronically institutionalized elderly men. J Am Geriatr Soc 1993;41:975–982.

48. Hennessey JV, Chromiak JA, DellaVentura S, et al. Growth hormone administration and exercise effects on muscle fibre type and diameter in moderately frail older people. J Am Geriatr Soc 2001;49:852–858.

49. Monson JP, Abs R, Bengtsson B-Å, et al. Growth hormone deficiency and replacement in elderly hypopituitary adults. KIMS Study Group. Clin Endocrinol (Oxf) 2000;53:281–289.

50. Herschbach P, Henrich G, Strasburger CJ, et al. Development and psychometric properties of a disease-specific quality of life questionnaire for adult patients with growth hormone deficiency. Eur J Endocrinol 2001;145:255–265.

51. Daughaday WH. The possible autocrine/paracrine and endocrine roles of insulin-like growth factors of human tumors. Endocrinology 1990;127:1–4.

52. Bengtsson B-Å, Edén S, Ernest I, Od'en A, Sjogren B. Epidemiology and long-term survival in acromegaly. A study of 166 cases diagnosed between 1955 and 1984. Acta Med Scand 1988;223:327–335.

53. Brunner JE, Johnson CC, Zafar S, Peterson EL, Brunner JF, Mellinger RC. Colon cancer and polyps in acromegaly: increased risk associated with family history of colon cancer. Clin Endocrinol Oxf 1990;32:65–71.

54. Ezzat S, Melmed S. Are patients with acromegaly at increased risk for neoplasia? J Clin Endocrinol Metab 1991;72:245–249.

55. Orme S, McNally R, Cartwright R, et al. Mortality and cancer incidence in acromegaly: a retrospective cohort study. J Clin Endocrinol Metab 1998;83:2730–2734.

56. Hankinson SE, Willett WC, Colditz GA. Circulating concentrations of IGF-I and risk of breast cancer. Lancet 1998;351:1373–1375.

57. Chan JM, Stampfer MJ, Giovanucci E. Plasma IGF-I and prostate cancer risk: a prospective study. Science 1998;279:563–566.

57a. Swerdlow AJ, Higgins CD, Ablard P, Preeze MA. Risk of cancer in patients treated with human pituitary GH in the UK, 1959–1985; a cohort study. Lancet 2002;360:273–277.

58. Cohn L, Feller AG, Draper MW, Rudman IW, Rudman D. Carpal tunnel syndrome and gynaecomastia during growth hormone treatment of elderly men with low circulating IGF-I concentrations. Clin Endocrinol Oxf 1993;39:417–425.

59. Growth Hormone Research Society. Consensus guidelines for the diagnosis and treatment of adults with growth hormone deficiency: summary statement of the Growth Hormone Research Society Workshop on Adult Growth Hormone Deficiency. J Clin Endocrinol Metab 1998;83:379–381.

60. Zadik Z, Chalew SA, McCarter RJJ, Meistas M, Kowarski AA. The influence of age on the 24-hour integrated concentration of growth hormone in normal individuals. J Clin Endocrinol Metab 1985;60:513–516.

61. Ho KY, Evans WS, Blizzard RM, et al. Effects of sex and age on the 24-hour profile of growth hormone secretion in man: importance of endogenous estradiol concentrations. J. Clin. Endocrinol. Metab. 1987;64:51–58.

62. Cook DM, Ludlum WH, Cook DM. Route of estrogen administration helps to determine growth hormone (GH) replacement dose in GH-deficient adults. J Clin Endocrinol Metab 1999;84:3956–3960.

63. Burman P, Johansson A, Siegbahn A, Vessby B, Karlsson F. Growth hormone deficient men are more responsive to GH replacement than women. J Clin Endocrinol Metab 1997;82:550–555.

64. Drake W, Coyte D, Camacho H, et al. Optimizing growth hormone replacement therapy by dose titration in hypopituitary adults. J Clin Endocrinol Metab 1998;83:9313–9319.

65. Hartman ML, Strasburger CJ, Selander KN, Kehely A, Hoffman AR, for the T002 Study Group. Efficacy and tolerability of an individualized dosing regimen for adult GH replacement therapy in comparison to fixed body weight-based dosing., Endocrine Society Annual Meeting, San Francisco, 2002, abstract OR24–1.

66. Hartman ML, Weltman A, Zagar A, Merriam GR, Hoffman AR. GH replacement improves aerobic fitness independently of dosing regimen and physical activity. J Growth Horm IGF Res, in press.

67. Corpas E, Harman SM, Blackman MR. Human growth hormone and human aging. Endocr Rev 1993;14:20–39.

68. Harman SM, Blackman MR. Growth hormone, IGF-I, gonadal steroids, and aging. Aging Milano 1992;4:257–259.

69. Degli Uberti EC, Ambrosio MR, Cella SG, et al. Defective hypothalamic growth hormone (GH)-releasing hormone activity may contribute to declining GH secretion with age in man. J Clin Endocrinol Metab 1997;82:2885–2888.

70. Russell-Aulet M, Jaffe CA, Demott-Friberg R, Barkan AL. In vivo semiquantification of hypothalamic growth hormone-releasing hormone (GHRH) output in humans: evidence for relative GHRH deficiency in aging. J Clin Endocrinol Metab 1999;84:3490-3497.

71. Rudman D, Shetty KR. Unanswered questions concerning the treatment of hyposomatotropism and hypogonadism in elderly men. J Am Geriatr Soc 1994;42:522–527.

72. Rudman D, Feller AG, Nagraj HS, et al. Effects of human growth hormone in men over 60 years old. N Engl J Med 1990;323:1–6.

73. Rudman D, Feller AG, Cohn L, Shetty KR, Rudman IW, Draper MW. Effects of human growth hormone on body composition in elderly men. Horm Res 1991;36:73–81.

74. Thompson JL, Butterfield GE, Marcus R, et al. The effects of recombinant human insulin-like growth factor-I and growth hormone on body composition in elderly women. J Clin Endocrinol Metab 1995;80:1845–1852.

75. Taaffe D, Pruitt L, Hintz R, Butterfield G, Hoffman A, Marcus R. Effect of recombinant growth hormone on the muscle strength response to resistance exercise in elderly men. J Clin Endocrinol Metab 1994;79:1361–1366.

76. Papadakis MA, Grady D, Black D, et al. Growth hormone replacement in healthy older men improves body composition but not functional ability. Ann Intern Med 1996;124:708–716.

77. Holloway L, Butterfield G, Hintz RL, Gesundheit N, Marcus R. Effects of recombinant human growth hormone on metabolic indices, body composition, and bone turnover in healthy elderly women. J Clin Endocrinol Metab 1994;79:470–479.

78. Marcus R, Butterfield G, Holloway L, et al. Effects of short term administration of recombinant human growth hormone to elderly people. J Clin Endocrinol Metab 1990;70:519–527.

79. Erdtsieck RJ, Pols HA, Valk NK, et al. Treatment of post-menopausal osteoporosis with a combination of growth hormone and pamidronate: a placebo controlled trial. Clin Endocrinol Oxf 1995;43:557–565.

80. Binnerts A, Wilson JH, Lamberts SW. The effects of human growth hormone administration in elderly adults with recent weight loss. J Clin Endocrinol Metab 1988;67:1312–1316.
81. Kaiser FE, Silver AJ, Morley JE. The effect of recombinant human growth hormone on malnourished older individuals. J Am Geriatr Soc 1991;39:235–240.
82. Chu L, Lam K, Tam S, et al. A randomized controlled trial of low-dose recombinant human growth hormone in the treatment of malnourished elderly patients. J Clin Endocrinol Metab 2001;86:1913–1920.
83. Münzer T, Harman SM, Christmas C, et al. Effects of GH and/or sex steroid administration on abdominal subcutaneous and visceral fat in healthy aged women and men. J Clin Endocrinol Metab 2001;86:3604–3610.
84. Christmas C, O'Connor KG, Harman SM, et al. Growth hormone and sex steroid effects on bone metabolism and bone mineral density in healthy aged women and men. J Gerontol A Biol Sci Med Sci 2002;57:M12–M18.
85. Merriam GR, Barsness S, Drolet G, et al. Responses to a GH-releasing hormone in normal aging: effects of gender and estrogen replacement, Endocrine Society Annual Meeting, Toronto, 2000, abstract 1634.
86. Weltman A, Weltman JY, Wideman L, et al. GH therapy for 1 year does not augment the effects of exercise training on fitness, strength, and function in healthy older adults., 11th International Congress of Endocrinology, Sydney, Australia, 2000.
87. Vitiello MV, Buchner DR, Cress ME, et al. GHRH effects on body composition and physical function in healthy older men and women. The Gerontologist 2001;41.
88. Edmond J, Busby-Whitehead MJ, Harman SM, et al. Effects of growth hormone and/or sex steroid administration on aerobic capacity in healthy elderly women and men., Endocrine Society Annual Meeting, 1999, abstract P2–530.
89. Blackman MR. Age-related alterations in sleep quality and neuroendocrine function. J Am Med Assoc 2000;284:879–881.
90. Vitiello MV, Schwartz RS, Buchner DR, Moe KE, Mazzoni G, Merriam GR. Treating age-related changes in somatotrophic hormones, sleep, and cognition. Dialogs in Clinical Neuroscience 2001;3:229–236.
91. Vitiello MV, Mazzoni G, Moe KE, et al. GHRH treatment may improve cognitive function in the healthy elderly. The Gerontologist 2000;40:39.
92. Abbasi AA, Rudman D. Observations on the prevalence of protein-calorie undernutrition in VA nursing homes. J Am Geriatr Soc 1993;41:117–121.
93. Gupta KL, Shetty KR, Agre JC, Cuisinier MC, Rudman IW, Rudman D. Human growth hormone effect on serum IGF-I and muscle function in poliomyelitis survivors. Arch Phys Med Rehabil 1994;75:889–894.
94. Martin FC, Yeo A-L, Sonksen PH. Growth hormone secretion in the elderly: aging and the somatopause. Ballière's Clin. Endocrinol. Metab. 1997;11:223-250.
95. Borst SE, Millard WJ, Lowenthal DT. Growth hormone, exercise, and aging: the future of therapy for the frail elderly. J Am Geriatr Soc 1994;42:528–535.
96. Slonim A, Bulone L, Damore M, Goldberg T, Wingertzahn M, McKinley M. A preliminary study of growth hormone therapy for Crohn's disease. N Engl J Med. 2000;342:1664–1666.
97. Bennett RM, Clark SC, Walczyk J. A randomized, double-blind, placebo-controlled study of growth hormone in the treatment of fibromyalgia. Am J Medicine 1998;104:227–231.
98. Horber FF, Haymond MW. Human growth hormone prevents the protein catabolic side effects of prednisone in humans. J Clin Invest 1990;86:265–272.
99. Gore DC, Honeycutt D, Jahoor F, Wolfe RR, Herndon DN. Effect of exogenous growth hormone on whole-body and isolated-limb protein kinetics in burned patients. Arch Surg 1991;126:38–43.
100. Maxwell H, Rees L. Recombinant human growth hormone treatment in infants with chronic renal failure. Arch Dis Child 1996;74:40–43.
101. Jenkins RC, Ross RJ. Growth hormone therapy for protein catabolism. Quart J Med 1996;89:813–819.
102. Mulligan K, Grunfeld C, Hellerstein MK, Neese RA, Schambelan M. Anabolic effects of recombinant human growth hormone in patients with wasting associated with the human immunodeficiency virus. J Clin Endocrinol Metab 1993;77:956–962.
103. Schambelan M, Mulligan K, Grunfeld C, et al. Recombinant human growth hormone in patients with HIV-associated wasting. A randomized, placebo-controlled trial. Ann Int Med 1996;125:873–832.
104. Lee PD, Pivarnik JM, Bukar JK, et al. A randomized, placebo-controlled trial of combined insulin-like growth factor I and low dose growth hormone therapy for wasting associated with human immunodeficiency virus. J.Clin Endocrinol Metab 1996;81:2968–2975.

105. Wanke C, Gerrior J, Kantaros J, Coakley E, Albrecht M. Recombinant human growth hormone improves the fat redistribution syndrome (lipodystrophy) in patients with HIV. AIDS 1999;13:2099–2103.
106. Gelato MC, Ross JL, Malozowski S, et al. Effects of pulsatile administration of growth hormone (GH)-releasing hormone on short term linear growth in children with GH deficiency. J Clin Endocrinol Metab 1985;61:444–450.
107. Thorner MO, Rogol AD, Blizzard RM, et al. Acceleration of growth rate in growth hormone- deficient children treated with human growth hormone-releasing hormone. Pediatr Res 1988;24:145–151.
108. Borges JL, Blizzard RM, Evans WS, et al. Stimulation of growth hormone and somatomedin C in idiopathic GH-deficient subjects by intermittent pulsatile administration of human pancreatic tumor GH-releasing factor. J Clin Endocrinol Metab 1984;59:1–6.
109. Corpas E, Harman SM, Pineyro MA, Roberson R, Blackman MR. Growth hormone (GH)-releasing hormone-(1-29) twice daily reverses the decreased GH and insulin-like growth factor-I levels in old men. J Clin Endocrinol Metab 1992;75:530–535.
110. Vittone J, Blackman MR, Busby-Whitehead J, Tsiao C, Stewart KJ, et al. Effects of single nightly injections of growth hormone-releasing hormone (GHRH 1-29) in healthy elderly men. Metabolism 1997;46:89–96.
111. Khorram O, Laughlin GA, Yen SSC. Endocrine and metabolic effects of long-term administration of [Nle27] growth hormone-releasing hormone (1-29)NH$_2$ in age-advanced men and women. J Clin Endocrinol Metab 1997;82:1472–1479.
112. Merriam GR, Barsness S, Drolet G, et al. Effects of GHRH treatment on 24-hour GH secretion, IGF-I, and body fat in healthy older men and women, Endocrine Society, San Diego, CA, 12–15 June, 1999.
113. Steiger A, Guldner J, Hemmeter U, Rothe B, Wiedemann K, Holsboer F. Effects of growth hormone-releasing hormone and somatostatin on sleep EEG and nocturnal hormone secretion in male controls. Neuroendocrinology 1992;56:566–573.
114. Kerkhofs M, Cauter Ev, Onderbergen Av, Caufriez A, Thorner MO, Copinschi G. Sleep- promoting effects of growth hormone-releasing hormone in normal men. Am. J. Physiol. 1993;264:E594–E598.
115. Chapman IM, Bach MA, van Cauter E, et al. Stimulation of the growth hormone (GH)- insulin-like growth factor I axis by daily oral administration of a GH secretagogue (MK-677) in healthy elderly subjects. J Clin Endocrinol Metab 1996;81:4249–4257.
116. Hensley S. Pfizer 'youth pill' ate up $71 million and died. Wall Street Journal, 2 May 2002.
117. Mericq V, Cassorla F, Salazar T, et al. Increased growth velocity during prolonged GHRP-2 administration to growth hormone deficient children. The Endocrine Society 1995, abstract OR30–33.
118. Mericq V, Cassorla F, Bowers CY, Avila A, Gonen B, Merriam GR. Changes in appetite and body weight in response to long-term oral administration of the ghrelin agonist GHRP-2 in GH-deficient children, International Conference on Pediatric Endocrinology, Montreal, Canada. Ped Res 2001;49:129A
119. Pasqualini T, Ferraris J, Fainstein-Day P, et al. Growth acceleration in children with chronic renal failure treated with growth hormone-releasing hormone (GHRH). Medicina (Buenos Aires) 1996;58:241–246.
120. Kelijman M, Frohman LA. Enhanced growth hormone (GH) responsiveness to GH-releasing hormone after dietary manipulation in obese and nonobese subjects. J Clin Endocrinol Metab 1988;66:489–494.
121. Cassorla F, Mericq V, Garcia H, et al. The effects of β-1-adrenergic blockade on the growth response to growth hormone (GH)-releasing hormone therapy in GH-deficient children. J Clin Endocrinol Metab 1995;80:2997–3001.
122. Mericq VG, Salazar T, Avila A, et al. Effects of eight months' treatment with graded doses of growth hormone (GH)-releasing peptide in growth hormone-deficient children. J Clin Endocrinol Metab 1998;83:2355–2360.
123. Liu L, Merriam GR, Sherins RJ. Chronic sex steroid exposure increases mean plasma GH concentration and pulse amplitude in men with isolated hypogonadotropic hypogonadism. J Clin Endocrinol Metab 1987;64:651–656.
124. Moe KE, Prinz PN, Larsen LH, Vitiello MV, Reed SO, Merriam GR. Growth hormone in postmenopausal women after long-term estrogen replacement therapy. J Gerontol Biol Sci 1998;53A.
125. Giudice LC. Insulin-like growth factors and ovarian follicular development. Endocrine Rev 1992;13:641–669.

II   PARATHYROID AND VITAMIN D

5

Therapy of Hypoparathyroidism and Vitamin D Deficiency

Eric S. Orwoll, MD

INTRODUCTION

Calcium is a critically important mineral necessary for both intracellular and extracellular processes. Calcium circulates in the blood in an ionized state, bound to albumin and other serum proteins, and chelated to citrate, sulfate, and lactate. Only the free, ionized form of calcium is biologically active. Generally, total serum concentrations of calcium reflect the ionized calcium available to cells. However, there are two clinically important exceptions to this rule: (1) alkalosis will decrease ionized calcium concentration because of an increase in the binding of calcium ions to albumin and (2) in many chronic illnesses, substantial reductions in serum albumin concentrations occur, and this may lower total serum calcium concentrations while the ionized calcium concentration remains normal. The circulating level of ionized calcium is maintained in the physiologic range through the concerted actions of parathyroid hormone (PTH) and 1,25-dihydroxyvitamin D, which mobilize calcium stores from bone and increase the efficiency of intestinal calcium absorption and renal calcium reabsorption. Hypocalcemia, in general, is an uncommon disorder. However, defects in the production or recognition of either PTH or 1,25-dihydroxyvitamin D, or a chronic deficiency of vitamin D, can precipitate hypocalcemia. Additionally, the removal of calcium from the circulation can occasionally exceed the capacity for correction by PTH and 1,25-dihydroxyvitamin D. In this section, the clinical presentations and appropriate therapeutic approaches for disorders associated with either deficient PTH or vitamin D action are discussed.

From: *Endocrine Replacement Therapy in Clinical Practice*
Edited by: A. Wayne Meikle © Humana Press Inc., Totowa, NJ

Table 1
Causes of Hypoparathyroidism

Dysembryogenesis
   Isolated
   DiGeorge syndrome
   Kearns–Sayre syndrome
   Kenny–Caffey syndrome
   Barakat syndrome
Destruction
   Surgical excision
   Autoimmune
   Metal overload (Fe, Cu)
   Radiation
   Granulomatous infiltration
   Neoplastic invasion
Deficient hormone secretion
   Maternal hyperparathyroidism
   Calcium receptor mutation
   Hypomagnesemia
Deficient hormone action
   Pseudohypoparathyroidism

HYPOPARATHYROIDISM

Differential Diagnosis

Hypoparathyroidism is a deficiency of effective parathyroid hormone *(1)*. A pathogenetic classification of disorders that can result in hypoparathyroidism is given in Table 1. The condition can arise from a failure of the glands to secrete the hormone or a failure of the tissues to respond to it (pseudohypoparathyroidism). The most common cause of hypoparathyroidism is surgical excision of or damage to the parathyroid glands as a result of total thyroidectomy, radical neck dissection, or repeated operations for primary hyperparathyroidism. The frequency of impaired parathyroid function following such operations is generally related to the amount of tissue resected and the experience and skill of the surgeon. In some cases, autotransplantation of parathyroid tissue at the time of neck surgery is indicated to prevent hypoparathyroidism.

The nonsurgical causes of parathyroid gland destruction are relatively uncommon. Malignant replacement of parathyroid tissue has been noted in patients with lymphoma and other neoplasms of the head and neck; however, functional impairment of the parathyroid glands is rare. Infiltrative diseases such as amyloidosis, hemochromatosis, or Wilson's disease have been associated with decreased parathyroid reserve, but clinically evident hypoparathyroidism is exceptional. High-dose radiation therapy for malignancies in the neck has been implicated as a cause of parathyroid insufficiency, but parathyroid tissue appears to be relatively radioresistant.

Congenital hypoplasia or agenesis of parathyroid tissue can result in a lifelong hypoparathyroid state. The parathyroid glands are derived from the third and fourth branchial pouches. Thus, hypoparathyroidism as a result of branchial dysembryogenesis is frequently associated with other branchial cleft abnormalities. The most common of these is DiGeorge syndrome, which may include thymic aplasia with defective cell-mediated immunity, cleft palate, facial abnormalities, and cardiac defects. These anomalies are frequently the result of a microdeletion on the long arm of chromosome 22. The mnemonic "catch 22" has been applied to this cluster of disorders (cardiac, abnormal facies, thymic aplasia, cleft palate, hypocalcemia and 22q deletion). All infants with congenital hypoparathyroidism should be evaluated for other occult anomalies (e.g., subclinical heart disease) and undergo cytogenetic analysis of chromosome 22. A negative result suggests another cause of hypoparathyroidism, although the possibility of as yet unknown deletions cannot be excluded. More commonly, hypoparathyroidism may develop in early childhood (between 6 mo and 20 yr of age; average age: 7–8 yr) and be accompanied by persistent mucocutaneous candidiasis and variable deficiencies of other endocrine glands, especially the adrenals and thyroids. This disorder may be sporadic or familial. Antibodies to endocrine tissue are a common feature of the disease, but it is uncertain as to whether these autoantibodies are of primary or secondary importance in the pathogenesis of the endocrine gland dysfunction.

Functional hypoparathyroidism can also develop as a consequence of altered regulation of parathyroid gland function. The calcium sensor in the parathyroid glands is responsible for monitoring serum ionized calcium concentrations. Hypercalcemia detected by the calcium sensor triggers an intracellular signaling cascade that results in a decrease in the synthesis and secretion of PTH. Recently, kindreds have been described with an inherited form of hypoparathyroidism that is the result of an activating mutation in the calcium receptor. As the calcium sensor is constitutively activated, affected subjects exhibit chronically suppressed PTH levels despite significant hypocalcemia. A much more common cause of functional hypoparathyroidism is magnesium deficiency. Hypomagnesemia both impairs PTH secretion and blunts its hypercalcemic effect. Hypomagnesemia may result from chronic alcoholism, malabsorption, excessive diuretic use, cis-platinum therapy, prolonged parenteral nutrition, hyperemesis, or an isolated defect in intestinal magnesium absorption. Patients with hypocalcemia as a result of hypomagnesemia are resistant to parenteral calcium and vitamin D therapy until magnesium concentrations are normalized and parathyroid gland function is restored. Interestingly, hypermagnesemia can also suppress PTH secretion and produce hypocalcemia. Acute alcohol intoxication has been demonstrated to produce a reversible impairment in PTH secretion accompanied by hypocalcemia and hypercalciuria. Occasionally, functional hypoparathyroidism occurs in infants born to mothers with primary hyperparathyroidism. Hypercalcemia in the mother results in enhanced placental transport of ionized calcium to the fetus and persistent hypercalcemia in the fetus leads to suppression of its parathyroid gland function. Hypocalcemia can last for up to 6 mo after birth.

Aside from conditions that impair PTH synthesis and release, hypoparathyroidism can also result from target-organ unresponsiveness. Albright initially described a syndrome of PTH resistance in 1941 and coined the term "pseudohypoparathyroidism" to describe this disorder. In these patients, exogenous administration of PTH fails to increase nephrogenous cyclic AMP and/or renal phosphate excretion (biomarkers of PTH action), suggesting that there is a defect in the PTH receptor signaling pathway. The incidence of pseudohypoparathyroidism is not known. Women are affected more commonly than men and both sporadic and familial forms exist. The mode of inheritance has varied in different families with evidence for autosomal-dominant, autosomal-recessive, and X-linked patterns being present in different kindreds. In some families, the defect has been localized to the stimulatory guanine nucleotide regulatory protein (G$_s$) that couples membrane receptors to adenylyl cyclase. This defect likely accounts for the variable resistance to other adenylyl cyclase-coupled hormone receptors, such as glucagon, gonadotropins and thyrotropin, that these patients manifest. Other possible molecular mechanisms responsible for the PTH resistance may reside in the PTH receptor itself or in the intracellular signaling pathway distal to cyclic AMP generation.

Clinical Features

The clinical manifestations of hypoparathyroidism depend on the severity and chronicity of the hypocalcemia and can range from a vague feeling of ill health to life-threatening neuromuscular and cardiovascular collapse. Neuromuscular complications are frequently seen in hypoparathyroidism, especially when serum calcium levels decrease acutely (e.g., immediately after neck surgery that affects the functioning of the parathyroid glands). Nervous tissue exposed to low calcium concentrations exhibits decreased excitation thresholds, repetitive responses to a single stimulus, reduced accommodation, and, in extreme cases, continuous activity (or tetany). The tetany may be latent or overt, and the symptoms in overt tetany can range from mild muscle cramps to frank seizures. Latent tetany may be demonstrated in otherwise asymptomatic patients by eliciting a Chvostek's sign or a Trousseau's sign. Chvostek's sign is performed by tapping on the facial nerve 2–3 cm anterior to the ear, evoking a contraction of the facial muscles and a drawing up of the lip. Trousseau's sign is a carpal spasm elicited by inflation of a blood pressure cuff to 20 mm Hg above the patient's systolic blood pressure for 3–5 min. Flexion of the wrist and metacarpophalangeal joints, extension of the interphalangeal joints, and adduction of the digits reflect the heightened irritability of the nerves to ischemia in the region below the cuff. Whereas upward of 10% of normal individuals will demonstrate a slightly positive Chvostek's sign, a positive Trousseau's sign is rarely seen in the absence of significant hypocalcemia. It should also be noted that significant hypocalcemia may be present in the absence of either Chvostek's or Trousseau's signs, particularly when hypocalcemia has been of gradual onset. Clinically, tetany usually begins with a prodrome of circumoral and facial paresthesias. Motor manifestations include stiffness and muscle cramps of the arms, legs, and feet that can progress to spontaneous carpopedal spasm. Other less common complications include abdominal cramps, urinary frequency, laryngeal stridor, bronchospasm, and, rarely, respiratory arrest.

Central nervous system manifestations of hypoparathyroidism can include mental retardation, psychosis, dementia and seizures of all types. Chronic hypocalcemia may be associated with extrapyramidal movement disorders, including classic parkinsonism. Such manifestations are presumed to be related in some way to the basal ganglia calcifications that are present in many patients. Anterior and posterior subcapsular cataracts, papilledema, dermatitis, and alopecia may also be present. The cardiovascular manifestations of hypocalcemia include arrhythmias, hypotension, and congestive heart failure. The electrocardiogram reveals a characteristic prolongation of the QT interval. The hypotension results from diminished smooth muscle tone and congestive heart failure from impaired myocardial contractility. The cardiovascular dysfunction is unresponsive to pharmacological interventions until the hypocalcemia is corrected. Abnormalities in tooth development are frequently observed in children with hypoparathyroidism. Depending on the age of onset of PTH deficiency, one may find defective enamel and root formation, dental hypoplasia or failure of adult teeth eruption. Untreated hypoparathyroidism during pregnancy has resulted in severe skeletal demineralization of the fetus and transient hypoparathyroidism in the newborn.

Patients with pseudohypoparathyroidism and deficient G_s activity exhibit a variety of phenotypic features that are not seen in other forms of hypoparathyroidism. These include short stature, obesity, round face, skeletal abnormalities (brachydactyly), and heterotopic calcifications. This constellation of somatic abnormalities has been termed "Albright's hereditary osteodystrophy" (AHO). The features of AHO may coexist with normal PTH responsiveness and this is termed "pseudohypoparathyroidism." Within a given family, affected individuals may show AHO with or without abnormal PTH responsiveness.

Therapy

The major goal of therapy in all hypoparathyroid states is to restore serum calcium and phosphorus to satisfactory levels so as to prevent symptoms of hypocalcemia and progression of long-term complications. The particular therapeutic approach depends on the severity of the hypocalcemia, the acuteness of onset, and the presence of symptoms. In acute, symptomatic hypocalcemia, intravenous administration of calcium salts is recommended. Available solutions include calcium chloride (272 mg of elemental calcium per 10-mL ampoule), calcium gluceptate (90 mg of elemental calcium per 5-mL ampoule), and calcium gluconate (90 mg of elemental calcium per 10-mL ampoule). Initial therapy for patients with severe symptoms (e.g., tetany) should ensure the rapid delivery of 250 mg of elemental calcium intravenously. Concentrated calcium solutions are quite caustic and may cause considerable local damage if they extravasate into soft tissue. It is preferable to dilute the calcium salt into 100 mL of a 5% dextrose solution (D_5W) and administer the initial dose over 15 min by a secure intravenous route. Calcium should always be administered very cautiously in patients receiving digitalis therapy, as hypercalcemia predisposes to digitalis intoxication and arrhythmias. If the hypocalcemia fails to resolve and symptoms continue or recur after the initial therapy, calcium can be administered by continuous intravenous infusion (e.g., 5–10 mg of elemental calcium/ kg body wt in 1 L of D_5W every 6 h). Serum calcium levels should be monitored frequently to maintain the serum calcium at 7–8.5 mg/dL. The cause of the hypocalcemia should be sought during this period and specifically treated, thus allowing intravenous calcium therapy to be discontinued. If magnesium depletion is suspected in the setting of hypocalcemia, a blood sample for magnesium determination should be obtained. Then, if renal function is intact, magnesium should be administered parenterally. If significant hypomagnesemia is documented, its cause should be evaluated and magnesium repletion (either parenterally or orally) should be continued until the serum value is normalized. Empiric magnesium therapy should not be considered in the presence of renal insufficiency.

The chronic hypoparathyroid states will require long-term therapy to maintain calcium levels. Theoretically, the most appropriate therapy for hypoparathyroidism would be physiologic replacement with PTH itself. Indeed, a recent study has demonstrated that once-daily sc administration of human PTH (1–34), which contains the biologically active region of PTH, may maintain calcium levels in the normal range throughout the day and reduce urinary calcium excretion (2). However, there are practical limitations to this approach, including the need to administer the hormone parenterally and the high cost of commercial preparations of PTH. Such treatment might become feasible in the

Table 2
Calcium Preparations for Oral Supplementation

Preparation	Common tablet size (mg)	Elemental calcium (%)	No. of tablets for 1500 mg calcium
Ca gluconate	1000	9	16
Ca lactate	650	13	18
Ca carbonate	650	40	6
	1300		3
Ca citrate	950	21	8

future as an alternative for patients poorly controlled by conventional regimens. Parathyroid autotransplantation has lowered the incidence of permanent hypoparathyroidism in selected patients. Unfortunately, the immunology of parathyroid transplantation is incompletely understood and the allograft success rate is too low to currently recommend this procedure on a routine basis (3,4).

Because of the absence of PTH and consequent hyperphosphatemia, little, if any, circulating 25-hydroxyvitamin D is converted to 1,25-dihydroxyvitamin D and there are low or undetectable serum levels of this metabolite in hypoparathyroidism. Although lowering of serum phosphate levels with diets low in phosphate (e.g., restricting dairy products and meat) and oral non-absorbable aluminum hydroxide gels (to bind intestinal phosphate) might be expected to increase the conversion of 25-hydroxyvitamin D to 1,25-dihydroxyvitamin D, such treatment has received little attention. Rather, treatment with supplemental calcium and vitamin D has been the mainstay of therapy (5).

Generally, at least 1 g/d of elemental calcium is required in hypoparathyroid patients under 40 yr of age and 2 g/d in patients over 40 yr. The amount of supplemental calcium necessary for adequate control may vary from 1 g/d (even in the absence of vitamin D supplements) in mild, partial hypoparathyroidism to 5–10 g/d (plus supplemental vitamin D) in more severe cases. Supplements can be provided by administering calcium as the gluconate, lactate, carbonate, or citrate salt (see Table 2). Calcium gluconate and lactate tablets contain relatively small quantities of elemental calcium, so that large numbers of tablets must be administered. Calcium carbonate preparations have the highest calcium content (on a weight-percent basis) and are therefore preferred by most patients. Calcium citrate may be of benefit for patients with hypercalciuria, because urinary excretion of citrate may prevent kidney stone formation. Oral calcium supplements are best absorbed in multiple small doses and in an acidic environment (e.g., with meals).

In patients with less severe parathyroid insufficency, oral calcium supplementation alone may be adequate. However, in most patients, therapy with vitamin D or one of its analogs is also required to prevent hypocalcemia. As indicated in Table 3, ergocalciferol (vitamin D_2) is the least expensive form of therapy. Many patients with hypoparathyroidism can be effectively (and inexpensively) treated with ergocalciferol supplements. Doses of 50,000 IU qod to 100,000 daily may be required, depending on the severity of hypoparathyroidism, the individual response, and the dose of calcium supplement. Generally, the ergocalciferol dose can be a stable foundation of therapy, and titration of the calcium supplement can be used to respond to the inevitable fluctuations in calcium control. It is ideal to identify a dose of ergocalciferol that allows the patient a modest requirement for calcium supplementation, as a need for large daily calcium doses soon becomes onerous.

Table 3
Characteristics of Commonly Used Vitamin D Preparations

Preparation	Physiologic dose[a] (µg)	Pharmacologic dose[b]	Onset of action (d)	Duration of action	Cost[c] ($)
Vitamin D$_2$ (ergocalciferol)	5–10	1–10 mg	10–14	4–12 wk	$7.00/100 (1.25 mg)
Dihydrotachysterol (DHT)	25–100	375–750 mg	4–7	1–4 wk	$94.02/100 (125 mg)
1,25[(OH)$_2$D] (calcitriol)	0.25–0.5	0.75–3.0 mg	1–2	2–5 d	$110.04/100 (0.25 mg) $175.98/100 (0.5 mg)

[a]Dosage for the treatment of nutritional deficiency.
[b]Dosage for the treatment of hypoparathyroidism.
[c]Average wholesale price (5a).
[d]25-Hydroxyvitamin D.

103

Importantly, the onset of the actions of ergocalciferol and the waning of its effects after a reduction in dose are usually quite delayed. Vitamin D is highly stored in adipose tissue and this depot is slow to accumulate and release its stores. This means that dose adjustments must be performed at 1- to 2-mo intervals, with careful assessments of biological response (serum calcium levels) before the next adjustment is made. These decisions can be challenging because of the variability in serum calcium levels in this situation. The careful identification of trends in serum calcium levels is required. The delayed onset of action and the delay in the reduction in action can be disadvantageous.

For these reasons, analogs with shorter half-lives and no requirement for renal 1-α hydroxylation (such as dihydrotachysterol and calcitriol) are preferred in some patients. Doses of calcitriol of 0.5–2.0 µg/d can provide rapid and stable control of hypocalcemia. The half-life of calcitriol is short, so dose adjustments can be made at 4- to 10-d intervals. However, calcitriol replacement is associated with more lability in serum calcium levels, and hypercalcemia is a more common complication. Therapy must be individualized in all cases of hypoparathyroidism (6). Because changes in calcium and vitamin D requirements may occur unpredictably during chronic treatment, routine monitoring of serum calcium levels is mandatory. Calcium should be measured weekly at the initiation of vitamin D therapy, during dosage adjustment, and at least every 3 mo during long-term follow-up. A single episode of vitamin D intoxication can irreversibly impair renal function.

A major impediment to restoration of normocalcemia with supplemental calcium and vitamin D analogs is the occurrence of hypercalciuria. As PTH is not present to maintain normal renal tubular reabsorption of calcium, enhanced absorption of calcium from the intestines initiated by calcium and vitamin D therapy results in an increased filtered load of calcium that is readily cleared through the kidney. Consequently, significant hypercalciuria may develop before serum calcium is normalized and can make the control of hypocalcemia more challenging. It may be necessary to accept a lower serum calcium concentration in order to limit the degree of hypercalciuria and the risks of nephrophthisis and nephrocalcinosis. Thiazide diuretics, which increase renal tubular calcium reabsorption, have been proposed as a means of reducing urine calcium in hypoparathyroidism with the added benefit of helping to restore eucalcemia (7,8). Although this approach is beneficial in some patients, the use of diuretics may be problematic in patients with concurrent adrenal insufficiency or impaired renal function. However, in patients with normal renal and adrenal function, thiazide diuretics in conjunction with calcium and vitamin D supplementation may provide a relatively inexpensive solution to the chronic hypercalciuria that is often encountered in this clinical setting.

Long-term restoration of serum calcium to normal or near-normal ranges usually results in improvements in the symptoms of hypoparathyroidism. Whether treatment of hypocalcemia in hypoparathyroidism affects the tendency to develop soft tissue calcification is unknown. The causation of the calcifications that occur in many tissues in untreated hypoparathyroidism is unclear and there is concern that higher than necessary calcium levels during therapy may contribute to the development or worsening of calcification. For that reason, the target of replacement therapy should be serum calcium levels at the lower levels of the normal range. This also minimizes the chance of developing hypercalcemia from excessive replacement doses of calcium and vitamin D. Other measures to avoid hypercalcemia include regular medication use and the avoidance of

Table 4
Causes of Vitamin D Deficiency

Decreased precursor vitamin D
    Malnutrition
    Malabsorption
    Sunscreen use
    Lack of sunlight exposure
    Antiseizure medications
Decreased conversion to active metabolites
    Liver disease
    Kidney disease
    Vitamin D-dependent rickets, type I
    Oncogenic osteomalacia
    X-Linked hypophosphatemic rickets
1,25-Dihydroxyvitamin D resistance
    Vitamin D-dependent rickets, type II

dehydration. Improved surgical techniques and the use of parathyroid autotransplantation surgery for disorders requiring extensive removal of thyroid or parathyroid tissue may lower the incidence of permanent hypoparathyroidism.

VITAMIN D DEFICIENCY

Differential Diagnosis

Dietary vitamin D_2 (ergocalciferol) is absorbed via the intestinal lymphatic system. Absorption takes place in the proximal small intestine and requires bile acids. Vitamin D_3 (cholecalciferol) is produced in the skin by photochemical synthesis from 7-dehydrocholesterol. Vitamins D_2 and D_3 exhibit little in the way of biologic activity. Both undergo hydroxylation in the liver to form 25-hydroxyvitamin D by action of the enzyme vitamin D-25 hydroxylase. 25-Hydroxyvitamin D serves as the primary storage form of vitamin D hormone. To become biologically active, 25-hydroxyvitamin D requires further hydroxylation to form 1,25-dihydroxyvitamin D by action of the enzyme 25-hydroxyvitamin D-1α-hydroxylase. This hydroxylation step takes place primarily in the kidney and is tightly regulated by circulating PTH, phosphate, and calcium levels. Thus, vitamin D deficiency can result from nutritional deprivation, inadequate sunlight exposure, impaired gastrointestinal absorption, reduced synthesis of 25-hydroxyvitamin D and/or 1,25-dihydroxyvitamin D or end-organ resistance to 1,25-dihydroxyvitamin D *(9)*. A pathogenetic classification of disorders that can result in vitamin D deficiency is given in Table 4.

Nutritional vitamin D deficiency is rare in the United States, because milk and cereals are commonly fortified with vitamin D_2. However, vitamin D deficiency can occur in alcoholics and the elderly because of their poor nutritional status and limited sunlight exposure. Gastrointestinal disease is now the predominant cause of vitamin D deficiency in the United States. Intestinal malabsorption syndromes that affect the small intestine (especially the duodenum and jejunum) are all associated with impaired vitamin D absorption as a result of either rapid transit or enhanced fecal loss of 25-hydroxyvitamin D because of impaired enterohepatic circulation. Similarly, patients with chronic severe parenchymal and cholestatic liver disease frequently exhibit vitamin D deficiency resulting from the associated malabsorption syndrome combined with a decreased hepatic capacity to convert vitamin D to 25-hydroxyvitamin D. Those patients who take phenobarbital or dilantin have increased activity of microsomal hydroxylases in the liver, and consequent accelerated metabolism of vitamin D can lead to functional vitamin D deficiency.

Renal disease is one of the most common causes of vitamin D deficiency. As kidney function declines, 1α-hydroxylase activity decreases, leading to reductions in circulating levels of 1,25-dihydroxyvitamin D and, consequently, impaired gastrointestinal calcium absorption. Additionally, phosphate excretion falls as renal function declines. Hyperphosphatemia then results in further decreases in the serum calcium level by chelating ionized calcium and inhibiting any remaining 1α-hydroxylase enzyme activity.

In rare instances, inborn errors of vitamin D metabolism can result in hypocalcemia. Patients with these disorders generally present early in life with hypocalcemia and skeletal abnormalities despite adequate vitamin D intake. Vitamin D-dependent rickets type I is an autosomal recessive disorder that stems from impaired renal 1α-hydroxylase activity. Affected patients have low concentrations of 1,25-dihydroxyvitamin D but respond to treatment with physiological doses of 1,25-dihydroxyvitamin D. In contrast, patients with vitamin D-dependent rickets type II have a variety of mutations in the vitamin D receptor, exhibit dramatically increased circulating concentrations of 1,25-dihydroxyvitamin D (as a consequence of their secondary hyperparathyroidism), and respond poorly even to pharmacological doses of 1,25-dihydroxyvitamin D. Patients with the more severe form of this disease frequently have alopecia.

Clinical Features

The clinical manifestations of vitamin D deficiency can include myotonia, muscle weakness, and, in severe cases, hypocalcemia and tetany. Additionally, skeletal abnormalities are also frequently present. The characteristic skeletal disturbance in vitamin D-deficient states is osteomalacia (literally, "soft bones"). The malacic bone results from impaired mineralization and is subject to distortion in shape and to fracture. When osteomalacia develops in young, actively growing children, it is referred to as rickets. If vitamin D deficiency is present during the first year of life, the characteristic features of rachitic bone can include widened cranial sutures, frontal bossing, posterior flattening of the skull ("craniotabes"), bulging of the costochondral junctions ("rachitic rosary"), indentation of the ribs at the diaphragmatic insertions ("Harrison's groove"), and enlargement of the wrists. After the first year of life, the deformities resulting from vitamin D deficiency are most severe in the long bones because of their rapid growth and weight-bearing function. The bony shafts of the long bones can be deformed (bowed) and subject to fracture. The ends of the long bones become enlarged and bowleg ("genu varum") or knock-knee ("genu valgum") deformities progressively worsen. In long-standing disease, there may be coxa vara and rachitic saber shins. Moderate deformities occurring before age of 4 may resolve with adequate vitamin D treatment, but those occurring later usually result in lasting deformity, compromised adult height or both.

The clinical features associated with osteomalacia in adults are subtler than those with rickets in children. In the mature, fully grown skeleton, bone turnover is less than 5% per year. Thus, a mineralization defect in adults must be present for several years to produce clinical manifestations. The characteristic symptom, if any, is pain when weight or pressure is applied to the affected bones. Low backache relieved by recumbency is one of the earlier complaints, but the pain may include other portions of the spine, ribs, and feet. Significant osteomalacia may be present without radiographic manifestations, but there is often a generalized decrease in bone mineral density. The most characteristic feature of adult osteomalacia is the pseudofracture (Looser's zone, Milkman's syndrome), a straight, transverse band localized, often symmetrically, at the concave ends of the shafts of long bones, ribs, scapulae, and pubic rami. The origin of these radiographic abnormalities is unknown, but they may arise from the pressure of overlying pulsating arteries. Skeletal fractures (sometimes superimposed on pseudofractures) can occur and usually unite very slowly. Long-standing disease can lead to bowing of long bones and distortion of the pelvic outlet (assuming a triangular appearance on standard anteroposterior views). Loss of vertebral height as a result of typical biconcave deformities can lead to kyphosis as a late manifestation. The skeletal deformities may be associated with other features of malnutrition and/or secondary hyperparathyroidism (e.g., subperiosteal resorption). Associated proximal weakness can contribute to a waddling gait or severe crippling.

Therapy

The goals of treatment in states of vitamin D deficiency are to (1) correct hypocalcemia, alleviate related symptoms, and prevent grand mal seizures and cataracts, (2) prevent the skeletal deformities of rickets and the occurrence of fragility fractures, (3) prevent toxicity (hypercalcemia, hypercalciuria, and their sequelae), and (4) promote normal growth and development in children. The choice of the vitamin D preparation used for therapy depends on the cost of the medication and associated illnesses that may influence vitamin D metabolism. Preparations of vitamin D and its metabolites that are available for clinical use in the United States are listed in Table 3. The table also lists the onset of optimal biologic activity, duration of effect after cessation of treatment, dosage forms available, and cost. The pharmacologic advantages and disadvantages of the drugs are listed in Table 5.

The precursor molecules, ergocalciferol (vitamin D_2) and cholecalciferol (vitamin D_3), are the least expensive. These compounds and 25-hydroxyvitamin D_3 (calcifediol) have the theoretical advantage that they are precursors of the other vitamin D metabolites, so that physiologic regulation may avert toxicity. A disadvantage of vitamin D_2 and D_3 is that they tend to be chemically unstable and lose activity during storage. They also tend to accumulate in fat and muscle during long-term administration so that the effect becomes cumulative. With both compounds, the therapeutic dose approaches the toxic dose, a long period is required for optimal biologic effect, and activity may persist after cessation of administration, a disadvantage in the event of intoxication. The advantages of dihydrotachysterol (DHT) and calcitriol (1,25-dihydroxyvitamin D_3) are that the onset of maximum biological activity is short and their effects last only a short period after cessation of treatment. Both are effective when 1α-hydroxylation of 25-hydroxyvitamin D is defective. However, both drugs are relatively expensive, and hypercalcemia can occur episodically in patients on long-term treatment. The hypercalcemia is easily managed by stopping the drug and it is prevented by reducing the dose.

Optimal management of vitamin D deficiency is dependent on its underlying cause and treatment must be individualized with regard to pathogenesis and severity of the disorder. For cases of nutritional vitamin D deficiency, ergocalciferol or cholecalciferol are reasonable initial choices: 400–800 IU of ergocalciferol will achieve normal circu-

Table 5

Advantages and Disadvantages of Vitamin D and Its Derivatives

Drug	Advantages	Disadvantages
Vitamin D_2	Inexpensive; precursor of vitamin D metabolites	Therapeutic dose approaches toxic dose; long period for onset of biologic effect; may not be effective, particularly when vitamin D metabolism is defective; unstable, undergoes oxidation, photochemical decomposition, and loss of activity with storage
Dihydrotachysterol	Does not require 1α-hydroxylation, can be used when this step is impaired; short period for onset of biologic effect; duration of effect after cessation usually short	Therapeutic dose approaches toxic dose; moderately expensive; 25-hydroxylation required for biologic effectiveness; may be ineffective in liver disease
1,25-dihydroxyvitamin D_3	Short period of onset for biologic effect; short duration of effect after cessation; can be highly effective when 1α-hydroxylation is impaired and may provide normal or near-normal growth	Expensive; toxicity may occur spontaneously

lating levels of 25-hydroxyvitamin D in most patients. In patients with more severe deficiency (associated with symptoms) a regimen of 50,000 U (1.25 mg) per day of ergocalciferol is frequently used at the beginning of therapy (i.e., the first 3–6 mo) to more rapidly increase systemic vitamin D levels. After that time, maintenance dosages should be reduced and titrated to maintain 25-hydroxyvitamin D levels of at least 30 mg/mL. The cause of vitamin D deficiency should provide guidance for the amounts of vitamin D supplementation required. Vitamin D deficiency associated with malabsorption may require pharmacologic amounts of ergocalciferol (10–100,000 U/d; 0.25–0.625 mg/d). In the presence of malabsorption, concurrent magnesium depletion must always be considered. Vitamin D_2 or D_3 may not be appropriate in some circumstances. If vitamin D deficiency is secondary to intestinal resection, malabsorption, or impaired enterohepatic circulation, calcitrol (0.5–2.0 µg/d) may be absorbed more readily. In the setting of defective renal hydroxylation of 25-hydroxyvitamin D (e.g., end-stage renal disease, type I vitamin D-dependent rickets), therapy with either DHT or calcitriol is required. In general, states of vitamin D deficiency in which renal 1α-hydroxylation is intact should not be treated with analogs such as DHT or calcitriol. These compounds bypass the renal site of feedback control of 1,25-dihydroxyvitamin D biosynthesis and thus carry a greater risk of inducing hypercalcemia.

In most patients with vitamin D deficiency (those with adequate renal function and 1α-hydroxylase activity) the object is to restore and maintain optimal serum 25(OH) vitamin D concentrations. Monitoring serum levels after vitamin D supplementation begins should provide an adequate guide for dose adjustments. Measures at 1- to 2-mo intervals until the desired levels are obtained should be sufficient, and periodic measures thereafter will ensure stable vitamin D nutrition has been achieved. Intoxication can be a problem with vitamin D or any of its metabolites *(10)*. Hypercalcemia and hypercalciuria result from increased intestinal absorption of calcium and mobilization of calcium from the skeleton and may lead to impairment in renal function, nephrocalcinosis, nephrolithiasis, urinary tract infections, and so forth. Patients with intoxication are often asymptomatic, but they may have anorexia, nausea, vomiting, weight loss, polyuria, polydipsia, and alterations in mental status. Children and infants often show listlessness and hypotonia. Intoxication can occur unexpectedly, possibly as a result of changes in diet, gastrointestinal absorption of calcium, or hydration status.

The treatment of intoxication is to stop vitamin D and any calcium supplement and ensure optimal extracellular volume status (sometimes with intravenous fluids). If intoxication is profound, a short course of steroids or bisphosphonates may be required, usually only when hypercalcemia is produced by the longer-acting sterols. Use of lower doses of the drugs after episodes of hypercalcemia will prevent recurrences.

REFERENCES

1. Nusynowitz ML, Frame B, Kolb FO. The spectrum of hypoparathyroid states: A classification based on physiologic principles. Medicine 1976;55:105–119.
2. Winer KK, Yanovski JA, Cutler GB. Synthetic human parathyroid hormone 1-34 vs calcitriol and calcium in the treatment of hypoparathyroidism. JAMA 1996;276:631–636.
3. Wozniewicz B, Migaj M, Giera B, et al. Cell culture preparation of human parathyroid cells for allotransplantation without immunosuppression. Trans Proc 1996;28:3542–3544.
4. Tolloczko T, Wozniewicz B, Sawicki A, et al. Clinical results of human cultured parathyroid cell allotransplantation in the treatment of surgical hypoparathyroidism. Trans Proc 1996;28:3545,3546.
5. Avioli LV. The therapeutic approach to hypoparathyroidism. Am J Med 1974;57:34–42.

6. Okano K, Furukawa Y, Morii H, Fujita T. Comparative efficacy of various vitamin D metabolites in the treatment of various types of hypoparathyroidism. J Clin Endocrinol Metab 1982;55:238–243.
7. Parfitt AM. The interactions of thiazide diuretics with parathyroid hormone and vitamin D. J Clin Invest 1972;51:1879–1888.
8. Porter RH, Cox BG, Heaney D, et al. Treatment of hypoparathyroid patients with chlorthalidone. N Engl J Med 1978;298:577–581.
9. Drezner MK. Disorders of vitamin D metabolism: rickets and osteomalacia. In: Manolagos SC, Olefsky JM (eds.) Metabolic Bone and Mineral Disorders., vol. 5. Churchill Livingstone, New York, 1988, pp. 103–129.
10. Davies M, Adams PH. The continuing risk of vitamin D intoxication. Lancet 1978;i:621–623.

III   THYROID

6

Recombinant Human Thyrotropin in the Management of Thyroid Carcinoma and Other Thyroid Disorders

Steven I. Sherman, MD
and Luis Lopez-Penabad, MD

INTRODUCTION

The introduction of recombinant human thyrotropin (thyroid-stimulating hormone or TSH) (rhTSH; thyrotropin alfa; Thyrogen®, Genzyme Corporation, Cambridge, MA) has permitted the development of new diagnostic and treatment strategies for patients with a variety of thyroid diseases *(1,2)*. Originally introduced as a diagnostic adjunct in the follow-up of patients with thyroid carcinoma, broader interest has led to testing of the hormone to facilitate radioiodine therapy for benign, malignant, and ectopic thyroid neoplasms. Optimal utilization of this new mode of hormone therapy requires careful consideration of the normal physiology of TSH action and the benefits and limitations of the agent.

From: *Endocrine Replacement Therapy in Clinical Practice*
Edited by: A. Wayne Meikle © Humana Press Inc., Totowa, NJ

PHYSIOLOGY OF THE TRH–TSH–THYROID AXIS

The circulating level of TSH is the primary regulatory influence on the production of thyroxine and tri-iodothyronine by the thyroid gland. Produced by thyrotroph cells of the anterior pituitary, TSH is a two-subunit glycoprotein, the specificity of which is conferred by its β-subunit; the human α-subunit is structurally similar to that of follicle-stimulating hormone, luteinizing hormone, and chorionic gonadotropin. Negative feedback by thyroid hormones influences TSH synthesis and release. The hypothalamic tripeptide thyrotropin-releasing hormone (TRH) stimulates TSH secretion and modulates thyrotroph response to altered thyroid hormone levels. In conjunction with the suppressive effects of dopamine, corticosteroids, somatostatin, androgens, and endogenous opioids, TRH may be responsible for establishing the set point for the negative feedback loop that controls thyroid hormone levels. Hypothalamic production of TRH itself is regulated by circulating thyroid hormones, as well as by multiple central nervous system factors. The metabolic clearance of TSH is affected by the specific glycosylation patterns on the protein, which, in turn, vary depending on the underlying thyroid hormone status. Thus, during periods of hypothyroidism, newly produced TSH is increasingly sialylated, which, in turn, leads to slower metabolic clearance of TSH and a greater effective stimulation of the thyroid gland *(3)*.

At the thyroid cell membrane, TSH binds to the TSH receptor to stimulate signal transduction cascades that eventually lead to increased hormone production and increased thyroid cell mass. The TSH receptor is a member of the seven-transmembrane domain receptor family. Two primary signaling pathways interact with the TSH receptor, a G-protein complex that stimulates production of cyclic AMP and an inosityl phosphate-3 complex that activates a tyrosine kinase cascade. Of the downstream effects of stimulation of these pathways in thyroid follicular cells, those relevant to the clinical uses of recombinant human TSH (rhTSH) include stimulation of iodine uptake, increased iodine organification and incorporation into thyroid hormones, and increased production and release of thyroglobulin. Whether TSH provides a direct mitogenic stimulus to human thyroid cells is unproven *(4,5)*, but prolonged elevation of TSH levels is associated with goiter formation and growth of TSH-responsive thyroid neoplasms.

DEVELOPMENT OF RECOMBINANT HUMAN THYROTROPIN

The initial development of rhTSH was driven by the need to improve the approach to diagnostic testing and treatment of patients with differentiated carcinoma derived from thyroid follicular epithelium (papillary and follicular carcinomas) *(6)*. Following near-total or total thyroidectomy to remove the primary focus of differentiated thyroid carcinoma, adjuvant ablation with radioiodine of residual thyroid tissue may have three benefits: (1) to destroy any residual microscopic foci of disease, (2) to increase the specificity of subsequent radioiodine scanning for detection of recurrent or metastatic disease by eliminating uptake by residual normal tissue, and (3) to improve the value of measurements of serum thyroglobulin as a tumor marker *(7)*. Radioiodine scans for localization of uptake prior to such therapy are commonly performed, using diagnostic activities of 2–5 mCi of [131]I. Between 24 and 96 h after the diagnostic dosing, whole-body scans and spot images of the neck and other areas of uptake are performed with a large field of view γ-scintillation camera. Most patients demonstrate significant uptake of radioiodine within the thyroid bed following thyroidectomy, presumably from normal residual uptake, but metastatic disease can also be commonly detected by such scans. Treatment planning for adjuvant radioiodine would then be based on the results of such scans. A scan is often performed within 7 d after administration of radioiodine for therapy. Such posttherapy scans can demonstrate foci of radioiodine uptake not identified on the lower activity diagnostic scans performed before therapy, but these findings detect previously undiagnosed distant metastatic disease in only 10% of patients (8). During longitudinal follow-up, periodic radioiodine scans can also be of benefit to detect residual or recurrent disease (9).

A complementary diagnostic tool for detection of differentiated thyroid carcinoma following initial therapy is measurement of the serum thyroglobulin concentration (10). Following successful thyroidectomy and radioiodine ablation of remnant and malignant thyroid tissue, endogenous thyroglobulin levels should not be measurable. Therefore, an elevated thyroglobulin level would provide indirect evidence of the presence of functional thyroid tissue or tumor. The sensitivity of thyroglobulin determinations is markedly increased when TSH levels are elevated (11,12), thus leading to the common practice of measuring thyroglobulin levels concomitant with performing radioiodine scanning (13). Although both radioiodine concentration and thyroglobulin production are differentiated functions often seen in thyroid carcinomas, they are not necessarily linked. Patients with metastatic or recurrent disease will often produce thyroglobulin but have negative diagnostic radioiodine scans, and the converse can also occur (14). In many of these cases, subsequent posttherapy imaging after ^{131}I treatment can reveal the foci of disease otherwise detected by thyroglobulin alone, but whether such high-dose scanning and therapy improves patient outcomes is controversial (15–17). Despite the sensitivity of thyroglobulin immunoassays, problems remain in their clinical application. In immunometric assays, reported thyroglobulin concentrations can be falsely lowered by circulating endogenous antibodies that bind thyroglobulin and prevent antigen interaction with the assay's antibodies (18). For the 25% of the thyroid cancer population with antithyroglobulin autoantibodies, serum thyroglobulin levels must be interpreted with caution. The persistence of these autoantibodies following thyroidectomy and radioiodine ablation may, in itself, indicate the presence of residual thyroid tissue and an increased risk for recurrence (19).

Because of the dependence of thyroid follicular cells on TSH to stimulate iodine uptake and thyroglobulin production, maintenance of adequately elevated serum levels of TSH has been a cornerstone of optimal disease detection and treatment regimens. To maximize iodine uptake for scanning and therapy, the patient's thyroid hormone levels should be allowed to decline sufficiently to allow the TSH concentration to rise to above 25–30 mU/L, a period of hormone withdrawal that typically lasts 4–5 wk (20). Such periods of iatrogenic hypothyroidism are often debilitating, and the common symptoms of fatigue, cold intolerance, constipation, and cognitive impairment are poorly tolerated by patients (21,22). These moderate symptoms can be ameliorated with the use of the shorter half-life tri-iodothyronine during the first few weeks of thyroid hormone withdrawal, but all hormone therapy needs to be discontinued for 2–3 wk to achieve sufficient TSH elevation (23). More extreme complications of short-term hypothyroidism can develop, such as decompensation of otherwise controlled congestive heart failure, renal insufficiency, sleep apnea, or neurologic dysfunction (24–27). For patients with metastatic tumor in critical locations such as the central nervous system, even several weeks of TSH elevation can lead to tumor growth and/or peritumoral edema and subsequent intracranial or spinal cord compressive symptoms (27–30).

To avoid these complications of iatrogenic hypothyroidism, exogenous administration of TSH derived from animal sources was attempted *(6,31)*. Despite initial success in augmenting radioiodine uptake into thyroid remnants and metastases *(32–35)*, repeated use of bovine thyrotropin led to occasional severe systemic allergic responses and serial use was associated with decreased efficacy *(36)*. Human cadaveric pituitary sources of thyrotropin were never used because of evolving concerns about transmission of Creutzfeld–Jakob disease *(37)*. Diagnostic testing with scans and thyroglobulin determination following partial thyroid hormone withdrawal has been shown to be effective, but the effectiveness of radioiodine therapy has not been tested *(38)*.

Thus, by the late 1980s, the usefulness of recombinant thyrotropin became apparent. Following identification of the DNA sequence for both subunits of human thyrotropin, Chinese hamster ovary cells were stably transfected with the coding sequences to yield recombinant human TSH *(3)*. Commercial production of large quantities was enabled by culture of the rhTSH-secreting clones on microcarrier beads and sequential purification of secreted hormone from the culture media *(39)*. Characterization of the product included demonstration of three- to fourfold less TSH receptor binding affinity and cAMP-stimulating bioactivity than human pituitary TSH because of increased sialylation of rhTSH. However, this glycosylation pattern also resulted in a twofold lower metabolic clearance rate similar to that seen in primary hypothyroidism, thus yielding potentially adequate bioactivity when integrated over the duration of action of the hormone *(3,40)*. After a single intramuscular injection of 0.9 mg, the peak concentration of rhTSH averaged 116 mU/L and the half-life averaged 22 h. Preclinical studies confirmed the biologic efficacy of rhTSH to stimulate thyroid iodine uptake and hormone production in monkeys and to increase in vitro human fetal thyroid cell doubling time *(41,42)*.

RECOMBINANT HUMAN THYROTROPIN IN MANAGEMENT OF DIFFERENTIATED THYROID CARCINOMA

Diagnostic Testing

The initial human clinical trial of rhTSH identified dosing regimens that stimulated radioiodine uptake and thyroglobulin production in 19 thyroid carcinoma patients with tolerable side effects *(43)*. Following thyroidectomy, patients began therapy with tri-iodothyronine to suppress endogenous TSH production. After a median hormone treatment duration of 5 wk, patients were administered varying intramuscular doses of rhTSH, 0.9–3.6 mg (10–40 U) daily for 1–3 consecutive days. Dose-limiting nausea occurred after single doses of 2.7 mg and 3.6 mg, along with mild dizziness, weakness, and headache. Diagnostic activities of ^{131}I were given 24 h after the last dose of rhTSH, and whole-body scans were performed after another 48 h. Preliminary efficacy analysis suggested adequate radioiodine uptake into the thyroid bed with all dose schedules tested, and metastatic disease in the chest was visualized even after a single 0.9-mg dose. Tri-iodothyronine was then discontinued, and TSH levels allowed to rise endogenously; when TSH exceeded 25 mU/L, scanning was repeated. Comparing the paired scans for each individual studied, three patients had better visualization of lesions on rhTSH scans compared with hormone withdrawal, whereas the reverse was true in another three patients. Thyroglobulin levels continued to rise in response to rhTSH injection at least 72 h after the last administered dose but failed to rise as dramatically as after withdrawal.

On the basis of these initial safety and dosing results, two phase III trials were performed that led to approval of rhTSH for use in the United States and, subsequently, other countries. In the first trial, 127 patients underwent radioiodine scanning following rhTSH injection (0.9 mg im daily for two doses) and again following thyroid hormone withdrawal; the sequence of testing was not randomized *(44)*. Of this cohort, 22% had previously undergone thyroidectomy without subsequent radioiodine, and the remainder had previously received at least one treatment with radioiodine. As in the earlier study, each individual's scans were compared in pairwise fashion, looking for concordance or discordance between the results of the rhTSH-stimulated and the subsequent withdrawal scans. In 51% of patients, both sets of scans were negative for radioiodine uptake in thyroidal tissue. The remaining patients had uptake either limited to the thyroid bed (35%), in extrathyroidal cervical locations (8%), or in extracervical sites (6%) on at least one set of scans. Among those patients with at least one positive scan, both sets of scans were considered concordant only in 66%, whereas the rhTSH-stimulated scans were considered superior in 5% and the withdrawal scans were considered superior in the remaining 29%. Including the patients with negative scans, the concordance rate rose to 83%. As expected, symptoms and signs of hypothyroidism were limited only to the withdrawal period of the study.

The superior imaging outcomes obtained after thyroid hormone withdrawal were attributed to several potential mechanisms. Because renal clearance of iodine is impaired in hypothyroidism, retention of radioiodine by whole body as well as remnant thyroid tissue is augmented following thyroid hormone withdrawal; thus, scanning in the euthyroid patient following rhTSH administration may yield scans that are relatively "count poor" and less informative compared with thyroid hormone withdrawal. Unfortunately, the administered activity of radioiodine used in the various participating centers in the study was not well standardized, thereby introducing another potential variable. Finally, the diagnostic utility of testing thyroglobulin levels following TSH stimulation in conjunction with radioiodine imaging was not uniformly considered in the study design.

These issues were addressed in the second, confirmatory phase III trial *(45)*. The study design used the same paradigm of sequential testing with rhTSH followed by thyroid hormone withdrawal as in the earlier trials, with several key differences. First, the activity of ^{131}I administered was standardized at 4 ± 0.4 mCi for each scan, and whole-body gamma camera imaging was performed for a minimum of 30 min or 140,000 counts to avoid "count poor" scans. In addition, patients were randomly assigned to one of two rhTSH treatment regimens: 117 patients who received two 0.9-mg doses separated by 24 h, and 112 patients who received three 0.9-mg doses, each separated by 72 h to maximize the duration of TSH stimulation. Finally, serum thyroglobulin levels were measured in every patient sequentially for up to 7 d after the last dose of rhTSH, as well as once after thyroid hormone withdrawal.

All outcomes were similar in the two arms of the study, despite the differences in rhTSH dosing, so results are presented combining the two arms. Seventeen percent of the patients had previously undergone thyroidectomy without subsequent radioiodine, and the remainder had previously received at least one treatment with radioiodine. As in the previous study, 51% of patients had negative scans after both rhTSH stimulation and withdrawal. Of the remaining patients who had at least one positive scan, both sets of scans were considered concordant in 77%, whereas the rhTSH-stimulated scans were considered superior in 7% and the withdrawal scans were considered superior in the remaining 16%. Including the patients with negative scans, the concordance rate rose to 89%. For the patients who were found to have metastatic disease outside the thyroid bed on either withdrawal scans or subsequent posttherapy scans, the concordance rate was only 74%.

One hundred five patients who had previously undergone radioiodine therapy and did not have detectable serum antithyroglobulin autoantibodies had serum thyroglobulin concentrations that were elevated to at least 2 ng/mL after thyroid hormone withdrawal. Of these patients, serum thyroglobulin was similarly elevated in 50% before and 87% after rhTSH, peaking at 72 h after the last injection. By combining the results of scans and thyroglobulin measurements, the ability of rhTSH to facilitate detection of thyroid tissue was considerably improved. Ninety-three percent of the patients with scans showing uptake only in the thyroid bed after thyroid hormone withdrawal had either a positive rhTSH-stimulated scan or thyroglobulin level greater than or equal to 2 ng/mL. A subgroup of 30 patients was defined as having metastatic disease on the basis of pathologic ^{131}I uptake outside the thyroid bed on any scan. Within this subgroup, scans or elevated thyroglobulin level were positive after rhTSH in all patients.

Following each patient's withdrawal scan, the clinician-investigator needed to decide whether to treat the patient with radioiodine. Only two patients who received radioiodine therapy as a result of their withdrawal scan or thyroglobulin level had no evidence of disease on the basis of their rhTSH studies. One patient was treated because of a thyroglobulin concentration of 5 ng/mL, but both the withdrawal and posttherapy scans were negative; in the other patient, the withdrawal scan showed only faint thyroid bed uptake and thyroglobulin levels were undetectable even after withdrawal.

The adverse event profile in the two phase III studies was relatively mild. Transient headache and nausea were most common, each occurring in fewer than 10% of patients. Antithyrotropin antibodies did not develop in any patient, in distinct contrast to the previous experience with bovine TSH.

In summary, these two large multicenter studies demonstrated that rhTSH was a safe and well-tolerated alternative to thyroid hormone withdrawal prior to radioiodine scanning and thyroglobulin testing. Although scans were slightly less likely to be positive after rhTSH than after withdrawal, the incorporation of thyroglobulin testing permitted rhTSH testing to be nearly as accurate as thyroid hormone withdrawal, without the symptoms of severe hypothyroidism. Based on these studies, the Food and Drug Administration (FDA) approved Thyrogen® (thyrotropin alfa) for use as an adjunctive diagnostic tool for serum thyroglobulin testing with or without radioiodine imaging in the follow-up of patients with well-differentiated thyroid cancer. Subsequent reports of postapproval experience yielded outcomes comparable to those of the formal trials (46–49). Imaging at other time-points, ranging from 24 to 144 h after ^{131}I administration, may also provide adequate visualization of rhTSH-stimulated uptake (50,51). An alternate approach to rhTSH scanning using the shorter half-life isotope ^{123}I has also been explored, with a promising suggestion of excellent imaging characteristics and lower unintended radiation dose during diagnostic testing (52).

The high percentage of metastatic disease patients with positive rhTSH-stimulated thyroglobulin levels led to the suggestion that thyroglobulin testing without scanning could obviate the need for routine scanning (53–55). In one study of 72 patients who had previously undergone thyroidectomy and radioiodine therapy and had undetectable thyroglobulin levels while taking thyroid hormone, the results of rhTSH-stimulated thyroglobulin testing were compared with results of subsequently performed withdrawal scans and thyroglobulin determinations (56). Nearly 57% of patients had an rhTSH-stimulated thyroglobulin level less than 1 ng/mL. Within this group of patients with negative rhTSH-stimulated thyroglobulin levels, 73% had both negative withdrawal levels and scans, 5% had both elevated withdrawal levels and scans, and the remainder had one positive withdrawal test. All positive withdrawal scans after a negative rhTSH-stimulated thyroglobulin test had uptake limited to the thyroid bed. On the other hand, all patients whose rhTSH-stimulated thyroglobulin level was at least 1 ng/mL had a similarly elevated withdrawal level, and 74% also had a positive scan. Based on these results, it was proposed that in patients with negative thyroglobulin levels on thyroid hormone therapy, rhTSH-stimulated thyroglobulin testing could be used to identify those patients who required further scanning and possible treatment.

To identify clinical factors that could distinguish patients in whom rhTSH-stimulated testing would be of greatest utility, we analyzed our experience with 157 patients who underwent scanning and had thyroglobulin levels measured during a 2-yr period at our institution (51). Clinical staging at the time of initial diagnosis was stage I in 50%, stage II in 15%, stage III in 22%, and stage IV in 13%, using American Joint Commission on Cancer classifications (57). Nearly all patients had been previously treated with one (67%) or more (28%) courses of radioiodine, with a median duration of 1.5 yr since the most recent therapy. However, 14% had not been treated with ^{131}I for at least 5 yr. Unstimulated thyroglobulin levels were less than 1 ng/mL in 60% of patients and between 1 and 2 ng/mL in another 10%. Based on diagnostic testing performed before rhTSH (including physical examination, serum thyroglobulin levels on thyroid hormone therapy, chest radiographs, and neck high-resolution ultrasonography), 68% of the patients were classified as disease-free by their treating clinicians. Following administration of rhTSH, whole-body scanning was positive in 22% of patients, 38% of whom had uptake outside the neck in distant metastatic sites. Scans were positive in about 25% of stage I and II patients, 40% of those in stage III, and 90% of those in stage IV. Of the patients with a baseline thyroglobulin level less than 1 ng/mL before rhTSH, 15% had positive rhTSH-stimulated scans. Whereas the frequency of positive scans remained about 15% for patients with baseline thyroglobulin levels between 1 and 30 ng/mL, rhTSH-stimulated scans were positive in approx 60% of those whose baseline levels were between 31 and 500, and positive in all those whose baseline levels were greater than 500. Only one patient (3%) had a positive scan more than 5 yr from the last radioiodine therapy. The univariate factors that predicted a positive rhTSH-stimulated scan included increasing age, higher disease stage, clinician's pretest suspicion of disease, increasing pre-rhTSH thyroglobulin level, and shorter time interval since previous ^{131}I therapy. However, multivariate analysis indicated that the only independent predictors of a positive scan were the pretest suspicion of disease, increasing pre-rhTSH thyroglobulin, and shorter time since previous therapy.

Stimulated thyroglobulin levels remained suppressed in 76% of those whose baseline levels were less than 1 ng/mL and rose to 1 ng/mL or higher in the remaining 24%. Among the 107 patients whose baseline unstimulated thyroglobulin was below 2.5 ng/mL (the FDA cutoff for a positive rhTSH test result), 26% had a stimulated thyroglobulin that rose above that level. Independent predictors for an abnormal thyroglobulin response were the clinician's pretest suspicion of disease and fewer than 5 yr since previous ^{131}I therapy. Combining both criteria for a positive rhTSH test (i.e., either a positive scan or a stimulated thyroglobulin of at least 2.5 ng/mL), the only factor that independently predicted a positive test was the clinician's assessment of whether disease was present before rhTSH testing (odds ratio = 9.6; $p < 0.001$).

Various strategies for incorporating use of rhTSH testing in the routine management of patients with differentiated thyroid carcinoma have been proposed by some of the leading investigators in the field (2,49,54,58). In general, these recommendations have suggested that rhTSH testing with both radioiodine scans and thyroglobulin measurements should be limited to those patients thought to be at low risk for a positive finding that would require treatment, based on the slightly lower sensitivity of rhTSH testing compared with withdrawal and the lack of formal trials demonstrating the efficacy of rhTSH-stimulated ^{131}I therapy (see section on Radioiodine Therapy). The persistent presence of antithyroglobulin autoantibodies may interfere with the critical measurement of thyroglobulin during rhTSH testing as well as indicate a higher risk for residual disease and, therefore, may be viewed as an indication to proceed directly to withdrawal testing as well.

Instead of using both scans and thyroglobulin testing, it has been proposed that the results of rhTSH-stimulated thyroglobulin determinations 6–12 mo after initial adjuvant radioiodine ablation be used to guide the decision of whether to proceed directly to hormone withdrawal and therapy (54). This approach depends on the supposition that high-dose radioiodine therapy for patients with a detectable thyroglobulin level regardless of the results of diagnostic scanning is beneficial. However well reasoned this rationale may seem, recent reports indicate that patient outcomes may not be improved by such empiric radioiodine therapy (16,59). Other arguments against a thyroglobulin-only approach to rhTSH testing include the following: (1) It would be contraindicated in patients with antithyroglobulin autoantibodies and (2) patients whose metastatic disease does not produce thyroglobulin might escape early detection (46).

In our institution, the outcomes of the phase III trials and the analysis of our subsequent experience have led us to use rhTSH testing commonly, but selectively. Patients without initial distant metastases (TNM T1–4 N0–1 M0) who are treated with adjuvant radioiodine undergo evaluation 6 mo later that includes measurement of serum thyroglobulin while taking thyroid hormone. A neck ultrasound is also performed at this time if disease had been found at surgery in locoregional nodes or extrathyroidal locations (T4 or N1). Testing with rhTSH is scheduled for 6 mo later if the thyroglobulin level is 2 ng/mL or less and the ultrasound is negative for residual disease. If these subsequent tests are negative, rhTSH testing can be repeated after another 12–24 mo. Alternatively, given the low likelihood of disease detection, repeat rhTSH testing can probably be deferred in patients with disease initially localized only within the thyroid after a single set of negative rhTSH-stimulated scans and thyroglobulin measurement has been obtained. Annual physical examination with thyroglobulin determination while taking thyroid hormone and periodic neck ultrasound (if disease outside the thyroid has been resected previously) can then suffice in long-term follow-up, reserving stimulated testing for those patients with an abnormality detected during routine monitoring.

On the other hand, a patient with initial distant metastatic disease, an elevated thyroglobulin level while taking thyroid hormone, or persistent antithyroglobulin autoantibodies proceeds directly to thyroid hormone withdrawal testing, given the concern for a possible false-negative rhTSH-stimulated scan. The presence of suspicious findings by ultrasound are evaluated first by fine-needle aspiration and consideration of additional surgery (60,61). If surgery is planned, rhTSH-stimulated testing can be quickly performed preoperatively to determine if the disease can be detected by these means, thus lending greater confidence in the negative predictive value of a subsequent postoperative scan and thyroglobulin level.

Advance planning for routine rhTSH testing facilitates efficient use of patient and clinic staff time, as well as permits patients to follow an iodine-restricted diet. For scheduling rhTSH testing, beginning the procedures on Monday generally allows all needed outpatient appointments to be completed by Friday. After ruling out pregnancy in women of reproductive age, we usually administer intramuscular doses of rhTSH, 0.9 mg, on Monday and Tuesday mornings. If other imaging tests are required, such as ultrasound or chest radiography, these are also scheduled during these 2 d. The diagnostic dose of ^{131}I is given on Wednesday, and whole-body imaging is performed 24 h later. If the scan is negative on Thursday, it can be repeated the next day when a signal-to-background ratio might be more conducive to detecting faint lesions (50,62). A serum thyroglobulin level is drawn on Friday as well. Scheduling of a physician visit to review the results of these tests can be arranged for the same day as the scan or for the following week, by which time thyroglobulin results are usually available.

Radioiodine Therapy

Early in the clinical trials of rhTSH, it became apparent that some patients might potentially benefit from receiving therapeutic doses of ^{131}I after rhTSH administration. A compassionate use program was introduced by Genzyme to facilitate the availability of the drug for those few patients who needed radioiodine therapy of thyroid carcinoma in the absence of endogenous hypothyroidism or TSH elevation. Initial cases were reported describing such patients and their response to therapy. In a patient with a history of seizures and headache because of growth or swelling of metastatic lesions located in the brain during thyroid hormone withdrawal, we performed scanning and therapy after rhTSH (29). Posttherapy imaging demonstrated excellent uptake into the cerebral lesions, without any of the complications of tumor enlargement experienced previously. In another of our early patients, we administered 300 mCi of ^{131}I for skeletal metastases of follicular carcinoma after rhTSH, and palpable skull lesions resolved within 6 mo of treatment. A patient with progressively debilitating metastatic follicular carcinoma involving bones and lungs was treated with more than 500 mCi ^{131}I after rhTSH, with symptomatic improvement and eventual resumption of normal activities of daily living (63). In a patient with hypopituitarism associated with an empty sella, failure to increase endogenous TSH levels before therapy was overcome by administration of rhTSH (64).

Since these early case reports, several series have described benefit from rhTSH-stimulated therapy. Postoperative adjuvant ^{131}I to ablate thyroid remnant was described as highly effective to eliminate thyroid bed uptake in subsequent scanning in two groups totaling 22 patients (65,66). However, the efficacy of this approach in comparison with traditional withdrawal has yet to be tested in randomized prospective trial. One limitation has been the concern that the kinetics of radioiodine uptake and retention might differ significantly between the euthyroid and hypothyroid states, producing very different estimates of the total radiation dose absorbed by the thyroid tissue. Initial evidence of faster whole-body clearance of iodine led to the use of high empiric ^{131}I activities in the first few reported cases (29,63). However, longer retention of ^{131}I by thyroid remnant after rhTSH, leading to a greater rather than lesser absorbed radiation dose, could result from the rapid decline of serum TSH levels after rhTSH injection (66). Thus, the effectiveness of an administered activity of ^{131}I to ablate a thyroid remnant might be greater after rhTSH than after withdrawal, necessitating clinical trials that incorporate calculation of radiation dose delivered by treatment. If such an effect were confirmed, then adjuvant radioiodine treatment after rhTSH would yield an enhanced target-to-background ratio that could lead to rhTSH-stimulation becoming the preferred method of preparation before remnant ablation.

In three small recent series of patients with metastatic or locally invasive disease treated with rhTSH-stimulated ^{131}I, posttherapy imaging generally confirmed effectiveness of the preparative regimen to deliver the radioisotope to the intended targets *(27,67,68)*. However, only one-third of the combined cohort of patients experienced significant reductions in serum thyroglobulin levels as a response to treatment, and objective reduction in tumor bulk was only occasionally seen. Further investigation will be necessary to determine optimal rhTSH and radioiodine dosing for such therapy. Given the effect of lithium carbonate to prolong radioiodine retention and thereby maximize the delivered radiation dose in some metastatic thyroid carcinomas, we administer this routinely before and during rhTSH-stimulated ^{131}I therapy for metastases *(69)*.

In patients with bulky metastatic bone disease, acute expansion of tumor has occurred nearly overnight *(30)*. Pretreatment with high doses of glucocorticoids may prevent this complication. Because radioiodine therapy itself has been associated with acute tumor hemorrhage in intracerebral lesions, higher doses of dexamethasone, 4–8 mg daily for 5–10 d, are provided to patients with known brain metastases *(27,29)*.

RECOMBINANT HUMAN THYROTROPIN IN MANAGEMENT OF NODULAR GOITER

Whether endemic resulting from iodine deficiency or sporadic, nontoxic goiter is characterized by gradual heterogeneous growth and nodule formation. With the emergence and subsequent growth of TSH-independent adenomas, nontoxic goiter can occasionally evolve toward toxic hyperthyroidism requiring treatment. In other patients, nontoxic goiter is a common cause of symptomatic compression of upper aerodigestive tract structures. Nonsurgical therapy for symptomatic goiter has traditionally been limited to levothyroxine suppression, with marginal efficacy in many. Following reports of goiter shrinkage after radioiodine therapy, a prospective randomized trial compared thyroid hormone suppression with radioiodine in 57 iodine-sufficient patients with sporadic nontoxic goiter *(70)*. At study entry, goiter volume in the cohort averaged about 60 mL by ultrasound, and 81% of the patients were symptomatic. A median ^{131}I activity of 24 mCi (range: 12–90 mCi) was administered to 29 patients, calculated to deliver 0.12 mCi/mL thyroid tissue. In contrast, a mean daily levothyroxine dose of nearly 0.15 mg suppressed serum TSH levels to about 0.02 mU/L in the remaining 28 patients. Radiodine caused a 38% reduction in thyroid volume after 1 yr and 44% after 2 yr of follow-up, with 97% experiencing a more than 13% shrinkage. Mild radiation thyroiditis occurred in 14% and transient TSH suppression in 28%. Hypothyroidism developed in 45% during the first year after radioiodine therapy. Thyroid hormone suppression, on the other hand, caused 7% and 1% reductions in thyroid volume after 1 and 2 yr, respectively. Only 43% of patients had more than 13% shrinkage, with a median change in these "responders" of only 23%.

Radioiodine treatment protocols for goiter generally are based on the measured uptake of ^{131}I and thyroid size, higher activities being required for larger goiters and those with lower uptake measurements. Therefore, it was conjectured that preradioiodine administration of rhTSH could lead to greater tracer uptakes and either improved effectiveness of therapy or the ability to administer lower activities of ^{131}I *(71)*. To test this hypothesis, 15 iodine-sufficient patients with nodular goiter underwent radioiodine uptake measurements before and after varying doses of rhTSH. Following a single dose of rhTSH, 0.01 mg administered 24 h before ^{131}I, 6- and 24-h radioiodine uptake measurements rose from 18% and 29% to 40% and 51%, respectively, compared with nonstimulated uptakes. Slightly greater enhancement of uptake was seen after 0.03 mg rhTSH, but with prolonged increases in serum-free T4 and T3 above baseline levels. In a subsequently reported extension of this study, 26 patients also underwent planar scanning before and after rhTSH *(72)*. The uptake into regions that were relatively photopenic before rhTSH increased 30% more than the overall thyroid uptake, whereas the regions of relatively high uptake at baseline increased 13% less than the overall gland. There was a slight, albeit significant, decrease in the overall regional heterogeneity as measured by the coefficient of variation of radiation counts per scintigraphic pixel.

Thus, rhTSH can augment radioiodine uptake into nontoxic nodular goiter. Whether pretreatment with rhTSH before ^{131}I will shrink goiter more effectively will require further study. One separate advantage, however, of decreased heterogeneity seen in radioiodine distribution after rhTSH might be reduced theoretical risk of mutagenicity of therapy *(73)*. Radioiodine treatment for toxic nodular goiter, an extreme example of heterogeneity of intrathyroidal radiation dose, has been associated with a significantly increased risk of subsequent mortality because of thyroid cancer more than 5 yr later; such increased risk was not seen following the more homogeneously delivered treatment in patients with Graves' disease *(74)*. If relatively hypofunctioning areas in nontoxic nodular goiter absorb less iodine and as a result are exposed to sublethal radiation doses, enhancement of regional uptake by rhTSH could obviate this heterogeneity and potentially reduce the long-term risk of such therapy.

OTHER APPLICATIONS OF RECOMBINANT HUMAN THYROTROPIN

The acute response of normal thyroid glands to rhTSH administration has been examined in several recent studies. In six normal subjects without any evidence of thyroid disease, thyroid hormone levels were measured after single administration of rhTSH, 0.9 mg *(75)*. A rapid 65% increase in serum T_3 was noted within 4 h, peaking at 8 h, 89% above baseline, and remaining elevated for 3 d. Serum T_4 levels rose more slowly but to a greater extent, increasing 34% by 8 h, peaking nearly 180% of baseline after 48 h, and remaining elevated for 4 d. Because of this acute thyrotoxicosis, endogenous TSH levels fell below normal once the exogenously administered rhTSH cleared the circulation. Responses in circulating thyroid hormone levels of similar magnitude were later reported following administration of higher doses, 0.3 and 0.9 mg, suggesting that maximal hormone release occurred with no more than 0.1 mg of rhTSH *(76)*. It was proposed that rhTSH could be considered for dynamic testing in cases of uncertain thyroid function, such as patients taking thyroid hormone of long duration, but for dubious indications or patients in whom the distinction between primary and central hypothyroidism is unclear. As a tool for physiologic investigation, it was also suggested that rhTSH could be used to determine whether thyroid responsiveness is normal in patients with nonthyroidal illness.

Another application of rhTSH that has been explored is the ability to overcome the suppressive effects of excess iodine ingestion on radioiodine uptake. Earlier in vitro experiments had provided evidence that TSH stimulation could reverse the acute Wolff–Chaikoff effect *(77)*. To test the hypothesis in human thyroids, nine normal euthyroid volunteers were iodide loaded with 15 mg daily for 7 d *(78)*. Iodine-123 uptakes measured before and after iodide ingestion demonstrated the expected 80% reduction in uptake. After administration of a single rhTSH dose, 0.9 mg, radioiodine uptake doubled within 16 h but remained one-third of that measured before iodide loading. Nonethless, the study supported the contention that rhTSH stimulation can partially overcome the suppression of iodide uptake, raising the possibility that iodine-induced hyperthyroidism such as seen as a complication of amiodarone treatment could be treated with radioiodine following rhTSH.

Radioiodine therapy has also been reported to be helpful in the management of patients with malignant struma ovarii, a rare ovarian teratoma consisting of ectopic thyroid tissue. A recent case report highlighted the use of rhTSH to enhance therapeutic radioiodine uptake in a woman with multiple hyperfunctioning hepatic metastases who was unable to increase her endogenous TSH *(79)*. Using lesion dosimetry to determine the minimal ^{131}I activity necessary to deliver 8000 cGy to the metastases, 65 mCi were administered following two doses of rhTSH, 0.9 mg each. The whole-blood radiation dose was acceptably low, 120 cGy. Partial tumor reduction was documented radiographically and the patient was able to be retreated with ^{131}I 6 mo later, now following thyroid hormone withdrawal having successfully ablated most of the thyroid hormone production by tumor foci. Thus, rhTSH facilitated delivery of a maximal therapeutic effect with minimization of whole-body radiation exposure.

FUTURE DIRECTIONS

Thyrotropin alpha as a first-generation rhTSH product has changed many traditional paradigms for the monitoring of patients with differentiated thyroid carcinoma within only 4 yr of its commercial introduction. Extensive multinational clinical experience has identified potential for new treatment strategies both adjuvant and therapeutic, and future formal clinical trials will likely substantiate these findings. Expanded indications in the treatment of benign goitrous disease may also result from further investigation using this drug.

Continuing research on the structure–function relationship between TSH and its receptor has identified particular structural domains critical to the high-affinity ligand interaction *(1,80)*. With this information, modified TSH molecules with greater affinity are under development that could lead to second-generation drugs of higher potency and effectiveness *(81)*. Further work extending this knowledge may lead to clinical development of TSH receptor antagonists of potential use in treatment of Graves' disease as well as suppression of differentiated thyroid carcinoma *(82)*. Finally, it can be readily anticipated that introduction of a nonparenteral mode of drug delivery would lead to even greater future acceptance of rhTSH among patients and clinicians.

REFERENCES

1. Weintraub BD, Szkudlinski MW. Development and in vitro characterization of human recombinant thyrotropin. Thyroid 1999;9:447–450.
2. Ladenson PW, Ewertz ME, Dickey RA. Practical application of recombinant human thyrotropin testing in clinical practice. Endocrine Practice 2001;7:195–201.

3. Thotakura NR, Desai RK, Bates LG, Cole ES, Pratt BM, Weintraub BD. Biological activity and metabolic clearance of a recombinant human thyrotropin produced in Chinese hamster ovary cells. Endocrinology 1991;128:341–348.

4. Derwahl M, Broecker M, Kraiem Z. Thyrotropin may not be the dominant growth factor in benign and malignant thyroid tumors. J Clin Endocrinol Metab 1999;84:829–834.

5. Kimura T, Van Keymeulen A, Golstein J, Fusco A, Dumont JE, Roger PP. Regulation of thyroid cell proliferation by TSH and other factors: a critical evaluation of in vitro models. Endocr Rev 2001;22:631–656.

6. Robbins J. Pharmacology of bovine and human thyrotropin: an historical perspective. Thyroid 1999;9:451–453.

7. Sherman SI, Gillenwater AM, Goepfert H. Advances in the management of cancer of the thyroid gland. Advances in Otololaryngology-Head and Neck Surgery 2000;14:75–106.

8. Sherman SI, Tielens ET, Sostre S, Wharam MD, Jr., Ladenson PW. Clinical utility of posttreatment radioiodine scans in the management of patients with thyroid carcinoma. J Clin Endocrinol Metab 1994;78:629–634.

9. Grigsby PW, Baglan K, Siegel BA. Surveillance of patients to detect recurrent thyroid carcinoma. Cancer 1999;85:945–951.

10. Spencer CA, LoPresti JS, Fatemi S, Nicoloff JT. Detection of residual and recurrent differentiated thyroid carcinoma by serum thyroglobulin measurement. Thyroid 1999;9:435–441.

11. LoGerfo P, Colacchio T, Colacchio D, Feind C. Effects of TSH stimulation on serum thyroglobulin in metastatic thyroid cancer. J Surg Oncol 1980;14:195–200.

12. Pacini F, Lari R, Mazzeo S, Grasso L, Taddei D, Pinchera A. Diagnostic value of a single serum thyroglobulin determination on and off thyroid suppressive therapy in the follow-up of patients with differentiated thyroid cancer. Clin Endocrinol 1985;23:405–411.

13. Sherman SI. Adjuvant therapy and long-term management of differentiated thyroid carcinoma. Semin Surg Oncol 1999;16:30–33.

14. Pacini F, Lippi F, Formica N, et al. Therapeutic doses of iodine-131 reveal undiagnosed metastases in thyroid cancer patients with detectable serum thyroglobulin levels. J Nucl Med 1987;28:1888–1891.

15. Wartofsky L, Sherman SI, Gopal J, Schlumberger M, Hay ID. The use of radioactive iodine in patients with papillary and follicular thyroid cancer. J Clin Endocrinol Metab 1998;83:4195–4203.

16. Pacini F, Agate L, Elisei R, et al. Outcome of differentiated thyroid cancer with detectable serum Tg and negative diagnostic 131I whole body scan: comparison of patients treated with high 131I activities versus untreated patients. J Clin Endocrinol Metab 2001;86:4092–4097.

17. Pineda JD, Lee T, Ain K, Reynolds JC, Robbins J. Iodine-131 therapy for thyroid cancer patients with elevated thyroglobuiln and negative diagnostic scan. J Clin Endocrinol Metab 1995;80:1488–1492.

18. Mariotti S, Barbesino G, Caturegli P, et al. Assay of thyroglobulin in serum with thyroglobulin autoantibodies: an unobtainable goal? J Clin Endocrinol Metab 1995;80:468–472.

19. Spencer CA, Takeuchi M, Kazarosyan M, et al. Serum thyroglobulin autoantibodies: prevalence, influence on serum thyroglobulin measurement, and prognostic significance in patients with differentiated thyroid carcinoma. J Clin Endocrinol Metab 1998;83:1121–1127.

20. Schlumberger M, Tubiana M, De Vathaire F, et al. Long-term results of treatment of 283 patients with lung and bone metastases from differentiated thyroid carcinoma. J Clin Endocrinol Metab 1986;63:960–967.

21. Dow KH, Ferrell BR, Anello C. Quality-of-life changes in patients with thyroid cancer after withdrawal of thyroid hormone therapy. Thyroid 1997;7:613–619.

22. Dow KH, Ferrell BR, Anello C. Balancing demands of cancer surveillance among survivors of thyroid cancer. Cancer Pract 1997;5:289–295.

23. Goldman JM, Line BR, Aamodt RL, Robbins J. Influence of triiodothyronine withdrawal time on ^{131}I uptake postthyroidectomy for thyroid cancer. J Clin Endocrinol Metab 1980;50:734–739.

24. Ambrosino N, Pacini F, Paggiaro PL, et al. Impaired ventilatory drive in short-term primary hypothyroidism and its reversal by L-triiodothyronine. J Endocrinol Invest 1985;8:533–536.

25. Donaghue K, Hales I, Allwright S, et al. Cardiac function in acute hypothyroidism. Eur J Nucl Med 1985;11:147–149.

26. Punzengruber C, Weissel M. Influence of L-thyroxine on cardiac function in athyreotic thyroid cancer patients-an echophonocardiographic study. Klin Wochenschr 1988;66:729–735.

27. Pellegriti G, Scollo C, Giuffrida D, Vigneri R, Squatrito S, Pezzino V. Usefulness of recombinant human thyrotropin in the radiometabolic treatment of selected patients with thyroid cancer. Thyroid 2001;11:1025–1030.
28. Goldberg LD, Ditchek NT. Thyroid carcinoma with spinal cord compression. Jama 1981;245:953,954.
29. Chiu AC, Delpassand ES, Sherman SI. Prognosis and treatment of brain metastases in thyroid carcinoma. J Clin Endocrinol Metab 1997;82:3637–3642.
30. Robbins RJ, Voelker E, Wang W, Macapinlac HA, Larson SM. Compasionate use of recombinant human thyrotropin to facilitate radioiodine therapy: case report and review of the literature. Endocrine Prac 2000;6:460–464.
31. Stanley MM, Astwood EB. The response of the thyroid gland in normal human subjects to the administration of thyrotropin, as shown by studies with I-131. Endocrinology 1949;44:49–60.
32. Catz B, Petit D, Starr P. The diagnostic and therapeutic value of thyrotropin hormone and heavy dosage scintigrams for the demonstration of thyroid cancer metastases. Am J Med Sci 1959;237:158–164.
33. Sturgeon CT, Davis FE, Catz B, Petit D, Starr P. Treatment of thyroid cancer metastases with TSH and I-131 during thyroid hormone medication. J Clin Endocrinol Metab 1953;13:1391–1407.
34. Pfannenstiel P, Sitterson BW, Andrews GA. Use of thyrotropin hormone (TSH) for demonstration and postoperative treatment of thyroid cancer with radioiodine. Res. Rep. ORINS-49. US AEC Oak Ridge Inst Nucl Stud 1964;17:72–78.
35. Benua RS, Sonenberg M, Leeper RD, Rawson RW. An 18 year study of the use of beef thyrotropin to increase I-131 uptake in metastatic thyroid cancer. J Clin Endocrinol Metab 1964;5:796–801.
36. Melmed S, Harada A, Hershman JM, Krishnamurthy GT, Blahd WH. Neutralizing antibodies to bovine thyrotropin in immunized patients with thyroid cancer. J Clin Endocrinol Metab 1980;51:358–363.
37. Law A, Jack GW, Tellez M, Edmonds CJ. In-vivo studies of a human-thyrotrophin preparation. J Endocrinol 1986;110:375–378.
38. Guimaraes V, DeGroot LJ. Moderate hypothyroidism in preparation for whole body 131I scintiscans and thyroglobulin testing. Thyroid 1996;6:69–73.
39. Cole ES, Lee K, Lauziere K, et al. Recombinant human thyroid stimulating hormone: development of a biotechnology product for detection of metastatic lesions of thyroid carcinoma. Biotechnology (NY) 1993;11:1014–1024.
40. Szkudlinski MW, Thotakura NR, Bucci I, et al. Purification and characterization of recombinant human thyrotropin (TSH) isoforms produced by Chinese hamster ovary cells: the role of sialylation and sulfation in TSH bioactivity. Endocrinology 1993;133:1490–1503.
41. Huber GK, Fong P, Concepcion ES, Davies TF. Recombinant human thyroid-stimulating hormone: initial bioactivity assessment using human fetal thyroid cells. J Clin Endocrinol Metab 1991;72:1328–1331.
42. Braverman LE, Pratt BM, Ebner S, Longcope C. Recombinant human thyrotropin stimulates thyroid function and radioactive iodine uptake in the rhesus monkey. J Clin Endocrinol Metab 1992;74:1135–1139.
43. Meier CA, Braverman LE, Ebner SA, et al. Diagnostic use of recombinant human thyrotropin in patients with thyroid carcinoma (phase I/II study). J Clin Endocrinol Metab 1994;78:188–196.
44. Ladenson PW, Braverman LE, Mazzaferri EL, et al. Comparison of administration of recombinant human thyrotropin with withdrawal of thyroid hormone for radioactive iodine scanning in patients with thyroid carcinoma. N Engl J Med 1997;337:888–896.
45. Haugen BR, Pacini F, Reiners C, et al. A comparison of recombinant human thyrotropin and thyroid hormone withdrawal for the detection of thyroid remnant or cancer. J Clin Endocrinol Metab 1999;84:3877–3885.
46. Durski JM, Weigel RJ, McDougall IR. Recombinant human thyrotropin (rhTSH) in the management of differentiated thyroid cancer. Nucl Med Commun 2000;21:521–528.
47. Robbins RJ, Tuttle RM, Sharaf RN, et al. Preparation by recombinant human thyrotropin or thyroid hormone withdrawal are comparable for the detection of residual thyroid carcinoma. J Clin Endocrinol Metab 2001;86:619–625.
48. David A, Blotta A, Bondanelli M, et al. Serum thyroglobulin concentrations and 131-I whole-body scan results in patients with differentiated thyroid carcinoma after administration of recombinant human thyroid-stimulating hormone. J Nucleic Med 2001;42:1470–1475.
49. Haugen BR, Ridgway EC, McLaughlin BA, McDermott MT. Clinical comparison of whole-body radioiodine scan and serum thyroglobulin after stimulation with recombinant human thyrotropin. Thyroid 2002;12:37–43.
50. Sarkar SD, Afriyie MO, Palestro CJ. Recombinant human thyroid-stimulating hormone-aided scintigraphy: comparison of imaging at multiple times after I-131 administration. Clin Nucl Med 2001;26:392–395.

51. Lopez-Penabad L, Ghori F, Sherman SI. Diagnostic utility of recombinant human TSH testing during long-term follow-up of patients with differentiated thyroid carcinoma, 10th Annual Meeting of the American Association of Clinical Endocrinologists, San Antonio, Texas, 2001.
52. Gulzar Z, Jana S, Young I, et al. Neck and whole-body scanning with 5-mCi dose of (123)I as diagnostic tracer in patients with well-differentiated thyroid cancer. Endocr Pract 2001;7:244–249.
53. Pacini F, Lippi F. Clinical experience with recombinant human thyroid-stimulating hormone (rhTSH): serum thyroglobulin measurement. J Endocrinol Invest 1999;22:25–29.
54. Schlumberger M, Ricard M, Pacini F. Clinical use of recombinant human TSH in thyroid cancer patients. Eur J Endocrinol 2000;143:557–563.
55. Mazzaferri EL, Kloos RT. Is diagnostic Iodine-131 scanning with recombinant human TSH useful in the follow-up of differentiated thyroid cancer after thyroid ablation? J Clin Endocrinol Metab 2002;87:1490–1498.
56. Pacini F, Molinaro E, Lippi F, et al. Prediction of disease status by recombinant human TSH-stimulated serum Tg in the postsurgical follow-up of differentiated thyroid carcinoma. J Clin Endocrinol Metab 2001;86:5686–5690.
57. Beahrs OH, Henson DE, Hutter RVP, Myers MH. Manual for Staging of Cancer. Philadelphia: J.B. Lippincott, 1992.
58. Mazzaferri EL, Kloos RT. Using recombinant human TSH in the management of well-differentiated thyroid cancer: current strategies and future directions. Thyroid 2000;10:767–778.
59. Fatourechi V, Hay ID, Javedan H, Wiseman GA, Mullan BP, Gorman CA. Lack of impact of radioiodine therapy in TG-positive, diagnostic whole- body scan-negative patients with follicular cell-derived thyroid cancer. J Clin Endocrinol Metab 2002;87:1521–1526.
60. Franceschi M, Kusic Z, Franceschi D, Lukinac L, Roncevic S. Thyroglobulin determination, neck ultrasonography and iodine-131 whole-body scintigraphy in differentiated thyroid carcinoma. J Nucleic Med 1996;37:446–451.
61. Krishnamurthy S, Bedi DG, Caraway NP. Ultrasound-guided fine-needle aspiration biopsy of the thyroid bed. Cancer (Cytopathology) 2001;93:199–205.
62. McDougall IR, Weigel RJ. Recombinant human thyrotropin in the management of thyroid cancer. Curr Opin Oncol 2001;13:39–43.
63. Rudavsky AZ, Freeman LM. Treatment of scan-negative, thyroglobulin-positive metastatic thyroid cancer using radioiodine 131-I and recombinant human thyroid stimulating hormone. J Clin Endocrinol Metab 1997;82:11–14.
64. Colleran KM, Burge MR. Isolated thyrotropin deficiency secondary to primary empty sella in a patient with differentiated thyroid carcinoma: an indication for recombinant thyrotropin. Thyroid 1999;9:1249–1252.
65. Perros P. Recombinant human thyroid-stimulating hormone (rhTSH) in the radioablation of well-differentiated thyroid cancer: preliminary therapeutic experience. J Endocrinol Invest 1999;22:30–34.
66. Robbins RJ, Tuttle RM, Sonenberg M, et al. Radioiodine ablation of thyroid remnants after preparation with recombinant human thyrotropin. Thyroid 2001;11:865–869.
67. Luster M, Lassmann M, Haenscheid H, Michalowski U, Incerti C, Reiners C. Use of recombinant human thyrotropin before radioiodine therapy in patients with advanced differentiated thyroid carcinoma. J Clin Endocrinol Metab 2000;85:3640–3645.
68. Lippi F, Cappezzone M, Angelini G, Taddei D, Molinaro E, Pinchera A. Radioiodine treatment of metastatic differentiated thyroid cancer in patients on L-thyroxine, using recombinant human TSH. Eur J Endocrinol 2001;144:5–11.
69. Koong SS, Reynolds JC, Movius EG, et al. Lithium as a potential adjuvant to 131I therapy of metastatic, well differentiated thyroid carcinoma. J Clin Endocrinol Metab 1999;84:912–916.
70. Wesche MFT, Buul MCT, Lips P, Smits NJ, Wiersinga WM. A randomized trial coomparing levothyroxine with radioactive iodine in the treatment of sporadic nontoxic goiter. J Clin Endocrinol Metab 2001;86:998–1005.
71. Huysmans DA, Nieuwlaat W-A, Erdtsieck RJ, et al. Administration of a single low dose of recombinant human thyrotropin significantly enhances thyroid radioiodine uptake in nontoxic nodular goiter. J Clin Endocrinol Metab 2000;85:3592–3596.
72. Nieuwlaat W-A, Hermus AR, Sivro-Prndelj F, Corstens FH, Huysmans DA. Pretreatment with recombinant human TSH changes the regional distribution of radioiodine on thyroid scintigrams of nodular goiters. J Clin Endocrinol Metab 2001;86:5330–5336.
73. Gorman CA, Robertson JS. Radiation dose in the selection of 131I or surgical treatment for toxic thyroid adenoma. Ann Intern Med 1978;89:85–90.

74. Ron E, Doody MM, Becker DV, et al. Cancer mortality following treatment for adult hyperthyroidism. Cooperative Thyrotoxicosis Therapy Follow-up Study Group. JAMA 1998;280:347–355.

75. Ramirez L, Braverman LE, White B, Emerson CH. Recombinant human thyrotropin is a potent stimulator of thyroid function in normal subjects. J Clin Endocrinol Metab 1997;82:2836–2839.

76. Torres MS, Ramirez L, Simkin PH, Braverman LE, Emerson CH. Effect of various doses of recombinant human thyrotropin on the thyroid radioactive iodine uptake and serum levels of thyroid hormones and thyroglobulin in normal subjects. J Clin Endocrinol Metab 2001;86:1660–1664.

77. Sherwin JR, Tong W. The actions of iodide and TSH on thyroid cells showing a dual control system for the iodide pump. Endocrinology 1974;94:1465–1474.

78. Lawrence JE, Emerson CH, Sullaway SL, Braverman LE. The effect of recombinant human TSH on the thyroid (123)I uptake in iodide treated normal subjects. J Clin Endocrinol Metab 2001;86:437–440.

79. Rotman-Pikielny P, Reynolds JC, Barker WC, Yen PM, Skarulis MC, Sarlis NJ. Recombinant human thyrotropin for the diagnosis and treatment of a highly functional metastatic struma ovarii. J Clin Endocrinol Metab 2000;2000:237–244.

80. Szkudlinski MW, Fremont V, Ronin C, Weintraub BD. Thyroid-stimulating hormone and thyroid-stimulating hormone receptor structure-function relationships. Physiol Rev 2002;82:473–502.

81. Leitolf H, Tong KP, Grossmann M, Weintraub BD, Szkudlinski MW. Bioengineering of human thyrotropin superactive analogs by site- directed "lysine-scanning" mutagenesis. Cooperative effects between peripheral loops. J Biol Chem 2000;275:27,457–27,465.

82. Zhang M, Tong KP, Fremont V, et al. The extracellular domain suppresses constitutive activity of the transmembrane domain of the human TSH receptor: implications for hormone-receptor interaction and antagonist design. Endocrinology 2000;141:3514–3517.

7

Thyroid Hormone Replacement Therapy for Primary and Secondary Hypothyroidism

David S. Cooper, MD

INTRODUCTION: DEFINITIONS, ETIOLOGIES, AND DIAGNOSIS OF PRIMARY AND SECONDARY HYPOTHYROIDISM

Primary hypothyroidism is defined as a deficiency of thyroid hormone as a result of intrinsic failure of the thyroid gland. This leads to low levels of circulating thyroxine, insufficient levels of thyroid hormone in target tissues, and typical symptoms, signs, and laboratory abnormalities. When severe or long standing, the clinical diagnosis is straightforward, confirmed by the finding of elevated serum levels of thyrotropin (TSH) and depressed serum concentrations of free-thyroxine (fT4) or the free-T_4 estimate (free-T_4 index or FTI). Circulating serum tri-iodothyronine (T_3) concentrations are generally low or low normal. It is a relatively common disorder, affecting 1–3% of the population. The annual incidence is approx 1–2 per 1000 women and 1 per 10,000 men, with higher rates in older individuals *(1)*. Autoimmune (Hashimoto's) thyroiditis is the cause of spontaneous primary hypothyroidism in the vast majority of cases. Postablative hypothyroidism after therapy for hyperthyroidism or thyroid surgery is the second most common

From: *Endocrine Replacement Therapy in Clinical Practice*
Edited by: A. Wayne Meikle © Humana Press Inc., Totowa, NJ

cause. Drugs may also precipitate primary hypothyroidism, especially in people with underlying autoimmune thyroid disease (i.e., positive antithyroid antibodies). Lithium and iodine-containing drugs such as the antiarrhythmic amiodarone frequently lead to hypothyroidism in such individuals. Rare congenital causes of primary hypothyroidism include thyroid agenesis or maldevelopment and a variety of hereditary intrathyroidal enzyme deficiencies or thyroglobulin biosynthetic abnormalities probably the result of specific genetic mutations.

The mildest form of primary hypothyroidism has been termed "subclinical hypothyroidism." Subclinical hypothyroidism is said to exist when serum fT4 levels fall but remain within the broad range of normal (2,3). Because of the exquisite sensitivity of the pituitary to subtle changes in fT4 levels, TSH secretion increases in response to these lower, albeit "normal" fT4 concentrations. Therefore, subclinical hypothyroidism is defined biochemically by a normal serum fT4 or fT4 estimate, a normal serum T_3 concentration, and an elevated serum TSH concentration. In this situation, the serum TSH level is usually less than 20 mU/L. Obviously, the diagnosis of subclinical hypothyroidism cannot be made if only the serum fT4 or FTI is assessed. Subclinical hypothyroidism is generally associated with few symptoms or signs of hypothyroidism and minimal biochemical changes (e.g., serum lipid levels) (2). Nevertheless, many experts feel that subclinical hypothyroidism may be associated with both subtle symptoms and mild dyslipidemia that could be detrimental to the patient (3). Subclinical hypothyroidism is likely the precursor to overt hypothyroidism in some cases, particularly in individuals with high titers of antithyroid antibodies. Subclinical hypothyroidism is far more common than overt hypothyroidism, affecting approx 5% of people; it is particularly prevalent in women over age 60, in whom the frequency has approached 20% in some surveys (4). The same factors that are associated with the development of overt hypothyroidism (autoimmune thyroiditis and other autoimmune diseases, postablation, and certain drugs) are also associated with subclinical hypothyroidism.

Secondary hypothyroidism is defined as a deficiency of thyroid hormone resulting from a lack of thyroidal stimulation by pituitary TSH. Generally, secondary hypothyroidism indicates the presence of significant underlying hypothalamic or pituitary disease. Secondary hypothyroidism is uncommon, but the actual prevalence is not known. The diagnosis may be more difficult than in the case of primary hypothyroidism, because serum TSH levels may not always be low. Thus, if the physician simply relies on the serum TSH as the sole laboratory test to screen for hypothyroidism, the diagnosis will be missed. On the other hand, if both the fT4 or FTI and the TSH are measured, the diagnosis should be entertained if the fT4 or FTI is low and the TSH level is either normal or low. In very rare cases, the TSH levels may be at the upper end of the normal range or slightly elevated, a situation which can masquerade as subclinical hypothyroidism. The "normal" TSH levels in secondary hypothyroidism are the result of the elaboration by the pituitary gland of a TSH molecule with normal immunoactivity but depressed bioactivity, possibly related to alterations in TSH glycosylation (5,6). It is often difficult to distinguish between hypothalamic and pituitary disease on clinical grounds. Stimulation with the hypothalamic peptide thyrotropin-releasing hormone (TRH) may be useful, as patients with pituitary disease usually do not respond or respond poorly to TRH, whereas those with hypothalamic disease respond, albeit with a delayed rise in serum TSH. However, with the almost ubiquitous use of magnetic resonance imaging (MRI) to establish the site and type of disease, TRH testing is rarely needed.

The following discussion focuses on the use of thyroid hormone in the management of patients with primary and secondary hypothyroidism. There have been several recent reviews of this topic (7–9). Although thyroid hormone can be used to treat goiter and thyroid nodules (so-called "suppression" therapy), this indication is beyond the scope of this review, as are the nuances of thyroid hormone therapy in patients with differentiated thyroid cancer.

THYROID HORMONE PREPARATIONS

When one speaks of "thyroid hormone," one generally means the sodium salt of levothyroxine (L-T4). However, the United States Pharmacopoeia lists five thyroid hormone preparations: synthetic L-T4, synthetic liothyronine (L-T3), liotrix (a fixed combination of synthetic L-T4 and L-T3 in a 4:1 ratio), as well as desiccated thyroid, manufactured from the thyroids of slaughterhouse animals, and purified animal thyroglobulin (10). L-T4 is the treatment of choice for the long-term management of primary and secondary hypothyroidism. L-T3 has specific, narrow, and self-limited indications, including suppression testing and in the preparation of thyroid cancer patients for radio-iodine scanning or therapy. Because of its relatively short half-life of 1 d, its use leads to variable serum hormone levels throughout the day. Liotrix and desiccated thyroid, although still available in pharmacies, are obsolete forms of therapy; patients taking either of these two drugs should be switched to L-T4 using the guidelines presented in the following section. Purified animal thyroglobulin (Proloid) is no longer available in the United States or Canada.

Thyroxine is one of the most frequently prescribed medications in the United States, with more than 18 million prescriptions for the various preparations written annually (11). Another study revealed that 6.9% of an unselected cohort of older adults were taking thyroid hormone (12).

THYROXINE PHARMACOLOGY (SEE TABLE 1)

The average daily secretion rate of thyroxine by the thyroid gland is in the range of 90 µg, but the usual requirement for orally administered L-T4 is 100–200 µg/d (13). This indicates that the gastrointestinal absorption of L-T4 is considerably less than 100%. Studies using simultaneous oral and iv thyroxine have indicated that L-T4 is 60–80% absorbed, with large individual differences (50–100%) in apparently healthy people (14). There is no absorption of orally administered L-T4 from the stomach, and the main absorptive sites appear to be the proximal and mid-jejunum. Progressively decreasing degrees of absorption occur along the distal bowel and proximal colon, but there are no reports of L-T4 malabsorption in colectomized individuals (14). People over age 70 yr may have a slight (10%) decrease in L-T4 absorption that is probably not clinically significant (15). Thyroxine absorption is greater if the drug is given on an empty stomach (16), and food may also delay absorption (17). Hypothyroidism may lead to a slight increase in thyroxine absorption (18).

FACTORS AFFECTING L-T4 ABSORPTION OR METABOLISM

A variety of intestinal diseases have been associated with increased L-T4 requirements, including sprue, Crohn's disease, and short-bowel syndromes (19–21). Chronic

Table 1
Conditions That May Affect L-T4 Requirements

Increased requirements
  Physiologic states
    Pregnancy
    Infancy and childhood
  Gastrointestinal disease
    Malabsorption (sprue, regional enteritis)
    Cirrhosis
    Pancreatitis
  Drugs that interfere with absorption
    Cholestyramine and colestipol
    Sucralfate
    Aluminum hydroxide
    Ferrous sulfate
    Calcium
    Lovastatin
  Drugs that block T4 to T3 conversion
    Amiodarone
  Drugs that accelerate L-T4 disappearance
    Phenytoin
    Carbamazepine
    Phenobarbital
    Rifampin
    Sertraline
  Drugs that increase thyroid-binding globulin
    Estrogen
  Dietary factors that interfere with absorption
    Soy-based infant formula
    Fiber supplements
Decreased requirements
  Physiologic
    Aging
  Drugs that decrease thyroid-binding globulin
    Exogenous androgen use

pancreatitis and cirrhosis have also been reported to cause L-T4 malabsorption (14). A factitious form of malabsorption termed "levothyroxine pseudomalabsorption" has been reported in patients with psychiatric disease, in whom normal L-T4 absorption is found when it is directly assessed (22). Drugs that interfere with thyroxine absorption include the bile acid sequestrant cholestyramine and possibly others (23,24) aluminum hydroxide (25), ferrous sulfate (26), sucralfate (27), and calcium supplements (28). Soy-based infant formulas and diets enriched with fiber supplements (29) have also been reported to lead to higher than expected thyroxine dosing.

After ingestion, serum thyroxine levels rise 10–15%, peaking at 2–4 h (30,31). Serum T_3 levels generally do not change after L-T4 administration, because of the slow conversion of T_4 to T_3 in peripheral tissues. Thus, exogenous L-T4 provides a steady source of T_3, similar to what is seen after endogenous T_4 secretion and deiodination.

Certain drugs accelerate thyroxine metabolism in the liver by inducing mixed-function oxygenase enzyme systems. Patients taking phenytoin *(32)*, carbamazepine (Tegretol) *(33)*, rifampin *(34)*, and possibly sertraline (Zoloft) *(35)* will often require an increased L-T4 dose. Patients taking amiodarone, a potent inhibitor of T_4 to T_3 conversion may also require an increase in dosage because of difficulty in normalizing serum TSH levels, likely the result of the blockade of intrapituitary T_4 to T_3 conversion *(36)*. Patients receiving exogenous estrogen have recently been reported to have increased thyroxine requirements, likely the result of increased circulating thyroid-binding globulin (TBG) levels, causing a decrease in free thyroxine that cannot be compensated for in a hypothyroid individual *(37)*. On the other hand, patients treated with androgen for breast cancer have been reported to require a 25–50% decrease in L-T4 dose, possibly related to a decrease in serum TBG concentrations, with subsequent increases in serum fT4 levels *(38)*.

REPLACEMENT THERAPY IN PRIMARY HYPOTHYROIDISM

Based on the criterion of normalization of serum TSH concentrations, the average L-T4 replacement dose is approx 1.6 µg/kg ideal body weight *(13)*. The dose is 10–40% lower in the elderly because of decreases in thyroxine turnover with age *(39,40)*, and it is significantly higher in infants and children (10–15 µg/kg in infants and 2–3 µg/kg in children) *(41)*. The reasons for these markedly increased requirements are not known, but probably reflect increased thyroxine turnover in children. The dose to normalize the serum TSH level may differ depending on the etiology of the hypothyroidism; all else being equal, the L-T4 dose in patients with primary or postsurgical hypothyroidism may be 20% greater than the dose in patients with postablative Graves' disease, presumably because of the continued presence of autonomously functioning thyroid tissue in the latter situation *(42)*.

Given the fact that the distribution of serum TSH levels is not Gaussian, but is skewed to the left, it is reasonable to strive for a serum TSH level in the lower one-half of the normal range (0.5–2.5 or 3 mU/L in an assay where the normal range is 0.5–5 mU/L). In the average otherwise healthy patient, the full replacement dose (1.6 µg/kg) can be given at the outset, without building the dosage up slowly. In extremely obese individuals, the dose should probably be based on lean body mass *(7)*. With this in mind, the average woman will require a dose in the range of 100–125 µg/d, and 125–175 µg/d will be needed for the average man. Because serum TSH levels fall at a rate of approx 50% per week *(43)*, it is usually recommended that serum TSH levels not be checked for 4–6 wk after therapy is initiated, especially if the serum TSH is extremely elevated at the start. Also, L-T4 has a serum half-life of about 6 d, and five half-lives are required for any drug to reach steady state levels in the blood. If the serum TSH level is persistently elevated after 8–12 wk of therapy, the L-T4 dose should be increased by 25 µg and the TSH reassessed after an additional 6–8 wk.

Clinical improvement generally begins after a few days to a few weeks, but complete recovery may require several months of therapy. Once the proper dose has been established, it should not change unless clinical circumstances change (e.g., introduction of an interfering drug, weight loss or gain, aging, pregnancy [*see* below]). In stable patients, serum TSH can be checked annually to assure compliance; it is usually not necessary to monitor the fT4 or FTI unless the TSH becomes abnormal *(44)*. If the fT4 or FTI is measured, it is often in the upper end of the normal range or may be even slightly above normal. This is likely the result of the need for a higher serum T_4 and fT4 to generate adequate T_3 in the absence of the thyroid gland. In normal individuals, approx 20% of circulating T_3 is derived from the thyroid itself, whereas 80% comes from the conversion of T_4 to T_3 peripherally. In treated primary hypothyroidism, a higher serum T_4 level is required to compensate for the loss of the thyroidal component of the daily T_3 production. Thus, serum T_3 and TSH values are almost always normal in L-T4 treated patients with so-called "euthyroid hyperthyroxinemia."

Noncompliance always should be considered in patients in whom the dose seems inappropriately large, assuming other factors that increase L-T4 dose requirements can be ruled out (see above and below). Patients with fT4 levels that are high-normal or elevated who also have elevated TSH levels most likely are taking their medications sporadically, especially in anticipation of a physician visit or laboratory testing. Because of its long half-life, thyroxine may be given once weekly to extremely noncompliant patients (45).

Overreplacement with thyroxine, as judged by a suppressed serum TSH concentration, should be avoided, particularly in older patients. Some (e.g., see refs. 46 and 47) but not all (48,49) studies have concluded that postmenopausal women on suppressive doses of L-T4 are at risk for lower bone mineral density compared to age-matched control women. Two meta-analyses have also shown similar findings in postmenopausal, but not premenopausal, women (50,51), and a recent study also documented higher fracture rates in women with suppressed serum TSH values (52). Estrogen use may attenuate the effect of excess thyroid hormone on bone turnover (53). In addition, a long-term prospective study examining the risk of atrial fibrillation found that patients with suppressed serum TSH levels (serum TSH <0.1 mU/L), (the majority of whom were taking L-T4) had an almost threefold elevation in the risk of atrial fibrillation over a 10-yr follow-up period compared to patients with either normal, slightly elevated, or slightly low serum TSH levels (54). Therefore, it behooves the clinician to carefully titrate the L-T4 dose against the serum TSH to be sure that it remains within the range of normal. Suppression of the serum TSH and, by inference, an adverse effect on the skeleton and heart, can be seen with changes in L-T4 dosage as small as 25 μg/d (55).

Patients taking desiccated thyroid or T_4/T_3 combinations should be switched to L-T4. Although it has been a traditional concept that 1 grain of desiccated thyroid is approximately equal to 100 μg of L-T4, this conversion often leads to excessive L-T4 dosing. Practically speaking, it is better to simply stop the desiccated thyroid and start L-T4 at a dose commensurate with the patient's weight, as described earlier. A recent small randomized double-blind, controlled trial suggested that patients receiving a combination of synthetic T_4 and T_3 noted statistically significantly improved cognitive function and mood compared to when they were receiving L-T4 alone (56). Although this report has rekindled interest in combination therapy with L-T4 plus T_3, this cannot be recommended for routine management without larger confirmatory studies. There is no evidence of benefit from thyroxine therapy in patients with fatigue, cold intolerance, weight gain, and other symptoms who have normal thyroid function (57).

BRAND NAME OR GENERIC THYROXINE?

There continues to be great controversy concerning the possible differences in potency and reliability of brand name (proprietary) versus generic thyroxine preparations (58).

With ever-increasing demands for cost containment, the pressure to prescribe less expensive L-T4 preparations has increased. Since 1983, all thyroxine products have been required to contain 90–110% of the stated tablet content, measured by high-pressure liquid chromatography. Although the proprietary products have consistently met this standard, there are troubling reports of departures from these standards with both generic products *(59)* and brand name products *(60)*, although the prevalence of this problem is not known. In addition, differences in thyroxine bioavailability, which is related to tablet solubility and composition rather than to hormonal content, may exist. The inert ingredients (called "excipients," including lactose, corn starch, talc) that permit a tablet to be formed into a specific shape and to have a particular consistency may be important in this regard. Neither the United States Pharmacopoeia nor the Food and Drug Administration (FDA) have specific guidelines for demonstrating thyroxine bioequivalence among various products. Furthermore, FDA guidelines for bioequivalence of drugs are based on the demonstration of similar acute pharmacokinetic profiles (i.e., area under the curve and maximal concentration after dosing) rather that the more relevant physiological parameter of serum TSH. Thus, although several recent studies have claimed that some L-T4 preparations are "bioequivalent" *(61,62)*, others have suggested differences *(63)*.

Methodological problems exist, and published and unpublished data on TSH levels show considerable individual variability after switching from one product to another *(61)*. In 1998, the FDA required all thyroxine manufacturers to submit New Drug Applications (NDAs), with documentation of tablet composition and stability. This should enable direct bioavailability comparisons to be made among the various products, as there will be, for the first time, FDA-approved thyroxine. However, the FDA still has not implemented a TSH-based criterion for interchangability.

One can be reasonably sure that serum levels of thyroxine and TSH will be stable if a patient consistently takes branded L-T4 manufactured by the same company. Unfortunately, if generic thyroxine is prescribed, the patient may receive thyroxine made by a different manufacturer each time a prescription is filled. Thus, it appears that the only way to be sure of consistency is to prescribe proprietary thyroxine. There are considerable cost differences among the various proprietary products. Switching from one brand to another is not recommended, and current guidelines published by the American Thyroid Association recommend that TSH levels be checked if thyroxine brands are changed *(64)*.

OTHER CONSIDERATIONS

Subclinical Hypothyroidism

There continues to be controversy over whether subclinical hypothyroidism represents a disease that requires therapy or a clinically insignificant set of laboratory abnormalities *(3,65–67)*. In the view of many experts, therapy is usually indicated for three reasons. First, several studies have shown that "subclinical" hypothyroidism may actually be associated with mild symptoms or subtle cognitive deficits consistent with hypothyroidism that are reversed with L-T4 therapy *(3,65,68–70)*. Second, there may be improvements in serum lipids, especially when serum TSH values are greater than 10–12 mU/L and serum cholesterol is >240 mg/dL *(70,71)*. Finally, patients, particularly the elderly, are at risk for the development overt hypothyroidism at a rate of 5–20% per year, especially, but not exclusively, in patients with positive antithyroid antibodies

(72,73). In subclinical hypothyroidism, most patients' TSH serum levels can be normalized with modest L-T4 doses, in the range of 50–100 µg/d. Indeed, it has been shown that the final replacement dose of L-T4 correlates with the pretreatment TSH level *(74)*. The arguments against therapy are cost, the danger of overtreatment leading to iatrogenic thyrotoxicosis, and the lack of unequivocal evidence showing benefit.

Pregnancy

At least 50–75% of pregnant hypothyroid women will require an increase in their L-T4 dose during pregnancy *(75,76)*. Possible reasons include increased thyroxine-binding globulin levels, transplacental passage of T_4, and placental deiodination of T_4. In one study, the mean daily increment required to normalize the serum TSH was 37 µg/d *(75)*; in another, it was 52 µg/d *(76)*. Increases in L-T4 requirements may begin in the first trimester, so that serum TSH should be checked at the end of the first trimester and every 6–12 wk thereafter. Some experts advise an increase in thyroxine dose of 25 µg/d as soon as pregnancy is diagnosed. After delivery, the L-T4 dose returns to the prepartum level, and overreplacement will ensue if the dose is not decreased at the time of delivery.

Transient Hypothyroidism

Patients with postpartum thyroiditis or subacute thyroiditis may have transient hypothyroidism as part of the evolution of their illness *(77)*. The majority of patients have mild hypothyroidism and remain asymptomatic. Occasionally, however, the hypothyroidism is severe enough to warrant treatment with L-T4. In this situation, treatment is continued for 3–6 mo and is then discontinued. In most instances, a euthyroid state will be found; however, approx 25% of patients with postpartum thyroiditis will require continued L-T4 therapy because of permanent impairment in thyroid function. The vast majority of patients with Hashimoto's thyroiditis have permanent hypothyroidism, but a small fraction (in the range of 10%) may have recovery of thyroid function *(78,79)*. However, most experts do not recommend a trial discontinuation of thyroxine in patients with long-standing typical primary hypothyroidism.

L-T4 Therapy in Patients with Ischemic Heart Disease

In the elderly (over age 65) or in patients with significant cardiac disease, it is prudent to begin with lower doses of L-T4 and to build up the dose gradually ("start low, go slow"). L-T4 therapy may increase myocardial oxygen requirements by enhancing myocardial contractility and heart rate. Theoretically, however, L-T4 therapy would also simultaneously decrease systemic vascular resistance and end-diastolic volume, both of which would tend to decrease myocardial oxygen consumption *(80)*. Indeed, the rate of development of angina was <5% in a large retrospective study of older hypothyroid individuals *(81)*. In the same study, 16% of patents with preexisting angina had a worsening of symptoms with thyroid hormone, whereas 38% had improvement or disappearance of symptoms. This study was published in an era before β-blockers, calcium channel blockers, and TSH assays.

Nowadays, it is possible to treat virtually all hypothyroid patients with coexisting cardiac disease effectively. It is appropriate to initiate therapy with L-T4 doses of 12.5–25 µg/d, with titration by 25 µg increments every 6–8 wk until the serum TSH levels are within the normal range. Occasional patients cannot be fully replaced with thyroxine because of exacerbation of angina, despite maximal antianginal medical therapy. In such patients, coronary revascularization or angioplasty should be considered. In hypothyroid patients who are in emergent need of myocardial revascularization or angioplasty because of myocardial infarction or crescendo angina, it is probably safer to proceed with the procedure rather than attempt to replace them with L-T4, because the surgical mortality in untreated hypothyroidism is no higher than in euthyroid individuals *(82,83)* and because the myocardium may be further jeopardized while waiting for the patient to achieve a euthyroid state *(84)*. However, perioperative morbid events (e.g., ileus, hyponatremia) do occur more frequently in hypothyroid patients *(83)* than in euthyroid controls.

Myxedema Coma

Myxedema coma represents the ultimate degree of hypothyroidism and results in death in at least 50% of cases *(85)*. Often, patients are elderly and are either undiagnosed or have discontinued L-T4 therapy for a protracted period of time. The management of myxedema coma is beyond the scope of this chapter because the correction of abnormalities related to profound hypothyroidism (CO_2 retention, hyponatremia, ileus, sepsis, etc.) is at least as important as therapy with thyroid hormones. There is controversy about the best treatment of myxedema coma because of its rarity and the lack of controlled clinical trials. Most clinical reviews (e.g., *see* refs. *85* and *86*) recommend a 300- to 500-µg intravenous bolus of L-T4, which will raise the serum concentration of T_4 to normal levels (based on a T_4 volume of distribution of 0.1 L/kg body wt, 500 µg will raise the serum T_4 concentration by about 7 µg/dL). Patients appear to have few adverse cardiovascular effects, despite receiving what seem to be very large L-T4 doses *(87)*. Because patients are critically ill, conversion of T_4 to T_3 in peripheral tissues will be diminished. Some feel that this is a beneficial protective mechanism; others have advocated the use of T_3 in this situation to more quickly treat the underlying hypothyroidism *(88,89)*. A recent retrospective analysis, however, showed that mortality was higher in patients over age 55 yr receiving daily L-T4 doses greater than 500 µg or daily T_3 doses above 75 µg *(90)*.

In the absence of a consensus, it is reasonable to recommend initial therapy with a bolus of intravenous L-T4, followed by daily intravenous L-T4 in doses of 75–125 µg/d. The intravenous route is preferred because of uncertain L-T4 absorption in any severe illness; the intravenous dose should be 20% lower than the oral dose, as oral L-T4 is only 60–80% absorbed. If a clinical response fails to occur after a few days, intravenous T_3 can be added in doses of 5 µg every 6 h or 10 µg every 8 h. Oral L-T4 can be resumed when gastrointestinal function has returned to normal. As noted earlier, scrupulous attention to the host of attendant medical problems is of vital importance, and most authorities recommend the use of stress doses of glucocorticoids.

Thyroxine "Allergy"

Occasional patients develop anxiety, palpitations, sweating, and other symptoms suggestive of hyperthyroidism on doses of L-T4 that do not produce biochemical hyperthyroidism. Typically, these complaints develop early in the course of treatment. The best way of dealing with these symptoms is to decrease the L-T4 dose and to progress with smaller and slower dose increments. A recent article suggested that patients poorly tolerant of thyroxine may be iron deficient, and that iron replacement therapy enabled patients to receive thyroxine therapy without any problems *(91)*. True allergy to L-T4 has been documented in one case report *(92)*, but numerous instances of urticaria or rash, possibly related to tartrazine or other dyes, have been reported *(93)*. The 50 µg tablets do not contain any dye and could be substituted if dye allergy is suspected. Lactose is present in thyroxine and many other drugs as a diluent. It is unlikely that the small amount of lactose present in a single tablet would cause problems even in lactose-sensitive individuals.

Treatment of Secondary Hypothyroidism

The treatment of secondary hypothyroidism is less straightforward than that of primary disease. First, the presence of coexistent secondary adrenal insufficiency must be considered and if present, glucocorticoid therapy should be initiated first. In addition, serum TSH levels cannot be used as a benchmark for the adequacy of therapy; it is reasonable to strive to keep the fT4 or FTI in the upper half of the normal range and to monitor the patient's clinical response. The replacement dose of L-T4 in central hypothyroidism will be roughly the same as would be calculated in a patient with primary hypothyroidism *(94)*.

REFERENCES

1. Vanderpump MPJ, Tunbridge WMG, French JM, et al. The incidence of thyroid disorders in the community: a twenty-year follow-up of the Whickham Survey. Clin Endocrinol (Oxf) 1995;43:55–68.
2. Wiersinga WM. Subclinical hypothyroidism and hyperthyroidism. I. Prevalence and clinical relevance. Neth J of Med 1994;6:197–204.
3. Cooper DS. Subclinical hypothyroidism. N Engl J Med 2001;345:260–265.
4. Canaris GJ, Manowitz NR, Mayor GM, Ridgway EC. The Colorado thyroid disease prevalence study. Arch Intern Med 2000;160:526–534.
5. Faglia G, Bitensky L, Pinchera A, Ferrari C, Parachi A, Beck-Peccoz P, et al. Thyrotropin secretion in patients with central hypothyroidism: evidence for reduced biological activity of immunoreactive thyrotropin. J Clin Endocrinol Metab 1979;48:989–998.
6. Beck-Peccoz R, Amir S, Menezes-Ferreira MM, Faglia G, Weintraub BD. Thyrotropin secretion in patients with central hypothyroidism: evidence for reduced biological activity of immunoreactive thyrotropin. J Clin Endocrinol Metab 1985;312:1085–1090.
7. Mandel SJ, Brent GA, Larsen PR. Levothyroxine therapy in patients with thyroid disease. Ann Intern Med 1993;119:492–502.
8. Roti E, Minelli R, Gardini E, Braverman LE. The use of misuse of thyroid hormone. Endocrine Rev 1993;14:401–423.
9. Toft AD. Thyroxine therapy. N Engl J Med 1994;331:174–180.
10. USP Dispensing Information: Volume 1—Drug Information for Health Care Professionals. Micromedex Thompson Healthcare Englewood, CO, 2001.
11. Kaufman SC, Gross GP, Kennedy DL. Thyroid hormone use: trends in the United States from 1960 through 1988. Thyroid 1991;1:285–291.
12. Sawin CT, Geller A, Hershman JM, Castelli W, Bacharach P. The aging thyroid: the use of thyroid hormone in older persons. JAMA 1989;261:2653–2655.
13. Fish LH, Schwartz HL, Cavanaugh J, Steffes MW, Bantle JP. Replacement dose, metabolism, and bioavailability of levothyroxine in the treatment of hypothyroidism. Role of triiodothyronine in pituitary feedback in humans. N Engl J Med 1987;316:764–70.
14. Choe W, Hays MT. Absorption of oral thyroxine. The Endocrinologist 1993;5:222–228.
15. Hays MT, Nielsen KRK. Human thyroxine absorption: age effects and methodological analyses. Thyroid 1994;4:55–64.
16. Wenzel KW, Kirscheiper HE. Aspects of the absorption of oral l-thyroxine in normal man. Metabolism 1977;26:1–8.
17. Benvenga S, Bartolone L, Squadrito S, Lo Giudice F, Trimarchi F. Delayed intestinal absorption of levothyroxine. Thyroid 1995;5:249–53.

18. Read DG, Hays MT, Hershman JM. Absorption of oral thyroxine in hypothyroid and normal man. J Clin Endocrinol Metab 1970;30:798,799.
19. Azizi F, Belur R, Albano J. Malabsorption of thyroid hormones after jejunoileal bypass for obesity. Ann Intern Med 1979;90:941,942.
20. Bevan JS, Munro JF. Thyroxine malabsorption following intestinal bypass surgery. Int J Obes 1986;10:245,246.
21. Stone E, Leiter LA, Lambert JR, Silverberg JDH, Jeeyeebhoy KN, Burrow GN. L-Thyroxine absorption in patients with short bowel. J Clin Endocrinol Metab 1984;59:139–141.
22. Ain KB, Refetoff S, Fein HG, Weintraub BD. Pseudomalabsorption of levothyroxine. JAMA 1991;266:2118–2120.
23. Northcutt RC, Stiel JN, Hollifiels JW, Stant EG. The influence of cholestyramine on thyroxine absorption. JAMA 1969;208:1857–1861.
24. Harmon SM, Siefert CF. Levothyroxine-cholestyramine interaction reemphasized. Ann Intern Med 1991;115:658,659.
25. Sperber AD, Liel Y. Evidence for interface with the intestinal absorption of levothyroxine sodium by aluminum hydroxide. Arch Intern Med 1992;152:183,184.
26. Campbell NR, Hasinoff BB, Stalts H, Rao B, Wong NC. Ferrous sulfate reduces thyroxine efficacy in patients with hypothyroidism. Ann Intern Med 1992;117:1010–1013.
27. Sherman SI, Tielens E, Ladenson PW Sucralfate causes malabsorption of L-thyroxine. Am J Med 1994;96:531–535.
28. Singh N, Singh PN, Hershman JM. Effect of calcium carbonate on the absorption of levothyroxine. JAMA 2000;283:2822–2825.
29. Liel Y, Harman-Boehm I, Shany S. Evidence for a clinically important adverse effect of fiber-enriched diet on the bioavailability of levothyroxine in adult hypothyroid patients. J Clin Endocrinol Metab 1996;80:857–859.
30. Browning MC, Bennet WM, Kirkaldy AJ, Jung RT. Intra-individual variation of thyroxine, triiodothyronine, and thyrotropin in treated hypothyroid patients: implications for monitoring replacement therapy. Clin Chem 1998;34:696–699.
31. Ain KB, Pucino F, Shiver TM, Banks SM. Thyroid hormone levels affected by time of blood sampling in thyroxine-treated patients. Thyroid 1993;3:81–85.
32. Faber J, Lumholtz IB, Kirkegaard C, Poulsen S, Jorgensen PH, Siersback-Nielsen K, et al. The effects of phenytoin (diphenylhydantoin) on the extrathyroidal turnover of thyroxine, 3,5,3'-triiodothyronine, 3,3',5'-triiodothyronine, and 3'5'-diiodothyronine in man. J Clin Endocrinol Metab 1985;61:1093–1099.
33. DeLuca F, Arrigo T, Pandullo E, Siracusano MF, Benvenga S. Changes in thyroid function tests induced by 2 month carbamazepine treatment in L-thyroxine-substituted hypothyroid children. Eur J Pediatr 1986;145:77–79.
34. Isley WL. Effect of rifampin therapy on thyroid function tests in a hypothyroid patient on replacement L-thyroxine. Ann Intern Med 1987;107:517,518.
35. McCowen KC, Garber JR, Spark R. Elevated serum thyrotropin in thyroxine-treated patients with hypothyroidism given sertraline. N Engl J Med 1997;337:1010,1011.
36. Figge J, Dluhy RG. Amiodarone-induced elevation of thyroid stimulating hormone in patients receiving levothyroxine for primary hypothyroidism. Ann Intern Med 1990;113:553–555.
37. Arafah BM. Increased need for thyroxine in women with hypothyroidism during estrogen therapy. N Engl J Med 2001;344:1743–1749.
38. Arafah BM. Decreased levothyroxine requirement in women with hypothyroidism during androgen therapy for breast cancer. Ann Intern Med 1994;121:247–251.
39. Rosenbaum RL, Barzel US. Levothyroxine replacement dose for primary hypothyroidism decreases with age. Ann Intern Med 1982;96:53–55.
40. Sawin CT, Herman T, Molitch ME, London MH, Kramer SM. Aging and the thyroid. Decreased requirement for thyroid hormone in older hypothyroid patients. Am J Med 1983;75:206–209.
41. Fisher DA. Management of congenital hypothyroidism. J Clin Endocrinol Metab 1991;72:523–529.
42. Bearcoft CP, Toms GC, Williams SJ, Noonan K, Monson JP. Thyroxine replacement in post-radioiodine hypothyroidism. Clin Endocrinol (Oxf) 1991;34:115–118.
43. Ridgway EC, McCammon JA, Benotti J, Maloof F. Acute metabolic responses in myxedema to large doses of intravenous L-thyroxine. Ann Intern Med 1972;77:549–555.
44. Helfand M, Crapo LM. Monitoring therapy in patients taking levothyroxine. Ann Intern Med 1990;113:450–454.

45. Stefan K, Grebe G, Cooke RR, Ford HC, Fagerstrom JN, Cordwell DP, et al. Treatment of hypothyroidism with once weekly thyroxine. J Clin Endocrinol Metab 1997;82:870–875.

46. Paul TL, Kerrigan J, Kelly AM, Braverman LE, Baran DT. Long-term L-thyroxine therapy is associated with decreased hip bone density in premenopausal women. JAMA 1988;259:3137–3141.

47. Stall GM, Harris S, Sokoll LJ, Dawson-Hughes B. Accelerated bone loss in hypothyroid patients overtreated with contemporary preparations. Ann Intern Med 1990;105:11–15.

48. Greenspan SL, Greenspan FS, Resnick NM, Block JE, Friedlander AL, Genant HK. Skeletal integrity in premenopausal and postmenopausal women receiving long-term L-thyroxine therapy. Am J Med 1991;91:5–14.

49. Franklyn JA, Betteridge J, Daykin J, Holder R, Oates GD, Parle JV, et al. Long-term thyroxine treatment and bone mineral density. Lancet 1992;340:9–13.

50. Faber J, Galloe AM. Changes in bone mass during prolonged subclinical hyperthyroidism due to L-thyroxine treatment: a meta-analysis. Eur J Endocrinol 1994;130:350–356.

51. Uzzan B, Campos J, Cucherat M, Nony P, Boissel JP, Perret GY. Effects on bone mass of long-term treatment with thyroid hormones: a meta-analysis. J Clin Endocrinol Metab 1996;81:4278–4289.

52. Bauer DC, Ettinger B, Nevitt MC, Stone KL for the Study of Osteoporotic Fractures Research Group. Risk for fracture in women with low serum levels of thyroid-stimulating hormone. Ann Intern Med. 2001;134:561–568.

53. Schneider DL, Barrett-Connor EL, Morton DJ. Thyroid hormone use and bone mineral density in eldery women. JAMA 1994;271:1245–1249.

54. Sawin CT, Geller A, Wolk PA, et al. Low serum thyrotropin concentration as a risk factor for atrial fibrillation in older persons. N Engl J Med 1994;331:1249–1252.

55. Carr D, McLeod DT, Parry G, Thornes HM. Fine adjustment of thyroxine replacement dosage: comparison of the thyrotrophin releasing hormone test using a sensitive thyrotropin assay with measurement of free thyroid hormones and clinical assessment. Clin Endocrinol (Oxf). 1988;28:325–333.

56. Bunevicius R, Kazanavicius G, Zalinkevicius R, Prange AJ Jr.. Effects of thyroxine as compared with thyroxine plus triiodothyronine in patients with hypothyroidism. N Engl J Med 1999;340:424–429.

57. Pollock MA, Sturrock A, Marshall K, et al. Thyroxine treatment in patients with symptoms of hypothyroidism but thyroid tests within the reference range: randomised double blind placebo controlled crossover trial. BMJ 2001;323:891–895.

58. Oppenheimer JH, Braverman LE, Toft A, Jackson, IM, Ladenson, PW. Thyroid hormone treatment: when and what? J Clin Endocrinol Metab 1995;80:2873–2883.

59. Dong BJ, Brown CH. Hypothyroidism resulting from generic levothyroxine failure. J Am Board Fam Pract 1991;4:167–170.

60. Peran S, Garriga MJ, Morreale de Escobar G, Asuncion M, Peran M. Increase in plasma thyrotropin levels in hypothyroid patients during treatment due to a defect in the commercial preparation. J Clin Endocrinol Metab 1997;82:3192–3195.

61. Escalante DA, Arem N, Arem R. Assessment of interchangeability of two brands of levothyroxine preparations with a third generation TSH assay. Am J Med 1995;98:374–378.

62. Dong BJ, Hauck WW, Gambertoglio JG, Gee L, White JR, Bubp JF, et al. Bioequivalence of generic and brand-name levothyroxine products in the treatment of hypothyroidism. JAMA 1997;277:1205–1213.

63. Berg JA, Mayor GH. A study in normal human volunteers to compare the rate and extent of levothyroxine absorption from Synthroid and Levoxine. J Clin Pharmacol 1992;32:1135–1140.

64. Singer PA, Cooper DS, Levy EG, Ladenson PW, Braverman LE, Daniels G, et al. Treatment guidelines for patients with hyperthyroidism and hypothyroidism. JAMA 1995;273:808–812.

65. Cooper DS. Subclinical hypothyroidism: a clinician's perspective. Ann Int Med 1998;129:135–138.

66. McDermott MT, Ridgway EC. Subclinical hypothyroidism is mild thyroid failure and should be treated. J Clin Endocrinol Metab 2001;86:4585–4590.

67. Chu JW, Crapo LM. Treatment of sublinical hypothyroidism is seldom necessary. J Clin Endocrinol Metab 2001;86:4591–4599.

68. Cooper DS, Halpern R, Wood LC, Levin AA, Ridgway EC. Thyroxine therapy in subclinical hypothyroidism. A double-blind, placebo-controlled trial. Ann Intern Med. 1984;101:18–24.

69. Nystrom E, Caidahl K, Fager G, Wikkelso C, Lundberg PA, Lindstedt G. A double-blind cross-over 12 month study of L-thyroxine treatment of women with 'subclinical' hypothyroidism. Clin Endocrinol (Oxf) 1988;29:63–75.

70. Meier C, Staub J-J, Roth C-B, et al. TSH-controlled L-thyroxine therapy reduces cholesterol levels and clinical symptoms in subclinical hypothyroidism: a double-blind, placebo-controlled trial (Basel Thyroid Study). J Clin Endocrinol Metab 2001;86:4860–4866.

71. Danese MD, Ladenson PW, Meinert CL, Powe NR. Effect of thyroxine on serum lipoproteins in patients with mild thyroid failure: a quantitative review of the literature. J Clin Endocrinol Metab 2000;85:2993–3001.

72. Vanderpump MP, Tunbridge WM, French JM, et al. The incidence of thyroid disorders in the community: a 20 year follow-up of the Whickham survey. Clin Endocrinol (Oxf) 1995;43:55–68.

73. Rosenthal MJ, Hunt WC, Garry PJ, Goodwin JS. Thyroid failure in the elderly. Microsomal antibodies as discriminant for therapy. JAMA 1987;258:209–213.

74. Kabadi UM. Optimal daily levothyroxine dose in primary hypothyroidism. Its relation to pretreatment thyroid hormone indexes. Arch Intern Med 1990;149:2209–2212.

75. Mandel SJ, Larsen PR, Seely EW, Brent GA. Increased need for thyroxine during pregnancy in women with primary hypothyroidism. N Engl J Med 1990;323:91–96.

76. Kaplan MM. Monitoring thyroxine treatment during pregnancy. Thyroid 1992;2:147–152.

77. Singer PA. Thyroiditis acute, subacute, and chronic. Med Clin North Am 1991;75:61–77.

78. Takasu N, Yamada T, Takasu M, Komiya I, Nagasawa Y, Asawa T, et al. Disappearance of thyrotropin-blocking antibodies and spontaneous recovery from hypothyroidism in autoimmune thyroiditis. N Engl J Med 1992;326:513–518.

79. Comtois R, Faucher L, Lafleche. Outcome of hypothyroidism caused by Hashimoto's thyroiditis. Arch Intern Med 1995;155:1404–1408.

80. Klein I, Ojamaa K. Thyroid hormone and the heart. Am J Med 1996;101:459,460.

81. Keating FR, Parkin TW, Selby JB, Dickinson LS. Treatment of heart disease associated with myxedema. Prog Cardiovasc Dis 1960;3:364–381.

82. Weinberg AD, Brennan MD, Gorman CA, Marsh HM, O'Fallon WM. Outcome of anesthesia and surgery in hypothyroid patients. Arch Intern Med 1983;143:893–897.

83. Ladenson PW, Levin AA, Ridgway EC, Daniels GH. Complications of surgery in hypothyroid patients. Am J Med 1984;77:261–266.

84. Hay ID, Duick DS, Vliestra RE, Maloney JD, Pluth JR. Thyroxine therapy in hypothyroid patients undergoing coronary revascularization: a retrospective analysis. Ann Intern Med 1981;95:456–457.

85. Pittman CS, Zayed AA. Myxedema coma. Curr Ther Endocrinol Metab 1997;6:98–101.

86. Ringel MD. Management of hypothyroidism and hyperthyroidism in the intensive care unit. Crit Care Clin 2001;17:59–74.

87. Kaptein EM, Quion-Verde H, Swinney RS, Egodage PM, Massry SG. Acute hemodynamic effects of levothyroxine loading in critically ill hypothyroid patients. Arch Intern Med 1986;146:662–666.

88. Pareira VG, Haron ES, Lima-Neto N, Medeiros-Neto GA. Management of myxedema coma: report on three successfully treated cases with nasogastric or intravenous administration of triiodothyronine. J Endocrinol Invest 1982;5:331–334.

89. Chernow B, Burman KD, Johnson DL, McGuire RA, O'Brian T, Wartofsky L, et al. T3 may be a better agent than T4 in the critically ill hypothyroid patient: evaluation of transport across the blood-brain barrier in a primate model. Crit Care Med 1983;2:99–104.

90. Yamamoto T, Fukuyama J, Fujiyoshi A. Factors associated with mortality of myxedema coma: report of eight cases and literature survey. Thyroid 1999;9:1167–1174.

91. Shakir KM, Turton D, Aprill BS, Drake AJ III, Eisold JF. Anemia: a cause of intolerance to thyroxine sodium. Mayo Clin Proc 2000;75:189–192.

92. Shibata H, Hayakawa H, Hirukawa M, Tadokoro K, Ogata E. Hypersensitivity caused by synthetic thyroid hormones in a hypothyroid patient with Hashimoto's thyroiditis. Arch Intern Med 1986;146:1624,1625.

93. Magner J, Gerber P. Urticaria due to blue dye in Synthroid tablets. Thyroid 1994;4:341.

94. Banovac K, Carrington SAB, Levis S, Fill MD, Bilsker MS. Determination of replacement and suppressive doses of thyroxine. J Intern Med Res 1990;18:210–218.

8

Thyroid Hormone Therapy of Congenital and Acquired Hypothyroidism in Children

Stephen LaFranchi, MD

CONTENTS

INTRODUCTION: EPIDEMIOLOGIES, ETIOLOGIES, AND DIAGNOSIS OF PRIMARY AND SECONDARY HYPOTHYROIDISM IN INFANTS AND CHILDREN

Congenital Hypothyroidism

Congenital hypothyroidism occurs in approx 1/3000 to 1/4000 newborn infants *(1)*. There is some racial and ethnic variation in incidence. Congenital hypothyroidism is more common in the white population, 1/4000, as compared to the black population, 1/32,000, and it occurs most commonly in the Hispanic population, 1/2000*(2)*. The majority of cases, approx 85%, are sporadic, whereas 15% are hereditary. The most common etiology is some form of thyroid dysgenesis: aplasia, hypoplasia, or an ectopic gland. Thyroid ectopia accounts for approximately two-thirds of dysgenesis, and so worldwide (in areas of iodine sufficiency), it is the most common etiology of congenital hypothyroidism. There is an approx 2/1 female preponderance for ectopia, although the ratio is more even for aplasia *(3)*. A small percent of cases, 3% or so, have been shown to result from mutations in transcription factors that play a role in thyroid gland morphogenesis and differentiation, such as PAX-8, TTF-1, and TTF-2 *(4–6)*. Rare cases are the result of "loss of function" mutations of thyroid-stimulating hormone (TSH) *(7,8)* or the

From: *Endocrine Replacement Therapy in Clinical Practice*
Edited by: A. Wayne Meikle © Humana Press Inc., Totowa, NJ

TSH receptor *(9,10)*. However, in the majority of cases, the underlying cause of thyroid dysgenesis remains unknown. Hereditary causes of congenital hypothyroidism include one of the inborn errors of thyroid hormone synthesis or secretion, including defects in iodine trapping, oxidation and organification, coupling, abnormal thyroglobulin, defective proteolysis and secretion, and a deiodinase defect. Specific genes and mutations have now been identified for each of these autosomal recessive disorders *(11)*. Familial cases may be the result of maternal antibody-mediated congenital hypothyroidism *(12,13)*. This condition, occurring in approx 1/100,000 newborns, is a transient disorder that resolves as the infant metabolizes the maternal thyrotropin receptor blocking antibody (TRB-Ab) *(14,15)*. In areas of iodine deficiency, endemic goiter remains the most common cause of congenital hypothyroidism. Exposure of infants, especially preterm infants, to iodine, as in topical antiseptics, may lead to iodine excess and transient hypothyroidism *(16)*.

The vast majority of infants with congenital hypothyroidism are now detected through newborn screening programs. Screening for congenital hypothyroidism was developed in the mid-1970s *(17)*, and is now routine in all 50 states, Canada, and most developed countries in the world. Thyroid screening tests use heel-prick blood spotted on a filter paper card, obtained between 2 and 5 d of age. In North America, most programs initially measure a serum T_4 concentration; serum TSH is measured in infants with T_4 below a set cutoff, usually the 10th percentile. Physicians of infants with a low filter paper T_4 and an elevated TSH concentration are notified. The infant is immediately recalled, and a serum sample is obtained to confirm the diagnosis, showing a subnormal T_4 (or free T_4) and elevated TSH. One should keep in mind that the normal ranges for thyroid function tests are different for infants compared to children and adults. Results should be compared to age-specific normal ranges *(18)*. From 1 to 2 wk of age, the normal range for T_4 is 8–16 µg/dL, for free T_4 it is 1.6–3.8 ng/dL, and for TSH it is 1.7–9.1 mU/L. Imaging studies may be undertaken to try and determine the underlying cause *(19)*. Thyroid ultrasound is the least invasive, but it may not always identify ectopic glands *(20)*. Thyroid scintigraphy, using either technetium pertechnetate 99m or iodine-123, is more accurate but involves small amounts of radioactivity. Most consider imaging studies optional, as they generally do not change management. In infants born to mothers with known autoimmune thyroid disease, it is worthwhile measuring TRB-Ab in mother and infant, as infants positive for this maternal antibody will have a transient form of congenital hypothyroidism *(15)*.

Congenital hypopituitary hypothyroidism is less common, occurring in 1/50,000 to 1/100,000 newborns. Congenital TSH deficiency usually occurs with other pituitary hormone deficiencies (e.g., growth hormone deficiency). It is also associated with other congenital syndromes, particularly midline defects, such as septo-optic dysplasia or mid-line cleft lip and palate defects, and may follow birth trauma or asphyxia. A few screening programs follow up infants with persistently low screening T_4 concentrations and so detect infants with congenital TSH deficiency *(21)*. Infants may also be discovered because of symptoms or signs of other pituitary hormone deficiencies. Serum thyroid function tests typically show a low free T_4 and either "normal" or subnormal TSH concentration. A low T_4 combined with a normal TSH is not adequate to make this diagnosis, as these findings may be explained by low serum thyroxine-binding globulin (TBG) or other binding proteins. Infants with congenital TSH deficiency should undergo clinical and biochemical evaluation for other pituitary hormone deficiencies. They should also undergo a careful eye exam and magnetic resonance imaging (MRI) of the brain to search for midline defects, such as absence of the septum pellucidum or corpus callosum.

Acquired Hypothyroidism

Acquired hypothyroidism occurs in approx 1/500 school children *(22)*. There is a female preponderance, with a peak in the adolescent age range. The most common cause of acquired hypothyroidism in children is chronic lymphocytic thyroiditis (Hashimoto's thyroiditis). Approximately 2.4% of school-age girls and 1.2% of boys have antithyroid antibodies *(23)*. Autoimmune thyroid disease (AITD) is associated with certain chromosomal disorders, including trisomy 21 *(24,25)*, Turner *(26,27)*, and Klinefelter syndromes *(28)*. It may also occur as part of an autoimmune polyglandular syndrome *(29)*. Other, less common causes of acquired hypothyroidism include excess iodine ingestion, which may be contained in expectorants or kelp-derived "health supplements," iodine deficiency in parts of the world where this is endemic, after radiation, as for tumors of the head and neck *(30,31)*, and after radioiodine treatment or thyroidectomy, as for Graves' disease or thyroid carcinoma *(32)*. It may also occur with diseases that infiltrate the thyroid gland, such as Langerhan cell histiocytosis and cystinosis. A recently recognized cause is seen in infants and children with large hepatic hemangiomas, which contain high levels of type 3 deiodinase, so converting T_4 to reverse T_3 and T_3 to T_2 *(33)*. Serum thyroid function tests show a low free T_4 or T_4 and elevated TSH concentration. Children with a normal free T_4 or T_4 in the face of an elevated TSH concentration have subclinical hypothyroidism. Again, one must keep in mind that the normal range for thyroid function tests is somewhat different from adults, and results must be compared to age-related norms *(18)*. Between 1 and 10 yr, the serum T_4 range is approx 6.4–14.2 µg/dL, the free T_4 is 0.8–2.1 ng/dL, and TSH is 0.7–6.4 mU/L. The most useful test to search for an underlying etiology is measurement of antithyroid antibodies. Antithyroid peroxidase and antithyroglobulin are positive in approx 85% of children with AITD. Imaging studies are generally not indicated. If hypothyroidism is associated with a goiter, ultrasound examination is more accurate than physical examination in determining size and consistency *(34)*. With AITD, ultrasonography will show variable areas of hypoechogenicity, whereas scintigraphy will show variable or "patchy" uptake of the radionuclide.

Acquired hypopituitary hypothyroidism is relatively rare. It is most commonly caused by hypothalamic–pituitary tumors (craniopharyngioma most common) or the treatment used for these tumors, including surgery or radiation therapy. Less commonly, it may occur after meningoencephalitis or serious head trauma. Serum thyroid function tests show a low free T_4 and either "normal" or subnormal TSH concentration.

THYROID HORMONE PREPARATIONS

Thyroid hormone preparations available for treatment include thyroxine (levothyroxine sodium) (L-T4), tri-iodothyroinine (liothyronine) (L-T3), liotrix (a fixed combination of L-T4 and L-T3 in a 4:1 ratio), and desiccated thyroid hormone, obtained from animal thyroid glands and containing T_4 and T_3. L-T4 is the treatment of choice for congenital or acquired hypothyroidism in children. L-T3, with its short half-life, is generally limited to use in children undergoing thyroid hormone withdrawal in preparation for a radionuclide uptake and scan or a treatment dose. There is some discussion about whether L-T4 treatment normalizes tissue T_3 levels in all organs in hypothyroid individuals. There is some animal data to suggest that in thyroidectomized rats only the combination of T_4 and T_3 replacement, and not T_4 alone, results in euthyroidism in all tissues *(35)*. This may depend on which organs derive T_3 from the circulation vs locally produced T_3 by deiodination of T_4. Patients with hypothyroidism on L-T4 replacement with a normal free T_4 and TSH may still complain of features, which may potentially be explained by tissue hypothyroidism. One study in hypothyroid adults showed improvement in some measures of cognitive function and mood with the combination of T_4 and T_3 vs T_4 alone *(36)*. However, until more is known about combination replacement therapy, L-T4 remains the treatment of choice in children.

THYROXINE PHARMACOLOGY IN INFANTS AND CHILDREN

The T_4 production rate is higher in newborns and infants compared to children and adults. The estimated daily T_4 production rate on a weight basis is 10–15 µg/kg in the newborn, 7–9 µg/kg in the first year, 3-5 µg/kg at 1–3 yr, 2–3 µg/kg at 3–9 yr, and 1–2 µg/kg in adults *(37)*. Several factors appear to be responsible for the higher T_4 production rate: an increased iodide clearance rate (three times higher in infants than adults), higher thyroxine turnover, and a shorter thyroxine half-life (5 d in children, 6 d in adolescents, and 6.7 d in adults *[37]*). The thyroid gland by necessity is more active in infancy and childhood, and this may, in part, explain the somewhat higher serum T_4, free T_4, and TSH concentrations. These factors also appear to explain why the thyroxine replacement dose is higher on a weight basis in infancy and childhood.

Thyroxine is absorbed primarily from the small intestine. In adults, approx 60–80% of ingested thyroxine is absorbed *(38)*. Serum thyroxine concentrations in any particular patient will depend on the integrity of the intestinal system and simultaneous ingestion of agents that inhibit thyroxine absorption. Hypothyroid infants or children with short-bowel syndrome, disorders of malabsorption (e.g., celiac disease or pancreatic insufficiency) or inflammatory bowel disease (e.g., Crohn's disease or ulcerative colitis) will likely need higher thyroxine replacement doses. Agents known to bind thyroxine and inhibit absorption include iron, soy protein *(39)*, and calcium. Thus, if hypothyroid infants are receiving multivitamins with iron, L-T4 and the multivitamins should be given 3 h apart. If infants need to be on a soy formula, the L-T4 tablet should be crushed and mixed with water and given halfway between feeds. For a more complete list of conditions that may affect L-T4 requirements, including drugs that block T_4 to T_3 conversion, and drugs that accelerate L-T4 turnover, see Table 1 in Chapter 7.

REPLACEMENT THERAPY IN CONGENITAL HYPOTHYROIDISM

The goals of treatment in infants with congenital hypothyroidism are to assure normal growth and development, with psychometric outcome similar to genetic potential. The fetal hypothalamic–pituitary–thyroid axis begins to produce significant amounts of thyroid hormone by mid-gestation. Fetal thyroid hormone plays a significant role in fetal neurodevelopment. In the hypothyroid fetus, transfer of maternal thyroid hormone may ameliorate some of the deleterious effects of hypothyroidism on the developing brain. Studies show that approximately one-third of maternal thyroxine crosses to the fetus at term *(40)*. This maternal contribution is metabolized and disappears in the first few weeks after delivery. Studies of psychometric outcome show that the longer it takes to correct the hypothyroxinemia after birth, the greater risk to subsequent neurodevelopment. In general, the results of newborn screening tests are available by 1–3 wk after delivery. Treatment should be started as soon as the confirmatory serum sample is obtained, pending results. It is important to choose an initial starting dose that will normalize serum T_4 or free T_4 as rapidly as possible as the maternal thyroxine disappears.

Initial L-T4 Starting Doses

Studies in newborn animals show that the majority of brain T_3 is derived from local intracellular deiodination of circulating T_4. For this reason, L-T4 is the treatment of choice. An initial starting dose of 10–15 µg/kg/d will raise the T_4 or free T_4 into the normal range by 3–7 d of treatment (41,42). Because L-T4 comes as 25- or 50-µg tablets, this usually means 37.5–50 µg daily for term infants. The higher starting dose should be used in infants with more severe hypothyroidism, as judged by lower serum T_4 concentrations (43). For example, a 3.5-kg infant with a serum T_4 <5 µg/dL should be started on 50 µg daily (14.3 µg/kg/d). Only L-T4 tablets should be used. Currently, there are no approved liquid preparations in the United States, and thyroid suspensions prepared by individual pharmacists may result in unreliable dosing. The L-T4 tablet should be crushed and mixed with a small volume (a few cubic centimeters) of breast milk or water and fed to the infant with a spoon or plastic syringe. As described in the previous section, tablets should not be mixed with soy protein or any preparation containing iron as these will bind the thyroxine and inhibit absorption.

Treatment Objectives

The objectives of treatment are to raise the serum T_4 or free T_4 as rapidly as possible into the upper part of the normal range while normalizing serum TSH concentrations. Again, one must bear in mind that the serum T_4 or free T_4 concentration is higher for infants and children. The serum T_4 or free T_4 should become normal within 1–2 wk, whereas the TSH will usually normalize after 1 mo of treatment. Using the above L-T4 starting doses, in the first few weeks after treatment the serum T_4 and free T_4 may be elevated above the normal range, whereas the serum TSH remains normal or even somewhat elevated. After the first few weeks of treatment and normalization of the serum T_4 or free T_4, the L-T4 dose should be adjusted to assure biochemical and clinical euthyroidism. The L-T4 dose gradually decreases on a weight basis; see Table 1. In the first year of life, the T_4 target range is 10–16 µg/dL, whereas the free T_4 target is approx 1.4–2.3 ng/dL. Infants who have serum T_4 concentrations <10 µg/dL in the first year of life will have lower IQs compared to infants with serum T_4 maintained >10 µg/dL (44,45). At the same time, overtreatment for prolonged periods of time should be avoided. Persistently high serum T_4 concentrations may accelerate brain development and cause it to finish prematurely (46), and it may result in disorders of temperament and attention span 47,48) and premature craniosynostosis. In this context, studies using starting L-T4 doses of 10–15 µg/kg/d did not show any harmful effects on linear growth or skeletal maturation (49).

Although the serum TSH normalizes in a few weeks to months in most infants, some may have a high TSH concentration (10–20 mU/L) despite serum T_4 or free T_4 concentrations in the upper part of the normal range. This "thyroid hormone resistance" may be the result of fetal hypothyroidism leading to a resetting of the pituitary-thyroid feedback

Table 1
Recommended L-Thyroxine Treatment Doses
in Infants and Children

Age	Na L-Thyroxine ($\mu g/kg/d$)
Initial starting dose	10–15
1–6 mo	6–10
6–12 mo	5–8
1–3 yr	4–6
3–10 yr	3–4
>10 yr	1.75–3

axis. Studies show that some degree of this resistance may be seen in up to 40% of infants <1 yr, but it decreases to 10% in older children *(50)*.

Treatment of infants with congenital hypopituitary hypothyroidism follows the same principles as for infants with primary congenital hypothyroidism. The initial starting L-T4 dose can be judged based on the pretreatment serum T_4 or free T_4 concentration. Although these infants may be as hypothyroid as infants with primary hypothyroidism, often they do not have a complete deficiency of thyroid hormone and they are diagnosed after a month of age, so the starting L-T4 starting dose may be more in the range of 6–10 µg/kg/d. They should be monitored as carefully as infants with primary hypothyroidism *(see* the following subsection). Serum TSH measurements, however, will not be useful in judging L-T4 dosage. The treatment goal should be to keep the serum T_4 or free T_4 in the upper part of the normal range for age.

Monitoring

Clinical evaluation should be performed at the usual well-baby check-ups, but laboratory testing may be carried out at more frequent intervals to ensure optimal T_4 dosage. The American Academy of Pediatrics (AAP) recommends measurement of serum T_4 or free T_4 and TSH *(51)*:

- At 2 and 4 wk after the initiation of L-T4 treatment
- Every 1–2 mo in the first year of life
- Every 2–3 mo in between 1 and 3 yr of life
- Every 3–12 mo thereafter until growth and puberty are complete
- Two weeks after any change in dose (first 2 yr of life)
- At more frequent intervals when compliance is questioned or abnormal results are obtained

Assessment of Permanent vs Transient Hypothyroidism

Not all infants detected by newborn screening will have permanent hypothyroidism; studies show that approximately 10% will have transient hypothyroidism. Potential causes of transient hypothyroidism include maternal TRB-Ab transfer and exposure to high doses of iodine. In cases where maternal TRB-Ab is thought to be the cause of the hypothyroidism, it is prudent to treat infants until the antibody has been excreted, which usually occurs by 3–6 mo of age. After 6 mo of age, L-T4 treatment can be discontinued and thyroid function checked in 2 and 4 wk. If the T_4 or free T_4 and TSH concentrations remain normal, the infant can be monitored carefully off treatment. A similar strategy can be followed in infants whose hypothyroidism is thought to be the result of iodine exposure.

Permanent hypothyroidism may be confirmed by thyroid radionuclide scanning that shows an ectopic gland or absent thyroid tissue, confirmed by ultrasound examination, or studies that show one of the inborn errors of thyroid hormone synthesis or secretion. In addition, if the serum TSH concentration rises to >20 mU/L after the first 6 months of life because of insufficient L-T4 treatment, permanent hypothyroidism is confirmed. If permanent hypothyroidism is not established, L-T4 treatment can be discontinued after age 3 yr, an age when the brain no longer has a critical dependence on thyroid hormone. Measurement of serum T_4 or free T_4 and TSH after 30 d off L-T4 will separate permanent from transient hypothyroidism. If the T_4 or free T_4 are low and TSH is elevated, treatment is reinstituted. If thyroid function tests are normal, transient hypothyroidism is presumed. These children should still be examined periodically, and if they have any suspicious clinical features of hypothyroidism, such as slowing of growth, thyroid function tests should be performed. If the results are inconclusive, one may want to consider imaging studies if these have not been performed to look for a thyroid abnormality. Even if none is found, these children should undergo careful follow-up and subsequent retesting until the picture is clarified.

REPLACEMENT THERAPY IN ACQUIRED HYPOTHYROIDISM

The treatment of choice for acquired hypothyroidism in children is L-thyroxine (L-T4). For reasons described previously, the L-T4 dose is higher on a weight basis than in adults (see Table 1 for recommended dosing). The goals of treatment are to restore normal growth and development, including pubertal development in adolescent children. In most children, it is safe to start at full-replacement doses. One exception is children with significant growth retardation and delayed skeletal maturation owing to long-standing hypothyroidism. Such children may undergo rapid bone age advancement after L-T4 treatment is started, especially if they are adolescents and enter puberty. These children may not reach an adult height normal for their genetic potential (52). It is therefore recommended to start such children on a reduced dose and gradually increase to full replacement, although there are no studies to show that this improves adult height. Such a strategy must be balanced against leaving a child partially hypothyroid until full replacement is reached. Therefore, it is prudent to reach full replacement by 3–6 mo after diagnosis. Linear growth velocity and skeletal maturation should be monitored carefully, at roughly 4- to 6-mo intervals. If rapid bone age advancement occurs, resulting in decreased adult height potential, and the child is pubertal, treatment with gonadotropin-releasing hormone agonists to temporarily halt puberty and thus prolong the growing period may be considered.

Serum free T_4 (or T_4) and TSH should be monitored at appropriate intervals, approximately two to three times a year. The objectives of treatment are to keep the free T_4 (or T_4) in the upper half of the normal range for age and the TSH in the lower half of normal. The total L-T4 dose will gradually increase with age (although it will decrease on a weight basis). It is important to avoid overtreatment, as this may be associated with craniosynostosis in infants with open sutures, behavior problems in school-age children (53), and, potentially, decreased bone mineral density in adolescents (54).

Not all children with AITD will have permanent hypothyroidism. Studies show that approx 20% will recover to euthyroidism over several years (55,56). It is recommended that treatment be continued until growth and puberty are complete. L-T4 treatment can then be discontinued for a month, serum free T_4 or T_4 and TSH measured, so allowing separation of permanent from transient cases.

L-T4 treatment of children with acquired hypopituitary hypothyroidism is similar to children with primary hypothyroidism. Only measurement of serum free T_4 or T_4 is useful in monitoring treatment. The target free T_4 or T_4 range is the same as children with primary hypothyroidism (i.e., the upper half of the normal range for age).

OTHER TREATMENT CONSIDERATIONS

Prenatal Treatment of a Hypothyroid Fetus

Rarely, hypothyroidism may be suspected or diagnosed in a fetus prenatally. This may be the result of a maternal or fetal thyroid disturbance. Examples include inadvertent radioiodine treatment of a pregnant woman who has thyroid cancer or Graves' disease, antithyroid drug treatment of a pregnant woman, AITD with transplacental passage of TRB-Ab from mother to fetus, and recurrence of an inborn error of thyroxine synthesis or secretion with subsequent pregnancies. In some of these conditions, adjusting the mother's treatment can reduce the risk of fetal hypothyroidism (e.g., treating a woman with Graves' disease with the lowest dose of antithyroid drug that controls her hyperthyroidism). In others, such as low maternal TRB-Ab concentration or a less severe inborn error, the risk of injury from hypothyroidism to the developing fetal brain is judged to be minimal or reversible with correction of the hypothyroidism immediately after birth. However, in some cases (e.g., with maternal RAI exposure after a point that the fetal thyroid is capable of trapping iodine) a judgment may be made that the effects of the fetal hypothyroidism are likely to cause some irreversible injury to the fetal brain. In these rare cases, clinicians have elected to treat the fetus.

If L-T4 treatment is planned, it may be wise to monitor fetal thyroid function by cordocentsis. Case studies report successful treatment of fetal hypothyroidism by intra-amniotic injections of approx 500–1000 µg weekly until delivery (57). These dose calculations are based on the estimated concentration of amniotic fluid L-T4 and the amount of fluid swallowed daily by the fetus. These doses have been shown to normalize fetal serum T_4 and TSH concentrations.

Hypothyroxinemia in a Preterm Infant

The fetal hypothalamic–pituitary–thyroid axis begins to produce significant amounts of thyroid hormone from mid-gestation. Fetal serum T_4 and free T_4 concentrations gradually rise, and at term, they are similar to levels seen in children and adults (58). In infants born prematurely, the serum T_4 concentration is directly proportional to gestational age or birth weight (59). Infants who are born at 26–30 wk will have very low serum T_4 concentrations, in the range of 2–4 µg/dL. Over the first few weeks of life, these infants have serum T_4 concentrations that are lower than their in utero counterparts (60). There are several reasons for this, including loss of the maternal thyroxine contribution, immaturity at all levels of the hypothalamic–pituitary–thyroid axis, poor nutrition and low iodine intake, immature liver function with decreased TBG production, and other acute morbidities of prematurity that lead to the nonthyroidal illness syndrome. Preterm infants have many clinical features that might be ascribed to hypothyroidism, and they are at higher risk for adverse neurodevelopmental outcomes. In general, the serum TSH is not elevated. Some clinicians believe that this is just the normal "physiologic state" of the premie, whereas others have wondered whether these infants might have transient hypopituitary hypothyroidism.

For the above reasons, investigators have wondered whether some preterm infants might benefit from thyroid hormone replacement until they are term postnatally and their hypothalamic–pituitary–thyroid axis matures. Several studies have been carried out to examine the effects of L-T4 treatment. Although it is beyond the scope of this chapter to review all of the data, briefly, on balance, most studies do not show benefit of L-T4 treatment of preterm infants in reducing morbidity, mortality, or enhancing neuro-development. Van Wassenaer et al. treated 200 infants <32 wk gestation in a double-blind, placebo-controlled trial. Treated infants received L-T4, 8 µg/kg/d for the first 6 wk of life. Follow-up psychometric testing at 2 and 5 yr of age has now been published. As a group, the mean IQ in the L-T4-treated and placebo groups were not different. However, when the subgroup of infants <28 wk gestation were analyzed, there was a statistically significant 18-point higher IQ in the treated group, whereas in the subgroup 28–32 wk, the IQ was 12 points lower in the treated group (61). These findings persisted at the 5-yr follow-up (62). The investigators speculated that the very premature babies, <28 wk, may, in fact, not be physiologically normal and may benefit from treatment, whereas infants 28–32 wk are more mature, do not benefit from replacement, and may be harmed by too high a T_4 level.

It is the opinion of this clinician that L-T4 treatment of preterm infants should not be considered routine until further studies are conducted. If van Wassenaer's findings are confirmed, L-T4 treatment of infants born <28 wk may be warranted.

Subclinical Hypothyroidism

L-T4 treatment is recommended in children with subclinical hypothyroidism (normal free T_4 or T_4 and elevated serum TSH concentration). This recommendation is made because the "normal" free T_4 or T_4 may not be normal for that child, there may be subtle clinical features that benefit from treatment, and if there is progression to overt hypothyroidism, the child will go untreated until this is recognized. Once growth and pubertal development are completed, L-T4 treatment can be discontinued for a month and thyroid function testing carried out to determine whether treatment should be continued or not.

REFERENCES

1. Fisher DA. Second international conference on neonatal thyroid screening: progress report. J Pediatr 1983;102:653,654.
2. Penny R, Hoffman P, Barton L. Congenital hypothyroidism in Spanish-surnamed infants in Southern California: increased incidence and clustering of occurrence. Am J Dis Child 1989;143:640,641.
3. Devos H, Rodd C, Gagne N, et al. A search for the possible molecular mechanisms of thyroid dysgenesis: sex ratios and associated malformations. J Clin Endocrinol Metab 1999;84:2502–2506.
4. Macchia PE, Lapi P, Krude H, et al. PAX8 mutations associated with congenital hypothyroidism caused by thyroid dysgenesis. Nat Genet 1998;19:83–86.
5. Clifton-Bligh RJ, Wentworth JM, Heinz P, et al. Mutation of the gene encoding TTF-2 associated with thyroid agenesis, cleft palate and choanal atresia. Nat Genet 1998;19:399–401.
6. Vilain C, Rydlewski C, Duprez L, et al. Autosomal dominant transmission of congenital thyroid hypoplasia due to loss-of-function mutation of PAX-8. J Clin Endocrinol Metab 2001;86:234–238.

7. Collu R, Tang J, Castagné J, et al. A novel mechanism for isolated central hypothyroidism: inactivating mutations in the thyrotropin-releasing hormone receptor gene. J Clin Endocrinol Metab 1997;82:1561–1565.

8. Medeiros-Neto G, Herodotou DT, Rajan S, et al. A circulating, biologically inactive thyrotropin caused by a mutation in the beta subunit gene. J Clin Invest 1996;97:1250–1256.

9. Doeker BM, Pfaffle RW, Pohlenz J, Andler W. Congenital central hypothyroidism due to a homozygous mutation in the thyrotropin beta-subunit gene follows an autosomal recessive inheritance. J Clin Endocrinol Metab 1998;83:1762–765.

10. Sunthornthepvarakui T, Gottschalk ME, Hayashi Y, Refetoff S. Resistance to thyrotropin caused by mutations in the thyrotropin-receptor gene. N Engl J Med 1995;332:155–160.

11. Pohlenz J, Rosenthal IM, Weiss RE, et al. Congenital hypothyroidism due to mutations in the sodium/iodide symporter. Identification of a nonsense mutation producing a downstream cryptic 3' splice site. J Clin Invest 1998;101:1028–1035.

12. Iseki M, Shimizu M, Oikawa T, et al. Sequential serum measurements of thyrotropin binding inhibitor immunoglobulin G in transient familial neonatal hypothyroidism. J Clin Endocrinol Metab 1983;57:384–387.

13. Pacaud D, Huot C, Gattereau A, et al. Outcome in three siblings with antibody-mediated transient congenital hypothyroidism. J Pediatr 1995;127:275–277.

14. Zakarija M, McKenzie JM, Eidson MS. Transient neonatal hypothyroidism: characterization of maternal antibodies to the thyrotropin receptor. J Clin Endocrinol Metab 1990;70:1239–1246.

15. Brown RS, Bellisario RI, Botero D, et al. Incidence of transient congenital hypothyroidism due to maternal thyrotropin receptor-blocking antibodies in over one million babies. J Clin Endocrinol Metab 1996;81:1147–1151.

16. Cosman BC, Schullmger JN, Bell JJ, et al. Hypothyroidism caused by topical povidone-iodine in a newborn with omphalocele. J Pediatr Surg 1988;23:356–358.

17. Dussault JH, Coulombe P, Laberge C, et al. Preliminary report on a mass screening program for neonatal hypothyroidism. J Pediatr 1975;86:670–674.

18. Nelson JC, Clark SJ, Borut DL, et al. Age-related changes in serum free thyroxine during childhood and adolescence. J Pediatr 1993;123:899–905.

19. Muir A, Daneman D, Daneman A, et al. Thyroid scanning, ultrasound and serum thyroglobulin in determining the origin of congenital hypothyroidism. Am J Dis Child 1988;142:214–216.

20. Takashima S, Nomura N, Tanaka H, et al. Congenital hypothyroidism assessment with ultrasound. AJNR Am J Neuroradiol 1995;16:1117–1123.

21. Hanna CE, Krainz PL, Skeels MR, et al. Detection of congenital hypopituitary hypothyroidism: ten-year experience in the Northwest Regional Screening Program. J Pediatr 1986;109:959–964.

22. Rallison ML, Dobyns BM, Meikle AW, et al. Natural history of thyroid abnormalities: prevalence, incidence, and regression of thyroid diseases in adolescents and young adults. Am J Med 1991;91:363–370.

23. Rallison ML, Brown BM, Keating R, et al. Occurrence and natural history of chronic lymphocytic thyroiditis in childhood. J Pediatr 1975;86:675–682.

24. Pueschel SM, Pezzallo JC. Thyroid dysfunction in Down syndrome. Am J Dis Child 1985;139:636–639.

25. Rubello D, Pozzan GB, Casara D, et al. Natural course of subclinical hypothyroidism in Down's syndrome: prospective study results and therapeutic considerations. J Endocrinol Invest 1995;18:35–40.

26. Gruneiro de Papendieck L, Iorcansky S, Coco R. High incidence of thyroid disturbances in 49 children with Turner syndrome. J Pediatr 1987;111:258–261.

27. Chiovato L, Larizza D, Bendinelli G, et al. Autoimmune hypothyroidism and hyperthyroidism in patients with Turner's syndrome. Eur J Endocrinol 1996;134:568–575.

28. Kondo T. Klinefelter syndrome associated with juvenile hypothyroidism due to chronic thyroiditis. Eur J Pediatr 1993;152:540.

29. Neufeld M, MacLaren N, Blizzard R. Autoimmune polyglandular syndromes. Pediatr Ann 1980;9:154–162.

30. Samaan NA, Schultz PN, Yang KP, et al. Endocrine complications after radiotherapy for tumors of the head and neck. J Lab Clin Med 1987;109:364–372.

31. Ogilvy-Stuart AL, Shalet SM, Gattamaneni HR. Thyroid function after treatment of brain tumors in children. J Pediatr 1991;119:733–737.

32. Safa AM, Schumacher OP, Rodriguez-Autunez A. Long-term follow-up results in children and adolescents treated with radioactive iodine for hyperthyroidism. N Engl J Med 1975;292:167–171.

33. Huang SA, Tu HN, Harney JW, et al. Severe hypothyroidism caused by type 3 iodothyronine deiodinase in infantile hemangiomas. N Engl J Med 2000;343:185–189.

34. Gutekunst R, Hafermann W, Mansky T, Scriba PC. Ultrasonography related to clinical and laboratory findings in lymphocytic thyroiditis. Acta Endocrinol (Copenh) 1989;121:129–135.

35. Escobar-Morreale HF, del Rey FE, Obregon MJ, de Escobar GM. Only the combined treatment with thyroxine and triiodothyronine ensures euthyroidism in all tissues of the thyroidectomized rat. Endocrinology 1996;137:2490–2502.

36. Bunevisius R, Kazanavicius G, Zalinkevicius R, Prange AJ. Effects of thyroxine as compared with thyroxine plus triiodothyronine in patients with hypothyroidism. N Engl J Med 1999;340:424–429.

37. Fisher DA, Brown RS. Thyroid physiology in the perinatal period and during childhood. In: LE Braverman and RD Utiger, eds. Werner & Ingbar's The Thyroid: A Fundamental and Clinical Text, 8th ed., Lippincott Williams & Wilkins, Philadelphia, 2000, pp. 959–972.

38. Hays MT, Nielsen KR. Human thyroxine absorption: age effects and methodological analyses. Thyroid 1994;4:55–64.

39. Jabbar MA, Larrea J, Shaw RA. Abnormal thyroid function tests in infants with congenital hypothyroidism: the influence of soy-based bormula. J Am Coll Nutr 1997;16:280–282.

40. Vulsma, T, Gons, MH, de Vijlder, JJM. Maternal-fetal transfer of thyroxine in congenital hypothyroidism due to a total organification defect or thyroid agenesis. N Engl J Med 1989;321:13–16.

41. Germak JA, Foley TP, Jr. Longitudinal assessment of l-thyroxine therapy for congenital hypothyroidism. J Pediatr 1990;117:211–219.

42. Selva KA, Mandel S, Rien L, Nelson JC, LaFranchi SH. Replacement dose of l-thyroxine in congenital hypothyroidism. Pediatr Res 2001;49:10A.

43. Bongers-Schokking JJ, Koot HM, Wiersma D, et al. Influence of timing and dose of thyroid hormone replacement on development in infants with congenital hypothyroidism. J Pediatr 2000;136:292–297.

44. New England Congenital Hypothyroidism Collaborative. Characteristics of infantile hypothyroidism discovered on neonatal screening. J Pediatr 1984;104:539–544.

45. Heyerdahl S, Kase BF, Lie SO. Intellectual development in children with congenital hypothyroidism in relation to recommended thyroxine treatment. J Pediatr 1991;118:850–857.

46. Weichsel ME, Jr. Thyroid hormone replacement therapy in the perinatal period: neurologic considerations. J Pediatr 1978;92:1035–1038.

47. Rovet J, Ehrlich RM, Sorbara DL. Effect of thyroid hormone levels on temperament in infants with congenital hypothyroidism detected by screening of neonates. J Pediatr 1989;114:63–68.

48. Rovet J, Alvarez M. Thyroid hormone and attention in congenital hypothyroidism. J Pediatr Endocrinol Metab 1996;9:63–66.

49. Fisher DA, Foley BL, Early treatment of congenital hypothyroidism. Pediatrics 1989;83:785–789.

50. Fisher DA, Schoen EJ, LaFranchi S, et al. The hypothalamic-pituitary-thyroid negative feedback control axis in children with treated congenital hypothyroidism. J Clin Endocrinol Metab 2000;85:2722–2727.

51. American Academy of Pediatrics. Newborn screening for congenital hypothyroidism: Recommended guidelines. Pediatrics 1993;91:1203–1209.

52. Rivkees SA, Bode HH, Crawford JD. Long-term growth in juvenile acquired hypothyroidism: the failure to achieve normal adult stature. N Engl J Med 1988;318:599–602.

53. Rovet JF, Daneman D, Bailey JD. Psychological and psychoeducational consequences of thyroxine therapy for juvenile acquired hypothyroidism. J Pediatr 1993;122:543–549.

54. Saggese G, Bertellone S, Baroncelli GI, et al. Bone mineral density in adolescent females treated with l-thyroxine: a longitudinal study. Eur J Pediatr 1996;155:452–457.

55. Sklar CA, Qazi R, David R. Juvenile autoimmune thyroiditis: hormonal status at presentation and after long term follow-up. Am J Dis Child 1986, 140:877–880.

56. Moore DC. Natural course of 'subclinical' hypothyroidism in childhood and adolescence. Arch Pediatr Adol Med 1996;150:293–297.

57. Perelman AH, Johnson RL, Clemons RD, et al. Intrauterine diagnosis and treatment of fetal goitrous hypothyroidism. J Clin Endocrinol Metab 1990;71:618–621.

58. Thorpe-Beeston JG, Nicolaides KH, Felton CB, et al. Maturation of the secretion of thyroid hormone and thyroid-stimulating hormone in the fetus. N Engl J Med 1991;324:532–536.

59. Frank JE, Faix JE, Hermos RJ, et al. Thyroid function in very low birth weight infants: effects on neonatal hypothyroid screening. J Pediatr 1996;128:548–554.

60. Ares S, Escobar-Morreale HF, Quero J, et al. Neonatal hypothyroxinemia: effects of iodine intake and premature birth. J Clin Endocrinol Metab 1997;82:1704–1712.

61. Van Wassenaer AG, Kok JH, de Viljder JJM, et al. Effects of thyroxine replacement on neurologic development in infants born at less than 30 week's gestation. N Engl J Med 1997;336:21–26.

62. Van Wassenaer AG, Kok JH, Briet JM, et al. Thyroid function in preterm newborns;is T4 treatment required in infants <27 weeks' gestational age? Exp Clin Endocrinol Diabetes 1997;105:12–18.

9

Thyroid Hormone Replacement During Pregnancy

Amy E. Sullivan, MD and T. Flint Porter, MD

CONTENTS

INTRODUCTION

Thyroid metabolism plays an important role in reproductive processes and fetal development. Aberrant thyroid function can have profound effects on both maternal and fetal health. Hypothyoroidism is relatively common during pregnancy, but the diagnosis may be missed and treatment often problematic for several reasons. First, many of the classic signs and symptoms are considered typical of pregnancy. Second, the usually straightforward interpretation of thyroid function laboratory tests is made difficult by the physiologic effects of pregnancy on thyroid metabolism. Finally, obstetric abnormalities, such as gestational trophoblasic disease and hyperemesis gravidarum, may have profound effects on thyroid function.

THYROID FUNCTION

Physiologic Changes in Normal Pregnancy

Pregnancy-related changes in thyroid function are most likely the result of an increased thyroid hormone requirement critical for the normal embryonic period. Certainly, the very early presence of T_3 receptors in the fetal brain suggests the importance of thyroid hormone in neurological development *(1)*. Appropriate thyroid replacement in pregnancy requires a basic understanding of thyroid physiology and how it is affected by the pregnant state. Most thyroxine (T_4) and triiodothyronine (T_3) are bound to transporting proteins and circulate in the serum in their inactive forms. The majority of T_4 (70%) is bound to thyroxine-binding globulin (TBG), and most of the remainder to thyroxine-

From: *Endocrine Replacement Therapy in Clinical Practice*
Edited by: A. Wayne Meikle © Humana Press Inc., Totowa, NJ

binding prealbumin and albumin. A small fraction (0.02% of T_4 and 0.3% of T_3) circulates unbound and is biologically active.

The hyperestrogenic state of early pregnancy affects hormone binding by enhancing the overall production of TBG and promoting the formation of a more highly sialylated TBG isoform that is less readily cleared by the liver. Elevated TBG levels become detectable within the first several weeks of pregnancy, reaching a plateau at around 20 wk of gestation. In turn, there is a slight, transient decrease in free serum T_4 leading to the production of thyroid-stimulating hormone (TSH) and a compensatory increase in total T_4 production. All of this is usually clinically insignificant in the euthyroid pregnant woman.

Thyroid metabolism is also affected by the production of human chorionic gonadotropin hormone (hCG), which begins almost at the onset of pregnancy and peaks after approx 12 wk. There is marked structural homogeneity between hCG and the TSH molecule allowing for crossreactivity between hCG and the TSH receptor. Stimulation of the TSH receptor by the hCG mimics stimulation by TSH causing a mild and temporary increase in free T_4 and subsequent suppression of TSH. This is amplified by extraordinarily high hCG levels, common in the presence of multiple gestation, gesational trophoblastic disease, and hyperemesis gravidarum. Clinical manifestations of hyperthyroidism are not uncommon, but frank thyrotoxicosis is rarely seen *(2)*.

Euthyroid women are able to adapt to pregnancy without suffering any clinical repercussions. However, women with either intrinsic thyroid disease or iodine deficiency may develop overt clinical hypothyroidism. Women with mild or borderline thyroid pathology, unable to compensate for the increasing demands for thyroid production brought about by early pregnancy, may have normal TSH levels later in gestation, as both the demand for thyroid hormone diminishes and the hCG levels decrease *(3)*.

Fetal Thyroid Function

The fetal thyroid requirements are met by maternal thyroid production until about 10 wk of gestation. The traditional view that transplacental thyroid hormone transfer does not occur has been largely refuted. Although limited, transfer is demonstrated by detectable levels of T_4 in amniotic fluid as early as the fourth week of gestation *(4)*, and in umbilical cord blood samples from neonates with thyroid dysgenesis *(5)*. Reverse T_3 is also found in significant levels in amniotic fluid, metabolized from T_4 via the enzyme *5-deiodinase* found in fetal and placental tissues.

The development of the fetal hypothalamic–pituitary–thyroid axis begins as early as 8 wk gestation with the onset of TSH synthesis in the pituitary gland. Production is probably regulated by thyroid-releasing hormone (TRH) derived from placental tissue rather than the hypothalamus *(6)*. Indeed, anencephalic fetuses without hypothalamic TRH production are able to synthesize thyroid hormone *(7)*. In turn, the fetal thyroid gland begins to synthesize T_4 and T_3 after about 10 wk of gestation and, in doing so, becomes vulnerable to radioactive iodine and antithyroid medications.

The complete hypothalamic–pituitary–thyroid axis of the fetus is fully developed by 20 wk gestation. Fetal T_3 and T_4 levels rise progressively between 20 wk gestation and term, with a corresponding decline in fetal TSH levels in the third trimester. However, fetal TSH levels remain slightly elevated throughout the pregnancy in order to stimulate production of adequate amounts of thyroid hormone for the developing fetus. There is an abrupt increase in neonatal TRH, TSH, T_4, and T_3 within a few hours after birth.

Eventually, high levels of T_4 and T_3 inhibit pituitary gland production of TSH and levels diminish to a normal level by 10–14 d of life. Subsequently, T_4 and T_3 levels also return to normal.

HYPOTHYROIDISM IN PREGNANCY

Pregnancy Complications

Severe maternal hypothyroidism from iodine deficiency has been associated with severe neonatal hypothyroidism resulting in mental retardation and even overt cretinism *(5,8)*. Likewise, early studies of mild forms of maternal hypothyroidism reported a 50–60% incidence of neonatal mental and developmental delay and an increased incidence of congenital anomalies *(9–12)*.

Severe, untreated hypothyroidism has been associated with a number of complications in pregnancy, including fetal growth restriction, fetal demise, preeclampsia, placental abruption, and spontaneous miscarriage *(13,14)*. Table 1 summarizes the pregnancy outcomes of 50 patients with overt, untreated hypothyroidism and 57 patients with subclinical hypothyroidism. The rate of pregnancy-induced hypertension, intrauterine death, low birth weight, and placental abruption was significantly higher in the patients with uncontrolled hypothyroidism. However, favorable perinatal outcomes can be achieved with early diagnosis, effective and prompt treatment with L-thyroxine, antenatal surveillance, and early neonatal evaluation *(8,13–17)*. One small series of 11 pregnancies in 9 women with a mean TSH level at the first prenatal visit of 105 U/mL reported only slightly better perinatal outcomes when adequate treatment was given *(16)*. Only one intrauterine death occurred at 29 wk in an untreated mother with a serum TSH value of 293 U/mL. No other adverse perinatal events occurred that might be related to hypothyroidism. The live-born neonates were followed for 2.7 yr with normal developments.

Several studies have prompted some authorities to suggest universal screening for hypothyroidism in pregnant women. However, the link between maternal hypothyroidism and adverse fetal neurological development continues to be a hotly debated issue. One study of seven children born to hypothyroid mothers found no evidence of developmental delay between 1 mo and 2.5 yr of age *(16)*. Another study reported no difference in the IQ scores of 4- to 10-yr-old children of severely hypothyroid mothers who received treatment early in pregnancy, compared to their siblings who were born when the mothers were euthyroid *(18)*. A third reported that although children born to mothers with subclinical hypothyroidism had delayed mental development at 6 and 12 mo, no difference was noted at 24 mo compared to controls *(19)*.

These findings have not been supported by all investigators. Man compared the IQ scores of children born of hypothyroid mothers who did not receive adequate treatment to IQ scores of children born to hypothyroid mothers who did receive adequate treatment *(20)*. At 4 and 7 yr of age, the mean IQ score was lower in the offspring of the patients with hypothyroidism by six and five points, respectively, at the time that the testing was performed. Another group, studying both the cognitive and the psychomotor development of 220 infants born to women with serum free T_4 measurement in the lowest 10th percentile, had almost a sixfold increased incidence of psychomotor delay at 10 mo of age *(21)*. Haddow retrospectively evaluated more than 25,000 women for hypothyroidism based on serum TSH levels above the 98th percentile *(22)*. The children of the 62

Table 1

Pregnancy Outcomes in Patients with Uncontrolled vs Subclinical Hypothyroidism

	Overt hypothyroidism (n = 50)	*Subclinical hypothyroidism* (n = 57)
Pregnancy-induced hypertension	13 (26%)	9 (15%)
Placental abruption	3 (6%)	0
Hemorrhage	4 (8%)	2 (3.5%)
Stillbirths	4 (8%)	1 (1.7%)[a]
Congenital malformations	2 (4%)	0
Low body weight	10 (20%)	5 (8.7%)
Anemia	5 (10%)	1 (1.7%)

[a]Congenital syphilis.
Source: Data from refs. *13* and *14*.

women found to be hypothyroid underwent tests to evaluate intelligence, language skills, attention, reading ability, and visual–motor skills at age 7–9. Compared to controls, they did not perform as well. However, a statistically significant difference was seen for only one of two attention tests and in one of three language tests. Remarkably, when the offspring of inadequately treated hypothyroid mothers were evaluated separately, there was a significant difference in the mean IQ scores in this group compared to controls (100 vs 111). Nineteen percent of the children born to women who were not treated for hypothyroidism during pregnancy had IQ scores <85 compared to 5% of children whose mother's were euthyroid *(22)*.

Etiology

According to one study done by the World Health Organization (WHO) in 1998, greater than 30% of the world's population lives in areas of inadequate iodine supply *(23)*. Iodine deficiency is not common in North America; however, a recent National Health and nutrition survey demonstrated an increase in the number of women with low urinary excretion of iodine over the last 20 yr *(24)*. These levels were not low enough to reach even the "moderate" iodine deficiency as defined by the WHO study. Currently, several international health organizations recommend that all pregnant women consume 220 µg of iodine a day *(25)*. Women who are not pregnant should consume only 150 µg of iodine a day.

In North America, chronic autoimmune thyroiditis is by far the most common cause of hypothyroidism among women in the reproductive age group. There is a significantly smaller subset of patients who have been treated for Graves' disease and subsequently develop postablation hypothyroidism. In about 10% of patients, hypothyroidism is diagnosed for the first time during pregnancy. Women with only mild thyroid hormone deficiency may be asymptomatic until their thyroid function is challenged by pregnancy. Only 60% of patients have clinically significant symptoms; the others will be mildly symptomatic or completely asymptomatic *(13,14,16)*.

Primary hypothyroidism is the result of intrinsic thyroid disease and is most common during pregnancy. Secondary hypothyroidism, extremely rare in pregnancy, is defined as a defect at the level of the hypothalamus or pituitary. When seen, it is usually a result of a hypophysectomy for pituitary tumor, brain radiation, or hypothalamic disease.

Table 2
Medications That Interfere
with Thyroid Hormone

Interference with thyroid hormone synthesis
Methimazole
PTU
Iodine
Lithium
Increases thyroxine clearance
Carbamazipine
Phenytoin
Rifampin
Interference with absorption
Aluminum hydroxide
Cholestyramine
Ferrous sulfate
Sucralfate

There is almost always deficiency in other pituitary hormones and this often results in infertility. Several medications may also interfere with the production or absorption of thyroid hormone and may cause clinically overt hypothyroidism (*see* Table 2).

Thyroid malignancies are sometimes encountered during pregnancy and may be associated with hypothyroidism. Most are papillary or follicular lesions and no case of undifferentiated thyroid carcinoma has been reported. Pregnancy does not have any effect on the natural history of thyroid cancer. Likewise, thyroid cancer does not have any effect on the natural history of pregnancy.

Thyroid Function Tests

The cost-effectiveness and clinical utility of universal thyroid screening during pregnancy has been hotly debated but never established *(22)*. However, baseline thyroid function tests should be performed on those pregnant women with a history of thyroid disease or clinical findings suggestive of thyroid disorder. Results of thyroid function tests should be interpreted with caution because of the previously described changes in thyroid metabolism that accompany pregnancy.

The diagnosis of hypothyroidism during pregnancy is often confusing. The most sensitive test for primary hypothyroidism is a serum TSH level. In the nonpregnant state, primary hypothyroidism is suggested by an elevated TSH level in the presence of a low free T_4. However, because of the stimulating effects of both elevated estrogen and hCG during pregnancy, TSH levels may be slightly elevated in up to 15% of pregnant women who are euthyroid. Further, some women have serum TSH levels in the upper limits of normal or in the mildly elevated range despite the fact that they have compromised thyroid function.

Thyroid autoantibodies are often used to make the diagnosis of autoimmune thyroid disease, either Hashimoto's thyroiditis or Graves' disease. Several different categories exist, making the nomenclature of thyroid autoantibodies quite confusing. Anti-TPO antibodies (formerly termed "antimicrosomal antibodies") are detected in 90% of patients

Table 3
Clinical Scenarios for Testing for TSH Receptor Antibodies

Clinical suspicion of fetal or neonatal hyperthyroidism
    Previous pregnancy with fetal or neonatal hyperthyroidis
    Presence of fetal tachycardia
    Detection of a fetal goiter on ultrasound
Women with primary myxedema or Hashimoto's thyroiditis
    Previous pregnancy with neonatal hypothyroidism
Women in the postpartum period
    Infant born with neonatal hypothyroidism
    Neonatal thyroid gland is seen on ultrasound in a hypothyroid infant

with Hashimoto's thyroiditis. Antithyroglobulin antibodies (ATA) are seen in approx 75% of patients with Graves' disease. A third category of thyroid autoantibodies, TSH receptor antibodies, can either stimulate (thyroid-stimulating antibodies [TSAbs]) or inhibit (TSH-binding inhibitory imunoglobulins [TBIIs]) thyroid function. They are present in approx 90% of patients with Graves' disease but only 10% of patients with Hashimoto's thyroiditis (26).

All of the thyroid autoantibodies are of the IgG isotype and readily cross the placenta. Anti-TPO antibodies and ATAs are not toxic to the fetal thyroid gland and high cord blood titers are not associated with overt fetal hypothyroidism (26). However, high titers of TSH receptor antibodies are known to affect fetal thyroid function and have been associated with fetal goiter and hyperthyroidism. Their biological half-life is several months, and affected neonates have only transient hypothyroidism. Whether or not this transient neonatal hypothyroidism has any long-term effects is unknown.

Thyroid autoantibodies should not be used in screening for thyroid disorders, as they can be detected in 6–20% of all pregnant women (27,28). Instead, testing for TSH receptor antibodies should be limited to a few clinical scenarios (see Table 3).

Treatment

Many patients require a periodic increase in their thyroxine supplementation during pregnancy. Mandel reported that serum TSH levels increased steadily between 6 and 25 wk gestation in 12 hypothyroid women, 9 of whom became hypothyroid (29). In a larger series, 7 of 34 hypothyroid women demonstrated an elevation of serum TSH to the hypothyroid range and subsequently required an increase in their doses of thyroxine (30). These findings have been confirmed by others (31,32).

The development of more sensitive thyroid function tests (serum TSH and free T_4 assays) have made it easier to accurately monitor and appropriately treat hypothyroid women during pregnancy. Most hypothyroid women demonstrate an elevation in serum TSH levels early in pregnancy. However, they may not need an increase in their thyroxine dose until the second or third trimester. Changes should be based on the serum TSH level (33). Serum TSH and free T_4 levels should be checked at the first prenatal visit and 6 wk after adjusting the dose. If the initial thyroid function tests are normal, they should be repeated in the second trimester and then again early in the third trimester.

For patients diagnosed with hypothyroidism for the first time during pregnancy, L-thyroxine should be initiated at 150 µg/d and thyroid function tests should be checked

Table 4
L-Thyroxine Dosing

TSH level	Increase in L-thyroxine
<10 U/L	41 ± 24 µg/d
10–20 U/L	65 ± 22 µg/d
>20 U/L	105 ± 19 µg/d

Source: ref. *33.*

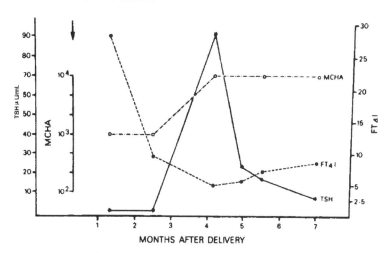

Fig. 1. Transient hyperthyroidism and hypothyroidism in the postpartum period in a patient with chronic autoimmune thyroiditis with spontaneous recovery. TSH, thyroid stimulating hormone; MCHA, microsomal hemagglutination antibodies; FT4I, free thyroxine index.

every 6 wk until normal. Testing should be repeated in each trimester and in the puerperium. Thyroxine supplementation should be adjusted as needed (*see* Table 4).

POSTPARTUM THYROID DYSFUNCTION

Postpartum thyroid dysfunction develops in approx 5–15% of women. Autoimmune thyroiditis (Graves' disease or Hashimoto's thyroiditis) typically improves during the third trimester of pregnancy, likely because of its relatively immunosuppressed state. However, exacerbation is not uncommon during the postpartum period when immune function returns to normal (*see* Fig. 1).

Women with postpartum thyroiditis usually present in the first 2–4 mo postpartum with symptoms of hyperthyroidism. These symptoms are often relatively mild and may be difficult to distinguish from physiologic postpartum fatigue and weight loss. Goiter is sometimes palpable and, occasionally, palpitations and even frank thyrotoxicosis develop. Rather than stimulation by autoantibodies, postpartum hyperthyroidism is the result of gland destruction identified histologically by a destructive lymphocytic infiltrate. In most patients hyperthyroidism is followed by a period of temporary hypothyroidism that is sometimes manifested as depression. This typically lasts several months and women frequently require treatment. Most women become euthyroid within about 8 mo when medication can be safely stopped. Up to 10% of women remain permanently hypothyroid and require long-term replacement (*34*).

REFERENCES

1. Ekins R. Roles of serum thyroxine-binding proteins and maternal thyroid hormones in fetal development. Lancet 1985;1:1129–1132.
2. Hershman JM, Higgins HP. Hydatidiform mole—a cause of clinical hyperthyroidism. Report of two cases with evidence that the molar tissue secreted a thyroid stimulator. N Engl J Med 1971;284:573–577.
3. Kamijo K, Saito T, Sato M, et al. Transient subclinical hypothyroidism in early pregnancy. Endocrinol Jpn 1990;37:397–403.
4. Contempre B, Jauniaux E, Calvo R, et al. Detection of thyroid hormones in human embryonic cavities during the first trimester of pregnancy. J Clin Endocrinol Metab 1993;77:1719–1722.
5. Vulsma T, Gons MH, de Vijlder JJ. Maternal-fetal transfer of thyroxine in congenital hypothyroidism due to a total organification defect or thyroid agenesis. N Engl J Med 1989;321:13–16.
6. Koivusalo F. Evidence of thyrotropin-releasing hormone activity in autopsy pancreata from newborns. J Clin Endocrinol Metab 1981;53:734–736.
7. Burrow G. Thyroid Function and Disease. WB Saunders, Philadelphia, PA, 1989, p. 292.
8. Buckshee K, Kriplani A, Kapil A, et al. Hypothyroidism complicating pregnancy. Aust NZ J Obstet Gynaecol 1992;32:240–242.
9. Man EB, Jones WS, Holden RH, et al. Thyroid function in human pregnancy. 8. Retardation of progeny aged 7 years; relationships to maternal age and maternal thyroid function. Am J Obstet Gynecol 1971;111:905–916.
10. Man EB, Holden RH, Jones WS. Thyroid function in human pregnancy. VII. Development and retardation of 4-year-old progeny of euthyroid and of hypothyroxinemic women. Am J Obstet Gynecol 1971;109:12–19.
11. Grennman GW, Gabrielson MD, Howard-Flanders J, Wessel MA. Thyroid dysfunction in pregnancy. N Engl J Med 1962:426–431.
12. Man EB. Maternal hypothyroxiinemia development of 4 and 7 year old offspring. In: Fisher DA, Burrows GN, eds. Perinatal Thyroid Physiology and Disease: Raven, New York, 1975, p. 177.
13. Davis LE, Leveno KJ, Cunningham FG. Hypothyroidism complicating pregnancy. Obstet Gynecol 1988;72:108–112.
14. Leung AS, Millar LK, Koonings PP, et al. Perinatal outcome in hypothyroid pregnancies. Obstet Gynecol 1993;81:349–353.
15. Montoro MN. Management of hypothyroidism during pregnancy. Clin Obstet Gynecol 1997;40:65–80.
16. Montoro M, Collea JV, Frasier SD, et al. Successful outcome of pregnancy in women with hypothyroidism. Ann Intern Med 1981;94:31–34.
17. Wasserstrum N, Anania CA. Perinatal consequences of maternal hypothyroidism in early pregnancy and inadequate replacement. Clin Endocrinol (Oxf) 1995;42:353–358.
18. Lui H, Momotani N, Noh JY, Ishikawa N, Takebe K, Ito K. Maternal hypothyroidism during early pregnancy and intellectual development of the progeny. Arch Intern Med 1994;154:785–787.
19. Smit BJ, Kok JH, Vulsma T, et al. Neurologic development of the newborn and young child in relation to maternal thyroid function. Acta Paediatr 2000;89:291–295.
20. Man EB, Brown JF, Serunian SA. Maternal hypothyroxinemia: psychoneurological deficits of progeny. Ann Clin Lab Sci 1991;21:227–239.
21. Pop VJ, Kuijpens JL, van Baar AL, et al. Low maternal free thyroxine concentrations during early pregnancy are associated with impaired psychomotor development in infancy. Clin Endocrinol (Oxf) 1999;50:149–155.
22. Haddow JE, Palomaki GE, Allan WC, et al. Maternal thyroid deficiency during pregnancy and subsequent neuropsychological development of the child. N Engl J Med 1999;341:549–555.
23. WHO U, and ICCIDD. Progress towards the elimination of iodine deficiency disorders (IDD), WHO, UNICEF , and ICCIDD, Geneva, 1999.
24. Hollowell JG, Staehling NW, Hannon WH, et al. Iodine nutrition in the United States. Trends and public health implications: iodine excretion data from National Health and Nutrition Examination Surveys I and III (1971-1974 and 1988-1994). J Clin Endocrinol Metab 1998;83:3401–3408.
25. Panel on Mocronutrients F, and Nutrition Board, Institute of Medicine. Dietary reference intakes for vitamin A, vitamin K, arsenic, boron, chromium, copper, iodine, iron, maganese, molybdenum, nickel, silicon, vanadium, and zinc. National Academy Press, Washington, DC, 2001.

26. Dussault JH, Letarte J, Guyda H, et al Lack of influence of thyroid antibodies on thyroid function in the newborn infant and on a mass screening program for congenital hypothyroidism. J Pediatr 1980;96:385–389.
27. Glinoer D, Soto MF, Bourdoux P, et al. Pregnancy in patients with mild thyroid abnormalities: maternal and neonatal repercussions. J Clin Endocrinol Metab 1991;73:421–427.
28. Stagnaro-Green A, Roman SH, Cobin RH, et al. Detection of at-risk pregnancy by means of highly sensitive assays for thyroid autoantibodies. Jama 1990;264:1422–1425.
29. Mandel SJ, Larsen PR, Seely EW, et al. Increased need for thyroxine during pregnancy in women with primary hypothyroidism. N Engl J Med 1990;323:9–96.
30. Pekonen F, Teramo K, Ikonen E, et al. Women on thyroid hormone therapy: pregnancy course, fetal outcome, and amniotic fluid thyroid hormone level. Obstet Gynecol 1984;63:635–638.
31. Kaplan MM. Monitoring thyroxine treatment during pregnancy. Thyroid 1992;2:147–152.
32. Girling JC, de Swiet M. Thyroxine dosage during pregnancy in women with primary hypothyroidism. Br J Obstet Gynaecol 1992;99:368–370.
33. Mandel SJ, Brent GA, Larsen PR. Levothyroxine therapy in patients with thyroid disease. Ann Intern Med 1993;119:492-502.
34. Tachi J, Amino N, Tamaki H, et al. Long term follow-up and HLA association in patients with postpartum hypothyroidism. J Clin Endocrinol Metab 1988;66:480–484.

IV   Diabetes

10

Diagnosis and Management
of Diabetes in Children

Dana S. Hardin, MD

INTRODUCTION

Diabetes mellitus is the most common endocrine/metabolic disorder of childhood, with important consequences for physical and emotional development. It is caused by a deficiency of insulin secretion (type 1 diabetes), or decreased insulin action (type 2 diabetes of youth), or both (*see* the section on other recognizable types of diabetes). Hyperglycemia, caused by abnormal metabolism of carbohydrates, is the hallmark finding of all types of childhood diabetes. In addition to hyperglycemia, untreated diabetes results in altered metabolism of protein and fat, which can negatively impact growth and development. Early detection and treatment of diabetes in children is imperative, and correct classification ensures that disease-specific therapy is utilized.

DIAGNOSTIC CRITERIA, SCREENING, AND CLASSIFICATION

Diabetes mellitus is not a single entity but a heterogeneous group of disorders with separate etiologic and pathophysiologic mechanisms. It is important for the clinician to adequately distinguish between these types of diabetes so that each child receives disease-specific medical management. The Expert Committee on the Diagnosis and Classification of Diabetes Mellitus Diabetes has proposed revised criteria for the diagnosis of diabetes (*1*). These diagnostic criterion have been previously outlined and do not differ for children or adolescents. It is important to note that similar to adults, hemoglobin A_{1c} (A_{1c}) is not recognized as a valid diagnostic tool. Although results from an oral

From: *Endocrine Replacement Therapy in Clinical Practice*
Edited by: A. Wayne Meikle © Humana Press Inc., Totowa, NJ

glucose tolerance test (OGTT) represent one of the three methods for establishing a diagnosis of diabetes, in most cases the diagnosis of diabetes in children can be made from clinical symptoms and casual blood glucose levels. In many cases, an OGTT is not necessary to establish the diagnosis of diabetes in children. Screening for type 1 diabetes is not recommended in nonsymptomatic children. However, screening of children/adolescents who are at high risk for type 2 diabetes (*see* the section on other recognized types of diabetes) is recommended *(2)*.

The Expert Committee recently revised classification of diabetes into four major types: type 1 diabetes, type 2 diabetes, other recognized types of diabetes, and gestational diabetes *(1)*. All but gestational diabetes are pertinent to children and adolescents and are defined in the following subsections.

Type 1 Diabetes

This type of diabetes is the most common form of childhood diabetes and is almost always the cause of diabetes in prepubertal children *(2)*. Type 1 diabetes is characterized by severe insulinopenia and dependence on exogenous insulin to prevent ketoacidosis and to preserve life. This condition has previously been referred to as insulin-dependent diabetes mellitus (IDDM) and has also been called "juvenile-onset" diabetes, because of its more common presentation during childhood. Although many patients present with significant ketosis, there may be a preketotic, non-insulin-dependent phase in the natural history of the disease. Type 1 diabetes is associated with certain human leukocyte antigens (HLAs), autoimmunity, and the presence of circulating antibodies to cytoplasmic and cell surface components of islet cells *(3,4)*.

Type 2 Diabetes

Type 2 diabetes, as it occurs in children, most commonly presents in pubertal adolescents who are obese and who have a strong history of type 2 diabetes in adult family members. It is more commonly seen in children from specific ethnic backgrounds *(5,6)*. Children with this type of diabetes are not insulin dependent, although they may use insulin for correction of symptomatic hyperglycemia. These patients do not tend to be ketosis prone; however, they may develop ketosis under special circumstances such as episodes of infection or stress and many have mild to moderate ketosis at initial presentation *(7)*. This type of childhood diabetes is most similar to type 2 diabetes found in adults; however, more research is needed to fully understand its pathogenesis and treatment.

Other Recognized Types of Diabetes

This category includes genetic defects of β-cell function including maturity onset diabetes of the young and atypical diabetes, formerly called diabetes type 1.5 *(8)*, genetic defects of insulin action (leprechaunism, type a insulin resistance, Rabson-Medenhall syndrome, lipoatrophic diabetes, and others), endocrinopathies, diabetes associated with genetic syndromes, disease of the exocrine pancreas (cystic fibrosis and pancreatectomy), and diabetes secondary to drugs, chemicals, and infection.

TYPE 1 DIABETES IN CHILDHOOD

Incidence and Prevalence

Early statistics suggest that prevalence of type 1 diabetes in the United States is 1–2/ 1000 schoolage children I. More recent data suggest there has been an increase in prevalence during the past few years, related to epidemiclike outbreaks *(10)*. The prevalence is highly correlated with age, ranging from 1/1430 children at 5 yr to 1/360 children by age 16 *(9)*. Prevalence throughout the world varies widely, being highest in northern Scandinavia and lowest in Japan *(10,11)*. Among the African-American population, the prevalence of insulin-dependent diabetes is 20–30% of that in American Caucasians *(11)*. Both the prevalence and incidence of type 1 diabetes mellitus (DM) in the United States are similar to those reported in Great Britain, parts of Sweden, and Australia *(10,11)*. Earlier studies of incidence rates shows a frequency of 12–16 new cases per 100,000 children per year *(12)*. In Caucasians, males have a higher incidence, and in non-Caucasians, the incidence in females is higher *(10)*. There is no correlation with socio-economic status *(13)*. Peaks of presentation occur in two age groups: ages 5–7 yr, and at the time of puberty *(14)*. These age-related peaks correspond in the former to the increased exposure to infectious agents accompanying the beginning of school *(15)*; in the latter, they likely secondary to peaks of growth hormone and sex steroids, both acting as insulin antagonists *(16,17)*.

Etiology, Genetics, and Pathogenesis

The ultimate cause of the clinical findings of type 1 diabetes is insulin deficiency. Basal insulin levels may be normal in newly diagnosed cases; however, insulin production in response to a variety of potent secretagogues is blunted and usually completely disappears over a period of months to years. Although the destruction of β-cells leads progressively to more severe insulin deficiency, some limited capacity for insulin secretion remains and may persist for a variable period of time, usually not exceeding 1–2 yr. This period of residual insulin secretion is known as "the honeymoon period" *(18)*. The mechanisms leading to pancreatic β-cell failure are incompletely understood, but they are related to an autoimmune destruction of pancreatic islets in predisposed individuals *(19,20)*. The histologic pancreatic changes are characterized by lymphocytic infiltration around the islets of Langerhans. Later, the islets become progressively hyalinized and scarred, a process suggesting an ongoing inflammatory response, possibly autoimmune in nature *(19,21)*. There is evidence to suggest that at least 80% of islet cell function must be lost before diabetes manifests *(22)*.

Investigations show a high prevalence of circulating antibodies directed against the cytoplasmic components of islet cells and against the cell surface components of β-cells *(23,24)*. These antibodies, listed in Table 1, are present in over 75% of cases at the clinical onset of disease. In the presence of complement, the antibodies have been shown to be cytotoxic to in vitro β-cells *(25)*. Similarly, T-lymphocytes from diabetics have been shown to be cytotoxic to human insulinoma cells in culture *(26)*. These findings suggest that type 1 diabetes, like other autoimmune diseases, is a disease in which autoantibodies, in concert with other factors, destroy their target cell—in this case, the insulin-producing islet cell of the pancreas *(27)*. Although the presence of islet cell antibodies (ICAs) in serum of unaffected individuals may vary with time, the persistence of ICAs appears to be a strong predictive factor for developing type 1 diabetes in nonaffected siblings *(28)*.

Type 1 diabetes has long been known to be associated with an increased prevalence of other autoimmune disorders such as Addison diṡease, Hashimoto thyroiditis, and pernicious anemia *(29)*. These autoimmune disorders, including type 1 diabetes, are associated with an increased frequency of certain histocompatibility antigens, in particu-

Table 1
Antibodies Associated with Type 1 Diabetes

Autoantigen	T-Cell reactivity	Description
GM2-1	?	Nonspecific; in all islet cells
Glutamic acid decarboxylase (GAD)	Positive	Present as GAD-65, GAD-67, and 64,000 M_r antibodies
Insulin	Positive	Insulin autoantibodies (IAAs)
ICA-69 (IPM-1)	?	Homologous with bovine serum albumin (BSA)
38,000 M_r	Positive	Secretory granule related
52,000 M_r	?	Rubella associated
Carboxypeptidase H	?	Secretory granule related
GLUT	?	Inhibition of glucose-stimulated insulin secretion

Source: Adapted from Diabetes and Complications, a CORE Curriculum for Diabetes Education, 4th ed. American Association of Diabetes Education, Washington, DC, 2001.

lar HLA-DR3 and HLA-DR4 (29–33). The HLA system is the major histocompatibility complex, located on chromosome number 6, consisting of a cluster of genes that code for transplantation antigens and that play a central role in the immune response (34,35). In type 1 diabetes, the inheritance of HLA-DR3 or HLA-DR4 confers a two- to threefold greater relative risk for developing the disease (34). When both DR3 and DR4 are inherited together, the relative risk for developing diabetes is 7- to 10-fold greater, suggesting that DR3 and DR4 are additive in their effect of conferring relative risk (33,35). More than 90% of Caucasian patients with type 1 diabetes possess DR3. However, not all have one of the HLA types that are more frequently associated with this disease. Studies of family pedigrees and HLA typing suggest that in Caucasians, the recurrence risk to siblings is of the order of 2–5%; the risk to offspring is also 2–5% (36). In American blacks, these risks are one-half to two-thirds of those in Caucasians (32).

Although genetics clearly confer susceptibility to diabetes, factors other than inheritance are involved in producing clinical disease. The concordance rate among identical twins is 50%, suggesting the participation of environmental factors (36,37). Previous epidemics of mumps, rubella, and the Coxsackie virus have been associated with subsequent increases in the frequency of type 1 diabetes (37,38). The occurrence of acute-onset diabetes induced by the coxsackie B4 virus has been documented (38,39). Thus, the best hypothesis for development of type 1 diabetes is that the inheritance of certain genes confers a predisposition for autoimmune disease. Once a predisposed child is exposed to a particular environmental trigger or trigger(s), autoantibody-mediated destruction of the β-cell begins and diabetes ultimately develops.

Metabolic Changes Associated with Uncontrolled Type 1 Diabetes

Insulin is one of the two major anabolic hormones of the body, and lack of insulin can cause multiple metabolic disturbances. Insulin serves an important role in preventing catabolic loss of protein from skeletal muscle (40). Thus, patients who are under-insulinized become catabolic and demonstrate wasting of muscle tissue. Furthermore, insulin is an antilipolytic hormone, and inadequate levels result in loss of subcutaneous fat. Many patients with diabetes present with acute loss of body weight that results from loss of both fat and muscle.

Although insulin deficiency is the primary defect in type 1 diabetes, elevation of classical stress hormones (epinephrine, cortisol, growth hormone, and glucagon) accelerate and exaggerate the rate and magnitude of the metabolic decompensation *(41,42)*. Excessive levels of epinephrine can further impair insulin secretion, and cortisol and growth hormone can antagonize insulin action. Hormonally mediated increase in hepatic glucose production (gluconeogenesis and glycogenolysis) contribute to hyperglycemia *(43,44)*. Glucosuria results when the renal threshold of 160–180 mg/dL is exceeded. The resultant osmotic diuresis produces polyuria, dehydration, and an increase in serum osmolarity. Serum glucose levels are commonly elevated to 600 mg/dL or higher, which further contributes to increased serum osmolarity. Compensatory polydipsia is triggered by the normal neurologic reaction to hyperosmolarity; however, patients typically cannot drink and retain enough fluid to correct osmolarity. Thus, hyperosmolarity contributes to clinical complications and has important implications for therapy.

The presence of insulin deficiency leads to lipolysis and impaired lipid synthesis, which can cause marked elevation in the plasma concentrations of free fatty acids. The hormonal interplay of insulin deficiency and increased glucagon shunts the free fatty acids to ketone body formation, and the rate of their formation exceeds the capacity for peripheral utilization. Accumulation of these ketoacids results in metabolic acidosis *(44)*. Ketones are readily excreted in the urine in association with cations, further compounding losses of water and electrolytes. Acetone, formed by nonenzymatic conversion of acetoacetate, is responsible for the characteristic fruity odor of the breath. Compensatory rapid deep breathing (Kussmaul respiration) develops in an attempt to excrete excess carbon dioxide and correct acidosis. Progressive dehydration, acidosis, and hyperosmolarity result in diminished cerebral oxygen utilization and consciousness gradually becomes impaired. If untreated, coma develops *(41)*. Thus, insulin deficiency produces a profound catabolic state that is worsened by normal counterregulatory hormone response. The clinical features of untreated diabetes can be explained on the basis of predictable alterations in metabolism. The severity and duration of the symptoms are a reflection of the degree of insulinopenia *(42)*.

Clinical Presentation

Generally, the diagnosis of type 1 diabetes can be established without the use of an oral glucose tolerance test because of the presence of recognizable signs and symptoms, in addition to hyperglycemia *(45)*. Most children present with a history of polyuria, polydipsia, and polyphagia. These symptoms may be present for days to weeks. Other common symptoms include dehydration, lethargy, weakness, and weight loss *(45,46)*. In younger children, parents may report the onset of enuresis in a previously toilet-trained child. In teenage girls, monilial vaginitis may occasionally be the presenting feature. Although documentation of glucosuria is the simplest screening test for diabetes, it is important to document hyperglycemia by blood glucose testing to establish the diagnosis of diabetes. Renal glucosuria in a child with vomiting and starvation ketosis may mimic the urinary findings of ketoacidosis. However, in these cases, blood glucose levels are normal, indicating that insulin therapy is not needed *(45)*.

Diabetic Ketoacidosis

Only a minority of children (40% or less) initially present with frank diabetic ketoacidosis (DKA); however, children age 5 or under are at higher risk *(45,46)*. Diabetic ketoacidosis can be said to exist when there is ketonemia (ketones strongly positive at greater than 1:2 dilution of serum), acidosis (pH 7.30 or less), glucosuria, and ketonuria *(47,48)*. Although most cases of DKA involve significant hyperglycemia (blood glucose level 300 mg/dL or more), patients with protracted poor oral intake and/or protracted vomiting may have low-normal glucose levels, yet still present with significant acidosis *(48)*. Diabetes ketoacidosis should be distinguished from other causes of acidosis, including lactic acidosis, salicylate intoxication or other ingestions, and from overwhelming sepsis *(45)*. Nonketotic hyperosmolar coma is rare in children, but may occur *(45)*.

Clinical symptoms associated with ketoacidosis can include vomiting, leukocytosis, and abdominal pain. Abdominal pain can be severe, but generally resolves after several hours of rehydration and insulin therapy. An isolated elevation of serum amylase may occur but may not indicate the existence of pancreatitis *(45,46)*. Additional amylase levels and elevation of serum lipase must be obtained to document the existence of pancreatitis. Symptoms of severe, untreated ketoacidosis can include Kussmaul respiration, obtundation, and coma. Serum sodium concentration may be normal or low. It is important to note that elevation of serum glucose can falsely lower sodium values depending on the assay used. Despite large deficits of potassium and phosphate, serum concentrations of these ions are not uniformly reduced prior to initiation of therapy; however, they often manifest once insulin therapy is initiated *(45,47)*.

Precipitating factors of DKA include stress such as trauma, infections, and vomiting. Recurrent episodes of ketoacidosis in established diabetics usually imply nonadherence to therapy *(45)*. Children with more than two episodes of ketoacidosis should receive psychosocial evaluation. Additionally, increasing the frequency of outpatient contact with the physician and diabetes team can help some patients improve. However, If these efforts do not result in positive change, the case should be reported to local child protection agencies.

Medical Management of DKA in Children

COMPLICATIONS

With appropriate therapy, complications of DKA are uncommon in children. Iatrogenic complications include hypoglycemia, hypokalemia from inadequate potassium replacement and hypocalcemia from too vigorous use of phosphate. The major complication of concern in children treated for DKA is cerebral edema. Although the etiology is poorly understood, studies suggest its occurrence is related to rapid change in osmolarity, sodium, and glucose *(45,49,50)*. Cerebral edema generally develops in patients several hours after the institution of therapy and often after clinical and biochemical indices suggest improvement. Clinical symptoms of increased intracranial pressure include headache, deterioration in level of consciousness, and development of fixed dilated pupils. Once clinically obvious, this complication has a high morbidity and mortality. Treatment with mannitol, 0.25 g/kg, given as an intravenous "push" and repeated 5–10 min as needed *(51)*, should be instituted as soon as possible to reduce cerebral edema. The incidence of cerebral edema can be reduced by age-appropriate DKA management, by the prevention of DKA through increasing public awareness to promote early diagnosis, and by avoidance of recurrent episodes of DKA through effective patient–family education and support.

FLUIDS AND ELECTROLYTES

Children differ little from adults in the basic pathophysiologic disturbances, clinical features, and trends in the treatment of DKA *(45)*. However, what distinguishes the child from the adult is the greater need for precision in fluid and insulin management and the need to provide close monitoring with individualization of therapy. The initial metabolic stabilization of a child with DKA is achieved by a combination of fluid and electrolyte therapy and insulin administration. The extent of metabolic decompensation must be assessed by estimating the degree of dehydration and noting whether there is an alteration in the conscious state. A biochemical confirmation of the presence of DKA must be sought by measurement of blood glucose and serum pH. Serum electrolytes, including calcium, magnesium and phosphorus, should be checked, as well as blood urea nitrogen (BUN) and creatinine, for an estimate of renal function. Further evaluation such as bacterial cultures and a chest radiograph may be indicated, depending on the patient's history. Repeated measurements of blood glucose and pH should be obtained hourly if intravenous insulin is utilized. In general, serum electrolytes should be obtained at 4- to 6-h intervals depending on the initial and subsequent levels. Occasionally, certain electrolyte values may need to be obtained as often as every 2 h (e.g., in a child presenting with hyperkalemia). The maintenance fluid requirement of a child changes as the child grows, but is constant when expressed per unit of surface area. It is not constant when expressed per unit of body weight. A rate of 1500 cm^3/m^2/d is accepted as maintenance fluid requirement (51). In contrast, dehydration is expressed as a percentage of body weight. In general, clinical assessment usually underestimates the degree of dehydration in children; however, most children with DKA may be assumed to have lost at least 10% of body weight. The total fluid to be administered is the sum of maintenance and estimated dehydration plus ongoing losses. Fluid replacement is generally begun intravenously at twice maintenance (3000 cm^3/m^2/24 h) and is extended over 24–36 h to reduce the likelihood of a too-rapid drop in plasma osmolarity. To further reduce the potential for developing cerebral edema, the initial replacement fluid consists of normal saline (0.9%), which is continued for the first 6 h. Initiation of insulin therapy and correction of acidosis may be followed by sharp reduction in the serum potassium because of shifts of this ion to the intracellular compartment. Potassium therapy is initiated once urine output is established and is generally provided as one-half chloride and one-half phosphate. This helps prevent excess chloride, which may aggravate acidosis (52), and also prevents decreased phosphate levels. Provision of phosphate promotes the formation of 2,3-diphophoglycerate, which permits the oxygen dissociation curve to shift to the right, thus facilitating the release of oxygen to tissues and the correction of acidosis (53). Both hypophosphatemia and hypomagnesemia have been associated with resistance to insulin action (54); thus, adequate replacement is essential. Although phosphate therapy is necessary, it is important to be aware of the potential for precipitating hypocalcemia through excessive use of phosphate. Therefore, serum calcium should be measured periodically. Hypocalcemia requires appropriate treatment with calcium gluconate.

INSULIN

Fluid and electrolyte therapy often result in clinical and biochemical improvement, even before the initiation of insulin therapy (45). However, the provision of insulin is essential to restore normal intermediary metabolism and to hasten the correction of acidosis. The preferred method of insulin delivery is continuous low-dose insulin infusion (an insulin "drip") using a starting dose of 0.1 U/kg/h. The starting dose should be less for children less than 8 yr, but generally should not be lower than 0.05 U/kg/h. A priming dose is unnecessary and can lower the glucose level more rapidly than desired

(55). The decline in serum glucose should be no greater than 80–100 mg/dL/h. The insulin infusion rate should be adjusted by no more than 10% per hour and should be increased to improve persistent acidosis. Typically, acidosis persists longer than the hyperglycemia and it is important to continue insulin administration at a rate of 0.05–1.0 U/kg/h to avoid worsening of ketosis. This can safely be accomplished by adding dextrose to the infusate. In general, dextrose should be added once the serum glucose level falls below 300 mg/dL. An increase in dextrose, rather than decrease in insulin, is always preferred during acidosis. Quick response to hourly monitoring of serum or whole-blood glucose levels will avoid hypoglycemia and will prevent too rapid a fall in plasma osmolarity. Once blood glucose levels fall below 200 mg/dL, the dextrose infusion should be adjusted to maintain glucose levels of 100 and 160 mg/dL.

Once acidosis is resolved, the insulin infusion may be discontinued and subcutaneous insulin may be administered. The dose may be approximated by calculating the total daily insulin requirement from the insulin infusion rate, or in the case of an established patient, the child may be returned to his or her home dose. Persistent hyperglycemia and electrolyte deficiency reduce insulin sensitivity *(56)*; thus, insulin needs may decrease after several days following an episode of ketoacidosis. Care should be taken to adequately reduce insulin if necessary.

USE OF BICARBONATE

Provision of fluid and insulin are generally adequate to correct diabetes-mediated metabolic acidosis, and, in general, bicarbonate is not recommended. One concern over the use of bicarbonate includes the potential for overcorrection causing alkalosis. This can lead to lactic acidosis and rapid hypokalemia. However, the most important concern is that bicarbonate may lead to cerebral acidosis *(56)* and possibly cerebral depression *(50,57)*. Studies of adult patients have demonstrated that use of bicarbonate did not improve outcome and caused increase risk for cerebral depression *(57)*. Thus, bicarbonate is generally not recommended for treatment of children with diabetes-mediated acidosis. Despite these issues, in some centers, bicarbonate is used to help correct severe acidosis.

Daily Medical Management of Children with Type 1 Diabetes

INSULIN DOSING AND ADJUSTMENT

In general, a child who is prepubertal and no longer making any endogenous insulin, requires approx 1.0 U of insulin per kilogram per day. During puberty, a dose as high as 1.5 U/kg/d may be needed to maintain good glycemic control *(45)*. A newly diagnosed patient who is metabolically stable will typically require slightly less insulin until the honeymoon period is over. In preadolescents, we generally start the daily dose at 0.7 U/kg/d; adolescents are generally started 0.8–1.0 U/kg/d. The insulin dose is adjusted as needed. It should be noted that in a newly diagnosed child, 4–7 d may be required for the insulin needs to stabilize. Children may be sent home with mild hyperglycemia, but they should always be ketone free prior to discharge. Blood sugar levels often change when the child is in the home environment because of improved exercise and return to normal diet; therefore, frequent contact with the family is indicated for several weeks. Use of supplemental insulin for hyperglycemia should only be started once a clear pattern for glycemic control is established. If started too soon, adjustments to the baseline insulin dose may be made unnecessarily.

Table 2
Types of Human Insulin and Duration of Action

Insulin preparation	Onset of action	Peak	Maximum duration
Rapid acting			
Humalog™ (lispro)	20–30 min	30–90 min	4–6 h
aspart			
Short acting			
regular	30–60 min	2–3 h	6–8 h
Intermediate acting			
NPH	2–4 h	6–10 h	14–18 h
lente	3–4 h	6–12 h	16–20 h
Long acting			
ultralente	6–10 h	10–16 h	20–24 h
Insulin glargine	1 h 10 min	No peak	24+ h

There are many types of insulin and potential insulin regimens available for treating children with diabetes, and therapy should be individualized. However, there are several principles that should guide the clinician in choice of therapy. These include (1) a regimen that allows the child to obtain good glycemic control (in general, this can only be accomplished by use of multiple injections), (2) basal and meal coverage should be provided, (3) the regimen should as closely as possible fit the patient's lifestyle, and (4) the regimen should confer as low a risk as possible for the development of hypoglycemia. Commonly used insulin regimens for children include (1) neutral protamine Hagedorn (NPH) given at breakfast and at bed with either regular or Humalog given at meals, (2) use of lente insulin in the same way as NPH given with regular or Humalog, or (3) ultralente insulin given at breakfast and supper with either regular or Humalog given at meals. Some physicians, including this author, have mixed Humalog with regular to improve postprandial glucose levels. However, there is no specific data available on the effect of mixing these types of insulin. Recently, physicians have been using the new insulin Lantus™ in the treatment of pediatric (mostly adolescent) patients. However, specific studies detailing the efficacy of this insulin are lacking in people under the age of 18 yr. Table 2 summarizes the commercially available human-derived types of insulin. There is increased risk of developing anti-insulin antibodies from animal insulin (58); thus, these insulins are rarely used in children.

Use of the Insulin Pump

The insulin pump, also called continuous subcutaneous insulin infusion or CSII, was originally pioneered in the late 1970s and has documented efficacy in the treatment of children and adolescents (59). The major advantage of the pump is the ability to easily provide bolus insulin for all meals and snacks without the need for an additional injection. This allows great flexibility in the child's diet. The insulin pump also provides flexible basal insulin rates resulting in therapy that provides the closest approximation to a normal pancreas. This allows the patient flexibility in activity and accommodates hormonally mediated changes in glucose levels, such as occurs with cortisol secretion in the early morning. Despite these obvious advantages, this mode of therapy has only recently experienced growing use in children. Reasons for lack of use may include the lack of publications comparing efficacy of pump therapy to multiple daily insulin injections, lack of experience by physicians and nurses, and the cost of the equipment *(60)*. To combat these problems, pump manufacturers have published several instruction manuals and have begun offering classes to health care providers that provide "hands-on" experience. Investigators at Yale, a pioneering site for pump use, have recently published results from a clinical trial demonstrating improved A_{1c} levels in adolescents treated with CSII, compared to those treated with multiple daily injections *(61)*. This is the first study to compare the pump to intensive insulin treatment. Currently, most Diabetes Centers select potential pump candidates from their older patients, who are considered to be the most adherent to therapy. However, some clinicians report improved A_{1c} levels in previously nonadherent to therapy adolescents. Recently, several centers have begun utilizing CSII in children under the age of 5, particularly for improvement in first-morning blood glucose levels *(62)*. Although there are no specific studies to document predictors of success, experience suggests that important predictors include the child's desire to participate in his or her own care and the child's, not just the parent's, desire to use pump therapy. Another important predictor is the child's and parent's ability to count carbohydrates. Training classes for patients and parents are very useful prior to pump placement, and frequent follow-up for several weeks is imperative.

When calculating insulin rates for use with the pump, calculate the total daily dose of insulin and subtract 20%. This new dose will be the total daily dose of insulin to be provided by the pump in 24 h. In general, 40–50% of the daily total should be provided as the basal infusion rate, and the rest should be divided as bolus doses with meals and snacks *(63)*. Calculation of the patient's sensitivity factor and response to carbohydrate load prior to institution of the pump is helpful. Serum glucose levels should be checked frequently during the first 24–48 h of CSII and should include postprandial glucose readings, as well as premeal values. More than one basal dose is likely to be necessary to maximize glucose control.

MONITORING GLUCOSE IN CHILDREN

The Diabetes Control and Complications Trial (DCCT) has demonstrated that good glycemic control reduces the risks of diabetes complications *(64)*. Thus, physicians treating children with diabetes have the enormous responsibility of maintaining as near-normal glucose control as is compatible with the physical and psychological well-being of each child. Optimizing therapy for the diabetic child cannot be accomplished without frequent monitoring of blood glucose levels, and both children and their parents should be taught how to perform self-blood glucose monitoring (SBGM) *(65)*. Ideally, glucose levels should be monitored before meals and before bed. Occasionally, middle of the night levels should be obtained to determine the presence of nocturnal hypoglycemia or to distinguish the cause of early morning hyperglycemia. It is important that caregivers and patients monitor blood sugar levels over time and adjust insulin based on a pattern, rather than changing insulin doses in reaction to isolated values that are out of the desired target range. There are many excellent glucose meters and lancet devices from which to choose. It is especially important that the lancet device provide a comfortable finger prick.

Measurement of glycosylated hemoglobin (A_{1c}) in blood is a useful index of control and provides a measure of the average blood glucose concentration over the preceding 2–3 mo *(66)*. The results are not invalidated by an isolated episode of hyper- or hypogly-

Table 3
Target Blood Glucose Levels for Children

Age (yr)	Before eating (no food for 2 h)		Bedtime (before bedtime snack)	
	(mg/dL)	(mmol/L)	(mg/dL)	(mmol/L)
<5 yr	90–180	5.0–10.0	120[a]–180	6.6–10.0
5–12 yr	80–180	4.4–10.0	100[a]–160	5.5–8.8
12 and over	80–120	4.4–6.7	100[a]–140	5.5–7.8

[a]If blood glucose is less than lower limit, add 15 g of carbohydrate to bedtime snack.

cemia; thus, A_{1c} is superior to random or fasting blood glucose measurements. Children should have an A_{1c} level checked every 3–4 mo in conjunction with their routine outpatient clinic visit. Both the value and its interpretation for glucose control should be provided to families in written form.

TARGET GLUCOSE LEVELS

The American Diabetes Association (ADA) has listed recommended glycemic control for nonpregnant individuals (2). Their position is based on the findings of decreased complications in tightly controlled patients as reported by the DCCT (64). Although this group documented that treatment regimens that reduced the average A_{1c} level to approx 7% were associated with fewer long-term microvascular complications, there were no children in the trial and relatively few adolescents. Thus pediatric diabetes centers have developed target glucose levels that vary by the age of the child and relation to meals. These are depicted by Table 3.

MONITORING FOR COMPLICATIONS AND ASSOCIATED MORBIDITY

The diabetic child should have yearly measurement of thyroid function, including free thyroxine and thyroid-stimulating hormone. These may be checked sooner in a symptomatic child. Although thyroid disease is the most likely autoimmune complication, diabetic children can also develop Addison's disease. Routine measure of cortisol is not necessary, but clinicians should rule out the development of adrenal insufficiency in any child in whom hypoglycemia is a frequent problem despite insulin reduction. Routine measurement of antithyroid or antiadrenal antibodies is generally unlikely to prove cost-effective.

In general, the occurrence of retinopathy or nephropathy in the pediatric population is rare with most cases occurring after puberty. The ADA currently recommends that annual screening for these complications begins at age 10 (2). However, there is evidence to suggest that prepubertal duration of diabetes may be a determining factor in the development of complications (2). Thus, most pediatric centers check prepubertal children for complications if the diabetes has been present for 5 yr. The screening method of choice for retinopathy is a dilated eye examination by an ophthomologist who is knowledgeable about both pediatric eye disease and diabetes. The screening method of choice for nephropathy is a "spot" urine albumin level. If urine albumin is greater than 30 µg/mg creatinine, a 24-h urine collection is undertaken. Routine urinalysis as the initial screening tool for nephropathy is generally not utilized in pediatrics. Retinopathy and nephropathy should be treated as soon as possible in pediatric patients. Micro-albuminuria as indicated by 24-h collection greater than 30 mg/dL indicates the need for treatment *(67)*. This is generally provided by an angiotensin-converting enzyme (ACE) inhibitor such as Captopril.

SPECIFIC GLUCOSE PATTERNS

Hypoglycemic Reactions. The definition of hypoglycemia varies with age. In a term infant, the blood sugar less than 45 mg/dL is considered low. By 1 yr of age, a blood sugar of 55 mg/dL is low, and in school-age children, a blood sugar less than 65 mg/dL is abnormally low *(68)*. All diabetic children experience a hypoglycemic reaction during the course of their disease; however, these episodes can be extremely frightening to both child and parent. The earliest signs and symptoms are those resulting from an outpouring of counterregulatory hormones. These include trembling, shaking, sweating, apprehension, hunger, and tachycardia. Once cerebral glucopenia occurs, other symptoms such as drowsiness, mood or personality changes, and mental confusion develop. If hypoglycemia is untreated, seizures and coma can occur. Each child may experience different signs and symptoms and teaching a patient and family how to recognize early symptoms of hypoglycemia is an imperative part of the early education process. Common causes of hypoglycemia in children include inadequate carbohydrate intake through missing meals or planned snacks, exercise in the absence of increasing carbohydrate intake, unrecognized evolution of the honeymoon phase after initial diagnosis, and errors in insulin dosage.

Hypoglycemia should be treated by quickly raising the blood glucose level using a carbohydrate-containing snack or drink providing 15 g of carbohydrate. It is important that families are instructed to retest the child's blood sugar in 15–20 min. Carbohydrate may be repeated if the blood sugar level is still low; however, it is important not to overcorrect hypoglycemia. Correction using ingested carbohydrate is preferable in the conscience patient; however, parents and teachers should also be instructed in the use of glucagon HCl (0.3–0.1 mg/kg, maximum 1-mg dose) given intramuscularly *(51)*. Glucagon is particularly useful when the patient is losing consciousness, unconscious, or is vomiting. Unfortunately, emesis is a common side effect of glucagon. Patients should be instructed to notify the physician should they have an unexplained, or severe, episode of hypoglycemia, so that the insulin dose can be adjusted prior to the next outpatient clinic visit. If exercise has been the precipitating factor, the patient should be instructed to take additional carbohydrates prior to exercise, and if hypoglycemia persists, then reduce the appropriate insulin dose by 10–20%. It should be noted that hypoglycemia should be verified by checking a glucose level as soon as possible. This is important to document severity and so that patients who do not have true hypoglycemia do not receive treatment. In patients who have had consistently high blood sugar levels, symptoms from release of counterregulatory hormones may occur in response to rapid lowering of glucose into the normal range *(69)*. However, the blood glucose levels would not meet the criteria for hypoglycemia, and treatment would only cause hyperglycemia.

Somogyi Phenomenon. Hypoglycemic episodes that manifest in the late night or early morning and that alternate with hyperglycemia should arouse the suspicion of the Somogyi phenomenon. This syndrome has been described as "hypoglycemia begetting hyperglycemia" and is also called "rebound hyperglycemia." The Somogyi phenomenon is caused by an outpouring of counterregulatory hormones in response to insulin-induced hypoglycemia *(69,70)*. Cortisol and growth hormone act as insulin antagonists. Hyperglycemia is also caused when hypoglycemia causes increased endogenous hepatic glucose production. This liver release of glucose is unrestrained and often results in hyperglycemia, rather than simple correction of hypoglycemia *(71,72)*. Symptoms of the Somogyi phenomenon may include early morning sweating, night terrors, and headaches. Appropriate treatment consists of reducing the dose of the evening intermediate-acting insulin.

Dawn Phenomenon. The early morning rise in blood glucose may also be the result of waning activity of biologically available insulin unrelated to the action of counterregulatory hormones *(73)*. This is called the Dawn phenomenon. Normal children are able to increase their insulin secretion to compensate for the nocturnal surges in cortisol and growth hormone that antagonize insulin action. However, the diabetic child is unable to mount an appropriate increase in insulin secretion. Thus, the peak in these counterregulatory hormone levels causes a rapid rise in the blood glucose concentration between 2 AM and 6 AM, in the absence of antecedent hypoglycemia *(73)*. Recognition of this condition requires measurement of blood glucose between 2 AM and 6 AM. Unfortunately, the Dawn phenomenon may be difficult to manage. Increase in the dose of intermediate-acting insulin could result in hypoglycemia. Thus, moving the administration time of the intermediate insulin is, in general, the best solution. Management of the Dawn phenomenon is a definite benefit of the insulin pump because the pump provides ability to set multiple basal rates to give the appropriate insulin dose at the appropriate time.

Medical Nutrition Therapy for Children with Type 1 Diabetes

The nutritional requirements of diabetic children are similar to those of healthy non-diabetic children of similar age, sex, weight, and activity, eating the foods of their own cultural, social, and ethnic background *(74,75)*. Thus there is no special diet for the diabetic child; rather, there are nutritional requirements that must be met for optimal growth and development *(75)*. For example, children require slightly more protein than adults. Daily provision of 1.2 g protein/kg of body wt meets the needs of most children and adolescents; however, very athletic children may have slightly higher needs. Meeting appropriate calorie intake is important. Table 4 provides a list of caloric guidelines by gender and age group. The distribution of these calories should comprise approx 50–55% carbohydrate, less than 30% fat, and 15–20% protein. The total daily caloric intake is generally divided to provide 20% at breakfast, 20% at lunch, and 30% at dinner, leaving 30% of calories to be given with snacks *(76)*. Young children generally require three snacks in addition to meals. These are given mid-morning, mid-afternoon, and evening. Older children often do not need a mid-morning snack, and these calories may be moved to another meal. In general, pubertal adolescents tend to eat large mid-afternoon snacks. These calories may be best taken from dinner. Although appropriate calorie intake should be the starting point for management, the needs of each child must be separately and individually planned and adjusted.

Many patients and families report that dietary change is the hardest component of diabetes management *(77)*. Recognition of the role of carbohydrates in changing glycemic control has greatly influenced the current management of children. Previous dietary recommendations for diabetic children have stressed regularity of the eating pattern which was matched according to the chosen insulin regimen *(74)*. However, prior to developing diabetes, many children have had a dietary intake that was quite flexible. Prescribing a restrictive or nonflexible diet imposes unnecessary stress; therefore, it is

Table 4
Calorie Requirements for Children

Age (gender)	Calories per kg	Average
0–6 mo (both)	108	650
6 mo–1 yr (both)	98	850
1–3 yr (both)	109	1300
7–10 yr (both)	90	1800
11–14 yr (girls)	47	2000
11–14 yr (boys)	55	2500
15–18 yr (girls)	40	2200
15–18 yr (boys)	45	3000

Source: Adapted from Food and Nutrition Board,
National Academy of Sciences–National Research
Council. Recommended Dietray Allowances, 10th ed.
National Academy Press, Washington, DC, 1989.

important that children and parents be rapidly taught the principles of carbohydrate counting. Generally, the first stage teaches recognition of carbohydrates (75). A fixed insulin regimen based on a set carbohydrate intake per meal is then prescribed by the physician. It is important that the child's actual diet be carefully considered before the fixed carbohydrate diet is implemented. This stage of managing dietary intake can be discouraging for children if it represents significant change from their usual intake. The next stage of teaching should encompass quantification of carbohydrate, called "carbohydrate counting." Once patients learn to do this, they can rapidly pass to level-three education, dosing rapid or short-acting insulin based on carbohydrate intake. Once this stage of learning is accomplished, the amount of carbohydrate at a given meal or snack can be changed. This method of dosing insulin is the most physiologic and allows normal flexibility in the child's diet. Furthermore, such a plan does not foster rebellion and stealth in obtaining desired food. Flexible carbohydrate intake with insulin dosing based on carbohydrate quantity is especially helpful for adolescents who tend to have erratic eating habits. This method lends itself well to insulin pump therapy.

Exercise

Exercise is an integral component of growth and development. No form of exercise, including competitive sports of any kind, should be forbidden to the diabetic child. Furthermore, the physiologic and psychologic benefits of exercise suggest that exercise should be greatly encouraged in diabetic children. Although the physiologic adaptation in energy homeostasis associated with exercise in normal and insulin-dependent diabetic adults has been extensively investigated (79,80), direct information in children is lacking. The major complication of exercise in diabetes is the occurrence of hypoglycemic reactions during or shortly after vigorous exercise. In the diabetic child, there are two major contributing factors to hypoglycemia with exercise. The first is improved insulin sensitivity, which is a well-documented benefit of exercise (78). The duration of improved sensitivity, and therefore the risk of hypoglycemia, may vary depending on the intensity of exercise and the duration of the exercise. To best determine the management, the child's blood sugar should be monitored immediately prior to the event, midway during the activity, immediately after the event and 4–6 h after the event. Once the blood sugar pattern is known, the clinician will be able to determine how best to prevent the occurrence of hypoglycemia. Prevention should include reduction of the appropriate insulin dose, increased carbohydrate intake, or both. Another cause of hypoglycemia during exercise is an increased rate of insulin absorption from its injection site because of increased blood flow in the exercising limbs (81). Thus, one approach to minimize hypoglycemia is to choose an injection site least likely to be affected by the exercise. However, from the practical point of view, exercise usually involves all limbs, with an increased blood flow throughout the body. Through careful blood sugar monitoring and planning of exercise, children can avoid hypoglycemia. It is important that families recognize the risk while also understanding the importance of exercise in their child's well-being and normal development.

Managing Concurrent Illness or Surgery in a Child with Type 1 Diabetes

Infections are no more common than in a diabetic child than in a nondiabetic child; however, insulin needs increase during infection. If these increased needs are not met, the risk of ketoacidosis is high. Families should be taught that during an illness, they should monitor the child's urine for the presence of ketones, regardless of the blood sugar level. Additional insulin should be administered for either hyperglycemia, ketosis, or both. Typically, 10–20% of the total daily insulin dose should be administered in the form of rapid- or short-acting insulin before each meal. Patients who are vomiting should be advised not to discontinue insulin injections. If vomiting precludes ingestion of clear liquids, admission to the hospital for intravenous therapy with glucose and electrolytes is warranted. Patients and families should receive education regarding "sick day" management and should have their insulin supplemental dose recalculated for them at each outpatient visit.

Most surgeries require that the patient fast; thus, insulin adjustments are needed. If surgery is elective, the patient should be instructed on insulin adjustment and, if possible, the physician should speak to the anesthesiologist. Typically, the intermediate- or long-acting insulin dose is cut in half on the morning of surgery. The blood glucose concentration should be monitored at periodic intervals before, during, and after surgery so that glucose levels remain approx 100–160 mg/dL. Rapid- or short-acting insulin is given subcutaneously, every 3–4 h as needed to maintain euglycemia. For prolonged or complex surgery, it may be preferable to administer insulin intravenously. Whenever possible, the surgery should be scheduled for early morning so that insulin adjustments need only be made for the day of surgery. An exception is for children treated with Lantus™, given before bedtime. Because of its long-acting nature, the biological effects of this insulin would be present throughout the day of surgery. Thus, the dose given the night before surgery should be halved. Intravenous fluids should be provided during the surgery and should be continued until the patient is awake and capable of eating. The rate of infusion should provide maintenance fluid requirements, plus estimated losses during surgery. Whenever possible, the fluids should not contain greater than 5% dextrose. During the post-op period, correction of hyperglycemia using rapid-acting insulin may be necessary. Return to the normal insulin dosing schedule should be done when the patient is eating normally.

If emergency surgery is required, and the patient has taken his or her normal daily insulin dose, frequent monitoring of blood glucose levels is indicated. Adjustment of an intravenous infusion of dextrose and insulin should be conducted as needed to maintain blood glucose levels at 100–160 mg/dL.

Long-Term Outcome and Future Directions for Type 1 Diabetes

As the diabetic child progresses to adulthood, the risk of diabetes-related complications increases. Statistics compiled by the National Diabetes Data Group indicate that retinopathy is present in 20% of type 1 diabetics after 10 yr and in 45–60% after 20 yr of disease *(82)*. The incidence of proliferative retinopathy increases progressively with increasing duration of disease. Diabetic nephropathy has an incidence of 40% after 25 yr of diabetes *(83)*. Emphasis should be placed on securing full insurance coverage for all diabetes supplies and for patient education, including psychological counseling if indicated. Only by thorough education and patient empowerment can complications be minimized.

Although specific data for children is missing, the bulk of clinical, experimental, and biochemical studies strongly suggest an association between control and later development of complications, although genetic predisposition or resistance to development of these complications also plays a role *(84)*. Recent improvements in insulin delivery, home glucose monitoring, and new emphasis on improving glycemic control are likely to improve the long-term outlook for children diagnosed with type 1 diabetes. National databanks that carefully review patients' progress would be helpful in documenting improvement in complications and comorbidity.

The ability to identify autoantibodies present in high-risk individuals and the protracted course of islet destruction have directed research aimed at preventing the clinical onset of disease by arresting the ongoing destruction of islets through immunologic suppression *(85,86)*. Among the first trials were those using cyclosporin *(87)*. Recently, the National Institutes of Health has targeted prevention as a major goal by sponsoring TrialNet, a group of investigators who will select the best prevention-trial medications and coordinate implemetation of these trials.

Transplantation of whole pancreas or islet cells has been successfully utilized in adults *(88,89)* but the immunosuppressive therapy required has thus far precluded its use in growing children. Transplantation of isolated fetal pancreatic islets to enhance growth potential, and their culture prior to transplantation, may overcome the problems of rejection and of adequate islet tissue.

TYPE 2 DIABETES IN CHILDREN AND ADOLESCENTS

Incidence and Prevalence

The prevelance of type 2 diabetes in children ranges from 4.1 per 1000 of 12- to 19-yr-olds to 50.9 per 1000 in 15- to 19-yr-old Pima Indians in Arizona. The disease is reported in many populations, including Asia and the Middle East *(6)*. This form of diabetes most commonly occurs after the onset of puberty. Among children in the United States, the mean age at diagnosis is 12–14 yr of age. Girls are more often affected than boys. Evidence clearly suggests that certain children are at greater risk than others for developing this condition. Risk factors include obesity, family history of type 2 diabetes, exposure to diabetes *in utero*, and signs of insulin resistance *(6,7)*. Evidence also suggests that certain ethnic groups are at higher risk. These include American Indians, Mexican-Americans, African-Americans, and Tongan-Americans *(5,6)*.

Etiology and Pathogenesis

To date only a few studies have been conducted evaluating the cause of type 2 diabetes as it presents in children and adolescents. These studies suggest that the etiology is similar to type 2 diabetes in adults, with one likely cause being insulin resistance. Studies have demonstrated high fasting and postmeal insulin levels in affected and high-risk children (90,91). Our group recently documented insulin resistance in a small number of adolescents with type 2 diabetes using a hyperinsulinemic euglycemic clamp (92). Although insulin resistance has often been viewed to be the principal cause of type 2 diabetes in adults, recent publications suggest that beta cell dysfunction also plays a role (93–95). Current theory suggests that β-cell secretion, although higher than in nonaffected individuals, is inadequate to meet the increased needs conferred by insulin resistance, and eventually β-cells produce little insulin (94). In children, evidence suggests that β-cell function persists. but similar to adults, it is inadequate to control hyperglycemia. We used a Sustacal™ Challenge test to document continued beta cell function 1 yr after diagnosis (92).

Obesity seems to be the universal environmental trigger for the onset of type 2 diabetes (96–98). However, the relative contribution of genetics and environment to the development of obesity is unknown. Each of the ethnic groups noted to be at high risk for development of type 2 diabetes also carries a large incidence of obesity (99). Multiple studies in adults (100,101) have documented less insulin sensitivity in obese individuals. Studies by our group (102) and others (103) have demonstrated the heritability of insulin sensitivity. Thus, it is possible that these children inherit the propensity for both insulin resistance and obesity, which places them at risk for development of type 2 diabetes. However, there is little doubt that the environment plays a pivitol role in the development of obesity. Unfortunately, the incidence of obesity in children is ever increasing, with recent reports suggesting doubling of the incidence in the past 20 yr (104).

Clinical Presentation

Presenting symptoms in most children and adolescents include polyuria, polydipsia, hyperglycemia, and dehydration. Ketoacidosis may be present (6). Although a history of weight loss may be illicited on patient interview, the weight loss may not have been noticed or, if noticed, may not have caused concern. Some patients complain of fatigue or abdominal pain. Adolescent females may have a monilial vaginal infection. Some patients may be diagnosed by screening tests performed by their physician upon recognition of multiple risk factors.

Although its occurrence is rare, occasionally some of the patients may present with nonketotic hyperosmolar coma. In this condition, the glucose is greater than 500 mg/dL and serum osmolality exceeds 300 mOsm/kg. Ketones are absent in serum and urine (45,105).

Medical Management of Type 2 Diabetes Presenting in Children and Adolescents

The first line of therapy for type 2 diabetes in children is prevention. Early recognition of clinical risk factors should prompt thorough discussion with parents and patient regarding the need to prevent development of type 2 diabetes. Of particular importance is a dietary evaluation. In children with body mass index (BMI) greater than 28, weight loss management should be instituted *(106)*. Weight reduction should occur using calorie reduction, with the weight loss goal of 1–2 lbs/wk. In actively growing children, depending on the degree of obesity, a weight-maintenance diet may be adequate because the natural obtainment of height can normalize the BMI. Calorie reduction should not be more than 10–20% of the child's normal intake during the first few weeks *(107)*. Marked reduction in calories will likely result in nonadherence to the program. In many families with obese children, fat intake is excessive. Children at high risk for development of type 2 diabetes are also at high risk for development of Syndrome X *(108)*. Clearly, these children should take less than 30% of their total calories from fat.

Increasing exercise is the second major component for prevention of type 2 diabetes. Many obese children are significantly deconditioned and unable to participate in vigorous activity until reconditioning occurs. Furthermore, if exercise has not been a regular habit for these children, they are likely to become discouraged in the face of too vigorous a change. For these reasons, increasing activity should occur in stages. The earliest phases should include a walking program, with later progression to swimming, running, and team sports. It is important that the psychological and physical benefits of exercise be stressed by the physician and the health care team. The home environment may be preclusive to outdoor exercise. In these situations, the health care team should help families pursue possible exercise locations, including the school or community youth center.

Once a child develops hyperglycemia, pharmacologic therapy is indicated in addition to dietary management. Very few studies have been done evaluating medical therapy for children with type 2 diabetes. Metformin has been approved by the Food and Drug Administration (FDA) for use in children, and one group has published a relatively large study of is efficacy *(109)*. Although this study documented safety, the protocol was designed using Metformin as monotherapy of any patient whose A_{1c} was less than 12%. The trial was ended early secondary to many patients requiring insulin "rescue." Our group has recently published results from our clinic using Metformin and insulin therapy *(110)*. In our clinic, we generally start insulin on any patient whose blood glucose level is greater than 300 mg/dL or in any patient with acidosis at the time of presentation. Metformin is added once the blood sugar is less than 300 mg/dL, and insulin is weaned by 20% per day once low normal blood sugar levels develop. Metformin is used as initial monotherapy only in those patients whose initial blood glucose levels are less than 300 mg/dL, if that patient has a normal pH. We documented efficacy of Metformin used as monotherapy or in addition to insulin and we found no major side effects from the drug *(110)*. Other oral agents have been used, but, to date, no published results exist for these. One new study that is promising is an evaluation of Glucovance™, a combination insulin sensitizer and insulin-secretion aide. More studies are needed to best determine management of type 2 diabetes in children, but particular emphasis should be placed on weight loss management and prevention of obesity.

The fluid and electrolyte management of hyperosmolar coma is similar to that for ketoacidosis. However, insulin should be given with extreme caution to prevent a rapid fall in glucose and osmolality. Generally insulin is given once the blood glucose level has remained stable for several hours following the initial fall from intravenous fluid administration. More aggressive use of insulin can induce cerebral edema *(46)*.

OTHER RECOGNIZED TYPES OF DIABETES

Transient Diabetes of the Newborn

Onset of persistent insulin-requiring diabetes before the age of 6 mo is most unusual and is called transient diabetes mellitus of the newborn. This syndrome is rare, with an incidence of 1/4000 *(111)*, and is distinct from type 1 diabetes because it is not associated with HLA haplotypes and no evidence exists of autoimmunity *(111,112)*. Recent research suggests that this syndrome is the result of an imprinted gene for diabetes (chromosome 6) mapping to 6q24 *(113)*.

The onset is generally during the first week of life. Its duration is self-limited, lasting only several weeks to months before spontaneous resolution *(114,115)*. It generally occurs in infants who are small for gestational age *(114)* and is characterized by hyperglycemia with minimal or no ketonemia or ketonuria *(115)*. Although the basal insulin concentration is normal, the insulin secretory response to glucose or tolbutamide is low or absent *(115)*. Following spontaneous recovery, the insulin responses to these same stimuli are brisk and normal. Once the disease is recognized, therapy with insulin is mandatory. Treatment with a long-acting insulin such as Ultralente results in dramatic improvement and accelerated growth and weight gain. Attempts at gradually withdrawing the insulin therapy may be made as soon as recurrent hypoglycemia becomes manifest or after 2 mo of age *(114)*. Transient diabetes of the newborn should be distinguished from severe hyperglycemia occurring in diseases associated with abnormalities of the central nervous system and disturbances of electrolytes. These patients are usually older infants rather than newborns, and they respond promptly to rehydration with a minimal requirement for insulin *(116)*.

Transient diabetes is associated with an increased risk for development of type 2 diabetes *(117,118)*, and there have been a few case reports documenting persistence and development of permanent type 1 diabetes. However, permanent diabetes has not recurred in any affected infant who has recovered.

Genetic Defects of β-Cell Function

MATURITY-ONSET DIABETES OF THE YOUNG

The term "maturity-onset diabetes of the young" (MODY) refers to a type of diabetes syndrome chracterized by an age of onset less than 25 yr, the correction of fasting hyperglycemia without insulin for at least 2 yr following diagnosis, nonketotic disease, and an autosomal dominant mode of inheritance *(119)*. The striking distinguishing feature of MODY is the strong family history. The incidence varies from 0.14% in Germany to 10% in Caucasian-French families. Less than 5% of diabetes in children is caused by MODY *(120)*.

To date, research suggests that mutations in five genes cause MODY. These genes encode hepatocyte nuclear factor-α, (MODY 1), glucokinase (MODY 2), hepatocyte nuclear factor-1α (MODY 3), insulin promotor factor-1 (MODY 4), and hepatocyte nuclear factor-1β (MODY 5) *(120,121)*. MODY 2 accounts for most of the cases in children, and MODY 1, 2, or 3 account for most cases occurring in Caucasians *(120,122)*. There are no statistically significant associations between this type of diabetes and specific HLAs, autoimmunity, or islet-cell antibodies *(122)*.

The diagnosis of MODY can be made through a careful review of the patient's clinical course, severity of hyperglycemia, and family history. The disease is slowly progressive and may be asymptomatic, with some individuals who do not require insulin even after many years of follow-up. Many patients are only diagnosed by oral glucose tolerance testing. In approximately one half of the affected families, there is direct vertical transmission through three generations, and 50% of tested siblings have impaired glucose tolerance *(119)*. MODY can be ruled out in any patient who has islet cell autoantibodies. Testing for MODY mutations is expensive and, thus, should be reserved only for those patients strongly believed to be affected. Distinguishing MODY from type 2 diabetes presenting in childhood is best done through identification of the risk factors for type 2 diabetes, particularly obesity, and through comparison of the clinical course.

Maturity-onset diabetes of the young in children and adolescents can often be managed thorough diet and oral medication. Insulin therapy should be started if glycemic control cannot be maintained or if growth is not normal on conservative management *(123)*.

Atypical Diabetes Mellitus

This is a subtype of MODY which occurs in approx 10% of African-Americans with youth-onset diabetes *(8)*. The patients present with acute-onset diabetes often associated with weight loss, ketosis, and ketoacidosis. Months to years following diagnosis, a non-insulin-dependent clinical course develops. It is at this time that the disease can be distinguished from type 1 diabetes. Approximately 50% of patients with atypical diabetes are obese *(120)*. In this specific type of diabetes, significant ketoacidosis can be found at time of presentation, but the patient rapidly becomes non-insulin-dependent. This type of diabetes has been predominantly described in black adolescents *(8)*. Further studies will need to be done to determine if this type of diabetes is in any way related to type 2 diabetes presenting in children.

Diabetes Secondary to Disease of the Exocrine Pancreas

PANCREATECTOMY

Diabetes resulting from partial or total removal of the pancreas should be treated with exogenous insulin. The most common cause for this in children is partial removal of the pancreas secondary to persistant neonatal hyperinsulinism.

CYSTIC FIBROSIS-RELATED DIABETES

People with cystic fibrosis (CF) have a high incidence of diabetes and abnormal glucose tolerance. This type of diabetes is called CF-related diabetes (CFRD) to reflect its unique nature and emphasize the need for disease specific management. Recent evidence suggests that 15% of adult patients have CFRD and as many as 75% have abnormal glucose tolerance *(124)*. The incidence is expected to increase secondary to improved patient longevity and the result of increased emphasis on screening for diabetes in this population. The North American CF Foundation has recently emphasized the importance of recognizing and treating this disease, and in 1998 it sponsored a consensus consortium to standardize diagnosis and management *(125)*. Although more outcome studies are needed, the current body of literature suggests that CFRD is associated with worsened morbidity and morality *(126,127)*. Furthermore, microvascular diabetes complications have been well reported to occur in these patients *(128,129)*. Insulin deficiency has been well recognized as on cause of CFRD *(125)*. However, the defect in insulin secretion occurs at an early age *(128)*, whereas CFRD generally does not develop until adolescence or early adulthood *(124)*. Recent research has also described the con-

Table 5
Glucose Tolerance Categories in Cystic Fibrosis

	Abbreviation	Fasting blood glucose (mg/dL)	2-h postprandial glucose (mg/dL)
Normal glucose tolerance	NGT	<126	<150
Impaired glucose tolerance	IGT	<126	151–200
CF-Related diabetes without fasting hyperglycemia	CFRD w/o FH	<126	>200
CF-Related diabetes with fasting hyperglycemia	CFRD w/ FH	>126	>200

tribution of insulin resistance and high hepatic glucose production as contributing causes to development of CFRD (129–131).

Current management recommendations for CFRD includes only insulin management (125). However, this may be revised once more studies have been completed. When implementing insulin therapy, several things need to be considered. In general, these patients tend to have the most problem with postprandial hyperglycemia; thus, emphasis should be placed on premeal insulin. Insulin Lys-Pro is an excellent choice if patients do not choose to snack between meals or if they undergo exercise between meals. However, in patients who frequently snack, a mixture of Lys-Pro and regular insulin may be necessary to avoid additional injections at time of snack. Long-acting insulin is often not necessary to achieve euglycemia; however, when needed, ultralente is an excellent choice because of its basal nature. Patients with CFRD often do not experience early warning sings of hypoglycemia; thus, emphasis should be placed on hypogycemia avoidance. Intermediate-acting insulins can be associated with hypoglycemia unless meal/snacks are appropriately timed. An intermediate-acting insulin mixed with regular insulin is the best choice for patients who require nighttime enteral feedings.

People with CF have high energy expenditure resulting in calorie requirements 130–150% of the Recommended Daily Allowance for age-matched children and adults (132). Furthermore, malnutrition has been associated with worsened morbidiity and mortality (133). Thus, diabetes management should not interfere with nutrition (125). Given the unique dietary need of people with CF, in general the best way to manage CFRD is to teach carbohydrate counting with flexible dosing of rapid or short-acting insulin based on carbohydrate intake. Our group has had excellent results with use of the insulin pump in this population.

The 1998 consensus participants have recognized four categories of glucose tolerance in CF. These are provided in Table 5. A fifth category, transient CFRD, can occur with or without fasting hyperglycemia. Currently, treatment is recommended only for those who have fasting hyperglycemia in addition to postprandial hyperglycemia (CFRD with FH). Some practices, including ours, currently offer insulin to patients without fasting hyperglycemia, but high postprandial glucose levels (CFRD w/o FH), if, additionally, the patient has difficulty with weight loss or worsened pulmonary function. Studies by our group (134) and others (135) have documented protein catabolism in people with CF. Insulin is an anticatabolic hormone (40). Given the documentation of insulin deficiency in these patients, use of insulin in those with declining clinical status and paucity of muscle tissue makes empiric sense. Research is underway to determine whether or not treatment of patients without fasting hyperglycemia should be recommended. Research evaluating safety and efficacy of oral agents is also underway.

Genetic Defects in Insulin Action

LEPRECHAUNISM

Leprechaunism has also been called Donahue syndrome and Rabson–Medenhall Syndrome. It is a rare disorder characterized by intrauterine and postnatal growth impairment, diminished fat and muscle mass, characteristic facies, abnormal gonadal function, hyperinsulinemia, and early death *(136)*. Abnormalities of the insulin receptor gene cause this syndrome *(137)*. Early in the course of disease, these patients have high circulating insulin levels. Recent research has suggested that the progression of disease is the result of the decline in insulin levels *(138)*.

TYPE A SYNDROME OF INSULIN RESISTANCE

This form of insulin resistance is associated with abnormalities of the insulin receptor *(139)*. Type A occurs in females generally between the ages of 8 and 16 yr and is characterized by the presence of acanthosis nigricans, virilization, and amenorrhea (often associated with polycystic ovaries), hyperglycemia, and high circulating levels of insulin. The concentration of insulin receptors on circulating monocytes is reduced and antibodies to the insulin receptor are not found in the serum. Further studies are needed to determine the relationship between this form of diabetes and type 2 diabetes presenting in children and adolescents.

LIPODYSTROPHY

Familial lipodystrophy (congenital generalized lipodystrophy) is an extremely rare autosomal recessive disease affecting all ethnic groups. Patients have nearly complete absence of adipose tissue from birth *(140)*. They have accelerated growth, voracious appetite increased basal metabolic rate, and advanced bone age. Acanthosis nigricans is common, and severe hyperinsulinemia and high serum triglyceride concentrations are present during infancy *(141)*. Adolescent patients often develop eruptive xanthomas and acute pancreatitis. Fatty infiltration of the liver occurs and can cause cirrhosis. Severe insulin resistance occurs with resultant hyperglycemia *(142)*. Children with this syndrome are best managed with high-dose insulin therapy. However, studies are needed to determine safety and efficacy of oral agents.

Genetic Syndromes

A number of rare genetic syndromes is associated with increased incidence of diabetes or carbohydrate intolerance. These syndromes represent a broad spectrum of diseases, including Werner or Cockayne syndromes and Prader–Willi syndrome. The cause of each syndrome is unique to the disease and discussion is beyond the scope of this chapter. Treatment is with insulin, dietary managment, or oral agents, depending on the syndrome.

Diabetes Associated with Endocrinopathies

States of excess of counterregulatory hormones, such as acromegaly and Cushing syndrome can lead to insulin resistance and subsequent glucose intolerance. The mechanisms by which this occurs have been discussed in the subsection on metabolic changes associated with uncontrolled type 1 diabetes. Medical management includes treating the underlying endocrinopathy and treatment with exogenous insulin. Insulin needs may be high secondary to the underlying insulin resistance.

Diabetes Secondary to Drugs and Chemicals

Certain drugs and chemicals cause hyperglycemia. Thiazide diuretics and β-blockers, used to treat children with heart problems, do so through reduction in total-body potassium with subsequent decreased insulin secretion. The effect is dose dependent and reveres by potassium replacement *(143)*. Protease inhibitors, used to treat children with human immunodeficiency virus (HIV) infection, have been found to cause hyperglycemia. The cause seems to be from induction of insulin resistance *(144)*. Some atypical antipsychotic agents cause hyperglycemia, but are rarely used in children.

Chemotherapeutic agents administered to either treat cancer or to prevent rejection following organ transplant are associated with hyperglycemia *(145)*. Many of these agents decrease insulin action, including high-dose corticosteroids, tacrolimus, cyclosporin, and gusperimus *(145)*. The chemotherapeutic agent L-aspariginase, often used to treat acute lymphocytic leukemia, interferes with insulin secretion *(146)* Treatment for chemotherapeutic-induced diabetes is always exogenous insulin administration.

PSYCHOLOGICAL ASPECTS OF DIABETES MANAGEMENT

Neither type 1 or type 2 diabetes has been associated with any specific personality disorders or psychopathology; however, psychological counseling is often necessary because many patients have difficulty adjusting to the disease. Diabetes in a child affects the lifestyle and interpersonal relationship of the entire family unit *(147,148)*. Feelings of anxiety and guilt are common in parents. Overprotection on the part of parents is frequent and is not in the best interests of the patient. Perception of the likelihood of developing complications and of decreased life-span in type 1 diabetes fosters parental anxiety. Some parents also have additionally anxiety regarding the potential risk of their other children developing the disease. Similar feelings are observed in families with other chronic disorders.

Diabetic children and teens often have problems with denial and anger, and feelings of being different or of being alone are common. These feelings find expression in nonadherence to therapy, including nutrition and insulin therapy, or noncompliance with self-monitoring. Signs of extreme anger and denial can include deliberate overdosing with insulin resulting in hypoglycemia, and omission of insulin, resulting in ketoacidosis. Psychological counseling is always indicated when these problems are noted.

The key to improving psychological well-being is patient and family education. It is particularly important to foster the perception of the child as normal. Parents should be encouraged to allow their children to participate in all social activities. Nutrition management that promotes flexibility is particularly helpful in teenagers. Peer discussion groups led by local associations are excellent venues for discussing the common feelings of isolation and frustration. Summer camps allow children an excellent opportunity for learning and sharing under expert supervision. The company of many peers with similar problems permits the development of newer insights for the diabetic child.

In addition to the problems faced by other diabetics, children with type 2 diabetes have some unique challenges. Most are significantly obese and have low self-esteem, in part, because of their weight. The child's recognition of their obesity further contributes to feelings of isolation and to sadness. Many of these children have sought comfort for feelings of sadness by overeating. Thus, impacting change for these children needs to targeted at improving self-esteem and finding new ways to cope with stress rather than overeating. Furthermore, many of these children come from families where overweight and obesity is common, in part as a result of poor dietary habits and inactivity. Thus, change must involve the entire family.

Children who have secondary diabetes suffer the emotional trauma of their primary disease, in addition to the new burden of developing diabetes. The diabetes team needs to be cognizant of these feelings and work hand-in-hand with the child's primary pediatrician and other subspecialty teams in order to effectively impact change.

CONCLUSION

The endocrinologist faces many challenges when treating children with diabetes. Each type of childhood diabetes must be managed in a disease-specific manner. Effective communication, patience and a multidisciplinary team approach are the keys to success.

REFERENCES

1. The Expert Committee on the Diagnosis and Classification of Diabetes Mellitus. Report of the Expert Committee on the diagnosis and classification of diabetes mellitus. American Diabetes Association: Clinical Practice Recommendations 2002. Diabetes Care 2002;25(1):S5–S20.
2. American Diabetes Association. Position Statement: Standard of medical care for patients with diabetes mellitus. American Diabetes Association: Clinical Practice Recommendations 2002. Diabetes Care 2002;25(1):S33–S49.
3. Nerup J, Mandrup-Poulsen T, Molvig J. The HLA-IDDM association: Implications for etiology and pathogenesis of IDDM. Diabetes Metab Rev 1987;3:779.
4. Riley WI, Winter WE, Mclaren NK. Identification of insulin-dependent diabetes mellitus before onset of clinical symptoms. J Pediatr 1988;112:314.
5. American Diabetes Association. Type 2 diabetes in children and adolescents. Diabetes Care 2000;23:381–389.
6. Fagot-Campagna, Pettit, DJ, Egelgan, MM, et al. Type 2 diabetes among North American children and adolescents an epidemiologic review and public health perspective. J. Pediatr 2000;136:664–672.
7. Fagot-Campagna, A, Narayan, KMV. Type 2 diabetes in children. Br Med J 2001;322:377.
8. Winter WE, Maclaren NK, Riley WJ, et al. Maturity-Onset diabetes of youth in Black Americans. N Engl J Med 1987;316:285.
9. Kyllo CJ, Nuttall FQ. Prevalence of diabetes mellitus in school-age children in Minnesota. Diabetes 1978;27:57.
10. Kenny, S.J., Aubert, RE, Geiss, LS. Prevalence and incidence of insulin dependent diabetes mellitus. National Instutues of Health Proceedings, 2001.
11. Calnan M, Peckham CS. Incidence of insulin dependent diabetes in the first 16 years of life. Lancet 1977;1:589.
12. Holmgren G, Samuelson G, Hermansson B. The prevalence of diabetes mellitus: A study of children and their relatives in a northern Swedish county. Clin Genet 1974;5:465.
13. Cowie, CC, Eberhardt, MS. Sociodemographic characteristics of persons with diabetes. Proc Natl Instit Health.
14. LaPorte RE, Fishbein HA, Drash AL, et al. The incidence of insulin dependent diabetes mellitus in Allegheny County, Pennsylvania (1965–1976). Diabetes 1981;30:279.

15. LaPorte RE, Dorman JS, Orchard TJ. Preventing insulin dependent diabetes mellitus: the environmental challenge. Br Med J 1987;295:479.

16. Bloch CA, Clemons P, Sperling MA. Puberty decreases insulin sensitivity. J Pediatr 1987;110:481.

17. Amiel SA, Sherwin RS, Simonson DC, et al. Impaired insulin action in puberty. A contributing factor to poor glycemic control in adolescents with diabetes. N Engl J Med 1986;315:215.

18. Craighead JE. Current views on the etiology of insulin-dependent diabetes mellitus. N Engl J Med 1978;299:1439.

19. MacCuish AC, Irvine WJ. Autoimmunological aspects of diabetes mellitus. Clin Endocrinol Metab 1975;4:435.

20. Drash AL. The etiology of diabetes mellitus. N Engl J Med 1978;300:1211.

21. Atkinson, MA, Mclaren, NK. The pathogenesis of insulin-dependent diabetes mellitus. N Engl J Med 1994;331:1428.

22. Martin, S, Pawlowski, B, Greulich, B, et al. Natural course of remission in IDDM during 1st year after diagnosis. Diabetes Care 1992;15(1):66–74.

23. Neufeld M, MacLaren NK, Riley NJ, et al. Islet cell and other organ-specific antibodies in U.S. Caucasians and blacks with insulin-dependent diabetes mellitus. Diabetes 1980;29:589.

24. Irvine WF, McCallum CF, Gray RS, et al. Pancreatic islet-cell antibodies in diabetes mellitus correlated with the duration and type of diabetes, coexistent autoimmune disease and HLA type. Diabetes 1977;26:138.

25. Dobersen MJ, Scharff JE, Ginsberg-Fellner F, et al. Cytotoxic autoantibodies to beta cells in the serum of patients with insulin dependent diabetes mellitus. N Engl J Med 1980;303:1493.

26. MacLaren NK, Huang SW, Fogh J. Antibody to cultured human insulinoma cells in insulin-dependent diabetes. Lancet 1975;1:997.

27. Huange SW, MacLaren N. Insulin-dependent diabetes: A disease of autoaggression. Science 1976;192:64.

28. Tam AC, Dean BM, Schwarz G, et al. Predicting insulin-dependent diabetes. Lancet 1988;1:845.

29. Nerup F, Platz P, Ortved-Anderson O, et al. HLA antigens and diabetes mellitus. Lancet 1974;2:864.

30. Rubinstein P, Suciu-Foca N, Nicholson JF. Genetics of juvenile diabetes mellitus. N Engl J Med 1977;297:1036.

31. Deschamps I, Lestradet H, Bonati C, et al. HLA genotype studies in juvenile insulin-dependent diabetes. Diabetologia 1980;19:189.

32. Rotter JI, Hodge SE. Racial differences in juvenile-type diabetes are consistent with more than one mode of inheritance. Diabetes 1980;29:115.

33. Rotter JI, Rimoin DL. Heterogeneity in diabetes mellitus-update 1978. Diabetes 1978;27:599.

34. Rosenberg LE, Kidd KK. HLA and disease susceptibility: A primer. N Engl J Med 1977;297:1060.

35. Pyke DA. Diabetes: The genetic connections. Diabetologia 1979;17:333.

36. Gamble DR. An epidemiological study of childhood diabetes affecting two or more siblings. Diabetologia 1980;19:341.

37. Fleegler FM, Rogers KD, Drash AL, et al. Age, sex and season of onset of juvenile diabetes in different geographic areas. Pediatrics 1979;63:374.

38. Yoon JW, Austin M, Onodera T, Notkins AL. Virus-induced diabetes mellitus: Isolation of a virus from the pancreas of a child with diabetic ketoacidosis. N Engl J Med 1979;300:1173.

39. Rayfield EJ, Seto Y. Viruses and the pathogenesis of diabetes mellitus. Diabetes 1978;27:1126.

40. Fukagawa, NK, Minaker, LL, Rowe, JW, et al. Glucose and amino acid metabolism in aging man. Differential effects on insulin. Metabolism 1988;37:371–377.

41. Schade DS, Eaton RP. The temporal relationship between endogenously secreted stress hormones and metabolic decompensation in diabetic man. J Clin Endocrinol Metab 1980;50:131.

42. Felig P, Wahren J, Sherwin R, et al. Insulin, glucagon, and somatostatin in normal physiology and diabetes mellitus. Diabetes 1976;25:1091.

43. Raskin P, Unger RH. Hyperglucagonemia and its suppression: Importance in the metabolic control of diabetes. N Engl J Med 1978;299:433.

44. Cryer PE, Gerich JE. Glucose counter-regulation, hypoglycemia, and intensive therapy in diabetes mellitus. N Engl J Med 1985;313:232.

45. Levy-Marshall C, Patterson CC, Green A, EURODIAB ACE Study Group. Geographical variation of presentation at diagnosis of type 1 diabetes in children: the EURODIAB Study. DIabetalogia 2001;44:B75–B80.

46. Sperling MA. Diabetic ketoacidosis. Pediatr Clin N Am 1984;31:591.
47. Foster DW, McGarry JD. The metabolic derangements and treatment of diabetic ketoacidosis. N Engl J Med 1983;309:159,.
48. Kreisberg RA. Diabetic ketoacidosis: New concepts and trends in pathogenesis and treatment. Ann Intern Med 1978;88:681.
49. Carroll MF, Schade DS. Ten pivotal questions about diabetic ketoacidosis. Answers that clarify new concepts in treatment. Postgrad Med 2001;110(5):89–95.
50. Duck SC, Wyatt DR. Factors associated with brain herniation in the treatment of diabetic ketoacidosis. J Pediatr 1988;113:10.
51. Siberry GK, Iannone R (eds.). The Harriet Lane Handbook, 15th ed. Mosby, St. Louis, MO, 2000.
52. Hammeke M, Bear R, Lee R, et al. Hyperchloremic metabolic acidosis in diabetes mellitus. Diabetes 1978;27:16.
53. Harris GD, Fiordalisi I, Finberg L. Safe management of diabetic ketoacidemia. J Pediatr 1988;113:65.
54. Kanter Y, Gerson JR, Bessman AN. 2,3-Diphos- phoglycerate, nucleotide phosphate, and organic and inorganic phosphate levels during the early phases of diabetic ketoacidosis. Diabetes 1977;26:429.
55. Low-dose insulin infusion in the treatment of diabeteic ketoacidosis: bolus versus no bolus. J. Pedatr 1980;96(1):36–40.
56. Harris GD, Fiordalisi I Harris WL, et al. Minimizing the rjisk of brain herniation during treatment of diabetic ketoacidemia: a retropective and prospective study. J Pediatr 117:22.
57. Morris LR, Murphy MB, Kitabchi AE. Bicarbonate therapy in severe diabetic ketoacidosis. Ann Intern Med 1986;105(6):836–840.
58. Witters LA, Ohman JL, Weir GC, et al. Insulin antibodies in the pathogenesis of insulin allergy and resistance. Am J Med 1977;63:703.
59. Bougneres PF, LaJ1dier F, Lemmell C, et al. Insulin pump therapy in young children with type I diabetes. J Pediatr 1990;105:212.
60. Tamborlane, WV, Press, CM. Insulin infusion pump treatment of type 1 diabetes. Pediatr. Clin N Am 1984;31(3):721–734.
61. Boland EA, Grey M, Oesterle A, et al. Continuois subcutaneous insulin infusion. A new way to lowr risk of sever hypoglycemia, imporve metabolic control, and enhance coping in adolecents with type 1 diabetes. Diabetes Care 1999;22(11):1779–1784.
62. Tamborlane WV, Press CM. Insulin infusion pump treatment of type I diabetes. Pediatr Clin N Am 1984;31:721.
63. Minimed. Fredrickson, ed. Establishing and verifying basal rates. The insulin pump therapy book. Insights from the experts. Minimed, 1995.
64. The DCCT Research Group. The effect of intensive treatment o diabetes on the development and progression of long-term complications in sinuslin-dependent diabetes mellitus. N Engl J Med 1993;329:977–986.
65. Sonksen PH, Judd SL, Lowy D. Home monitoring of blood-glucose: Method for improving diabetic control. Lancet 1978;1:729.
66. Goldstein DE, Walker B, Rawlings SS, et al. Hemoglobin Alc levels in children and adolescents with diabetes mellitus. Diabetes Care 1980;3:503.
67. Mogensen CW. Mangement of diabetic renal involvement and disease. Lancet 1988;1:867.
68. Sperling, MA. Hypoglycemia, In: Behrman, Kliegman, Arvin, eds. Nelson Textbook of Pediatrics, 15th ed. Saunders, Philadelphia, 1996.
69. Santiago JV, Clarke WL, Shah SD, Cryer PE. Epinephrine, norepinephrine, glucagon, and growth hormone release in association with physiological decrements in the plasma glucose concentration in normal and diabetic man. J Clin Endocrinol Metab 1980;51:877,.
70. Rosenbloom AL, Giordano BP. Chronic over-treatment with insulin in children and adolescents. Am J Dis Child 1977;131:881.
71. Gale EAM, Kurtz AB, Tattersall RB. In search of the Somogyi effect. Lancet 1980;2:279.
72. Bolli G, Gottesman I, Campbell P, et al. Glucose counter-regulation and waning of insulin in the Somogyi phenomenon. N Engl J Med 1984;311:1214.
73. Campbell P, Bolli G, Cryer P, et al. Pathogenesis of a dawn phenomenon in patients with insulin-dependent diabetes mellitus. N Engl J Med 1985;312:1473.
74. Bantle JP. The dietary treatment of diabetes mellitus. Med Clin N Am 1988;72:1285.

75. Franz MJ, ed. A Core Curriculum for Diabetes Education, 4th ed. American Association of Diabetes Educators, 2001.

76. Tamborlane W, Held N. Diabetes. In: Tamborlane W, ed. The Yale Guide to Children's Nutrition. Yale University Press, New Haven, 1999.

77. Weinger K, O'Donnell KA, Ritholz MD. Adolescent views of diabetes-related parent conflict and support: A focus group analysis. J Adoles Health 2001;9:330–336.

78. Hardin DS, Azzarelli B, Edwards J, et al. Mechanisms of enhanced insulin sensitivity in endurance trained athletes. J Clin Endocr Metab 1995;80:2437–2446.

79. Landt KW, Campaigne BN, James FW, et al. Effects of exercise training on insulin sensitivity in adolescents with type I diabetes. Diabetes Care 1985;5:461–465.

80. Horton ES. Exercise and diabetes mellitus. Med Clin N Am 1988;72:1301.

81. Zinman G, Murray FT, Vranic M, et al. Gluco-regulation during moderate exercise in insulin treated diabetics. J Clin Endocrinol Metab 1977;45:641.

82. Diabetes in America: Diabetes Data Compiled 1984. US Department of Health and Human Services Publication No. 85-1468 (NIH). US Government Printing Office, Washington, DC, 1985.

83. Leslie ND, Sperling MA. Relation of metabolic control to complications in diabetes mellitus. J Pediatr 1986;108:491.

84. Skyler JS. "Control" and diabetic complications. Diabetes Care 1978;3:204.

85. Winter WE, Maclaren NK. Type I insulin dependent diabetes: An autoimmune disease that can be arrested or prevented with immunotherapy? Adv Pediatr 1985;32:159.

86. Cudworth AG, Gorsuch AN, Wolf E, Festeinstein H. A new look at HLA genetics with particular reference to type-1 diabetes. Lancet 1979;2:389.

87. Bougneres PF, Carel JC, Castano L, et al. Factors associated with early remission of type I diabetes in children treated with cyclosporine. N Engl J Med 1988;318:663.

88. Sutherland, DER, *Goetz* FC, Chin PL, et al. Pancreas transplantation. Pediatr Clin N Am 1984;31:735.

89. Lacy PE, Davie *JM*. Transplantation of pan- creatic islets. Annu Rev Immunol 1984;2:183,.

90. Haffner, SM, Stern, MP, Hazuda HP. Hyperinsulinemia in a population at high risk for non-insulin-dependent diabetes mellitus. N Engl J Med 1986;315:220–224.

91. Pinhas-Hamiel O, Dolan LM, Daniels SR. Increased inscidenc e of non-insulin dependent diabetes mellitus among adolescents. J Pediatr 1996;12:608–615.

92. Haffner SM, Mithinea H, Gaskel SP, Stern MD. Decreased insulin secretion and increased insulin resistance are independently related to the 7 year risk of NIDDM. Diabetes 1995;49:1386–1391.

93. Hardin DS, Yafi M, Brosnan P. Clinical characteristics of patients with type 2 diabetes of youth. Diabetes 2001;50(2):225.

94. Polonsky KS, Sturis J, Bell GT. Non-insulin dependent diabetes mellitus-A genetic program failure of the beta cell to compensate for insulin resistance N Engl J Med 1999;334:777–783.

95. Caprio S, Sherwin R, Evans K, Belous A, Tamborlane W. Early phase insulin secretion is normal in obese adolescents with impaired glucose tolerance. Diabetes 2002;50(2):224.

96. Deitz WH. Overweight and precursors of type 2 diabetes mellitus in children and adolescents. J Pediatr 2001;138:453,454.

97. Deckelbaum RJ, Williams CL. Childhood obesity: the health issue. Obesity Res 2001;9:239S–243S.

98. Bjorntorp P. Hazards in subgroups of human obesity. Eur J Clin Invest 1984;14:239–241.

99. Triano RP, Flegal KM. Overweight children and adolescents: Description epidemiology, and demographics. Pediatrics 1998;101:497–504.

100. Ludwik B, Nolan JJ, Baloga J, Saks D, Olefsky J. Effects of obesity on insulin resistance in normal subjects and patients with NIDDM. Diabetes 1995;44:1121–1125.

101. Kolterman OG, Insel J, Olefshy JM. J Clin Invest 1980;65:1272–1284.

102. Hardin DS, Maianu L, Sorbel J. Genetic factors are more important than environment in determining insulin sensitivity, muscle GLUT4 content and related metabolic factors in normal twins. Diabetes 1994;43:73.

103. Vaag A, Henriksson JE, Madsbad S, et al. Insulin secretion, insulin action, and hepatic glucose production in identical twins discordant fro NIDDM. J Clin Invest 1995;95:690–698.

104. Mokdad AH, Serdula MK, Dietz WH, et al. The spread of the obesity epidemic in the United States. JAMA 1999;282:1519–1522.

105. Waldhausl W, Kleinberger G, Korn A, et al. Severe hyperglycemia: effects of rehydration on endocrine derangements and blood glucose concentration. Diabetes 1979;28:577.

106. Johnson WG, Hinkle LK, Carr RE, et al. Dieteary and exercise interventions for juvenile obesity: long-term effect of behavioral and public health models. Obesity Res 1997;5:257–261.
107. Dietz WH, Gortmaker SL. Preventing obesity in children and adolescents. Annu Rev Public health 2001;22:337–353.
108. Hardin DS, Hebert JD, Bayden T, Dehart M, Mazur L. Treatment of childhood syndrome X. Pediatric 197;100:1–4.
109. Jones KE, Arslanian S, Peterkova VA, et al. Effect of metformin in pediatric patients with type 2 diabetes: a randomized controlled trial. Diabetes Care 2002;25:89–94.
110. Zhurick-Yafi M, Brosnan P, Hardin DS. Treatment of type 2 diabetes of youth. J Pediatr Endocr Diabetes, in press.
111. Shield JPH, Howell WM, Temple KM. Neonatal diabetes. Diabetes Care 1997;20:1045,1046.
112. Shield JPH, Gardner RJ, Wadswroth EJK, et al. Antiopathology and genetic basis of neonatal diabetes. Arch Dis Child 1997;76:F39–42.
113. Temple IK, Gardner RJ, Mackay DJG, et al. Transient Neonatal Diabetes. Widening the understanding of the etiopathogenesis of diabetes. Diabetes 2000;49:1359–1366.
114. Schiff D, Colle E, Stern L. Metabolic and growth patterns in transient neonatal diabetes. N Engl J Med 1972;287:119.
115. Pagliara AS, Karl IE, Kipnis DB. Transient neo-natal diabetes: delayed maturation of the pancreatic beta cell. J Pediatr 1973;82:97.
116. Daugberg PS. A case of permanent diabetes in a neonate. Dan Med Bull 1981;28:216.
117. Shield JPH, Baum JD. Is transient neonatal diabetes a risk factor for diabetes in later life? Lancet 1993;341:683.
118. Temple JK, James RS, Crolla JA, et al. An imprinted gene(s) for diabetes? Nat Genet 1995;9:110–112.
119. Hattersley AT. Maturity-onset diabetes of the young. Balliere's Clin Pediatr 1996;4:663–680.
120. Winter WE, Kakamura M, House DV. Monogenic diabetes melltus in youth the MODY syndromes. Pediatr Endocr 1999;28:765–785.
121. Velho G, Lathrop GM, Froguel P. A gene for maturity onset diabetes of the young (MODY) maps to chromosome 12Q. Nat Genet 1995;9:418–423.
122. Velho G, Froguel P. Genetic, metabolic and clinical characteristics of maturity onset diabetes of the young. Eur J Endocrinol 1998;138:233–239.
123. Guazzarotti L, Bartolotta E, Chiarelli F. Maturity Onset diabetes of the young.(MODY): a new challenge for pediatric diabetologists. J Pediatr Endocr Metab 1999;12:487–497.
124. Moran A. Abnormal glucose metabolism in cystic fibrosis. J Pediatr 1998; 133:10–17.
125. Moran A, Hardin D, Rodman, et al. The diagnosis, management and treatment of patients with cystic fibrosis related diabetes. Res Clin Prac 1999;45:61–73.
126. Finkelstein SM, Wielinski CL, Ellitt, GR. Diabetes mellitus associated with cystic fibrosis. J Pediatr 1988;112:373– 377.
127. Lanng S, Thoresteinsson B. Lund-Andersen C, et al. Diabetes miltus in Danch cystic fibrosis patients. Prevalence and late diabetic complications. Acta Paediatr Scand 1994;83:72–77.
128. Mohan V, Alagappan V, Snehalatha C, et al. Insulin and C peptide responses to glucose laid in cystic fibrosis. Diabetes Metab 1985;11:376–379.
129. Hardin DS, Leban A, Lukenbaugh S. Seigheimer, DK Insulin resistance is associated with decreased clinical status in cystic fibrosis J Pediatr 1997;6:948–956.
130. Hardin DS, Leblanc A, Para L, Seilheimer DK. Hepatic insulin resistance and defects in substrate utilization in cystic fibrosis. Diabetes 1999;48:1082–1087.
131. Austin A, Kahan SC, Orenstein D, et al. Roles of insulin resistance and beta cell dysfunction in the pathogenesis of glucose intolerance in cystic fibrosis. J Clin Endocr Metab 1994;79:80–85.
132. Zemel BS, Kawchak DA,Cnaan A, et al. Prospective evaluation of resting energy expenditure, nutritional status, pulmonary function, and genotype in children with cystic fibrosis. Pediatr Res 1996;40:578–586.
133. Kraemer R, Ruderberg A, Hadorn B, Rossi E. Relative underweight in cystic fibrosis and its prognostic value. Acta Paediatr Scand 1978;67:33–35.
134. Hardin DS, Lebanc A, Lukenbaugh S, et al. Increased rates of proteolysis associates with insulin resistance in cystic fibrosis. Pediatris 1998;10:948–946.
135. Zipf WB, Kien CL, Horswill CA, McCoyu KS. Effects of feeding on daily protein turnover balance (DPTB) in cystic fibrosis (CF). Pediatr Res 1991;30:178.

136. Geffner ME, Kaplan SA, Bersch N, et al. Leprechaunism: in vitro insulin action despite genetic resistance. Pediatr Res 1987;22:286.

137. Acillii D. Molecular defects of the insulin receptor gene. Diabetes Metab Rev 1995;11:47–62.

138. Longo N, Wang Y, Pasquali M. Progressive decline in insulin levels in Rabson-Mendenhall syndrome. J Clin Endocr Metab 1999;84:2623–2629.

139. Flier JS, Kahn CR, Roth J. Receptors, antireceptor antibodies and mechanisms of insulin resistance. N Engl J Med 1979;300:413.

140. Seip M, Trygstad O. Generalized lipodystrophy, congenital and acquired (lipoatrophy). Acta Paediatr 1996;413:2–28.

141. Seip M. Liposdystrophy and gigantism with associated endocrine manifestations: a new diencephalic syndrome. Acta Paediatrica 1959;48: 555–574.

142. Copeland K, Nair KS, Kaplowitz PD, et al. Discordant metabolic actions of insulin in extreme lipodystrophy of childhood. J Clin Endocri Metab 1993;77:1240–1245.

143. Helderman JH, Elahi D, Anderson DK. Prevention of the glucose intolerance of thiazide diuretics by maintanence of body potassium. Diabetes 1983;32:106–111.

144. Walli RK, Herfort O, Michi GM. Treatment with protease inhibitors associated with peripheral insulin resistance and impaired oral glucose tolerance in HIV-1 invecte patients. AIDS 1998;12:F167–173.

145. Jindal RM, Sidner RA, Milgrom ML. Post-transplant diabetes mellitus. The role of immunosuppression. Drug Exp Drug Safety 1997;16(4).

146. Charan VD, Desai N, Singh AP, Choudhry VP. Diabetes mellitus and pancreatitis as a complication of L-asparaginase therapy. Indian Pediatr 1993;30(6):809,810.

147. Jacobson AM, Leibovich JB. Psychological issues in diabetes mellitus. Psychosomatics 1984;25:7.

148. Cerreto MC, Travis LB. Implications of psychological and family factors in the treatment of diabetes. Pediatr Clin N Am 1984;31:689.

11 Treatment of Type 2 Diabetes

Insulin and Oral Agents that Augment Hormone Synthesis and Action

Donald A. McClain, MD, PhD

CONTENTS

INTRODUCTION

Two recent developments have served to refocus attention on the treatment of type 2 diabetes mellitus. First, the prevalence of the disease is increasing at an alarming rate, including in pediatric populations. Second has been the demonstration that intensive pharmacotherapy of the disease has a dramatically beneficial effect on its outcome. Control of hyperglycemia is not the only goal of therapy. In fact, the control of associated obesity, hypertension, and dyslipidemia may be as beneficial, if not more so, for long-term outcomes than is the regulation of glycemia. Furthermore, there well may be shared features in the pathogenesis of these and other comorbidities associated with the "metabolic syndrome," making a separation of their treatment from those aimed at normoglycemia *per se* somewhat artificial. For example, most treatments that augment insulin action will lower serum triglycerides, other drugs may have direct cardiovascular effects that contribute to their overall beneficial effect, and certain antihypertensives can affect glucose homeostasis. However, this chapter will focus only on achieving normoglycemia. For further details on integrated diabetes care, such as surveillance and treatment of complications, or nutritional recommendations, the reader should consult more comprehensive sources such as the *Clinical Practice Recommendations* of the American Diabetes Association, published annually as a supplement to the journal *Diabetes Care* or available at their website (www.diabetes.org). The reader is also encour-

From: *Endocrine Replacement Therapy in Clinical Practice*
Edited by: A. Wayne Meikle © Humana Press Inc., Totowa, NJ

aged to consult the many excellent texts and review articles available on specific aspects of treatment or agents mentioned below.

OVERVIEW OF THE PATHOGENESIS OF HYPERGLYCEMIA AND TREATMENT GOALS IN TYPE 2 DIABETES MELLITUS

The cause of most cases of type 2 diabetes mellitus remains obscure. It is clear that type 2 diabetes is not a single disease. Multiple (and distinct) genetic entities have been elucidated wherein type 2 diabetes results from mutations in the insulin receptor, glucokinase, or a number of transcription factors expressed in the liver and in the β-cells. However, the genetic underpinnings of "typical" type 2 diabetes are not yet known. An association of a genetic variation in the calpain-10 gene with diabetes in a Hispanic population was recently reported (1). Although at this time verification of the association in other populations and the mechanism for the association are still lacking, the finding may provide the first explanation for a significant fraction of the genetic risk for type 2 diabetes. The extraordinarily high prevalence of the disease in some communities suggests further that the condition may represent a "normal" evolutionary adaptation to specific environmental conditions rather than a disease caused by a collection of "bad" genes. The largest predisposing factor for type 2 diabetes remains caloric excess and/or obesity. The importance of excess nutrients in the genesis of type 2 diabetes is underlined by the fact that the pathophysiologic hallmarks of that disease—insulin resistance and β-cell failure—not only contribute to but can also *result from* excess glucose and lipids. The processes by which these nutrients exert their adverse effects—so-called "glucose toxicity" (2) and "lipotoxicity" (3)—are not fully understood. Diabetes is also characterized by abnormalities in several metabolic pathways and in several organs, and this multitude of abnormalities may be more easily explained in terms of a common mechanism involving normal physiologic responses to the availability of excess nutrients.

Regardless of the primary cause of type 2 diabetes, it is clear by the time the disease manifests itself clinically that the hyperglycemia results from the following:

- Abnormalities in insulin secretion
- Excessive hepatic glucose production
- Resistance to the action of insulin in skeletal muscle and fat tissue

The complex interrelationships among these abnormalities have made it impossible to assign primacy or causality to any one of them. In fact, a viable and parsimonious hypothesis is that all of these hallmarks of diabetes may, in fact, be natural, physiologic, and, in some cases, even adaptive outcomes of ingesting too many calories (4). Nevertheless, the conceptual framework of the pathogenic triad of liver, β-cell, and muscle/fat has great usefulness in directing and understanding the useful therapies for the disease. The multipartite pathogenic scheme also explains the rationale for effective polypharmacy. The exceptions to effective drug combinations can be late in the natural history of the disease when β-cell failure results in a lack of efficacy of the insulin secretagogues, or where specific combinations have not been approved by the Food and Drug Administration (FDA). Additional targets for therapy include the gastrointestinal (GI) tract (the proximal source for the excess calories, although nutrient absorption is not intrinsically abnormal in diabetes) and the central nervous system (the ultimate culprit responsible for overeating). Useful therapies aimed at the former mechanism exist and will be described, although effective and safe treatments for the latter are still elusive.

The guiding principle of therapy at this time is that whatever the fundamental cause of type 2 diabetes, it is *hyperglycemia* that has been shown to be detrimental. It is management of hyperglycemia, even at the expense of hyperinsulinemia, that has been shown to decrease and/or delay diabetic complications *(5–7)*. A major question remaining is what degree of normalization of glycemia should be sought when treating type 2 diabetes. Obviously, this decision needs to be tailored to the individual patient. Extremely tight metabolic control appropriate for a 20-yr-old with a good support system would likely prove prohibitively dangerous for a bed-ridden 80-yr-old. However, there is an increasing awareness that the closer one approaches normoglycemia, both in the fasting and postprandial states, the lower one's risk of diabetic complications.

With rapidly acting insulins and drugs designed to focus on postprandial glycemia, it becomes more important to monitor not only fasting glucose but 1- or 2-h postprandial glucose as well. In fact, there are suggestions that focusing on postprandial glucose is more effective in lowering hemoglobin A_{1c} (HbA_{1c}) than strategies that consider only the fasting glucose levels *(8)*. There are also strong indications that isolated postprandial hyperglycemia may be a significant risk factor for diabetic complications, particularly coronary heart disease and stroke. The data on which we base our current treatment guidelines—and on which we base the definition of diabetes itself—reveal the levels of glycemia that confer a significant risk of diabetic complications. These data (such as were gathered in the Diabetes Control and Complications Trial) are most precise for microvascular disease such as retinopathy and are responsible for the definition of diabetes as a fasting blood glucose in excess of 7 mmoles/L. However, there are data to suggest that the risk of macrovascular disease—heart attack and stroke—may be established at even lower levels of glycemia than for microvascular disease:

- Isolated postprandial hyperglycemia confers significant cardiovascular risk in females *(9)*.
- Postchallenge glucose levels, even in the nondiabetic range, are a significant risk factor for cardiovascular disease in men *(10)*.
- HbA_{1c} levels, even in nondiabetic men and throughout the range of normal values, are positively correlated with the risk of cardiovascular disease *(11)*.
- World Health Organization criteria for diabetes (focusing on postprandial glucose values) identify many more individuals at risk for cardiovascular disease than the American Diabetes Association criteria (focusing on fasting glucose values) *(12)*.

Thus, there are several indications that isolated postprandial or postchallenge glycemia, even in ranges not defined as diabetic, is a risk factor for macrovascular disease in persons with diabetes. Given the fact that heart attacks and strokes are the major cause of mortality in diabetes, it would seem prudent to recommend that the goal of therapy in diabetes should be normalization of fasting glucose and postprandial glucose excursions, with the significant caveat that this be done in a manner that avoids or minimizes dangerous hypoglycemia. Recently, the American Association of Clinical Endocrinologists has adopted guidelines essentially recommending normalization of glucose where feasible in persons with diabetes. Those goals are for the HbA_{1c} to be less than 6.5%, fasting glucose to be less than 110 mg/dL, and 2-h postprandial glucose to be less than 140 mg/dL. Goals set by the American Diabetes Association are somewhat less stringent, targeting a HbA_{1c} of 7.0%. Strategies to achieve these goals are considered below. In addition, the importance of adjunct therapy to address other cardiovascular risk factors (LDL cholesterol, blood pressure, tobacco use, obesity, and triglycerides) cannot be overemphasized.

THERAPY OF DIABETES: ORAL AGENTS

General Principles

It is very clear that the single largest risk factor for most cases of typical type 2 diabetes is obesity. Weight loss remains the treatment of choice for the disease, and it is best accomplished with a combination of diet and exercise. Even when pharmacological treatment becomes necessary, weight loss must be emphasized and re-emphasized to the patient as a means of lowering subsequent risk and increasing the efficacy of therapy. This is particularly important because a major side effect of many treatments for diabetes is weight gain: If excess calories continue to be ingested, most antidiabetic therapies will result in the successful deposition of those excess calories as fat. Even more effective would be *prevention* of obesity, especially as type 2 diabetes is becoming established as a disease in children and adolescents. Successful diet therapy, exercise programs, and confronting public policy problems—abolition of physical education and recess programs in schools combined with the students' easy access to soft drinks and high-fat foods, for example—would be infinitely superior to disease management.

There are insufficient data to support a single optimal drug regimen or even a stepped algorithm for management of diabetes. This probably reflects disease heterogeneity as well as heterogeneity of drug metabolism and target-cell responsiveness. Specific situations may exist that favor a certain agent or disqualify another, and these will be described with each agent. Cost, another significant factor, will not be considered in this review because of the rapid changes anticipated as agents lose patent protection and new agents are developed. In general, most diabetologists would support the following guidelines:

- If the patient has had prolonged and severe hyperglycemia—the all-too-typical patient who presents with many months of polyuria and polydipsia and significant weight loss—it is advantageous to intensively treat him or her with insulin for a period of 1 to 2 wk to break the vicious cycle of "glucose toxicity" (see the following subsection). This will increase the probability of a timely response to subsequently chosen oral agents. Diabetes education, initiation of diet therapy, screening for complications, and so forth can proceed in this period. A further advantage (unproven) of this approach is that it probably gives the patient a better appreciation for the seriousness of the condition than if he or she is handed a prescription and scheduled for a return visit in 6 mo. The obvious disadvantage of the approach is the time required and its cost.
- Start an oral agent and rapidly increase the dose until control is achieved. If control is not achieved, add a second oral agent whose action complements the first. For example, in an overweight individual with good renal function, a biguanide might be the first drug and an insulin secretagogue the second.
- If control is still not achieved, there are several options, including (1) adding a third oral agent; (2) substituting insulin for one of the oral agents, starting with a single bedtime dose and perhaps moving to multiple doses if necessary; or (3) switching exclusively to insulin.
- Evolution of the disease needs to be anticipated. The natural history of type 2 diabetes is that in most patients, glycemic control becomes more difficult over time, perhaps as β-cell function deteriorates. Thus, it is often the case that more drugs need to be added to the regimen over time. Weight loss or resolution of "glucose toxicity" can lead to the opposite, namely subtraction of drugs and improvement of β-cell function.

Until such a time as new tools and approaches such as pharmacogenetics allow us to identify subsets of individuals more or less likely to respond to a given agent, we are left

Table 1
Oral Agents for Therapy of Type 2 Diabetes

Oral agents	Brand names	Total daily dose (mg/d)	Dosing interval
Biguanides			
Metformin	Glucophage, generic	500–2550	bid–tid
Sulfonylureas			
Glimepiride	Amaryl	1–8	qd
Glipizide	Glucotrol, generic	2.5–40	qd–tid
extended release	Glucotrol XL	5–20	qd
Glyburide (glibenclamide)	Diabeta, generic	1.25–20	qd–bid
micronized	Glynase	0.75–12	qd–bid
	Micronase	1.25–20	qd–bid
Older agents: acetohexamide, chlorpropramide, tolazamide, tolbutamide			
α-glucosidase inhibitors			
Precose	Acarbose	75–300	tid/ac
Miglitol	Glyset	75–300	tid/ac
Glinides			
Nateglinide	Starlix	60–120	ac
Repaglinide	Prandin	1.5–12	ac
Thiazolidinediones			
Pioglitazone	Actos	15–45	qd
Rosiglitazone	Avandia	4–8	qd

with a process of trial and error to arrive at optimal therapy for any given individual. The bad news is that the process can be time and labor intensive; patients will likely need to be seen at frequent intervals (1–4 wk) during initiation of therapy. Furthermore, beyond the level of curing polyuria, the rewards are often not palpable to the patient; that is, the benefits of therapy show up more in statistical analysis of populations than in individual well-being. The good news, however, is that multiple effective, safe, and well-studied agents are available. Thus, it is generally possible to arrive at some agent or combination of agents that will control glycemia, and the data supporting a benefit for that effort are overwhelming. Currently available oral agents for the treatment of type 2 diabetes are listed in Table 1.

Biguanides

After centuries of use of related compounds as herbal folk cures for diabetes, the first biguanide to be used clinically was phenformin. Phenformin was introduced in the 1960s but withdrawn in the late 1970s because of dangers of lactic acidosis. The related compound metformin was subsequently used extensively in Europe with good efficacy and safety, but was not approved for use in the United States until 1993. Despite its long use, the molecular mechanism of its action is still only partially understood. Metformin appears to act primarily in reducing hepatic gluconeogenesis, a major determinant of fasting glucose concentrations in type 2 diabetes. Other effects of the drug are also consistently observed, including decreased insulin resistance and decreased blood levels of triglyceride and free fatty acids. It is unclear whether these effects of the drug are primary or perhaps secondary to decreases in glycemia.

CLINICAL EFFICACY

Metformin has been intensively studied and remains one of the most useful and safest compounds to treat type 2 diabetes. Numerous trials have demonstrated efficacy, most recently the landmark UKPDS (6). In most of the studies employing the drug, HbA_{1c} levels in treated patients have fallen 1–2%, and the UKPDS was able to show that this improvement in HbA_{1c} was associated with protection from diabetic complications. In addition, use of the drug is associated with improvements in lipid levels (10–20% reductions in triglycerides) and weight (loss of 1–4 kg). These effects are dose-responsive, increasing even beyond the currently approved maximum dose of 2550 mg/d.

USE IN COMBINATION WITH OTHER ANTIDIABETES DRUGS

Most studies of combination therapy have demonstrated that metformin is additive in improving glycemic control when used in conjunction with sulfonylureas, thiazolidine-diones, or insulin.

ADVERSE EFFECTS AND CAUTIONS

In general, metformin is safe if the precautions described below are followed. In particular, metformin does not by itself cause hypoglycemia. The most common side effects of metformin are gastrointestinal disturbances (diarrhea most frequently, but also nausea, vomiting, anorexia, and bloating). These are seen in up to 25–30% of patients in some trials, although a minority of those individuals is forced to discontinue the drug. In most individuals, the symptoms resolve spontaneously within a few weeks and upward titration of the dose (e.g., at weekly intervals) has been recommended to minimize those symptoms.

The most serious adverse effect of the drug, lactic acidosis, is also fortunately rare, occurring with a frequency of approx 1 case per 30,000–40,000 patient-years. In fact, there are data to suggest that lactic acidosis occurs with a similar frequency in diabetic individuals not on metformin, so the true incidence of *drug-induced* acidosis may be even lower than thought. Lactic acidosis occurs usually in the context of some serious intercurrent illness such as sepsis, severe congestive heart failure, or shock wherein lactate production will be increased. It is recommended that the drug not be used (or discontinued) in these situations.

Metformin is cleared by the kidneys and the chief contraindication to metformin use is renal insufficiency. The drug should not be used in patients with serum creatinine levels above 1.4–1.5. These levels of renal function are not uncommon in a diabetic population, and renal function can further deteriorate with dehydration, infections, heart disease, use of radiocontrast dye, or use of other medications (angiotensin-converting enzyme inhibitors, nonsteroidal anti-inflammatory drugs, antibiotics, etc.), all of which are seen frequently in the type 2 diabetes clinic. Caution, surveillance, and anticipation of these events is required. A good rule of thumb might be that if a patient is sick enough to be acutely hospitalized, then he or she is likely sick enough also to potentially get in trouble from metformin, either from the cause of hospitalization (e.g., cardiac disease) or complications (e.g., renal insufficiency). In such cases, the drug can be discontinued during hospitalization and therapy reinitiated once the underlying disease and renal function have stabilized. Insulin can be used in the interim.

Insulin Secretagogues

SULFONYLUREAS

The sulfonylureas have been in use for half a century and were the first agents approved for the treatment specifically of type 2 diabetes. They act by binding to a subunit (the sulfonylurea receptor, SUR) of the ATP-sensitive potassium (K_{ATP}) channel *(13)*. Sulfonylureas result in closure of the K_{ATP} channel and membrane depolarization, leading to calcium influx and a series of events that culminate in insulin secretion. This mimics the effects of a rise in the blood glucose concentration, whereby metabolism of glucose also leads to channel closure, perhaps signaled by a rise in the ATP/ADP ratio as the glucose is metabolized *(14)*.

FORMULATIONS AND EFFICACY

There are several formulations of sulfonylureas available for clinical use. All have approximately equal efficacy in terms of decreasing glycemia. First-generation sulfonylureas (chlorpropramide, tolazamide, and tolbutamide) are seldom now used because of side-effect profiles, unacceptably long duration of action, or low potency compared to the newer secretagogues (e.g., glimeperide, glipizide, and glyburide). Glipizide is available in an extended release formulation and glyburide in a micronized formulation. There are no compelling data that support superiority of any one of the newer sulfonylureas over the others. All have been shown to result in average decreases of HbA_{1c} levels of 1.5–2%, although this is highly dependent on the HbA_{1c} and glucose levels at initiation of therapy, adherence to a diet regimen, duration of disease, and a host of other variables. This decrease will result in a similar fraction of patients—30–60%—achieving "adequate" control of glycemia, although this number may be increased by first achieving glycemic control with insulin to break the vicious cycle of glucose toxicity and its effects on β-cell function. All formulations are also associated with "secondary failure" rates of several percent per year, that is, deterioration of glycemic control to unacceptable levels related to progression of the underlying disease processes.

SAFETY

The sulfonylureas have a long track record of safety with a low frequency of side effects, those being generally mild. The adverse effect of most concern is hypoglycemia. This is a direct consequence of the action of the drug to stimulate insulin secretion even when blood glucose levels are normal or low. Symptomatic hypoglycemia will occur in a few percent of patients per year. Event rates may be lower with glipizide compared to glyburide *(15)* or with glimepiride compared to either *(16)*. Serious hypoglycemia, defined as glucose low enough to require third-party intervention, occurs at a frequency of up to 1%, or 1 event per 100 patient-years. Events requiring hospitalization occur less frequently, approximately once in every 3000 patient-years, and deaths occur once in 30,000–50,000 patient-years. Not surprisingly, hypoglycemia is most often seen with missed/delayed meals, in the elderly, or in patients with otherwise well-controlled glycemia. Thus, in those subgroups, consideration should be given to use of shorter-acting insulin secretagogues such as the glinides (discussed next) or, in the case of the frail and/or elderly, to relaxation of glycemic goals.

The other common and well-described adverse effect of sulfonylureas is weight gain, approx 3 kg over the first year or two of therapy. Allergic reactions can be seen, and the drugs are contraindicated if there is a history of severe reaction to another sulfonylurea or related compound, including sulfa drugs. The drugs are not approved for use in pregnancy or dialysis, although metabolites of the newer sulfonylureas are mainly inactive and largely excreted in the bile.

There is general agreement that β-cell failure is the "straw that breaks the camel's back" in the evolution and clinical presentation of type 2 diabetes. That is, isolated insulin resistance is generally well tolerated and well compensated until β-cell failure ensues and insulin levels fall. The concept of "β-cell exhaustion" has been used to describe this event, and thus the concern has emerged that asking the β-cell to work even harder under the influence of a sulfonylurea might hasten the "exhaustion." Sulfonylureas can also lead to β-cell desensitization to these agents. However, studies suggest that control of diabetes by whatever means, including sulfonylureas, *prolongs* insulin secretory capacity (17). The likely explanation is that the β-cell failure observed in type 2 diabetes is actually the result of cumulative exposure to excess glucose or lipids—the "glucose toxicity" and "lipotoxicity" phenomena—rather than simple overwork. Furthermore, it should be re-emphasized that control of hyperglycemia—not maintenance of β-cell function—is the chief goal of therapy. Control of hyperglycemia, whether through the use of sulfonylureas or other agents, has been verified to be of benefit in preventing diabetic complications. This fact should also allay fears of the sulfonylurea causing a worsening of hyperinsulinemia, a factor that has been speculated to be linked to atherosclerosis. There is no evidence that hyperinsulinemia *per se* is detrimental, whereas there are very clear data that treatment of diabetes even at the cost of hyperinsulinemia improves outcome, at least in net.

One study of outcomes in patients treated with sulfonylureas, the University Group Diabetes Program (UGDP), demonstrated an increase in adverse cardiovascular events in patients treated with sulfonylureas (18). Although there is a potential rationale and mechanism for such effects—the presence of SURs and K_{ATP} channels in cardiac muscle (19)—there are several lines of evidence that counter the results of the UGDP:

- There were serious concerns about the statistical analysis of the UGDP study
- The universality of the adverse events has been questioned
- Several subsequent studies including the UKPDS (6,7) have not demonstrated increased coronary disease or mortality in sulfonylurea-treated groups compared to controls; on the contrary, there was a trend toward benefit that just missed being statistically significant.

Thus, the current recommendation of the American Diabetes Association is that there should be no restrictions on use of sulfonylureas based on the UGDP study.

GLINIDES

Recently, a new class of insulin secretagogues has been introduced. These include repaglinide and nateglinide and bind to the SUR but at a site distinct from the sulfonylureas. The main practical feature distinguishing them from the sulfonylureas is their rapidity of action, with peak levels being reached in 30–45 min and effective duration of action being 3–4 h. Nateglinide is somewhat more rapid than repaglinide in its action and comes closer to reproducing a physiologic insulin response to a meal. Thus, these medications are dosed before each meal. The drugs have been shown to have similar overall efficacy compared to sulfonylureas and can be rationally combined with other agents such as the biguanides.

If, conceptually, the sulfonylureas can be said to correspond to the use of longer-acting insulins, then the glinides are used more similarly to regular or short-acting insulins. Thus, a major advantage of these newer compounds is the same as using rapidly acting insulins before each meal: Meals can be delayed or even skipped with minimal risk of hypoglycemia and the patient can enjoy greater freedom and a lifestyle more consistent with the demands of a job or other activities. The ability to skip meals and minimize snacking is especially important in facilitating weight loss and allowing adherence to lower calorie diets. The short duration of action also leads to less hypoglycemia, corresponding to lower insulin levels in the fasted state compared to the sulfonylureas. The analogy of sulfonylureas and glinides with short- and long-acting insulins does not extend to a rationale for combination therapy, however: It is unlikely that a β-cell that is chronically stimulated by a sulfonylurea will have sufficient reserve to accommodate a further fully therapeutic burst of secretion in response to a glinide.

The drugs are not significantly cleared by the kidneys and can be used in renal and moderate hepatic insufficiency.

THIAZOLIDINEDIONES

Thiazolidinediones are a relatively new class of hypoglycemic agents that act by binding to the peroxisome proliferator activated receptor (PPAR). In particular, the PPAR-γ isoform is the target of these agents. Other isoforms exist, with the PPAR-α being the target of the fibrate class of lipid-lowering agents, and the PPAR-δ being less well characterized. All are members of the steroid superfamily of nuclear receptors. They form heterodimers with another nuclear receptor (RXR), bind to DNA, and regulate gene transcription. The precise identity of the endogenous ligand(s) for the PPARs is not known, although prostanoids and other fatty acid derivatives bind to the receptors, consistent with a role in nutrient sensing and in directing appropriate responses to those nutrients such as augmenting fat storage or metabolism.

The precise gene or tissue target that is responsible for the drugs' hypoglycemic action is similarly not known. The drugs were initially characterized as "insulin sensitizers" in that they augmented insulin-stimulated glucose disposal in skeletal muscle. Whether that is a direct effect on muscle or an indirect one mediated by the fat cell is not known. PPAR-γ was discovered and is relatively highly expressed in adipose tissue, and the receptor plays important roles in adipocyte function and differentiation. However, the receptor has also been detected at lower levels in other key tissues of glucose homeostasis such as muscle and the β-cell, and these may be important in directing some of the drugs' multiple effects. As is the case for all drugs that reverse hyperglycemia, it is difficult to determine whether some of the drugs' effects may be secondary events that reflect the interplay and cause-effect relationships among glycemia, insulin resistance, β-cell function, and hepatic glucose production.

The drugs also have potentially significant effects on parameters of cardiovascular risk. All currently used forms of the drugs, even those with high selectivity for PPAR-γ, raise high-density lipoprotein (HDL) cholesterol levels. Pioglitazone and troglitazone lower triglycerides, although rosiglitazone may increase triglycerides to a modest degree. However, these potentially beneficial effects are accompanied by modest increases in LDL cholesterol such that the HDL/LDL ratio remains generally unaffected. Other more direct effects on the vascular endothelium are currently under investigation.

Formulations and Efficacy. Three members of this class of drug—troglitazone, pioglitazone, and rosiglitazone—have been introduced, although troglitazone has since been withdrawn from the market because of associated deaths from liver failure (*see* subsection on safety). All have shown similar efficacy, with reductions of HbA_{1c} in the range of 1–2%. Consistent with the description of the agents as "insulin sensitizers," the drugs do not seem to be effective in the absence of insulin. However, in patients with some reserve of insulin secretion, they can be used as monotherapy. More often, the agents are used in combination with sulfonylureas, metformin, and/or insulin. All of these uses, as monotherapy or in combination with other agents, are rational, although not all have received FDA approval as of this writing, so the package inserts should be consulted for guidance.

Safety. The first thiazolidinedione to be approved by the FDA was troglitazone. However, there was a significant frequency of hepatotoxicity with this formulation and approx 100 people taking the drug died of liver failure. This reaction was felt to be idiosyncratic, although epidemiologic studies suggested the possibility that the incidence of liver failure might have proven to be time and dose related if the experience with troglitazone had been longer. Liver failure has not been noted in significant frequency with the newer formulations pioglitazone and rosiglitazone. Nevertheless, the screening of liver function tests is still recommended every 2 mo for the first year of treatment and periodically thereafter.

The other major adverse effects of the thiazolidinediones are weight gain and fluid retention. The former probably results mainly from improved insulin action, such as is seen also with insulin or sulfonylurea therapy. In addition, the thiazolidinediones' ability to promote fat-cell differentiation may play a role. Fluid retention can be serious in patients with clinical heart failure and should be monitored by history and physical exam.

Hypoglycemia is very rarely seen in monotherapy with thiazolidinediones as would be predicted from their effect in augmenting insulin action rather than insulin secretion. However, in combination with insulin or a sulfonylurea, the agents can precipitate hypoglycemia. Thus, when the agents are added to insulin, it may be advisable to decrease the insulin dose to some degree (e.g., 20–30%), especially if the patient is already near glycemic goals. In the patient with poorly controlled blood sugars this is rarely necessary, although patients should be reminded about hypoglycemic symptoms and appropriate treatment should hypoglycemia occur.

Other Uses of Thiazolidinediones. Troglitazone had been included as an arm in a large National Institute of Health (NIH)-sponsored trial to develop methods to prevent or delay the onset of type 2 diabetes, although that arm of the trial was dropped after a subject died of liver failure. There is a rationale for this potential use of the drug, but given the relative short time over which these agents have been used, it is urged that practitioners wait for the results of ongoing controlled trials and FDA approval before using the drugs for that purpose. Safety becomes an even more overwhelming concern when drugs are used for prevention of a disease as opposed to treatment. Similarly, the use of the drugs to treat the "insulin-resistance syndrome" before the onset of diabetes is not approved and has little basis in science or data. More data are available to support use of the thiazolidinediones in the polycystic ovary syndrome, but that is counterbalanced by issues of fetal safety. Again, therefore, it is urged that off-label use of these and all drugs be minimized until safety and efficacy are proven.

α-*Glucosidase Inhibitors*

Complex carbohydrates require digestion in the upper gastrointestinal tract prior to their absorption as monosaccharides. This is accomplished by several enzymes, including a family of α-glucosidases. Inhibitors of these α-glucosidases can improve glycemic control in type 2 diabetes, largely by delaying absorption of the complex carbohydrate portion of the meal. This leads to lower and slower postprandial glycemic excursions that can be better controlled by the typically sluggish insulin release characteristic of type 2 diabetes. In addition, delivery of nutrients to more distal portions of the small bowel may induce secretion of gut hormones such as glucagonlike peptide 1 (GLP-1), a so-called incretin that will augment insulin secretion in response to increases in glycemia. Acarbose was the first α-glucosidase inhibitor available for clinical use. It has been extensively studied and found to be both safe and effective. Several large studies have demonstrated that the drug leads to reductions of HbA_{1c} in the range of 1%. Its effects are additive with those of other hypoglycemic agents, including sulfonylureas, metformin, and insulin. Miglitol, another α-glucosidase inhibitor, has a similar safety and efficacy profile. The use of α-glucosidase inhibitors to prevent or delay onset of type 2 diabetes is being explored.

These agents are especially attractive because of their safety profiles. They do not cause significant weight gain or hypoglycemia. It should be noted, however, that in patients also taking other antidiabetic drugs, the α-glucosidase inhibitors could delay absorption of starch or fructose taken to reverse hypoglycemia. Thus, patients on α-glucosidase inhibitors should be cautioned to use only glucose for rapid reversal of hypoglycemia. Acarbose is not significantly absorbed into the circulation, so is unlikely to have systemic side effects. Miglitol can be absorbed systemically, but its safety is comparable to that of acarbose. Rare hepatotoxicity has been reported, almost exclusively in Japan, and there is some question of whether this is even a specific drug effect, but currently the FDA does recommend periodic (every 3 mo) monitoring of liver function tests. Drug interactions could theoretically occur in the intestine via delayed absorption, but this has not proven to be a significant problem in practice. The major side effect is flatulence, serious enough to prompt patients to discontinue the drug, although this can be minimized by careful upward titration of doses. This minimizes delivery of carbohydrate to the large intestine both by defining a dose that does not allow such spillover and also by allowing induction of α-glucosidases in the ileum where they are normally expressed only at low levels.

THERAPY OF DIABETES: INSULIN

The oral antidiabetic agents each target one of the major causes of hyperglycemia in type 2 diabetes (e.g., hepatic glucose production, insulin resistance, or β-cell insufficiency). One agent targets all three pathologic mechanisms simultaneously and that is obviously insulin itself. The main drawback to insulin therapy has generally been hesitation on the part of the patient to inject the drug, but a host of factors are making that less of an issue. Needles are sharper, glucose monitoring is easier and more reliable, and therapy can be significantly less expensive than two- or three-drug oral regimens. In the future, when insulin is delivered by other routes, or when continuous glucose monitors will be linked to insulin pumps to achieve normoglycemia with minimal hypoglycemia, insulin therapy will be even more advantageous. Currently available insulin formulations are listed in Table 2. Not listed are the available combinations of intermediate- and rapid-acting insulins such as neutral protamine Hagedorn (NPH) mixed with regular or lispro insulin in ratios of 50/50, 70/30, or 75/25.

Table 2
Human Insulin Preparations

	Brand names	Onset	Peak
Very rapid			
lispro	Humalog	5–15 min	1–2 h
aspart	Novolog	5–15 min	1–2 h
Rapid			
regular	Humulin R, Novolin R, Velosulin	30–60 min	2–4 h
Intermediate			
NPH	Humulin N, Novolin N	1–3 h	5–7 h
lente	Humulin L, Novolin L	1–3 h	4–8 h
Long-acting			
ultralente	Humulin U	2–4 h	8–14 h
Very long-acting			
glargine	Lantus	1–3 h	[a]

[a]Nearly steady state levels are maintained for approx 24 h, with little "peaking."

Physiologic insulin replacement in total insulin deficiency (e.g., type 1 diabetes) requires a rapidly absorbed bolus of insulin taken with meals and a steady baseline throughout the day, with some adjustments of dosing in the early morning hours, with exercise, or with intercurrent illness. Achieving euglycemia is difficult: Undershooting insulin requirements will result in hyperglycemia and overshooting will result in hypoglycemia. Insulin therapy in type 2 diabetes, however, is more forgiving in that there is often a significant degree of residual β-cell function. Thus, it is often the case that "unloading" the β-cell with as little as one injection per day of longer-acting insulin is sufficient to add to the amount of insulin being produced endogenously and to result in adequate glycemic control. Hence, therapy is often simpler and safer than in type 2 compared to type 1 diabetes, although even type 2 can progress to the stage where very little insulin secretory capacity remains and multi-injection therapy becomes necessary.

Significant insulin resistance can sometimes make therapy in type 2 diabetes more difficult. It is not uncommon to use hundreds of units of insulin per day to achieve adequate control in some cases. A further complication is the fact that suppression of hepatic glucose production is usually more sensitive to insulin than is disposal of a glucose load into muscle and fat. Thus, a regimen that normalizes fasting glucose may be woefully inadequate to control postprandial surges, and addition of mealtime boluses of more rapidly acting insulins can become necessary after all. Finally, it should be pointed out that there is a maximum for the rate of insulin-stimulated glucose disposal. As seen in glucose "clamp" studies, for example, there is a point where insulin action is maximized and a plateau of glucose uptake is reached. For nondiabetic individuals, it is difficult to exceed those rates in nonexperimental situations. However, in type 2 diabetes, the maximal glucose disposal rate is often as low as 100 mg/min/m^2 of body surface area, or less than 0.2 g/min (12 g/h) total. These maximal glucose disposal rates can be exceeded with intravenous infusions or even oral intake: Total parenteral nutrition schemes can employ high-dextrose solutions, and a typical soft drink contains 30–40 g of carbohydrate. Thus, it is quite possible in an insulin-resistant individual to achieve rates of glucose absorption that cannot be handled by insulin-dependent mechanisms, regardless of the dose of insulin that is given.

Adding Insulin to Oral Agents

As mentioned previously, declaring a patient as an oral agent "failure" and instituting insulin therapy may be done prematurely in some cases. In a newly diagnosed diabetic, the phenomenon of "glucose toxicity" may impair β-cell function and exacerbate insulin resistance to a degree such that oral agents may not be sufficient to induce adequate glycemic control. However, after a relatively short period of glycemic control (e.g., with insulin), glucose levels can often be maintained using those same "failed" oral agents without additional insulin. Ultimately, however, the natural course of type 2 diabetes in most individuals is characterized by progressive failure to maintain adequate insulin secretion and progressive worsening of glycemic control. Thus, in practice, insulin therapy is most often initiated after "failure" of one or more oral agents. Whether insulin is added to a treatment regimen after failure of one, two, or more agents is largely an individual decision based on patient preference, cost, and other factors such as the generosity and persuasiveness of the local pharmaceutical sales force. In the author's experience, the decision to start insulin is often inappropriately delayed by the patient's fears, unrealistic promises to (finally) start serious dieting, or the difficulty in obtaining diabetes education and instruction services in a smaller practice setting. All of these are unfortunate. Patients to whom insulin therapy is properly introduced often find that it is not such a "big deal," and neither is it prohibitively difficult in most office settings to educate a patient to start a single injection of insulin daily.

Most patients start insulin after having been on a combination of a sulfonylurea and metformin. In the absence of one drug being discontinued for a specific reason, there are no completely conclusive data as to which agent, if any, should be replaced with insulin. Both sulfonylureas and metformin have been shown to be efficacious in combination with single doses of insulin (e.g., *see* ref. *20*). In fact, the weight gain that usually accompanies insulin therapy is attenuated in insulin–sulfonylurea combinations and may be eliminated altogether in metformin–insulin combinations *(20)*. The latter study demonstrated better control in the insulin–metformin group, so if renal function allows, it may be generally better to proceed from metformin–sulfonylurea combinations to insulin–metformin regimens. Whether there exists for these regimens an optimal insulin formulation, dose, or schedule is not clear. Good results have been obtained with bedtime NPH insulin, morning NPH, or suppertime 70/30 insulin. The above-cited large comparative study concluded that bedtime NPH with metformin was optimal *(20)*. Other combinations—insulin with a thiazolidinedione or an α-glucosidase inhibitor, for example—are also rational and effective. As was the case for choosing an oral agent for initial therapy, there are many routes to control and no means currently of predicting which will be best for a given patient.

The required doses of insulin used in combination with oral agents are unpredictable and need to be tailored to the individual. In most type 2 diabetics with normal or increased weight, it is safe to begin at 20 U of NPH at bedtime. It is important to note, however, that the dose that is ultimately determined to be effective may easily be twice or three times that. Thus, it is important to make changes rapidly enough so that control is achieved in a reasonable amount of time. An effective way to do so is to allow the patient to adjust his or her dose at home. This should not be done too rapidly: Resolving glucose toxicity can lead to overshooting the proper dose, and one does not want to rely on single glucose determinations to dictate the therapy. One reasonable scheme is to make adjustments of 2 U at a time and to make those adjustments only every 3–4 d. For example, a patient may be instructed to increase his or her dose in that manner until a suitably safe target (e.g., a morning fasting glucose level of 140–160 mg/dL after bedtime NPH) is reached. Fine-tuning and tighter control can then proceed at the next visit to the practitioner.

Proceeding to Multiple Injections of Insulin

Once a target glucose level is achieved in response to the single injection of insulin, it is then necessary to decide if the overall glycemic control is adequate. In the case of bedtime NPH, after a target blood glucose value (110–140 mg/dL) is reached in the morning, it is simple then to check blood sugar values during the afternoon. If presupper glucose levels are adequately controlled, then the chosen regimen may be sufficient. Further checks of postprandial glucose levels and, after a suitable interval, HbA_{1c} levels will dictate if all of the goals for that individual have been met. If the initially chosen single-injection insulin regimen employs suppertime 70/30 insulin, bedtime hypoglycemia may limit dose increases so that morning goals cannot be safely met. If overall glycemic control is not adequate, additional injections of insulin will be added to the regimen. Generally, the first step will be to add a second injection of NPH; in the case where the first injection was at bedtime, the second will be before breakfast. If goals through the rest of the day are not met with two injections, it is probably best to proceed directly to full insulin replacement. This is best done with a scheme that provides a relatively steady baseline (ultralente insulin, insulin glargine, or two injections of NPH) plus bolus coverage with each meal (regular or a shorter-acting insulin such as lispro). As is the case for type 1 diabetes, once the patient has been deemed to be dependent on multiple injections for glycemic control, there is little to recommend simpler insulin regimens, such as twice daily injections of mixed NPH and regular. In this situation, trying to cover glycemic excursions at lunch with a morning dose of NPH insulin are restrictive and often result in late-morning hypoglycemia. This, in turn, necessitates snacking, resulting in weight gain and worsening control. Dose requirements are highly variable from individual to individual. The patient following simple dosage adjustment algorithms at home can often get close to the proper dose in a timely fashion. However, in such cases, it is safest and easiest to adjust the dose of only one component of the regimen at a time and to choose conservative goals so that hypoglycemia does not ensue.

It should be remembered that with the shorter-acting insulins, even four premeal glucose determinations per day do not necessarily inform us as to how high the postprandial excursions may have been. Goals for postprandial glucose levels and the risks of isolated postprandial hyperglycemia are still being evaluated, but the evidence at this time supports the potential dangers of excessive postprandial glucose excursions. In practice, it is often easier first to achieve the chosen goals for the fasting glucose values and then proceed with determining the precise dosing for control of postprandial glucose levels with the shorter-acting insulin. In this situation, patients should be taught how to vary the insulin dose based on carbohydrate content of the meal and other variables such as activity, intercurrent illness, and the level of glucose before the meal.

If it has been determined that a complex, multi-injection regimen is necessary for adequate glycemic control, the next question is when or whether to discontinue the oral agent(s) altogether. There are no conclusive data that allow us to make universal recommendations. In general, if the oral agent is a sulfonylurea, it makes somewhat less sense to maintain that agent if insulin is being replaced with multiple injections. Other agents, particularly metformin, acarbose, and thiazolidinediones, may help with maintaining glycemic control even in multi-injection regimens and may have other benefits (e.g., minimization of weight gain).

Adding Oral Agents to Insulin

To this point, the discussion has focused on adding insulin to oral regimens, but it may also be the case that oral agents can be added to insulin. Adding metformin, a thiazolidinedione, or acarbose to an inadequate insulin regimen may be sufficient to achieve control without resorting to more complex, multi-injection schemes. Adding a glinide with each meal to a twice-daily NPH regimen is also logical although unstudied and not FDA approved. A special situation is the patient not under control despite very large doses of insulin (hundreds of units daily). This group may include patients who are eating enough to exceed their maximal glucose disposal rates despite saturating doses of insulin. The thiazolidinediones may be particularly helpful in the presence of this degree of insulin resistance, perhaps by means of opening new fat depots for storage of the excess calories.

Dangers of Insulin Therapy

The chief danger of insulin therapy is hypoglycemia, which is seen at higher frequency than in therapy with sulfonylureas. However, this is still much less of a problem in type 2 than in type 1 diabetes. A VA Co-operative Study found, for example, that the rate of hypoglycemia with intensive treatment of type 2 diabetes was only 5% of that seen in intensive treatment of type 1 diabetes *(21)*. This is probably best explained by the fact that residual β-cell function in most cases of type 2 diabetes allows the final "filling in" of insulin requirements by endogenous insulin secretion, which is, of course, glucose dependent. As an aside, it should be pointed out that this same VA study encountered a higher rate of cardiac events in the intensively treated group. The etiology of this effect is not clear, and it was not seen in other studies of intensive management of type 2 diabetes, where, in fact, decreased rates of cardiac events resulted. However, it may argue for a slower approach to normoglycemia, especially in the more elderly type 2 diabetes population that is already highly likely to have at least some degree of coronary artery disease.

Special Situations for Insulin Therapy

Several special situations may call for temporary insulin therapy in type 2 diabetes in patients previously controlled with oral agents. These include the following:

- **Temporary situations of increased insulin demand.** Corticosteroid therapy may worsen insulin resistance. Insulin may be added temporarily, although it may also be possible to simply "wait out" the situation, especially for short courses of steroids, unless the hyperglycemia is resulting in other problems such as dehydration from polyuria. The latter can be a particular problem if the steroids are being used as part of a cancer chemotherapy routine and other agents being used are toxic and/or cleared by renal excretion. In this and other situations to follow, however, it is important to remember that the illness necessitating the steroids may also be one that affects appetite or ability to eat. If this is the case, it may be more prudent to treat with shorter acting insulins. For longer term steroid use, thiazolidinediones may be of benefit (*see* next section).

- **Infections.** Hyperglycemia may impair the body's ability to combat infections, and at the same time the cytokines being elaborated can impair glycemic control. With the same caveats of the previous example, in general it is recommended that glucose levels be maintained below 200 mg/dL during acute infections.
- Acute care of **diabetic ketoacidosis or nonketotic hyperosmolar hyperglycemia** generally requires insulin therapy.
- There is evidence that insulin/glucose infusions in **acute myocardial infarction** may limit infarct size and result in better long-term survival in some patients with type 2 diabetes (e.g., *see* ref. *22*). This is currently not universally practiced, but based on existing evidence it should be strongly considered. More recent data demonstrate similar beneficial effects of tight glycemic control in a broader spectrum of patients in the intensive care unit.
- In **pregnancy**, insulin is the only agent approved for diabetes treatment.

THERAPY DECISIONS IN SPECIAL SITUATIONS

There are several specific situations that frequently confront the physician caring for people with diabetes, some of which have been addressed in previous sections. These include the following:

- **Renal failure.** Insulin is an ideal solution to the patient with advanced renal disease. In particular, a flexible regimen that includes a rapidly acting insulin given with each meal will accommodate the fluctuations in appetite and scheduling that occur with end-stage renal disease and dialysis. Some of the newer sulfonylureas and glinides are largely cleared through the liver and do not have active metabolites that would accumulate in renal failure. These may be safe and effective in advanced renal disease, although their use in dialysis remains controversial, unproven, and/or unapproved.
- **The elderly.** Caution with all pharmacotherapy is called for in the elderly. Most of the dangers associated with the agents described in this chapter will increase in the elderly. For example, renal function may become tenuous and increasingly affected by a host of factors such as dehydration, urinary obstruction, or infection. Furthermore, loss of muscle mass may result in serum creatinine levels becoming less obvious as indices of renal failure. Surveillance, such as with metformin use, thus becomes even more critical than in the general population. Any agent that predisposes to hypoglycemia also becomes more of a danger in the elderly, particularly in those individuals who are less able to sense and respond appropriately to hypoglycemia. Therefore, as the therapies become more hazardous in the elderly, targets for therapy may need to be relaxed. Furthermore, it becomes less urgent to prevent diabetic nephropathy 10 yr hence in a person with another illness that confers an expectancy of survival less than that. Tight glycemic control may also be less important in those patients who, for whatever reason, may have had diabetes for decades but have no proteinuria or indications of cardiovascular disease. However, glycemic control may be associated with improved cognitive function in the elderly, and at the very least, it is important to minimize nocturia that can result in dehydration, dangerous nighttime excursions to the bathroom, or incontinence. Thus, treatment of diabetes in the elderly should proceed with caution but should not be ignored.
- **Children.** Type 2 diabetes is becoming increasingly prevalent in youth. Optimal therapies are still being investigated; weight loss and exercise remain the best option. When pharmacologic therapy is needed, consideration should be given to the fact that these children may be taking medications for the next 60 yr of their lives. Thus, proven remedies with long track records of safety (e.g., metformin, insulin secretagogues, or insulin) may be preferable until the newer drugs have been tested for longer periods.

- **Glucocorticoid use.** The use of insulin in cases of diabetes resulting from steroids has been considered in this chapter. In patients who will be on steroids for more prolonged periods, thiazolidinediones have been demonstrated to be effective in animal models *(23)*, although further investigation in humans is needed.

FUTURE THERAPIES

Assuming the physician, patient, and health care team are well informed and dedicated, it is usually possible to achieve adequate control of glycemia in most patients with type 2 diabetes, at least to current standards. However, some current evidence suggests that to impact cardiovascular disease risk more favorably, we may need to achieve even tighter levels of glycemic control in our patients. Achieving these more stringent goals will be more elusive and will be increasingly limited by the risk of hypoglycemia. New therapies and preventative strategies are therefore still needed, and among the most likely to succeed in the near future are the following:

- **Better drugs for weight control.** Knowledge about the mechanisms of appetite regulation by the central nervous system is increasing at a rapid pace, such that safe and effective appetite suppression may be feasible in the foreseeable future. Mechanisms to promote fat oxidation (e.g., through the manipulation of adrenergic tone in the adipocyte or the activity of uncoupling proteins) are also being pursued. This seems an almost necessary component of an effective antidiabetic armamentarium, especially in preventing the disease. Ultimately, without addressing decreased intake or increased burning of excess calories, it is difficult to imagine a strategy that will simply allow us to store excess calories without leading eventually to other problems such as weight gain or excess tissue levels of carbohydrate or lipid.
- **Drugs that can achieve glycemic control with less danger of hypoglycemia.** Agents that require sensing of hyperglycemia before the hypoglycemic action is initiated would be ideal. Incretins such as GLP-1 may prove useful in this regard. The other strategy to avoid hypoglycemia is to link therapy (e.g., insulin) to continuous blood glucose sensing, and that goal, too, is rapidly becoming a realistic possibility.
- **Drugs to prevent type 2 diabetes in subjects at risk.** At this time, these studies are largely focused on treatment of abnormal glucose homeostasis, using the agents already used for diabetes itself (metformin, thiazolidinediones), but at an earlier stage in the evolution of the disease. Many of these same agents are being investigated for safety and efficacy in dealing with other diabetes-related conditions such as the polycystic ovarian syndrome.
- Perhaps most important of all, **social and political solutions need to be found at the level of family, school, and community** to encourage less eating and more exercise.

REFERENCES

1. Horikawa Y, Oda N. Cox NJ, et al. Genetic variation in the gene encoding calpain-10 is associated with type 2 diabetes mellitus. Nat Genet 2000;26:163–175.
2. Rossetti L, Giaccari A, DeFronzo RA. Glucose toxicity. Diabetes Care 1990;13:610–630.
3. Lee Y, Hirose H, Ohneda M, . Beta-cell lipotoxicity in the pathogenesis of non-insulin-dependent diabetes mellitus of obese rats: impairment in adipocyte-beta-cell relationships. Proc Natl Acad Sci USA 1994;91:10,878–10,882.
4. McClain DA, Crook ED. Hexosamines and insulin resistance. Diabetes 1996;45:1003–1009.
5. The Diabetes Control and Complications Trial Research Group. The effect of intensive treatment of diabetes on the development and progression of long-term complications in insulin-dependent diabetes mellitus. N Engl J Med 1993;329:977–986.

6. UK Prospective Diabetes Study (UKPDS) Group. Effect of intensive blood-glucose control with metformin on complications in overweight patients with type 2 diabetes (UKPDS 34). Lancet 1998;352:854–865.

7. UK Prospective Diabetes Study (UKPDS) Group. Intensive blood-glucose control with sulphonylureas or insulin compared with conventional treatment and risk of complications in patients with type 2 diabetes (UKPDS 33). Lancet 1998;352:837–853.

8. Bastyr EJ 3rd, Stuart CA, Brodows RG, et al. Therapy focused on lowering postprandial glucose, not fasting glucose, may be superior for lowering HbA1c. IOEZ Study Group. Diabetes Care 2000;23:1236–1241.

9. Barrett-Connor E, Ferrara A. Isolated postchallenge hyperglycemia and the risk of fatal cardiovascular disease in older women and men. The Rancho Bernardo Study. Diabetes Care 1998;21:1236–1239.

10. Donahue RP, Abbott RD, Reed DM, et al. Postchallenge glucose concentration and coronary heart disease in men of Japanese ancestry. Honolulu Heart Program. Diabetes 198736:689–692.

11. Khaw KT, Wareham N, Luben R, et al. Glycated haemoglobin, diabetes, and mortality in men in Norfolk cohort of european prospective investigation of cancer and nutrition (EPIC- Norfolk). Br Med J 2001;322:15–18.

12. The DECODE study group. European Diabetes Epidemiology Group. Diabetes epidemiology: collaborative analysis of diagnostic criteria in Europe. Glucose tolerance and mortality: comparison of WHO and American Diabetes Association diagnostic criteria. Lancet 1999;354:617–621.

13. Ashcroft SJ, Ashcroft FM. The sulfonylurea receptor. Biochim Biophys Acta 1992;1175:45–59.

14. Matschinsky FM. Banting Lecture 1995. A lesson in metabolic regulation inspired by the glucokinase glucose sensor paradigm. Diabetes 1996;45:223–241.

15. Shorr RI, Ray WA, Daugherty JR, et al. Individual sulfonylureas and serious hypoglycemia in older people. J Am Geriatr Soc 1996;44:751–755.

16. Campbell RK. Glimepiride: role of a new sulfonylurea in the treatment of type 2 diabetes mellitus. Ann Pharmacother 1998;32:1044–1052.

17. Kosaka K, Kuzuya T, Akanuma Y, et al. Increase in insulin response after treatment of overt maturity-onset diabetes is independent of the mode of treatment. Diabetologia 1980;18:23–28.

18. Meinert CL, Knatterud GL, Prout TE, et al. A study of the effects of hypoglycemic agents on vascular complications in patients with adult-onset diabetes. II. Mortality results. Diabetes 197019:789–830.

19. Ashcroft FM, Gribble FM. Tissue-specific effects of sulfonylureas: lessons from studies of cloned K(ATP) channels. J Diabetes Complic 2000;14:192–196.

20. Yki-Jarvinen H, Kauppila M, Kujansuu E, et al. Comparison of insulin regimens in patients with non-insulin-dependent diabetes mellitus. N Engl J Med 1992;327:1426–1433.

21. Abraira C, Henderson WG, Colwell JA, et al. Response to intensive therapy steps and to glipizide dose in combination with insulin in type 2 diabetes. VA feasibility study on glycemic control and complications (VA CSDM). Diabetes Care 1998;21:574–579.

22. Diaz R, Paolasso EA, Piegas LS, et al. Metabolic modulation of acute myocardial infarction. The ECLA (Estudios Cardiologicos Latinoamerica) Collaborative Group. Circulation 1998;98:2227–2234.

23. Okumura S, Takeda N, Takami K, Yet al. Effects of troglitazone on dexamethasone-induced insulin resistance in rats. Metabolism 1998;47:351–354.

12 Management of Diabetes in Pregnancy

Kay F. McFarland, MD, Laura S. Irwin, MD, and Janice Bacon, MD

CONTENTS

INTRODUCTION

Diabetes increases the risks associated with pregnancy. During pregnancy retinopathy and nephropathy may worsen in women with pregestational diabetes *(1,2)*. Other maternal complications include increased frequency of hypoglycemia, preeclampsia, pyelonephritis, and polyhydramnios. The infant also faces challenges imposed by the abnormal

From: *Endocrine Replacement Therapy in Clinical Practice*
Edited by: A. Wayne Meikle © Humana Press Inc., Totowa, NJ

metabolic environment. Macrosomia, hypoglycemia, congenital anomalies, respiratory distress syndrome, hyperbilirubinemia, and hypocalcemia increase neonatal morbidity *(3–9)*. However, intensive glucose management minimizes complications and optimizes the outcome for the mother and the baby *(10–12)*.

CLASSIFICATION AND PREVALENCE

Gestational diabetes, carbohydrate intolerance first recognized during pregnancy, affects about 7% of pregnancies though the prevalence may range from 1 to 14% of pregnancies depending on the population studied and the diagnostic tests used *(13)*. The designation simply means that hyperglycemia first became evident during pregnancy and does not preclude the possibility that glucose intolerance antedated pregnancy. Also, the designation applies whether or not diabetes persists after pregnancy *(13)*. Subdividing gestational diabetes by treatment, *diet managed* or *insulin treated*, assists in timing the initiation of fetal surveillance and delivery.

The onset of diabetes prior to pregnancy, called *preexisting diabetes*, occurs much less frequently than gestational diabetes. Further classification of preexisting diabetes into *type 1*, insulin-sensitive diabetes, and *type 2*, insulin-resistant diabetes, predicts the lability of glucose fluctuations, with the widest excursions occurring in type 1 diabetes. Pregnancy sometimes accelerates diabetic renal disease and retinopathy, which add substantial risk to pregnancies associated with these complications. Therefore, *diabetes-related complications* warrant special notation. Some *complications of past pregnancies*, such a history of a stillbirth, also influence management of subsequent pregnancies. Therefore, classification of diabetes during pregnancy includes any diabetes-related complication or pregnancy-related complication, in addition to the designation: gestational diabetes (diet managed or insulin treated) or preexisting diabetes (type 1 or type 2).

PATHOPHYSIOLOGY

The placenta secretes insulin antagonistic hormones, including progesterone and human placental lactogen, which, along with elevated levels of prolactin and cortisol contribute to the insulin resistance found during pregnancy. Hyperglycemia results when insulin secretion does not increase sufficiently to counterbalance the increasing insulin resistance characteristic of the second half of pregnancy. Thus, gestational diabetes results from a combination of insulin resistance and impaired insulin secretion *(14–16)*.

The insulin resistance leads to more rapid mobilization of maternal fat, which increases plasma and urinary ketones during the fasting state. Glucose utilization by the fetus contributes to lower maternal fasting plasma glucose levels and activation of hepatic glucose production. When insulin secretion does not keep pace with the increasing insulin resistance, maternal hyperglycemia results and the fetus receives an overabundant supply of glucose. This causes increased fetal insulin production which leads to macrosomia.

Both diabetes and pregnancy alter counterregulatory hormonal responses to hypoglycemia. Also, the metabolic clearance rate of insulin decreases during pregnancy *(17)*. These changes contribute to a higher incidence of hypoglycemia in insulin-treated women during pregnancy *(18)*. Immediately after delivery of the placenta, progesterone and human placental lactogen levels fall and insulin requirements decline precipitously to levels present prior to pregnancy.

GLUCOSE LEVELS AND PREGNANCY OUTCOME

Elevated glucose concentrations negatively affect both maternal and infant outcomes. Macrosomia is the most common neonatal complication associated with gestational diabetes. Fetal size correlates with maternal glucose levels as early as the first trimester of pregnancy *(19)*. There is a significant relation between increasing maternal screening glucose levels and mean birth weight *(20)* and between postprandial glucose values and fetal abdominal circumference *(21)*. Persson and co-workers found that mothers with large-for-gestational-age infants had significantly higher fasting glucose levels during pregnancy weeks 27 to 32 than mothers of average size (for gestational age) infants *(8)*. Even in women without gestational diabetes, a continuum of risk related to maternal glucose levels exists for increased infant birth weight, an assisted delivery, congenital anomalies, and the likelihood of the baby being admitted to a special care nursery *(22–25)*.

Women who have abnormal glucose tolerance, also, are more likely to develop hypertension than those with normal glucose levels *(26)*. During pregnancy, the 2-h postprandial glucose level positively correlates with peak mean arterial pressure. Primiparous women with both gestational diabetes and preeclampsia are at increased risk of developing preeclampsia in a second pregnancy *(27)*.

In addition, diabetes during pregnancy increases the risk of fetal congenital abnormalities. Review of the Swedish Medical Birth Registry between 1987 and 1997, showed that women with preexisting diabetes had an infant malformation rate of 9.5% compared to 5.7% in the general population. The infants had an increased incidence of orofacial clefts, cardiovascular defects, esophageal/intestinal atresia, hyposapdias, limb reduction defects, spine malformations, and polydactyly *(28)*.

However, intensive glucose management instituted early in pregnancy significantly affects outcomes. During the Diabetes Control and Complication Trial, a multicenter study of the effect of intensive versus conventional management of type 1 diabetes, 180 women completed 270 pregnancies, which resulted in 191 total live births. The mean glycohemoglobin at conception differed between the intensively managed group and those using conventional therapy (7.4 vs 8.1%). After the onset of pregnancy, all women received intensive management and the glycohemoglobin averaged 6.6% in both groups. Eight congenital malformations occurred in women assigned to conventional therapy before conception and one occurred in the intensively treated group managed group (*p* = 0.06) Thirty spontaneous abortions occurred, 13.3% in the intensively and 10.4% in the conventionally treated group. Overall, there was no significant difference in outcome between the women using conventional therapy prior to pregnancy and those on intensive therapy. The study suggests that timely institution of intensive therapy is associated with rates of spontaneous abortion and congenial malformation similar to those in the nondiabetic population *(29)*.

PRECONCEPTION PLANNING FOR WOMEN WITH DIABETES

Counseling before pregnancy provides an opportunity to discuss the benefits of intensive diabetes management. Intensive therapy optimizes pregnancy outcomes and special prenatal care may reduce medical care costs *(30)*. The heightened fears surrounding diabetes during pregnancy calls for tact during the discussion of the risks associated with hyperglycemia during pregnancy. Nevertheless, women should know that high glucose levels during the first trimester increase the risk of congenital malformations and spontaneous abortion and that pregnancy may induce or aggravate preexisting hypertension. In more than 40% of women with renal insufficiency, pregnancy may induce permanent worsening of renal function *(31)*. Additional incentives for intensive management include the association of maternal hyperglycemia with fetal anomalies, macrosomia, and neonatal hypoglycemia. Before conception, hemoglobin A1χ levels should be as close to normal as possible and values less than 1% above the normal range are desirable *(32)*.

Couples need to decide what risks they are willing to accept to have a child. The women at highest risk are those with ischemic heart disease, proliferative retinopathy, and hypertension. Preconception counseling educates women with renal insufficiency about the possibility of more rapid deterioration of renal function during pregnancy. Women with vomiting or diarrhea associated with gastroenteropathy face the added risk of wide glucose swings resulting from variable food intake and absorption.

The preconception assessment should include a history and physical examination. Women with diabetes for more than 5 yr should have a dilated eye exam by an ophthalmologist. Appropriate laboratory tests include a hemoglobin A_{1c} to evaluate the mean glucose levels over the previous 2–3 mo, a urinalysis, serum creatinine, and 24-h urine albumin. A thyroid panel and EKG also may be indicated.

Management before pregnancy focuses on achieving as close to normal glucose levels as possible. This involves nutritional counseling, instruction about an exercise program, and details regarding insulin administration. A dietician can help patients devise meal plans to achieve or maintain ideal body weight and minimize hyperglycemia and insulin reaction. As women make positive changes for the sake of a future pregnancy, other health care issues such as smoking cessation and avoidance of alcohol may need attention.

PSYCHOSOCIAL ISSUES

Diabetes invariably intensifies emotional responses already heightened by pregnancy. Most women fear that diabetes will harm their baby and some worry about their own health. Glucose levels above the targeted range heighten a woman's fear and hypoglycemic reactions intensify anxiety. Hope and discouragement rise and plummet with glucose levels.

During the first trimester, vomiting may suppress the desire to eat and upset the regularity of meals, which may increase the frequency of hypoglycemia. Heightened insulin sensitivity, particularly in the last weeks of the first trimester, also, increase glucose variability. These accentuate the frequency of both hypoglycemic reactions and hyperglycemia. Frustration develops when glucose levels do not stay close to target goals. Financial worries may add to the distress and further influence diabetes management. Thus, emotional lability, variable coping resources, physiologic changes, and financial concerns all may negatively affect the ability to deal with medical recommendations.

Women often seek emotional support from family, friends, and, particularly, from members of the health care team. Fortunately, intensified management does not adversely affect mood, and women glean hope from normal glucose levels. Education, particularly about the favorable outcomes of most pregnancies complicated by gestational diabetes, provides reassurance.

In women with diabetic complications prior to pregnancy, fear of visual loss, or worsening renal insufficiency may sap energy and intensifies the anxiety normally accompanying pregnancy. This anxiety manifests differently in each individual. However, the psychological gains from near-normal glucose levels help buffer anxiety, although fear may resurface with each abnormal glucose check or hint of a complication.

Not all women are able to utilize the care given or conform to the rigorous schedule and multiple demands that a pregnancy complicated by diabetes demands. Each woman responds differently; thus guidelines and treatment regimens must be modified to take into account individual circumstances and limitations as well as medical needs. Individualization of care becomes essential to achieve the best possible glucose levels and pregnancy outcome.

SCREENING FOR GESTATIONAL DIABETES

Current guidelines recommend that all pregnant women over age 25 who do not have a prior history of glucose intolerance undergo screening for glucose intolerance. Also, those under age 25 should be tested if their weight is abnormal, they have a family history of diabetes, they have a history of a poor obstetric outcome, or if they are a member of a high risk ethnic population such as African-American, Hispanic-American, Native American, Asian-American, or Pacific Islander (33). Although other groups, such as women with polycystic ovarian disease (34,35), those who themselves were small at birth (less than the 10th percentile for gestational age) (36), and short women (37,38), have a higher risk of diabetes developing during pregnancy, there are no specific screening recommendations for these groups.

Screening, normally scheduled between 24 and 28 wk of gestation, involves the administration of a 50-g oral glucose solution with blood drawn for glucose measurement 1 h later. This screening test may be done at any time of the day, fasting or postprandial. When the plasma glucose exceeds 140 mg/dL (7.8 mmol/L), however, the women need to undergo a full 3-h glucose tolerance test. This two-tiered system identifies 80% of women with gestational diabetes. A screening value cutoff of greater than 130 mg/dL (7.2 mmol/dL) increases the diagnostic yield to 90%. Some prefer a one-tiered procedure that involves an initial glucose tolerance test without prior screening. This may be cost-effective in high-risk patients (13) and may necessitate less travel time (39).

GLUCOSE TOLERANCE TEST

The glucose tolerance test, performed after an overnight fast, involves measurement of a fasting plasma glucose and glucose levels at 1, 2, and 3 h after a 100-g oral glucose solution. Two values which equal or exceed 95 mg/dL (5.3 mmol/L) fasting, 180 mg/dL (10 mmol/L) at 1 h, 155 mg/dL (8.6 mmol/L) at 2 h, and 140 mg/dL (7.8 mmol/L) at 3 h confirm the diagnosis of gestational diabetes (33). Alternatively a 75-g 2-h glucose tolerance test may be used with the same values applied as for the 100 g glucose load (40).

TREATMENT GOALS

Discussion of the risks and benefits of intensive diabetes management assists in setting treatment goals. Prior to pregnancy recommended glycemic goals can be set at 80–110 mg/dL (4.4–6.1 mmol/L) fasting and <155 mg/dL (8.6 mmol/L) 2 h postprandially. However, these may require modification depending on the risk of hypoglycemia (32). Ideally, setting goals occurs prior to conception in women with type 1 or type 2 diabetes or immediately after diagnosis in those with gestational diabetes. During pregnancy goals include glucose levels as close to normal as possible with the least frequency of hypoglycemia. During the third trimester, the overall mean glucose level in women without diabetes is 75 mg/dL and the 1 h value is less than 105 mg/dL *(21)*.

GLUCOSE AND KETONE MONITORING

The results of self glucose monitoring provide a basis for determining the need for insulin therapy and for insulin dose changes *(41)*. A diabetes educator or pharmacist can familiarize the woman with the meter used for monitoring. The meters require periodic calibration using a reference solution and similar readings between meters used for home monitoring and those in the physician's office further verify meter and operator accuracy. A discrepancy of more than 15% between meters should prompt comparison of the code on the glucose strips and the meters. Next, the meters should be cleaned and a comparison test repeated. A continuing difference of more than 15% between meters necessitates comparison with a laboratory standard and replacement of the inaccurate meter(s).

Urine dipstick evaluation also should be done at each office visit to check for urinary tract infection, protein, and ketones. Skipped meals and inadequate caloric intake lead to increased utilization of fat for energy and ketonuria. Urine ketone testing, recommended for women with inadequate weight gain during pregnancy, provides a standard by which women can judge whether or not they have eaten enough. Trace urinary ketones usually do not require intervention. Moderate to large urinary ketones mean that the frequency and/or content of meals need modification.

DIABETES EDUCATION

In addition to verbal instruction, women welcome written material covering the essentials of diabetes care, including meal planning, insulin administration, and ways to balance exercise with meals and insulin. The frequency and timing of self glucose monitoring require consideration of each woman's schedule, type of diabetes, and financial resources. Education regarding preventive care, such as the need for periodic ophthalmologic examination, also necessitates individualized counseling. Women with diabetic retinopathy may have acceleration of their retinopathy during pregnancy, whereas women with diabetes first diagnosed during pregnancy do not need special ophthalmologic attention.

Insulin-treated women and their family members need to know the signs and symptoms of hypoglycemia and understand the importance of always keeping some source of sugar readily available. Women who take insulin should be instructed regarding the need to eat whenever glucose levels fall below 60 mg/dL or they sense a hypoglycemic reaction. Overtreatment of hypoglycemia causes rebound hyperglycemia and may contribute to poor glycemic control. Glucose tablets or gels work quicker than milk and result in a more consistent glycemic response without rebound hyperglycemia. Family members of women with type 1 diabetes need instruction regarding the use of glucagon for severe hypoglycemic reactions that result in unconsciousness.

NUTRITIONAL RECOMMENDATIONS

Individualized nutritional assessment becomes central for devising a diet plan that meets maternal and fetal needs and optimizes glycemia *(42)*. Cultural, economic, and educational factors influence dietary recommendations. In addition to appetite and weight assessments, blood glucose levels and the record of urinary ketones serve as guides to the individualized meal plan *(43)*.

Diabetes does not alter the general dietary recommendations for pregnancy, except that complex carbohydrates replace free sugars. Regular timing of meals and frequent snacks reduce the incidence of hypoglycemia. Women who use continuous subcutaneous insulin delivery by a pump have more flexibility with mealtimes and snacks than women who use injections. Consistency from day to day and minimizing the intake of sucrose assist in attaining glycemic goals. Limiting carbohydrate intake to 35–40% of calories may decrease maternal glucose levels and improve maternal and fetal outcomes *(44)*.

Weight gain recommendations, based on women's weight prior to pregnancy, vary from 15 lbs (7 kg) for obese women to 40 lbs (18 kg) for underweight women. A calorie intake sufficient to promote an average weight gain of 25–30 lbs usually prevents ketonemia. A dietician and diabetes educator can help the woman with diabetes devise creative meal plans suited to her preferences. The glycemic index defined as the percent increase in blood glucose after the ingestion of a food varies with both meal content and manner of preparation. Patients can determine how specific foods affect their glucose levels by frequent blood glucose monitoring. Insulin must balance the quantity of food, especially the carbohydrate intake. Three meals with three snacks are considered optimal and appropriate for nausea and vomiting associated with early pregnancy and also help avoid third-trimester early satiety.

Vitamin, mineral, and folate supplements help meet daily nutritional recommendations, as the typical American diet does not supply iron and folate needs. During pregnancy, the folate requirement more than doubles and the requirements for phosphorous, thiamine, and vitamin B_6 increase by 33–50% with lesser increases in protein, zinc, and riboflavin requirement. Calcium need increases by 33% to as much as 400% per day. Vitamin B_6, calcium, magnesium, iron, zinc, and copper intake often is deficient, with intakes less than 80% of the recommended daily requirements. Meats, poultry, fish, and dairy products, which are rich in these nutrients, help met these nutritional requirements *(42)*.

Artificial sweeteners, although not essential, help reduce consumption of simple sugars. Aspartic acid, a metabolite of aspartame, does not readily cross the placenta, and methanol levels rise only minimally. Phenylalanine, the third breakdown product of aspartame, does cross the placenta and fetal levels stay below toxic levels, even with twice the acceptable daily intake. Acesulfame-K and saccharin do not appear harmful during pregnancy *(42)*. Therefore, noncaloric sweeteners may be used in moderation *(45)*.

EXERCISE

Low- to moderate-intensity exercise may significantly decrease blood glucose levels in gestational diabetes *(46)*. However, exercise carries more potential risks during pregnancy than in nonpregnant adults. Physiologic changes during pregnancy such as increased laxity in joints, center of balance changes, plasma volume expansion, and progestational changes in venous compliance make injury, dehydration, and hypovolemia more likely.

An exercise program must be individualized. To avoid complications, the maternal heart rate should remain below 150 beats per minute. The "talk test" serves as a practical method to avoid overexertion. Other recommendations include limiting exercise to levels that do not cause exhaustion, maintaining good hydration and ventilation, and cessation of exercise if any pain or bleeding occurs. Although uterine activity may increase during exercise, overall exercise has not been associated with increased pregnancy risk *(47)*. Medical contraindications to exercise include preterm labor and hypertension, both of which may be increased in diabetes.

Although few studies assess the risks and benefits of exercise during pregnancy, the American Diabetes Association clinical practice recommendations indicate that women with gestational diabetes who do not have a medical or obstetrical contraindication may participate in an exercise program *(13)*. The therapeutic benefits still need defining, as a prospective randomized study of women with gestational diabetes showed that daily blood glucose levels, hemoglobin A_{1c}, use of insulin, and the incidence of newborn hypoglycemia were not different in women assigned to exercise compared to those in the no-exercise group *(48)*. On the other hand, Weller reports a 90% success rate in maintaining women with gestational diabetes on diet therapy and exercise without the need for insulin *(49)*.

INSULIN

Gestational diabetes often is managed by diet and exercise alone. However, insulin treatment is recommended if diet and exercise do not consistently maintain the fasting plasma glucose <105 mg/dL (5.8 mmol/dL) or the 2-h postprandial plasma glucose exceeds 120 mg/dL (6.7 mmol/L) *(13)*. Oral agents generally are not recommended. However, one randomized trial that compared insulin and glyburide treatment in women with gestational diabetes found that both forms of treatment produced similar perinatal outcomes *(50)*. Glyburide is not approved by the Food and Drug Administration (FDA) for the treatment of gestational diabetes and further studies are needed in larger patient populations to establish its safety *(13)*.

As pregnancy progresses, increasing production of placental hormones causes insulin resistance and increasing insulin need, often with a particularly large increase between 20 and 24 wk gestation. Insulin resistance makes hypoglycemia less frequent despite higher insulin doses. Usually during the second trimester and early third trimester, the insulin dose must be increased progressively to maintain near-normal glucose levels.

Human insulin, the least immunogenic insulin, comes in several modifications that alter absorption and duration of action. Regular insulin, usually taken 30–45 min before meals, begins acting 30–60 min after injection. To obtain normal postprandial glucose levels and avoid preprandial hypoglycemia, sometimes even 1 h needs to elapse between the injection of regular insulin and the meal. Also, because insulin absorption occurs more rapidly from the abdomen than from the legs or hips, using the abdomen for insulin injections before meals may help lower postprandial glucose concentrations. Insulin given four times rather than twice daily improved glucose levels and perinatal outcomes in one study *(51)*.

Lispro insulin begins working in minutes and lasts about 2 h. Injection just prior to meals offers convenience and effectively lowers 1 and 2 h postprandial glucose levels without leading to preprandial hypoglycemia. Even when taken 15 min after meals, lispro effectively lowers postprandial glucose levels. Although few studies are available to establish the safety of lispro insulin during pregnancy, treatment with lispro insulin does not appear to negatively affect diabetic retinopathy *(52)* or alter fetal outcomes *(53)*. Table 1 outlines insulin changes that may help regulate glucose levels.

Table 1
Insulin Dose Adjustments for Abnormal Glucose Levels[a]

Time	Glucose elevated	Glucose too low
Fasting	Increase PM NPH[b]	Decrease before supper/bedtime NPH
	Switch NPH from supper to bedtime	Increase bedtime snack
	Decrease bedtime snack	Decrease AM NPH
After breakfast	Increase AM regular/lispro	Decrease AM regular/lispro
	Change breakfast content	Decrease AM NPH
	Give injection in abdomen[c]	
	Switch regular to lispro[d]	
	Increase time interval between insulin (regular) injection and meal	
Before lunch	Increase AM regular/lispro	Decrease AM regular/lispro
		Decrease AM NPH
After lunch	Increase before lunch regular/lispro	Decrease before lunch regular/lispro
	Switch regular to lispro	Change or increase lunch content
	Change or decrease lunch content	Decrease AM NPH
	Increase AM NPH	Switch lispro to regular insulin
Before supper	Increase before lunch regular/lispro	Decrease before lunch regular/lispro
	Increase AM NPH	Decrease AM NPH
After supper	Increase before supper regular/lispro	Decrease before supper regular/lispro
	Change content of supper	Increase carbohydrates/calories at supper
	Give injection in the abdomen	
	Switch regular to lispro	
During night	Increase before supper/bedtime NPH	Decrease before dinner NPH or regular
		Add bedtime snack
		Move before supper NPH to HS

[a]Change dose by about 10%
[b]Wherever NPH appears in table lente may be substituted
[c]May apply to all after meal glucose elevations; abdominal injection decreases time for absorption
[d]Lispro is more rapidly absorbed with shorter duration of action than regular insulin
Source: Adapted from ref. 54.

A combination of neutral protamine Hagedorn (NPH) or lente insulin with regular or lispro insulin given before breakfast and supper often maintains glucose levels within the therapeutic range. Occasionally, high glucose levels after lunch necessitate a before lunch insulin dose. An elevated fasting level may require NPH or lente at bedtime.

In women with gestational diabetes, adjustment of insulin therapy according to postprandial rather than preprandial blood glucose levels improves glucose levels and decreases the risk of neonatal hypoglycemia, macrosomia, and cesarean delivery (55). When corticosteroids are used to enhance fetal lung maturity, the insulin requirement may dramatically increase after the steroid injection. Insulin resistance ends abruptly with delivery. Therefore, insulin rarely is given following the onset of labor.

Type 2 diabetes during pregnancy nearly always necessitates the use of insulin. At times the insulin dose may need to be reduced during the first trimester. A steady increase in insulin need begins during the second trimester. Usually, the insulin requirement does not increase during the last 4 wk of gestation. Intensive management enhances the ability to maintain glucose levels within the therapeutic goals, although rigid glycemic control should not be maintained at the cost of frequent, severe hypoglycemic reactions.

Insulin requirements often double or triple by the third trimester. After delivery the need for insulin declines dramatically. Exogenous insulin or oral hypoglycemic agents may not be needed for a variable period, sometimes up to several days. When glucose levels rise more than 150 mg/dL, insulin may be restarted at the dose used before pregnancy. Women who do not nurse may restart oral hypoglycemic agents rather than continue to use insulin, particularly if the oral agents maintained normal glucose levels prior to pregnancy. Within a few days after delivery, most women require a dose similar to that used prior to pregnancy.

Type 1 diabetes proves difficult to manage during pregnancy, because extreme insulin sensitivity leads to wide swings in glucose levels. Even with the same target glucose levels, average daily glucose levels are higher in women with type 1 diabetes than in those with type 2 diabetes. Also, the mean amplitude of glycemic excursion is wider in those with type 1 diabetes than in those with type 2 diabetes during pregnancy (56).

During the first trimester, nausea and vomiting change food intake and accentuate glucose variability. Even close attention to detail, multiple glucose checks, regular timing of meals, and consistent insulin administration cannot completely eliminate periodic high and low glucose levels (57). Frequent and severe hypoglycemic reactions occur most frequently between 9 and 16 wk gestation with the hypoglycemic episodes sometimes causing rebound hyperglycemia. However, several mild reactions per week may need to be tolerated.

In the second trimester, insulin need steadily increases with the greatest change occurring between 20 and 30 wk gestation. The insulin dose in more than 200 women with type 1 diabetes during pregnancy averaged an increase of 52 units per day. The degree of rise was positively related to maternal weight gain, particularly during the second trimester, and inversely related to diabetes duration. The dose was not related to level of glycemia, pregnancy complications, or pregnancy outcome. About 8% of women experience a fall in insulin requirement, which bears no relation to maternal characteristics or fetal outcomes. A decreased insulin requirement after 36 wk gestation does not indicate an adverse prognosis (58).

With delivery of the placenta, human placental lactogen, estrogen, and progesterone levels fall precipitously, leading to decreased insulin resistance and decreased insulin need. Growth hormone and gonadotropins remain suppressed. The result is a relative state of "panhypopituitarism," another reason that insulin need decreases. In addition, high prepartum insulin doses create stores of bound insulin that last for hours after the last injection.

Normally women take an insulin dose the evening prior to elective delivery and no insulin the morning of induction. Glucose levels are measured every 1–2 h during labor, and if the plasma glucose concentration rises to >140 mg/dL (7.8 mM), 1–4 U of insulin may be given hourly. However, most women do not need any insulin during active labor. If glucose levels fall below 70 mg/dL, 5% dextrose in water is given in place of the saline infusion. Other protocols for insulin and intravenous fluid administration may assist in management (59). Insulin pump therapy may be initiated during pregnancy and was associated in one study with maternal and perinatal outcomes and health care costs comparable to those among women who were already using the pump before pregnancy or who received multiple-dose insulin therapy (60).

Following delivery, insulin need falls precipitously. In order to anticipate when to restart insulin therapy, glucose checks should be done before meals and at bedtime. A preprandial value of 150 mg/dL (8.3 mmol/L) or more signals the need to restart insulin. The first dose should be slightly less than the prepregnancy dose. Subsequent dosage changes depend on glucose measurements done prior to meals and at bedtime.

The insulin dose used prior to pregnancy most closely approximates the dose needed after delivery. When the dose prior to pregnancy is not known, 0.5–0.7 units/kg body wt provides a reasonable starting dose. This may be divided into two doses, with two-thirds given before breakfast and one-third before supper. The morning dose may be divided into two-thirds intermediate-acting insulin and one-third short-acting insulin and the evening dose one-half short-acting and one-half intermediate-acting insulin.

HYPOGLYCEMIA

Intensive insulin therapy in type 1 diabetes significantly increases the risk of hypoglycemia. Severe hypoglycemia occurs three times more frequently with the use of three or more insulin injections per day compared to the use of one or two injections per day. Severe hypoglycemia occurs even more frequently during pregnancy, partly the result of diminished epinephrine and growth hormone responses to hypoglycemia (18). Clinically significant hypoglycemia requiring assistance from another person occurs in about 40% of pregnant women with type 1 diabetes (61).

Fortunately, severe hypoglycemia during the early weeks of embryogenesis is not associated with increased embryopathy. However, in women with recurrent episodes of hypoglycemia, the benefits of strict glycemic control must be weighed against the other hazards of hypoglycemia. Hypoglycemia becomes the limiting factor in the management of insulin-dependent diabetes.

Even when asymptomatic, those with diabetes should drink a carbohydrate-containing beverage or eat whenever glucose measurements register below 60 mg/dL. In addition, diabetes education should include instructions regarding measurement of glucose levels before driving. Driving should be postponed when glucose levels fall below 90 mg/dL. Table 1 outlines ways to adjust the insulin dose for low glucose levels.

PROGRESSION OF DIABETIC COMPLICATIONS DURING PREGNANCY

Diabetic retinopathy may worsen significantly during pregnancy. Some of the untoward ophthalmologic changes may be linked to the rapid normalization of glucose levels in women with previous chronic hyperglycemia. Also, hypertension is associated with progression of retinopathy during pregnancy.

Reduced creatinine clearance related to diabetic nephropathy increases pregnancy risks. When a reduction in renal function occurs during pregnancy, some women have continued deterioration of renal function postpartum (62). Women with an initial serum creatinine exceeding 1.5 mg/dL and/or proteinuria of more than 3 g in 24 h have an increased risk of early delivery, preeclampsia, cesarean delivery, and lower birth-weight infants. Women with an initial creatinine clearance greater than 90 mL/min and less than 1 g of urine protein per 24 h had less loss of renal function at follow-up (31). However, even microalbuminuria alters pregnancy risks by increasing preeclampsia in type 1 diabetes (63).

Fetal deaths are more common in women with renal disease and increase with the degree of renal dysfunction and proteinuria (64). Women with diabetes and hypertension are at high risk for a poor pregnancy outcome. These higher risks should be discussed when counseling women with renal disease who contemplate pregnancy. However, the outlook for a favorable outcome may be improving, as one study reported a 100% perinatal survival in 46 pregnancies complicated by diabetic renal disease *(31)*. Although about 10% of women with diabetes who do not have renal disease during pregnancy have diabetic nephropathy 10 yr after delivery, pregnancy and increasing parity do no appear to increase the overall risk for diabetic nephropathy *(65)*.

Proteinuria appearing during pregnancy is associated with the subsequent development of nephropathy. Kimmerle and co-workers studied the effect of diabetic nephropathy on the course of 36 pregnancies *(2)*. From the first to the third trimester, the percentage of women with proteinuria over 3 g/d increased from 14 to 53% and those treated with antihypertensive medication increased from 53 to 97%. There were no intrauterine or perinatal deaths, but one child died suddenly 4 wk postpartum. Of 36 newborns, 11 were born before wk 34 and had respiratory distress syndrome. Abnormal renal function in the first trimester, elevated diastolic blood pressure in the third trimester, and an elevated glycohemoglobin value were predictive of low birth weight.

FETAL SURVEILLANCE

Precise dating of the pregnancy assists in planning for delivery. A first-trimester ultrasound examination allows accurate dating and even some early detection of anomalies, whereas a second-trimester ultrasound offers more opportunity to detect anomalies. Maternal alpha-fetoprotein screening enables detection of neural tube defects *(66)*. This screening test is offered between 15 and 22 wk gestation and uses a standard curve for data interpretation. It is most sensitive for neural tube defect detection between 16–18 wk gestation. Diabetes may alter the ranges of normal, requiring an adjustment of the standard curve of up to 20% *(67)*. The addition of human chorionic gonadotropin and unconjugated estriol levels enhance detection of trisomy 21 *(66)*.

Serial ultrasonography may be necessary if fundal height measurements are abnormal for dates. Ultrasound may assist in diagnosing polyhydramnios, macrosomia, or intrauterine growth retardation, all or which are increased in diabetes *(66,68)*.

Fetal surveillance becomes important in the third trimester and consists of fetal movement assessment, nonstress tests, biophysical profiles, contraction stress tests, and umbilical artery Doppler velocimetry. Nonstress testing often begins at 32–34 wk gestation, although maternal or fetal complications may prompt testing as early as 26–28 wk gestation. Intrauterine fetal demise rates within 1 wk of a reassuring test are 1.9 per 1000 *(69)*.

The contraction stress test and the biophysical profile are even more reassuring, with fetal demise rates 0.3 per 1000 and 0.8 per 1000, respectively *(69)*. Umbilical artery Doppler velocimetry results are similar to the contraction stress test. The contraction stress test is time-consuming, labor intensive, potentially invasive, and may be contraindicated in some patients. The umbilical artery Doppler velocimetry requires advanced ultrasonographic techniques and equipment that may not be readily available. Because of this, the nonstress test and biophysical profile, performed biweekly, predominate.

DELIVERY AND POSTPARTUM CARE

Clinical factors including the type of diabetes, influence the timing of delivery. Delivery at 38.5–40 wk is the optimal time for most women with diabetes *(66)*. This maximizes cervical ripening and neonatal pulmonary status while minimizing fetal macrosomia, birth injury, and failed labor induction. Women with an unfavorable cervix may be followed expectantly, provided their glucose levels stay within the therapeutic range and fetal assessment remains reassuring.

Although preterm delivery may reduce macrosomia and intrauterine fetal demise, early delivery increases infant respiratory distress syndrome and other complications such as necrotizing entercolitis and cardiac hypertrophy. Elective delivery before 38.5 wk gestation requires documentation of fetal lung maturity based on the amniotic fluid lecithin/sphingomyelin ratio and the presence of phosphatidylglycerol (66). The interpretation of the lecithin/sphingomyelin ratio may differ between laboratories, although a ratio greater than 2 or 3 suggests pulmonary maturity. When lung maturity studies do not suggest fetal lung maturity and yet fetal surveillance is not reassuring, the risks of delivery must be weighed against the risks of delaying delivery. In gestations prior to 34 wk, corticosteriods may be considered to accelerate lung maturity (70). However, care must be taken, as corticosteriods can cause insulin resistance, and even precipitate diabetic ketoacidosis (66).

The route of delivery requires consideration. If a fetus can tolerate the labor process, maternal morbidity may be reduced by vaginal delivery. However, risks of cephalopelvic disproportion and shoulder dystocia exist, especially in the macrosomic fetus. Though controversy exists on any absolute weight limitation to vaginal delivery, cesarean delivery should be contemplated when the estimated fetal weight exceeds 4000 g and it should be the route of delivery if the estimated fetal weight exceeds 5000 g (71). The American Diabetes Association recommends delivery of women with gestational diabetes during the 38th wk to reduce the risk of increasing macrosomia (13).

RISK OF DEVELOPING DIABETES AFTER GESTATIONAL DIABETES

Women with gestational diabetes have an increased risk of gestational diabetes recurring in subsequent pregnancies. Gestational diabetes is more likely to recur in parous, obese women who had an early diagnosis of gestational diabetes and required insulin in the index pregnancy. Also, a shorter interval and a larger weight gain between pregnancies increases the risk of recurrence of gestational diabetes (72).

The percent of women with gestational diabetes who later develop type 2 or type 1 diabetes varies with the time of follow up, criteria used for initial diagnosis of gestational diabetes, and the criteria for diagnosis of type 2 diabetes. An elevated fasting glucose level, the diagnosis of diabetes before 22 wk gestation, or the need for insulin therapy during pregnancy increases the risk of diabetes developing postpartum (73,74). The risk of type 1 diabetes after gestational diabetes increases with the number of antibodies present at delivery (75). Based on the prevalence of antibodies to glutamic acid decarboxylase in women with gestational diabetes, about 1.7% will develop type 1 diabetes (76). Patients receiving at least 100 units per day of insulin have a 100% reported incidence of postpartum glucose intolerance (73).

Postpartum glucose screening is not needed for women managed by diet alone during pregnancy, because of the low incidence of postpartum glucose intolerance. The risk of developing diabetes postpartum increases continuously in relation to maternal glycemia during and after pregnancy (77). Long-term follow-up of women with previous gestational diabetes must be individualized.

Glucose measurements should be done if symptoms of hyperglycemia develop and periodically even in asymptomatic women. The fasting plasma glucose should be below 110 mg/dL. Two fasting values more than 126 mg/dL (7.0 mmol/dL) met the criteria for the diagnosis of diabetes *(33)*. Measures to prevent glucose intolerance postpartum include exercise and a well-balanced dietary plan aimed at maintaining normal weight.

CONTRACEPTION

The risks associated with diabetes during pregnancy usually outweigh the risks associated with most types of contraceptive use. Current contraception options include sterilization, oral hormone regimens, injectable hormone treatments, intrauterine devices, barrier methods, spermicides, and the rhythm method. Lifestyle, education, and a woman's ability to utilize a particular method influence the type of contraception recommended *(78)*. In addition, medical complications associated with diabetes such as hypertension, cardiac disease, and renal disease and the effectiveness of specific contraceptive methods affect contraception choice.

The *rhythm method*, the least effective means of contraception, involves estimating the fertile period from menstrual cycle lengths, examination of the cervical mucus, symptoms, and records of basal body temperature. Based on a 28-d cycle, the time for abstinence falls from cycle day 10 through cycle day 19. Pregnancy rates with the rhythm method range from as low as 2% to more than 80% per year *(79)*. Efficacy of this method is highly dependent on patient knowledge and adherence to the method *(80)*. Because of wide range of efficacy, this method is used when medical, moral, or religious reasons preclude other more effective and consistent options. Use of an ovulation predictor kit for detection of the preovulatory luteinizing hormone surge increases the accuracy of ovulation prediction. However, the added cost of the kit may limit repeated use *(81)*.

Latex condoms aid in the prevention of pregnancy and sexually transmitted diseases. The combined use of condoms and spermicides aid sexually transmitted disease protection, although correct use of latex condoms alone effectively prevent sexually transmitted diseases of bacterial and viral etiology *(82)*. The pregnancy rate for male condom use alone is 3.6 per 100 women-years *(83)*. New developments in male condom technology involves additional sizes ("magnum" or "maxi" brands) and new materials of polyurethane and silicon polymers. The female condom has not gained popularity largely because of the lack of availability, cost and decreased sensation *(84,85)*. Careful use, however, allows efficacy similar to other barrier methods.

Consistent use of a *diaphragm*, another barrier method of conception, is associated with low failure rates. The diaphragm should be fitted by experienced medical personnel to prevent displacement and urethral pressure. The diaphragm is filled with spermicidal jelly and left in place for at least 8 h after coitus. Additional spermicidal jelly must be placed intravaginally with each coitus. First-year failure rates are 6–12%, but they may decrease with user commitment and experience *(78)*. Diaphragm use may reduce the incidence of local and upper genital tract disease as a result, in part, of the simultaneous use of spermicides *(86)*. It is cost-effective.

The *intrauterine device* (IUD) is a popular and effective method of contraception. The copper intrauterine device offers 10 yr of contraception and relies on the slow metabolism of copper to prevent fertilization and implantation. The contraceptive action of all IUDs occurs in the uterine cavity and cervical mucus. IUDs are not abortifacients.

The levonorgestrel IUD was released in 2001. Its serum progestin concentrations are half those of contraceptive implants utilizing levonorgestrel. The increased endometrial exposure to levonorgestrel decreases menstrual blood loss and reduces dysmenorrhea. Thus, in women with anovulation and irregular bleeding related to chronic severe hyperglycemia, this device may provide an additional noncontraceptive benefit. The failure rate during first-year use approximates 3% (86). There is no increase in infections in women with diabetes compared to the general population (87). Contraindications for insertion of the device include suspicion of any of the following: pregnancy, malignancy, infection, and behavior suggesting a high risk for contracting a sexually transmitted disease.

The above-discussed contraceptive methods do not involve systemic medication. The remaining reversible contraceptive methods use exogenous hormones to alter ovulation or the endometrial and cervical environment. Hormones, however, may affect more than just reproductive function and the metabolic effects also need consideration especially in women with diabetes.

Oral contraceptive pills contain various combinations of estrogen and progestational agents. They alter ovulation, the endometrium, and cervical mucus and have other metabolic effects. Current contraceptives available contain 20–50 µg of ethinyl estradiol, but the most popular ones contain 20–35 µg of ethinyl estradiol combined with a variety of progestins including norethindrone, levonorgestrel, norgesterone, or ethynodiol diacetate. More recently formulated oral contraceptives contain ethinyl estradiol combined with newer progestins—desogestrel, norgestimate, or drospirenone.

Oral contraceptive pills contain monophasic, biphasic, or triphasic progestin preparations, and one of the newer pills has phasic ethinyl estradiol doses. The types of progestins used in oral contraceptives differ in their side-effect profiles. Side effects include weight gain, acne, nausea, breast tenderness, breakthrough bleeding, amenorrhea, and headache. Elevation of blood pressure may occur in less than 5% of women.

Oral contraceptive preparations containing only progesterone (norethindrone, levonorgestrel) are also available and are taken daily in a continuous fashion. When used correctly and consistently, failure rates are comparable to combination oral contraceptives (those containing estrogen and progesterone) (86). A contraceptive containing norethindrone and levonorgestrel appear particularly attractive for women who choose to breast feed, those with migraine, and women who are unable to tolerate estrogen-containing preparations.

Most women, including those with a history of gestational diabetes, and those with type 1 or type 2 diabetes, may safely use oral contraceptives, combination estrogen and progesterone pills, or those with progestin alone. Current "low-dose" oral contraceptives containing 20–50 µg of ethinyl estradiol with a progestin have less effect on carbohydrate metabolisms and lipid profiles than their predecessors containing 80 µg or greater of ethinyl estradiol. It has been shown in the past that even high dose oral contraceptives, however, do not alter a woman's chances of developing diabetes mellitus. Current use of low doses, therefore, does not alter future diabetic risk (88).

Women with altered glucose tolerance secondary to polycystic ovary syndrome but without diabetic or medical complications, such as hypertension or thromboembolic disease, should be reassured about the use of oral contraceptives. Oral contraceptive use blocks ovulation, thereby reducing ovarian testosterone production and assisting with disease management. Some women may be at an increased risk for development of type

2 diabetes while using progestin- only oral contraceptives, especially if breast-feeding follows a pregnancy complicated by gestational diabetes *(89)*.

Elevation of blood pressure may occur in a few women using oral contraceptives containing both estrogen and progesterone. This incidence is less than 5% *(90)*. Women with a history of hypertension may use oral contraceptives with regular blood pressure monitoring and maintenance of good blood pressure control.

Recent evidence is also reassuring with regard to oral contraceptive use and occurrence of stroke or myocardial infarction. Independent risk factors such as smoking or hypertension may alter this risk *(91)*. Women with long-standing diabetes mellitus should be evaluated for potential risk factors before initiating oral contraceptive therapy and be reassessed regularly.

Women with diabetic complications, however, including retinopathy, nephropathy, neuropathy, and poorly controlled hypertension or disease of greater than 20 yr duration, are generally directed to other forms of contraception. Oral contraceptives are not recommended.

Subcutaneous implants provide long-term sustained release hormonal contraception. The current product, *Norplant* consists of six silastic rods releasing levonorgestrel for continuous contraception up to 5 yr. New products in development release other progestins and will be biodegradable. The efficacy of these contraceptives approaches that of sterilization. They are more effective than oral contraception or barrier methods. Contraception results from anovulation, endometrial lining changes, and thickened cervical mucus. This method, like other progestin-only methods, is an excellent choice for women who are breast-feeding. Studies of the effects of levonorgestrel implants on carbohydrate metabolism, coagulation and lipid profiles demonstrate no major impact *(86)*.

Depo-medroxyprogesterone acetate, the most widely used injectable contraceptive, has a failure rate of less than 1.2 per 100 women-years. The injection is given every 12–14 wk, although elevated hormone levels may prevent ovulation for 7–9 mo after injection. Major side effects include irregular bleeding, weight gain, and delayed return to fertility. Depo-medroxyprogesterone does not significantly change glucose tolerance or increase thromboembolic events. The drug provides an effective contraceptive choice for women who cannot use estrogens.

A new contraceptive injectable preparation debuted in 2001. This monthly injection, Lunelle, utilizes 5 mg of estradiol cypionate combined with 25 mg of depo-medroxy-progesterone acetate. Its efficacy is the same as depo-medroxyprogesterone alone, but it decreases irregular bleeding or amenorrhea in most women and users should expect a regular monthly menses. This method also provides return to fertility sooner, approx 2–3 mo after discontinuation. It has no adverse affects on metabolic profiles, coagulation, or carbohydrate metabolism *(92)*.

Sterilization, a permanent method of contraception, has a risk equivalent to the risk of the surgical procedure performed. Diabetes does not alter the effectiveness of sterilization, but may increase surgical risks. Failure rates range from 7.5–36.5 per 1000 procedures *(93)*. The highest failure rate may occur utilizing a clip procedure and the lowest with unipolar cautery. Becuase of potential long-term complications of diabetes mellitus, especially renal, hypertensive, and cardiovascular, sterilization should be discussed with women who have completed childbearing.

LACTATION

Breast-feeding should be encouraged in women with diabetes managed by diet alone or with insulin. Insulin in breast milk is rendered inactive in the infant's gastrointestinal tract and, thus, does not adversely affect the infant. For women taking insulin, blood glucose monitoring with appropriate insulin and diet adjustment needs to be continued to prevent maternal hypoglycemia. The maternal use of oral hypoglycemic agents usually is considered a relative contraindication to breast-feeding.

Breast-feeding, even for a short time, has a beneficial effect on the mother's glucose and lipid levels. Epidemiological studies suggest that exposure of genetically susceptible infants to cow's milk before the age of 3 mo increases the risk of the child developing insulin-dependent diabetes. This provides another reason to favor breast-feeding *(94)*.

CONCLUSION

Diabetes mellitus complicates pregnancy and increases risks for mother and infant. Screening women with one or more risk factors at 24–28 wk gestation identifies those with gestational diabetes. Dietary measures are used initially and insulin is added if fasting glucose levels exceed 105 mg/dL or is 2-h postprandial glucose levels exceed 120 mg/dL. Results of glucose self-monitoring guide insulin modifications. Women with preexisting diabetes require intensive glucose management before conception to ensure the lowest incidence of congenital anomalies. Because of the greater risk for stillbirth and macrosomia associated with diabetes during pregnancy, fetal surveillance begins in the third trimester, with nonstress tests the most widely used. Ultrasound dating and determination of the lecithin/sphingomyelin ratio assist in timing delivery.

REFERENCES

1. McElvy SS, Demarini S, Miodovnik M, et al. Fetal weight and progression of diabetic retinopathy. Obstet Gynecol 2001;97:587–592.
2. Kimmerle R, Zass RP, Somville T, et al. Pregnancies in women with diabetic nephropathy: long-term outcome for mother and child. Diabetologia 1995;38:227–235.
3. Kitzmiller JL, Buchanan TA, Kjos S, et al. Pre-conception care of diabetes, congenital malformations, and spontaneous abortions. Diabetes Care 1996;19:514–541.
4. Casson IF, Clarke CA, Howard CV, et al. Outcomes of pregnancy in insulin dependent diabetic women: results of a five year population cohort study. BMJ 1997;315:275–278.
5. Hawthorne G, Robson S, Ryall EA, et al. Prospective population based survey of outcome of pregnancy in diabetic women: results of the Northern Diabetic Pregnancy Audit, 1994. Br Med J 1997;315:279–281.
6. Suhonen L, Hiilesmaa V, Teramo K. Glycaemic control during early pregnancy and fetal malformations in women with type I diabetes mellitus. Diabetologia 2000;43:79–82.
7. Mello G, Parretti E, Mecacci F, et al. Risk factors for fetal macrosomia: the importance of a positive oral glucose challenge test. Euro J Endocr 1997;137:27–33.
8. Persson B, Hanson U. Fetal size in relation to quality of blood glucose control in pregnancies complicated by pregestational diabetes mellitus. Brit J Obstet Gynaecol 1996;103:427–433.
9. Casey BM, Lucas MJ, McIntire DD, et al. Pregnancy outcomes in women with gestational diabetes compared with the general obstetric population. Obstet Gynecol 1997;90:869–873.
10. Adams KM, Li H, Nelson RL, et al. Sequelae of unrecognized gestational diabetes. Am J Obstet Gynecol 1998;178:1321–1332.
11. Reece EA, Lequizamon G, Homko C. Stringent controls in diabetic nephropathy associated with optimization of pregnancy outcomes. J Matern Fetal Med 1998;7:213–216.
12. McElvy SS, Miodovnik M, Rosenn B, et al. A focused preconceptional and early pregnancy program in women with type 1 diabetes reduces perinatal mortality and malformation rates to general population levels. J Matern Fetal Med 2000;9:14–20.
13. American Diabetes Association. Gestational diabetes mellitus. Diabetes Care 2001;24:S77–S79.
14. Xiang AH, Peters RK, Trigo E, et al. Multiple metabolic defects during late pregnancy in women at high risk for type 2 diabetes. Diabetes 1999;48:848–854.

15. Persson B, Edwall L, Hanson U, et al. Insulin sensitivity and insulin response in women with gestational diabetes mellitus. Hormone Metabol Research 1997;29:393–397.

16. Homko C, Sivan E, Chen X, et al. Insulin secretion during and after pregnancy in patients with gestational diabetes mellitus. J Clin Endocrol Metab 2001;86:568–573.

17. Bjorklund AO, Adamson UK, Lins PE, et al. Diminished insulin clearance during late pregnancy in patients with type 1 diabetes mellitus. Clin Sci 1998;95:317–323.

18. Rosenn BM, Miodovnik M, Khoury JC, et al. Counterregulatory hormonal responses to hypoglycemia during pregnancy. Obstet Gynecol 1996;87:568–574.

19. Rey E, Attie C, Bonin A. The effects of first-trimester diabetes control on the incidence of macrosomia. Am J Obstet Gynecol 1999;181:202–206.

20. Kieffer EC, Nolan GH, Carman WJ, et al. Glucose tolerance during pregnancy and birth weight in a Hispanic population. Obstet Gynecol 1999;94:741–746.

21. Parretti E, Mecacci F, Papini M, et al. Third-trimester maternal glucose levels from diurnal profiles in nondiabetic pregnancies: Correlation with sonographic parameters of fetal growth. Diabetes Care 2001;24:1319–1327.

22. Schaefer UM, Songster G, Xiang A, et al. Congenital malformations in offspring of women with hyperglycemia first detected during pregnancy. Am J Obstet Gynecol 1997;177:1165–1171.

23. Sacks DA, Greenspoon JS, Abu-Fadil S, et al. Toward universal criteria for gestational diabetes: the 75-gram glucose tolerance test in. Am J Obstet Gynecol 1995;172:607–614.

24. Moses RG, Calvert D. Pregnancy outcomes in women without gestational diabetes mellitus related to the maternal glucose level. Diabetes Care 1995;18:1527–1533.

25. Aberg A, Rydhstroem H, Frid A. Impaired glucose tolerance associated with adverse pregnancy outcome: a population-based study in southern Sweden. Am J Obstet Gynecol 2001;184:77–83.

26. Innes KE, Wimsatt JH, McDuffie R. Relative glucose tolerance and subsequent development of hpertension in pregnancy. Obstet Gynecol 2001;97:905–910.

27. Dukler D, Porath A, Bashiri A, et al. Remote prognosis of primiparous women with preeclampsia. European J Obstet Gynecol, Reprod Biology 2001;96:69–74.

28. Aberg A, Westbom L, Kallen B. Congenital malformations among infants whose mothers had gestational diabetes or preexisting diabetes. Early Human Development 2001;61:85–95.

29. Diabetes Control and Complications Trial Research Group. Pregnancy outcomes in the Diabetes Control and Complications Trial. Am J Obstet Gynecol 1996;174:1343–1353.

30. Herman WH, Janz NK, Becker MP, et al. Diabetes and pregnancy. Preconception care, pregnancy outcomes, resource utilization and costs. J Reprod Med 1999;44:33–38.

31. Gordon M, Landon MB, Samuels P, et al. Perinatal outcome and long-term follow-up associated with modern management of diabetic nephropathy. Obstet Gynecol 1996;87:401–409.

32. American Diabetes Association. Preconception care of women with diabetes. Diabetes Care 2001;24:S66–S68.

33. The Expert Committee on the Diagnosis and Classification of Diabetes Mellitus. Report of the expert committee on the diagnosis and classification of diabetes mellitus. Diabetes Care 2001;24:S5–S20.

34. Radon PA, McMahon MJ, Meyer WR. Impaired glucose tolerance in pregnant women with polycystic ovary syndrome. Obstet Gynecol 1999;94:194–197.

35. Anttila L, Karjala K, Penttila RA, et al. Polycytic ovaries in women with gestational diabetes. Obstet Gynecol 1998;92:13–16.

36. Plante LA. Small size at birth and later diabetic pregnancy. Obstet Gynecol 1998;92:781–784.

37. Jang HC, Min HK, Lee HK, et al. Short stature in Korean women: a contribution to the multifactorial predisposition to gestational diabetes mellitus. Diabetologia 1998;41:778–783.

38. Anastasiou E, Alevizaki M, Grigorakis SJ, et al. Decreased stature in gestational diabetes mellitus. Diabetologia 1998;41:997–1001.

39. Lavin JP, Lavin B, O'Donnell N. A comparison of costs associated with screening for gestational diabetes with two-tiered and one-tiered testing protocols. Am J Obstet Gynecol 2001;184:363–367.

40. Metzger BE, Coustan DR. Summary and recommendations of the Fourth International Workshop-Conference on Gestational Diabetes Mellitus. Diabetes Care 1998;21:B161–B167.

41. Laird J, McFarland KF. Fasting blood glucose levels and initiation of insulin therapy in gestational diabetes. Endocr Pract 1996;2:330–332.

42. Luke B, Murtaugh MA. Dietary management. In: Reece EA, Coustan DR, eds, Diabetes in Pregnancy. Churchill Livingstone, New York, 1995:191–200.

43. American Diabetes Association. Nutrition recommendations and principles for people with diabetes mellitus. Diabetes Care 2001;024:S44–S47.

44. Major CA, Henry MJ, DeVeciana M, et al. The effects of carbohydrate restriction in patients with diet-controlled gestational diabetes. Obstet Gynecol 1998;91:600–604.

45. Fagen C, King JD, Erick M. Nutrition management in women with gestational diabetes mellitus: a review by ADA's Diabetes Care and Education dietetic practice group. J Am Diet Assoc 1995;95:460–467.

46. Avery MD, Walker AJ. Acute effect of exercise on blood glucose and insulin levels in women with gestational diabetes. J Matern Fetal Med 2001;10:52–58.

47. Henriksson-Larsen K. Training and sports competition during pregnancy and after childbirth. Lakartidningen 1999;96:2097–2100.

48. Avery MD, Leon AS, Kopher RA. Effects of a partially home-based exercise program for women with gestational diabetes. Obstet Gynecol 1997;89:10–15.

49. Weller KA. Diagnosis and management of gestational diabetes. Am Fam Physician 1996;53:2053-2057;2061–2062.

50. Langer O, Conway DL, Berkus MD, et al. A comparison of glyburide and insulin in women with gestational diabetes mellitus. N Eng J Med 2000;343:1134–1138.

51. Nachum Z, Ben-Shlomo I, Weiner E, et al. Twice daily versus four times daily insulin dose regimens for diabetes in pregnancy: randomized controlled trial. BMJ 1999;319:1223–1227.

52. Buchbinder A, Miodovnik M, McElvy S, et al. Is insulin lispro associated with the development or progression of diabetic retinopathy during pregnancy? Am J Obstet Gynecol 2000;183:1162–1165.

53. Bhattacharyya A, Brown S, Hughes S, et al. Insulin lispro and regular insulin in pregnancy. Q J Med 2001;94:255–260.

54. Pasui K, McFarland KF. Management of diabetes in pregnancy. Am Fam Physician 1997;55:2731–2738, 2742–2744.

55. DeVeciana M, Major CA, Morgan MA, et al. Postprandial versus preprandial blood glucose monitoring in women with gestational diabetes mellitus requiring insulin therapy. N Engl J Med 1995;333:1237–1241.

56. Sacks DA, Chen W, Greenspoon JS, et al. Should the same glucose values be targeted for type 1 as for type 2 diabetics in pregnancy? Am J Obstet Gynecol 1997;177:1113–1119.

57. Rosenn BM, Miodovnik M, et al. Hypoglycemia: the price of intensive insulin therapy for pregnant women with insulin-dependent diabetes mellitus. Obstet Gynecol 1995;85:417–422.

58. Steel JM, Johnstone FD, Hume R, et al. Insulin requirements during pregnancy in women with type I diabetes. Obstet Gynecol 1994;83:253–258.

59. Jovanovic-Peterson L, Peterson CM. The art and science of maintenance of normoglycemia in pregnancies complicated by insulin-dependent diabetes mellitus. Endocr Pract 1996;2:130–143.

60. Gabbe SG, Holing E, Temple P, et al. Benefits, risks, costs, and patient satisfaction associated with insulin pump therapy for the pregnancy complicated by type 1 diabetes mellitus. Am J Obstet Gynecol 2000;182:1283–1291.

61. Rosenn BM, Miodovnik M. Glycemic control in the diabetic pregnancy: is tighter always better? J Matern Fetal Med 2000;9:29–34.

62. Prudy LP, Hantsch C, Molitch ME, et al. Effect of pregnancy on renal function in patients with moderate-to-severe diabetic renal insufficiency. Diabetes Care 1996:1067–1074.

63. Ekbom P, Damm P, Nogaard K, et al. Urinary albumin excretion and 24-hour blood pressure as predictors of pre-eclampsia in type I diabetes. Diabetologia 2000;43:927–931.

64. Holley JL, Bernardini J, Quadri KH, et al. Pregnancy outcomes in a prospective matched control study of pregnancy and renal disease. Clin Nephrol 1996;45:77–82.

65. Miodovnik M, Rosenn BM, Khoury JC, et al. Does pregnancy increase the risk for development and progression of diabetic nephropathy? Am J Obstet Gynecol 1996;174:1180–1189.

66. Moore JD. Diabetes in pregnancy. In: Creasy RK, Resnik R, eds. Maternal-Fetal Medicine. 4th edition. WB Saunders, Philadelphia, 1999, pp. 964–995.

67. Kramer RL, Yaron Y, O'Brien JE, et al. Effect of adjustment of maternal serum alpha-fetoprotein levels in insulin-dependent diabetes mellitus. Am J Med Genet 1998;13:176–178.

68. Sylvestre G, Divon MY, Onyeije C, et al. Diagnosis of macrosomia in the postdates population: combining sonographic estimates of fetal weight with glucose challenge testing. J Matern Fetal Med 2000;9:287–290.

69. American College of Obstetrics and Gynecology. Antepartum Fetal Surveillance. Washington, DC, 1999.

70. Gardner MO, Papile LA, Wright LL. Antenatal corticosteroids in pregnancies complicated by preterm premature rupture of membranes. Obstet Gynecol 1997;90:851–853.

71. American College of Obstetrics and Gynecology. Fetal Macrosomia. Washington, DC 2000.

72. Major CA, DeVeciana M, Weeks J, et al. Recurrence of gestational diabetes: who is at risk? Am J Obstet Gynecol 1998;179:1038–1042.

73. Greenberg LR, Moore TR, Murphy H. Gestational diabetes mellitus: antenatal variables as predictors of postpartum glucose intolerance. Obstet Gynecol 1995;86:97–101.

74. Buchanan BA, Xiang A, Kjos SL, et al. Gestational diabetes: Antepartum characteristics that predict postpartum glucose intolerance and type 2 diabetes in Latino women. Diabetes 1998;47:1302–1310.

75. Fuchtenbusch M, Ferber K, Standl E, et al. Prediction of type 1 diabetes postpartum in patients with gestational diabetes mellitus by combined islet cell autoantibody screening: a prospective multicenter study. Diabetes 1997;46:1459–1467.

76. Beischer NA, Wein P, Sheedy MT, et al. Prevalence of antibodies to glutamic acid decarboxylase in women who have had gestational diabetes. Am J Obstet Gynecol 1995;173:1563–1569.

77. Buchanan TA, Kjos SL. Gestational diabetes: risk or myth? J Clin Endocrinol Metabol 1999;84:1854–1857.

78. Trussell J, Vaughan B. Contraceptive failure, method-related discontinuation and resumption of use: results from the 1995 National Survey of Family Growth. Fam Plann Perspect 1999;31:64–72, 93.

79. Stanford JB, Thurman PB, Lemaire JC. Physicians' knowledge and practices regarding natural family planning. Obstet Gynecol 1999;94:672–678.

80. Sinai J, Jennings V, Arevalo M. The two-day algorithm: a new algorithm to identify the fertile time of the menstrual cycle. Contraception 1999;60:65–70.

81. Miller PB, Soules MR. The usefulness of a urinary LH kit for ovulation prediction during menstrual cycles of normal women. Obstet Gynecol 1996;87:13–17.

82. Davis KR, Weller SC. The effectiveness of condoms in reducing heterosexual transmission of HIV. Fam Plann 1999;31:272–279.

83. Poulter NR, Chang CL, Farley TM, et al. Reliability of data from proxy respondents in an international case-control study of cardiovascular disease and oral contraceptives. World Health Organization Collaborative Study in Cardiovascular Disease and Steroid Hormone Contraception. J Epidemiol Community Health 1996;50:674–680.

84. Trussell J. Contraceptive efficacy of the reality female condom. Contraception 1998;58:147,148.

85. Sapire KE. The female condom (Femidom)—a study of user acceptability. S Afr Med J. 1995;85:1081–1084.

86. Speroff L, Darney P. Barrier methods: a clinical guide for contraception. Lippincott, Williams & Wilkins, Philadelphia, 2001, pp. 259–295.

87. Kjos SL, Ballagh SA, LaCour M, et al. The copper T380A intrauterine device in women with type II diabetes mellitus. Obstet Gynecol 1994;84:1006–1009.

88. Troisi RJ, Cowie CC, Haris MI. Oral contraceptive use in glucose metabolism in a national sample of women in the U.S. Am J Obstet Gynecol 2000;183:389–395.

89. Kjos SL, Peters RK, Xiang A, et al. Contraception and the risk of type II diabetes mellitus in Latino women with prior gestational diabetes mellitus. JAMA 1998;280:533–538.

90. Chasan-Taber L, Willett WC, Manson JE, et al. Prospective study of oral contraceptives and hypertension among women in the United States. Circulation 1996;94:483–489.

91. Cardiovascular Disease and Steroid Hormone Contraception. Haemorrhagic stroke, overall stroke risk and combined oral contraceptives: results of an international, mutlticentre, case-controlled study. Lancet 1996;348:505–510.

92. Kaunitz AM, Garceau RJ, Cromie MA, Lumille Study Group. Comparative safety efficacy and cycle control of Lunelle monthly contraceptive injection and Ortho- Novum 7/7/7/ oral contraceptive. Contraception 1999;60:179–187.

93. Peterson HB, Xia Z, Hughes JM, et al. The risk of pregnancy after tubal sterilization: findings from the U.S. Collaborative Review of Sterilization. Am J Obstet Gynecol 1996;174:1161–1170.

94. Hammond-McKibben D, Dosch HM. Cow's milk, bovine serum albumin, and IDDM: can we settle the controversies? Diabetes Care 1997;20:897–901.

13

Insulin Pump Therapy in the Management of Diabetes

Raymond A. Plodkowski, MD
and Steven V. Edelman, MD

INTRODUCTION

Insulin therapy has been a constantly evolving science since its discovery by Macleod, Banting, and Best in 1921. The current state of the art in insulin delivery systems is via the insulin pump. It has been used to overcome limitations of intermittent subcutaneous insulin administration. The insulin pump delivers a continuous subcutaneous insulin infusion (CSII) and it is an excellent option for many patients to take control of their

From: *Endocrine Replacement Therapy in Clinical Practice*
Edited by: A. Wayne Meikle © Humana Press Inc., Totowa, NJ

Table 1
Patient Advantages of Insulin Pump Therapy

Improved quality of life because of increased self-reliance and control
Flexible lifestyle
Flexibility in meal timing and amounts
Fewer and less severe hypoglycemic reactions
Improved control with a variable work schedule
Improved control while traveling
Increased flexibility in exercise intensity and times

diabetes, reduce the excursions of daily glucose values, and improve their overall glucose control. Although the insulin pump may seem complex to the patient at first, he or she will quickly learn how to use the device. Most appropriately selected pump candidates are extremely pleased with the results. Physicians may be reluctant to prescribe insulin pumps because they are unfamiliar with the devices or there is a misconception that pumps create more work. In reality, insulin pump patients are easy to manage because they become self-sufficient in terms of self-care on a day-to-day basis. In this chapter, we discuss the benefits, indications, and practical guidelines for the use of insulin pumps.

From a patient's point of view, insulin pump therapy has several benefits, including a more flexible lifestyle while simultaneously enjoying improved glucose control. Insulin pump therapy allows for increased flexibility in meal timing and amounts, increased flexibility in the timing and intensity of exercise, improved glucose control while traveling across time zones or with variable working schedules, and a better quality of life in terms of self-reliance and control *(1)* *(see* Table 1).

IMITATING PHYSIOLOGIC INSULIN SECRETION VIA PUMPS

To understand the use of insulin pumps, the underlying physiology of insulin secretion should be considered. The goal of insulin pump therapy is to mimic the pancreas' normal insulin secretion as closely as possible. There are two main components to insulin secretion. A nondiabetic patient has an insulin surge after meals in order to control the postprandial glucose excursion that occurs. Patients with diabetes have an inadequate β-cell response and they require short-acting insulin before meals to mimic this surge. However, regular insulin's onset of action is slow at 30–60 min. Its peak action is also variable and occurs 2–4 h after injection. Newer insulin analogs improve this profile. Insulin Lispro and insulin aspart have an onset of action between 10 and 20 min and a peak between 30 and 90 min. Unfortunately, there is still a large amount of variability depending on injection technique and location. In addition, there is no mechanism for adjusting the profile of the insulin bolus once it is administered. An insulin pump involves a minimally invasive catheter that administers insulin to the same subcutaneous site for 3 d, which limits much of the variability associated with injections. The pump user also has the ability to adjust the time-action profile of the insulin boluses depending on the type, size, and length of the expected meal.

The second component to insulin replacement is the individual's basal insulin requirement. In addition to the postprandial surges of insulin, a constant basal insulin level is necessary over the entire 24-h period to maintain normal metabolic function and

Table 2
Physiologic Advantages of Insulin Pump Therapy

- A single subcutaneous infusion site is used for 72 h so there is less variation because of injection technique, as seen with multiple daily injections.
- Insulin boluses can be customized with regular, square-wave, and dual-wave infusion patterns for different types of meals.
- The unwanted peaks in insulin action seen with long-acting insulins such as NPH and ultralente are eliminated.
- Patients have the option to increase the basal rate in the early morning to compensate for the dawn phenomenon and periods of hyperglycemia.
- Patients can decrease the basal rate during periods of extended exercise.
- Patients have the ability to decrease the basal rate at night if he or she is prone to overnight hypoglycemia.

NPH, neutral protamine Hagedorn.

to prevent diabetic ketoacidosis. The usual approach to providing a basal insulin level involves the use of long-acting insulin. The two most popular long-acting insulins are NPH and ultralente. These insulins are composed of regular insulin mixed with the protein protamine and/or zinc. The protamine and zinc slow the absorption of the insulin. Unfortunately, the onset, peak, and duration of action are variable even within the same patient. Human ultralente has an onset of action that is approx 6–10 h and the peak is 10–16 h. Its duration of action is extremely variable from 18 to 24 h. NPH has an onset of action of 2–4 h, peak action of 6–10 h, and a duration of 10–18 h *(2)*. There is a new long-acting insulin analog, insulin glargine, that is a 24-h peakless basal insulin that helps address some of the unpredictability of the of older long-acting insulins. Unfortunately, there is still some variability depending on injection technique. In addition, its dose can not be adjusted once it is injected.

The insulin pump offers several distinct advantages because the pump user has the ability to program different basal rates at different times during the day. For example, some patients experience a significant "Dawn phenomenon," where the counterregulatory hormone, growth hormone, causes a rise in blood sugar in the early morning prior to waking. The insulin pump user has the option to program a slightly higher rate of insulin infusion for the early morning hours to address this rise in blood glucose. Patients who experience overnight hypoglycemia can program the pump to reduce the amount of basal insulin during the night. Finally, patients can use a temporary basal rate during strenuous exercise or illness *(see* Table 2).

CLINICAL STUDIES

Insulin pump therapy has become widespread, and clinical trials support its use. One of the greatest advantages over multiple daily injections is the elimination of unwanted peaks in insulin action that occur in many long-acting insulins such as NPH and ultralente. The ability to give a continuous infusion of short-acting insulin has a theoretical advantage. In a study by Bode et al., 255 type 1 diabetic subjects were studied who had experienced severe hypoglycemia, had a history of hypoglycemic unawareness, and/or had not achieved desirable levels of glycemic control (HbA$_{1c}$ >8.0%) after at least 1 yr of multiple daily injection (MDI) therapy *(3)*. The multiple daily insulin injections were stopped and all subjects were placed on subcutaneous insulin infusion via an insulin pump for 1 yr. The results showed a marked decrease in severe hypoglycemia from 138 to 22 events per 100 patient-years ($p = 0.0001$) during the year of the CSII treatment compared with the year of MDI therapy. Furthermore, patients with a baseline HbA$_{1c}$ greater than 8.0% had an improvement in the average HbA$_{1c}$ from 8.9 ± 0.8% to 8.1 ± 1.0% ($p = 0.0004$) after CSII treatment for 1 yr.

Using an insulin pump offers the opportunity to control blood glucose levels with less insulin. A study by Crawford et al. examined the total insulin dose when type 1 diabetic patients use CSII vs MDI therapy *(4)*. Because it is well established that insulin promotes weight gain, it benefits the patient to use the smallest amount of insulin possible to achieve the desired clinical effect. The results of the study showed that the daily total dose of insulin fell 18% ($p = 0.02$) in patients using CSII when compared to MDI while reducing HbA$_{1c}$ from 8.4 to 7.7% ($p < 0.01$). The patients' weight on CSII showed a decreasing trend of 0.2 kg compared with MDI; however, this was not statistically significant. This study showed that subjects using CSII therapy could use less insulin to maintain blood glucose control as measured by HbA$_{1c}$.

INSULIN PUMP THERAPY FOR INSULIN-REQUIRING PATIENTS WITH TYPE 2 DIABETES

Insulin pump therapy has been traditionally used for people with type 1 diabetes. People with type 1 diabetes usually do not have insulin resistance. Therefore, they require low basal rates and small insulin boluses. Because type 2 diabetics have the underlying defect of insulin resistance, in addition to β-cell failure, they have increased insulin requirements. Insulin pump therapy is extremely valuable in patients with insulin requiring type 2 diabetes who have not achieved glycemic control with subcutaneous injections, who are experiencing wide fluctuations in blood glucose levels complicated by hypoglycemia, or who are seeking a more flexible lifestyle. All of the above-discussed benefits that are enjoyed by patients with type 1 diabetes, also apply to people with type 2 diabetes. There are other potential advantages to pump therapy. A patient with type 2 diabetes should be treated with the minimal amount of insulin possible to improve glucose control because excess insulin administration could cause further weight gain. When the pump is used, the number of hypoglycemic events decreases. Therefore, there is less overeating to compensate for hypoglycemia, and weight gain may be less of an issue *(5)*.

Many older patients with the diagnosis of insulin-requiring type 2 diabetes have true late-onset type 1 diabetes. It has been documented in the literature that when large groups of patients with insulin-requiring type 2 diabetes mellitus were tested for anti-GAD antibodies (glutamic acid decarboxylase), approx 5–8% are positive. These individuals are thinner at the time of diagnosis and generally do not respond well to oral agents and require insulin, although they do not present in severe diabetic ketoacidosis *(5)*. This is another group that could potentially benefit from insulin pump therapy. In general, if a patient with insulin-requiring type 2 diabetes cannot achieve glycemic control with an intensive insulin injection regimen, then insulin pump therapy should be considered.

INSULIN PUMP PATIENT SELECTION

In general, any patient taking insulin with poor glycemic control and/or who is requesting a more flexible lifestyle should be considered for insulin pump therapy. Obviously, the patient has to be reliable because he or she must be able to perform frequent home glucose monitoring and have a fundamental understanding of diabetes and the importance of good control. The patient does not have to have a technical background to manage the pump's function. The patient only needs to understand some basic principals of operating and maintaining the insulin pump and related catheter care. Furthemore, there is no real age limit and patients who are between the ages of 8 and 80 yr can do well on pump therapy. In summary, good candidates for insulin pump therapy are patients who are interested in their diabetes and are reliable and compliant. Patients requesting insulin pump therapy, are probably good candidates, based on that fact they are interested and motivated.

One of the best techniques to determine if a patient is a good candidate for an insulin pump is to first prescribe an intensive insulin regimen. We usually prescribe insulin glargine or human ultralente as the basal insulin with insulin lispro or insulin aspart at mealtimes. An extra injection of insulin lispro or insulin aspart can be utilized at other times of the day for incidental hyperglycemia. This regimen requires home glucose monitoring at least four times a day and prepares that person for an easy conversion to an insulin pump if indicated. If the patient can perform this regimen and perform frequent home glucose monitoring reliably, then he or she will do well with insulin pump therapy.

DISADVANTAGES OF INSULIN PUMP THERAPY

In older text books, hypoglycemic unawareness is listed as a contraindication to insulin pump therapy because it was thought that any therapeutic regimen that improves glycemic control would increase the chance for hypoglycemia. Insulin pump therapy has been proven to reduce wide fluctuations in blood glucose values, including severe hypoglycemia. If a patient has hypoglycemic unawareness, it is important to set the patient's goals at a higher range to avoid severe hypoglycemia (6). For example, the goals of glycemic control for an individual with hypoglycemic unawareness should be between 120 and 180 mg/dL instead of the usual 70 to 140 mg/dL range used for individuals without hypoglycemic unawareness.

In our experience, patients with poor glycemic control frequently get skin infections and having a catheter or needle in the subcutaneous tissue over a long period of time increases the chance of having an infection. Therefore, in individuals who have frequent staphylococcosis skin infections, insulin pump therapy may be problematic. However, with the improved glycemic control that pump therapy can offer, many patients with a history of frequent skin infections no longer have this problem.

Another potential disadvantage of pump therapy is the risk of sudden extreme hyperglycemia and/or diabetic ketoacidosis, especially in type 1 diabetics. This is particularly true if the patient is using lispro or aspart insulin in the pump. Because only regular or fast-acting insulin is used, one can quickly develop extreme hyperglycemia and ketoacidosis if there is a prolonged interruption of insulin delivery. This can occur if there is a problem with the infusion line, depletion of a battery pack, or pump failure. Today's pumps are very reliable and failure is very unusual. This problem is easily counteracted by always carrying an extra bottle of insulin or an insulin pen containing regular, lispro, or aspart insulin.

Financial concerns are always an issue as the cost of insulin pump therapy with the accompanying supplies may be prohibitive if your patient does not have adequate insurance coverage. The pump itself costs $3500 to $5000 and the supplies, which include

Table 3
Disadvantages of Insulin Pump Therapy

* Risk of extreme hyperglycemia and diabetic ketoacidosis if pump or pump tubing fails
* Skin infections or abscesses at infusion site
* Initial high cost of pump and cost of maintenance supplies
* Problems at the airport security checkpoint
* Inconvenience of always having a bodily attachment

insulin infusion lines, syringes, tape, and batteries can total an additional $40–50 a month. Newer pumps will use standard AAA batteries, which should decrease the monthly cost a little. Most insurance companies will reimburse at least 80% of the pump's cost with appropriately applied pressure by you and your patient. Representatives from the three insulin pump companies also have special staff to help you submit the proper paperwork to insurance providers.

Many patients who travel frequently will have problems going through airport security station. Sometimes, but not always, the insulin pump sets off the metal detector alarm and they will have to explain that are on an insulin pump. Finally, some individuals get tired of having something connected to the body all of the time. When this occurs, we recommend a pump vacation, where the patient goes back to multiple daily injections for a few days to weeks. The disadvantages of insulin pump therapy are listed in Table 3.

MISCONCEPTIONS REGARDING INSULIN PUMP THERAPY

There are also many misconceptions about insulin pump therapy that you and your patients need to consider. Home glucose monitoring is still as important as ever with insulin pump therapy. Patients should be informed that frequent blood glucose measurements will be necessary, especially at the time of pump initiation. Later, when the patient is well adjusted on insulin pump therapy, the frequency of home glucose monitoring will be dependent on the variability of the patient's day-to-day activities. Many patients think that insulin pump therapy will allow them to eat anything they want at anytime. Although insulin pump therapy allows mealtimes and amounts to be more flexible, the patient must maintain some degree of dietary discretion in order to maintain or improve glycemic control. In addition, unwanted weight gain occurs in some individuals who start to overliberalize their diets despite good glycemic control. As mentioned earlier, insulin pump therapy is not contraindicated for people with hypoglycemic unawareness and insulin pumps are not only for individuals with type 1 diabetes.

HELPING PATIENTS DECIDE IF THE INSULIN PUMP
IS THE RIGHT THERAPY

An excellent way to help your patient decide if he or she would be an insulin pump candidate is to have the patient talk to people with personal experience. Have your patient check with the local American Diabetes Association or Juvenile Diabetes Foundation in your area to find a support group for people who use insulin pumps. Individuals in these groups can tell your patient the details of living with a pump on a day-to-day basis. In addition, insulin pump companies have information that they will send to your patient including video tapes and manuals. There are three insulin pump companies with

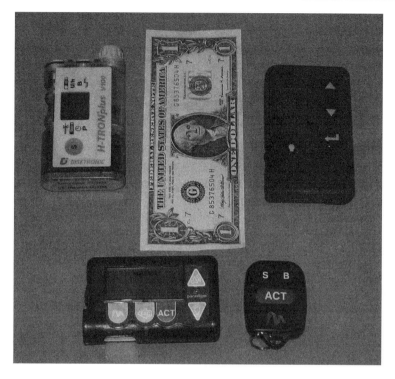

Fig. 1. Insulin pumps compared in size with a dollar bill. From left to right: Disetronic, Medtronic MiniMed, and Animas pumps.

excellent products (Medtronic MiniMed Inc., 1-800-933-3322, www.minimed.com; Disetronic Medical Systems, 1-800-280-7801, www.disetronic.com; and Animas Diabetes Care, LLC, 1-877-937-7867, www.animascorp.com).

Insulin pumps are now about the same size as a deck of cards or a beeper (*see* Fig. 1). They weigh approx 4 oz and can be put in a pocket, on a belt, in a specially designed bra, inside a sock or panty hose, and many other ingenious areas that patients have discovered. You can make an analogy between an insulin pump and an automatic, computerized, and mechanical insulin syringe that delivers insulin in a more physiologic fashion. Insulin pumps have a lever that mechanically pushes down a plunger of a large insulin syringe (up to 3.0 mL or 300 U of insulin) automatically 24 h/d (basal rate) and on demand before meals (bolus rate). The insulin then travels through a long infusion tube from the insulin syringe that is housed in the insulin pump, to the subcutaneous tissue via an implanted bent needle or a soft flexible catheter. The infusion lines now have a quick-release mechanism that can be temporarily disconnected from the insertion site (*see* Fig. 2). These quick-release catheters make showering, swimming, dressing, and other activities much more convenient.

Only regular or fast-acting insulin analogs are used in the insulin pumps. The basal rate of the insulin pump replaces the intermediate and longer acting insulins such as NPH, ultralente, or insulin glargine *(7,8)*. The boluses given before each meal are basically the same as with normal insulin injections of regular, lispro, or aspart. The majority of pump wearers insert the catheter or bent needle in the abdominal area, although the upper outer quadrant of the buttocks, upper thighs, and triceps fat pad of the arms can

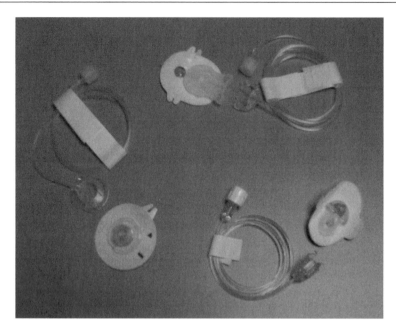

Fig. 2. Quick-release infusion lines from various manufacturers.

be used also (*see* Fig. 3). It is recommended that the syringe and the infusion set be filled and changed every 3 d. However, many patients use their infusion sets much longer (up to 6 d) before changing. Prolonged use of the infusion set at a single site greater than 3 d increases the likelihood of irritation or superficial abscess formation that may require antibiotic therapy and/or incision and drainage in the office setting. This scenario is very infrequent and most irritated sites improve on their own without the need for antibiotics or other interventions once the infusion set is removed. Insulin pumps have disposable batteries that last approx 5–8 wk. All three insulin pump brands have built in alarms to prevent inadvertent insulin delivery or to warn the patient if the insulin pump is empty or if the infusion set becomes clogged or dysfunctional.

INITIATING INSULIN PUMP THERAPY

Successful initiation of insulin pump therapy should be orchestrated by an educated and motivated health care, team including a physician, diabetes educator, registered dietitian, and a pump counselor. An inpatient ward was occasionally utilized in the past for starting insulin pump therapy. However, outpatient initiation of insulin pump therapy is a more realistic setting for integrating pump routines into an individual's lifestyle. The outpatient setting is also a necessity because of third-party reimbursement limitations. Before initiating insulin pump therapy, it is important to review several topics with the patient (*see* Table 4). The insulin pump companies have very knowledgeable profession-als (usually certified diabetes educators) that are available to help educate your patients on these important topics before, during, and after initiation of insulin pump therapy.

Initiating insulin pump therapy as an outpatient is feasible and only requires frequent contact with the patient for 2–3 d. After the patient has been educated to program the insulin pump and maintain the infusion lines, bolus and basal rates are determined and set. The patient is encouraged to follow his or her routine daily schedule with frequent

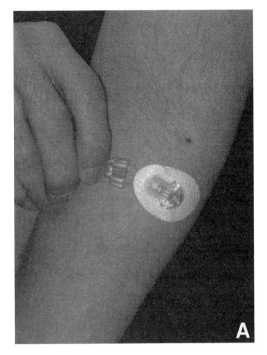

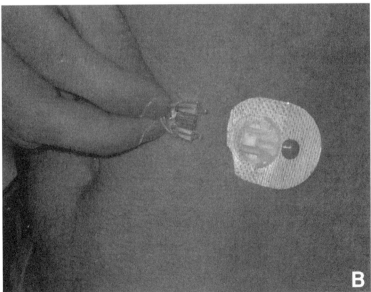

Fig. 3. Insulin pump infusion sites. (**A**) triceps fat pad; (**B**) abdominal fat pad.

home glucose monitoring. Blood glucose values should be obtained before and 1–2 h after each meal, at bedtime, and at 3 AM. These values will help you adjust the premeal bolus rates as well as the continuous basal rates during a 24-h period and assess if the patient needs any secondary basal rates to counteract the Dawn phenomenon for example.

Table 4
Topics to Discuss with the Pump Candidate Before Initiating Insulin Pump Therapy

- Basic operation of the pump including setting basal rate(s) and boluses
- Infusion set insertion and catheter care
- Targets for fasting and postprandial glucose values
- Prevention of hypoglycemia
- Prevention of diabetic ketoacidosis
- Sick-day rules
- Troubleshooting for unexplained hyperglycemia

The initial bolus and basal rates can be based on the patient's prior insulin regimen and/or by the 24-h insulin requirements. As mentioned earlier in the chapter, we put most of our patients on an intensive insulin regimen using insulin glargine once daily, or human ultralente prebreakfast and predinner with lispro or aspart insulin before each meal.

INSULIN PUMP BOLUS DOSE MANAGEMENT

When pump therapy is initiated, most patients can use the same insulin boluses he or she was using during MDI therapy. One of the distinct advantages of the insulin pump is the ability to modify the pattern of bolus administration. When a patient uses multiple daily injections, he or she is limited by the time-action profile of regular or the fast-acting lispro or aspart insulin. Some pumps have the ability to administer different types of boluses (see Fig. 4) The standard bolus has a quick rise and then fall of insulin administration. A "square-wave" bolus is characterized by a rapid-rise insulin, which is followed by sustained insulin administration and then a rapid fall in the insulin bolus. It provides insulin coverage in the event that the patient has an extended multicourse meal, buffet, high fat content meal (fat is absorbed slowly), or in patients with slow gastric emptying because of gastroparesis. Some pumps also have an option for a "dual-wave" bolus. This is a rapid peak bolus of insulin followed by a lower sustained insulin level, and then a rapid fall in administration. This is helpful in meals that contain both rapidly absorbed nutrients, such as fruit cocktail, followed by a multicourse meal. Patients can experiment and check their postprandial glucose measurements to see which type of bolus matches their eating style.

Another tool that can be utilized to tailor the bolus dose to a particular meal is carbohydrate counting. Because carbohydrates have a large effect on blood glucose excursions, estimating the amount of carbohydrates allows patients to more accurately approximate the size of the bolus with respect to the expected meal. There are different methods of carbohydrate counting, including gram counting and the older "exchange system." We prefer the gram counting method because it yields more accurate results (9). Patients should examine the "Nutrition Facts" label that is on all food packages as mandated by the Food and Drug Administration (see Fig. 5). First, the patient should determine the serving size and decide how many servings he or she is eating. Then, the patient should look at the "Total Carbohydrate" section of the label. The number of servings the patient is eating multiplied by the grams of carbohydrates per serving equals the total grams of carbohydrates consumed. When the patient is dining at restaurants or eating fast-food, they can use food lists, which give the nutritional content of foods. Several of the pump companies give away these guides and they can also be purchased

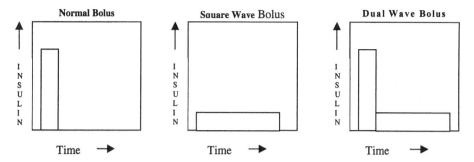

Fig. 4. Insulin bolus waves.

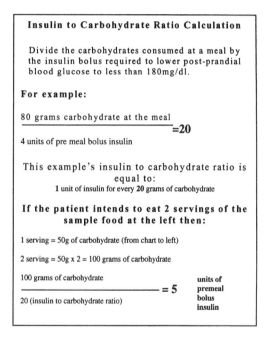

Nutrition Facts

Serving Size 2.5 oz.
Servings per container 3

Amount Per Serving

| Calories | 260 | |
| Calories from Fat | 25 | |

		% Daily Value*
Total Fat	2.5g	4
Saturated Fat	1g	5
Cholesterol	10mg	3
Sodium	560mg	23
Total Carbohydrate	50g	17
Dietary Fiber	1g	4
Sugars	7g	
Protein	11g	

*% Percent Daily Values Based on a 2,000 calories Diet.

Fig. 5. A "Nutrition Facts" label is on all food packages, as mandated by the Food and Drug Administration.

at bookstores. They are often extensive and they include food items at many common chain restaurants as well as popular meals from various types of cuisine. The next step is to determine your patient's insulin to carbohydrate ratio. Divide the grams of carbohydrates in a meal by the number of premeal insulin units that an individual requires to lower his or her post-prandial glucose to less than 180 mg/dL. For example, if a patient eats a 80-g carbohydrate meal and he or she typically requires 4 U of insulin to lower his or her blood sugar to the target range, then the insulin to carbohydrate ratio equals 1 U of insulin for every 20 g of carbohydrate. Therefore, if this patient has a 100-g carbohydrate meal, he or she divides 100 by 20 and thus the requirement is 5 U of insulin (*see* Fig. 5) Multiple pre- and postmeal blood glucose measurements are important to determine the most accurate insulin-to-carbohydrate ratio. With practice, patients can become very skilled in estimating the carbohydrate content of foods and this will be a valuable tool in further refining their insulin bolus regimen.

INSULIN PUMP BASAL RATE MANAGEMENT

To calculate the basal rate for a patient currently using multiple daily injections, simply take the daily insulin glargine dose or total daily ultralente dose and divide it by 24 h to calculate the initial basal rate. For example, a patient taking 10 U of ultralente in the morning and 14 U of ultralente in the evening would give a total of 24 U of insulin per day. Divide the 24 U by 24 h/d and this equals a basal rate of 1.0 U/h. If the patient has very good glucose control on the prior intensive insulin regimen with insulin glargine or ultralente, we reduce the basal rate by 10–20% because many individuals need less insulin when initiating pump therapy.

The basal rate can also be calculated by taking 50% of the total combined insulin requirements (including long- and short-acting insulins) of the patient and dividing it by 24 h. Once again, we usually reduce this rate by 10–20% if the patient's glucose control was fairly good prior to initiating insulin pump therapy. For example, if a patient's total daily combined insulin dose is 48 U of long- and rapid-acting insulin and the degree of control is quite poor, we would simply calculate the basal insulin dose as 24 U (50% of 48 U/d) divided by 24 h, equaling 1.0 U/h.

Calculation of the basal rate can also be estimated based on the patient's body weight. A conservative starting dose for the basal rate can be calculated by using 0.22 U/kg body weight per day. For example, if a patient weighs 75 kg, then the basal rate should be 0.7 U/kg (75 kg multiplied 0.22 U divided by 24 h). If there is a discrepancy in the estimated basal rate using these different techniques, the lower rate should be chosen for initiation of insulin pump therapy. It is also important to discontinue the patient's long-acting insulin at least 6–12 h before initiating pump therapy, depending on the type of long-acting insulin he or she is using.

VERIFYING THE BASAL RATE

To verify the overnight basal rate, the patient should avoid eating food after dinner and test the glucose value 2 h postdinner, at bedtime, at 3 AM, and the first thing in the morning. These values are very important to determine if the patient needs an increased basal rate in the early morning hours to counteract the Dawn phenomenon (the early morning resistance to insulin because of increased circulating growth hormone levels). In our experience, some patients will experience a rise in blood glucose values between 3 AM and 7 AM that require a 0.1–0.4 U/h increase in the basal rate during that time period. Occasionally, a patient may experience a decrease in basal insulin requirements between the hours of 12 midnight and 3 AM. In these patients, who are prone to nocturnal hypoglycemia, the basal rate can be decreased during this time period. The majority of pump users will achieve excellent glycemic control with three or less basal rates per day.

To evaluate the daytime and evening basal rates, instruct the patient to fast from the morning until dinnertime. If this is inconvenient, we suggest having the patient eat a very early breakfast, skip lunch, and monitor the blood sugars every 2–3 h up until dinnertime. An adequate basal rate will allow for ideal glucose control (between 70 and 110 mg/dL) while in the fasting state during the normal daily activities.

VERIFYING THE BOLUS DOSES

The premeal bolus insulin doses have usually been predetermined prior to insulin pump therapy based on the patient's MDI insulin regimen. The total daily dose of regular, lispro, or aspart insulin should be approx 50% of the total daily insulin requirements. Carbohydrate counting as detailed earlier will help to fine-tune the bolus doses. Many patients have been diabetic for several years and have a very good sense of how much insulin they need for any particular meal based on years of prior experience. In general, the premeal insulin dose should be based on prior experience, carbohydrate counting, the premeal glucose value, and any anticipated exercise after the ingestion of the meal.

1500 RULE

When suggesting supplemental regular, lispro, or aspart insulin to counteract an elevated blood glucose outside of mealtimes, one can use the "1500 rule." The 1500 rule, or sensitivity factor, gives an estimation of how much the patient's blood sugar will drop when given 1 U of regular, lispro, or aspart insulin. One simply takes the patient's total daily insulin requirements and divides 1500 by that number. For example, if a patient uses 50 U of insulin per day, 1 U regular, lispro, or aspart insulin of will lower the blood sugar by approx 30 mg/dL (1500 divided by 50). This particular patient would take an additional 1 unit extra of regular, lispro, or aspart insulin for every 30 mg/dL above the goal glucose value (i.e., 120 mg/dL). This sensitivity factor can change for an individual and, therefore, it is only meant to act as a guide.

Once the patient initiates pump therapy, he or she should make contact with the caregiver at least once every 24-h period in order to review the glucose values and to have any questions answered or concerns addressed that have arisen. The glucose values could be easily forwarded to the caregiver by facsimile or e-mail prior to the phone conversation. In most cases, after 2–3 d, the bolus and basal rates are fairly close to the ultimate final values and the patient can be seen in approx 2–4 wk after initiating therapy.

SPECIAL PRECAUTIONS AND EVERYDAY MANAGEMENT

One of the most important precautions for people utilizing insulin pump therapy is regarding unexplained severe hyperglycemia. Because there is no intermediate- or long-acting insulin in the patient's circulation, a disruption in the regular, lispro, or aspart insulin delivery can result in a fairly rapid rise in blood glucose concentration and subsequent development of diabetic ketoacidosis in type 1 diabetics. In general, we highly suggest using lispro or aspart in the insulin pump instead of regular insulin. The benefits of lispro or aspart insulin are an improved postprandial glucose value and a decreased incidence and severity of delayed hypoglycemia 3–5 h after a meal, and especially during exercise. However, there is a disadvantage to using lispro and aspart insulin for pump therapy that must be part of the pump candidate's education. If there is an unexpected discontinuation of insulin delivery (catheter dislodged, blockage, or the reservoir is empty), the patient will experience a more rapid rise in the blood glucose value because lispro and aspart are short acting. In addition, temporary pump discontinuation for showers, exercise, and so on can only be for a very short time, no longer than 45–60 min. The patient should be well trained in troubleshooting and should always carry a bottle of regular, lispro, or aspart insulin with a syringe or an insulin pen as a safety precaution.

We do not recommend initiating insulin pump therapy during pregnancy because a novice pump user would be at more risk for diabetic ketoacidosis than someone who is knowledgeable, comfortable, and had several months to years of experience with insulin pump therapy.

The new quick-release catheters help to solve the problems of showering, bathing, and dressing. However, if this type of catheter is not available, the pump can simply be put into a zip-lock bag and held in one hand or placed on a nearby shelf or soap dish during showering or bathing. Placement of the insulin pump during sleeping and sexual intimacy is usually not a problem with the exception of occasional entanglement in body parts. Many patients use the quick-release catheters to free themselves from the insulin pump during sexual intimacy or short periods of intensive exercise.

Traveling with an insulin pump is very convenient, especially when crossing many time zones and having erratic meal amounts, types, and times. As noted earlier, the only problem that may occur is going through the airport security. Many times, the insulin pump will trigger the airport security alarm and we would suggest taking all pens, coins, beepers, and any other metal off before going through the security. This may help your patients avoid a hand search or a delayed passage through security. A physician's letter may also help to facilitate the patient's way through security, especially after the unfortunate events of September 11, 2001.

Many patients enjoy a "pump vacation" from insulin pump therapy when they are participating in a water-sports weekend or just want to be totally free of the mechanical device connected to their body for a few days or weeks. In this case, we recommend that the patients go back to their previous intensive insulin regimen consisting long-acting insulin glargine or ultralente with lispro or aspart insulin before each meal. The same bolus insulin doses of lispro or aspart are used. To determine the amount of basal insulin, simply add up the total amount of basal insulin used in the pump over a 24-h period. Do not count the bolus doses in this calculation. The total will yield the amount of insulin glargine needed. If twice-a-day ultralente is used instead of insulin glargine, divide the total basal insulin by 2 and the patient would administer half of the ultralente dose in the morning and half in the evening. When your patient switches over to long-acting insulin glargine or ultralente, the patient continues the insulin pump basal rate for 3–4 h after the long-acting insulin is administered and then the pump is stopped (10). The reason for the overlap of therapy is that insulin glargine and ultralente are slow to start acting and blood glucose levels could rise excessively during this time.

FUTURE DEVELOPMENTS

In the future, insulin pump therapy will evolve into a closed-loop system. Currently, patients and physicians must interpret their blood glucose trends and adjust their basal insulin rates and boluses accordingly. As continuous glucose sensors are developed, they will be able to provide information to the insulin pump and automatically adjust insulin doses. Currently, there are minimally invasive glucose oxidase sensors that reside in the subcutaneous fat layer, similar to an insulin pump set. Medtronic MiniMed has a system where the patient wears the sensor continuously for 3 d (11). Then, the patient returns to the doctor's office and the information is downloaded to the computer for subsequent analysis. The glucose excursions and trends can be analyzed and then recommendations can be given to the patient. Numerous other companies are developing glucose sensing technology and the first real-time system available for patients in 2002 was the Glucowatch™ from Cygnus, Inc (12,13). There are several ongoing trials of real-time systems to determine if they are accurate and reliable enough for a closed-loop system. There are also indwelling glucose sensors that use electrochemical and optical sensors that are being developed for long-term use. The end of this evolution will probably be a system where the administration of insulin via an insulin pump will be completely controlled by a continuous glucose sensor and a computer algorithm. For now, the insulin pumps that are available are very reliable and offer an excellent alternative to multiple daily injections. They are simple to operate and they are very reliable. The insulin pump has improved the lives of many patients with type 1 and type 2 diabetes.

REFERENCES

1. Norby D. Intensive Insulin Therapy Using an Insulin Infusion Pump: A Guide to Develop a Protocol to Implement Insulin Pump Therapy. Disetronic Medical Systems, Inc., Minneapolis, 1995, pp. 33–52.
2. Skyler JS. Insulin treatment. In: Therapy for Diabetes Mellitus and Related Disorders. 3rd ed. American Diabetes Association, Alexandria, VA, 1998, pp. 186–203.
3. Bode BW, Steed RD, Davidson PC. Reduction in severe hypoglycemia with long-term continuous subcutaneous insulin infusion in type 1 diabetes. Diabetes Care 1996;19:324–327.
4. Crawford LM, Sinha RN, Odell RM, et al. Efficacy of insulin pump therapy: mealtime delivery is the key factor. Endocr Prac 2000;6:277,278.
5. Edelman, SV. Insulin pump therapy: a practical tool for treating persons with type 1 and insulin-requiring type 2 diabetes. In:Leahy JL, Clark NG, Cefalu WT, eds. Medical Management of Diabetes Mellitus. Marcel Dekker, New York, 2000, pp. 309–323.
6. Zinman B, Tildesley H, Chaisson JL, et al. Insulin Lispro in CSII: results of a double blind crossover study. Diabetes 1997;46:440–443.
7. Garg SK, Anderson JH, Gerard LA, et al. Impact of insulin lispro on HbA1c values in insulin pump users. Diabetes Obes Metabol 2000;2:307–311.
8. Bode BW, Strange P. Efficacy, safety, and pump compatibility of insulin aspart used in continuous insulin infusion therapy in patients with type 1 diabetes. Diabetes Care 2001;24:69–72.
9. Kulkarni K, Fredrickson L, Graff MR. Carbohydrate Counting: A primer for Insulin Pump Users to Zero in on Good Control. MiniMed Inc., Northridge, CA, 1999, pp. 6–19.
10. Edelman SV. Taking Control of Your Diabetes. 2nd ed. Professional Communications Inc., West Islip, NY, 2001, pp. 142,143.
11. Gross TM, Bode BW, Einhorn D, et al. Performance evaluation of the MiniMed continuous glucose monitoring system during patient home use. Diabetes Tech Therap 2000;2:49–56.
12. Pitzer KR, Desai S, Dunn T, et al. Detection of hypoglycemia with the Glucowatch Biographer. Diabetes Care 2001;24:881–885.
13. Tierney MJ, Tamada JA, Potts RO, et al. The Glucowatch Biographer: a frequent automatic and noninvasive glucose monitor. Ann Int Med 2000;32:632–641.

14 Detection and Management of Diabetes Mellitus During Glucocorticoid Therapy of Nonendocrine Disease

Susan S. Braithwaite, MD

CONTENTS

INTRODUCTION

For the patient who has preexisting type 1 or type 2 diabetes mellitus or the patient with new-onset diabetes during glucocorticoid therapy (steroid diabetes), glucocorticoid therapy of nonendocrine disease poses dilemmas. Glucocorticoid therapy exacerbates hyperglycemia, and tapering of a patient's glucocorticoid dose without adjustment of diabetes therapy may result in severe hypoglycemia. Nevertheless, beneficial glucocorticoid therapy should not be denied to patients having preexisting diabetes or developing steroid diabetes.

The goals of this chapter are to provide operational guidelines on how to detect steroid diabetes, prevent diabetic metabolic emergencies, meet standards of care with respect to chronic glycemic control for ambulatory patients, and achieve glycemic targets for hospitalized and surgical patients during glucocorticoid therapy. Many concepts about the general care of diabetes patients are applicable *(1–11)*. The chapter focuses on glucocorticoid therapy of nonendocrine disease for nonpregnant adults *(12–71)*. This chapter does not exhaustively discuss pathophysiology of steroid diabetes *(72–79)* or management of diabetes complicating organ transplantation *(80–111)*, glucocorticoid

From: *Endocrine Replacement Therapy in Clinical Practice*
Edited by: A. Wayne Meikle © Humana Press Inc., Totowa, NJ

therapy of children *(112–115)*, pregnancy *(116,117)*, endogenous Cushing syndrome *(118–121)*, megestrol therapy *(122)*, or adrenal insufficiency *(123,124)*.

LITERATURE REVIEW ON PATHOPHYSIOLOGY, INCIDENCE, AND COMPLICATIONS OF STEROID DIABETES

Pathophysiology and Incidence of Steroid Diabetes

In its mildest form, steroid diabetes results from peripheral insulin resistance (reduced clearance of glucose by adipocytes and myocytes) *(44,77 94)*. With increasing severity of steroid-induced diabetes or glucocorticoid-induced changes of diabetic control, and at higher doses of glucocorticoid, in humans there are observed defects in insulin secretion *(78)*, and increased hepatic glucose production occurs *(75,78,89)*. Genetically determined defects of insulin secretory capacity or impairment of β-cell function by cyclosporin or tacrolimus may enhance patient susceptibility to glucocorticoid-induced hyperglycemia *(79,104,107,109)*.

The reported frequency of steroid diabetes cannot be directly compared between series because of differences in definitions of diabetes, exclusion criteria for previously diabetic patients, and underlying illnesses and concomitant therapies. A sampling of published studies on incidence is presented in Table 1. Family history of diabetes, present in up to 33–80% of cases *(12,22,81–83,87,100)*, age *(38,95,96,115)*, and glucocorticoid dose *(12,22,38,56,87,96,100,106)* have emerged as possible predictors of steroid diabetes. Steroid diabetes, if it is to occur, usually appears early (e.g., within the first 30 d of treatment for chronic obstructive lung disease) *(68)*.

Most cases of posttransplant diabetes occur within the first year *(91–93,109)*, usually within the first 1–3 mo *(41,81–83, 87,90,95,108)*. Although the incidence of diabetes after renal transplant increased in the era following introduction of cyclosporin *(88)*, the trend has been offset by the development of glucocorticoid-sparing immunosuppression regimens *(90,106)*. The first recognition of diabetes or insulin requirement may follow intravenous bolus glucocorticoid therapy used in the treatment of acute rejection, especially if maintenance immunosuppression regimens are employed that use glucocorticoids sparingly *(80,82,95,108,109)*. Many liver-transplant recipients had preexisting diabetes in association with cirrhosis and do not experience worsening as a result of immunosuppression after successful transplantation *(103,110)*. However, the hyperglycemic hyperosmolar state (HSS) has been recognized following liver transplant *(97)*. Among heart-transplant recipients, posttransplant diabetes is common and may be related to rejection treatment *(100,108)*. Pancreas-transplant recipients may experience several abnormalities of glycemic control, including hypoglycemia resulting from systemic hyperinsulinemia or insulin-deficient diabetes as a result of rejection *(111)*. C-Peptide-positive pancreas-transplant recipients occasionally present with ketosis-resistant transplant diabetes or even HHS, and they do not invariably require insulin for long-term therapy.

Complications of Uncontrolled Steroid Diabetes

There is a paucity of objective data on chronic complications of diabetes among glucocorticoid-treated patients, but there is abundant evidence on the importance of metabolic control in other diabetic populations. Therefore, during long-term glucocorticoid therapy the prevention of diabetic microvascular complications is an appropriate concern.

Table 1
Frequency of Steroid Diabetes in Retrospective Series of Glucocorticoid-Treated Patients

Series	Medical condition	Patients in series	Steroid diabetes
1957 Ranney et al. (14)	Leukemia, lymphoma	34	5 (14.7%)
1961 Baldwin et al. (17)	Asthma	87	0 (0.0%)
1964 Keeney (21)	Asthma	25	1 (4.0%)
1966 Walsh and Grant (26)	Asthma	245	3 (1.2%)
1968 Smyllie and Connelly (32)	Respiratory disease	550	9 (1.6%)
1972 Lieberman et al. (38)	Asthma	50	14 (28.0%)
1973 Ruiz et al. (81)	Renal transplant	253	15 (5.9%)
1974 Hill et al. (82)	Renal transplant	31	12 (39.7%)
1975 Woods et al. (83)	Renal transplant	202	11 (5.4%)
1980 Gunnarsson et al. (85)	Renal transplant	114	52 (45.6 %)
1980 David et al. (41)	Renal transplant	286	31 (10.8%)
1983 Arner et al. (87)	Renal transplant	145	67 (46.2%)
1989 Shi and Zhang (55)	SLE, pemphigus, chronic nephritis	286	28 (9.8%)
1991 Sumrani et al. (91)	Renal transplant	337	39 (11.6%)
1993 Robert et al. (114)	Renal transplant, pediatric	700	8 (1.1%)
1996 Vesco et al. (95)	Renal transplant	1325	33 (2.5%)
1997 Hjelmesaeth et al. (96)	Renal transplant	167	31 (18.6%)
1999 Niewoehner et al. (68)	COPD	160	24 (15.0%)
2000 Covar et al. (115)	Asthma, pediatric	163	2 (1.2%)
2001 Nieuwenhuis and Kirkels (108)	Heart transplant	219	43 (19.6%)

Severe infection, sometimes leading to death, is a potential complication of transplant diabetes (85). In a series in which only 51.3% of renal-transplant recipients having transplant diabetes were treated with insulin, the incidence of infectious complications was significantly higher in the diabetic compared with the nondiabetic control group, and there were five sepsis-related deaths among the diabetic patients (91). Posttransplant diabetes or glucose intolerance is associated with a clustering of other cardiovascular risk factors and metabolic abnormalities (105). Observations on diabetic complications and cost of care provide strong support for the development of steroid-sparing immuno-suppressive regimens (98,101,106). The observations also should raise the question of whether undertreatment of transplant diabetes, or avoidance of insulin therapy specifi-cally, is partly responsible for the observed increase of infectious complications among diabetic transplant recipients.

Diabetic Metabolic Emergency During Glucocorticoid Therapy

In a series of 135 patients having HHS, use of corticosteroids was implicated as a possible contributory factor among 7% (51).

The literature was reviewed for cases of diabetic metabolic emergency occurring during glucocorticoid therapy, and these were classified as ketoalkalosis (1,2,118), hypoglycemia, ketoacidosis, or HHS. Ketoacidosis was identified if either the diagnosis was stated by the authors, could be inferred from the case description, or was documented by reported chemistries. Cases of ketonuria without ketoacidosis were not included here as examples of metabolic emergency. Because mixed pictures of ketoacidosis and diabetic hyperosmolar state were recognized, because classification of metabolic emergencies varied among authors, and because biochemical data was incomplete in many of the reviewed cases, it was difficult to apply a consistent classification rule. For that reason, the cases assigned to each category of metabolic emergency are specifically identified in Table 2, together with information on setting, duration of glucocorticoid therapy, and outcome, when determinable.

One case of diabetic ketoalkalosis probably was promoted by antecedent vomiting and several months of ambulatory corticotropin and glucocorticoid treatment *(15)*. One case of hypoglycemia was reported, occurring during sulfonylurea treatment of a patient who was first diagnosed with diabetes during replacement glucocorticoid therapy following adrenalectomy for breast cancer, with neuroglycopenia and fatal outcome during an intercurrent illness accompanied by reduced oral intake *(123)*. A case of insulin-induced hypoglycemia with seizure has been observed during ambulatory tapering of glucocorticoid therapy initiated in the hospital for obstructive airway disease (unpublished observation), but no cases of hypoglycemic emergency were discovered in the review of published literature about patients receiving glucocorticoid therapy for nonendocrine disease. In the literature reviewed, during glucocorticoid therapy the total numbers of cases discovered were 67 metabolic emergencies and 11 fatalities. The numbers of cases of each type of metabolic emergency were 1 ketoalkalosis, 1 severe hypoglycemia, 21 ketoacidosis, and 44 HHS. The numbers of fatalities in association with each were 1 with hypoglycemia, 2 with ketoacidosis, and 8 with HHS.

In the literature review (*see* Table 2), one case of HHS was precipitated by intra-articular injection of glucocorticoid *(53)* and one by alternate-day therapy in combination with hydrochlorothiazide *(47)*. Some cases of metabolic emergency occurred during hospitalization, sometimes for massive-dose therapy, or following anti-rejection therapy *(80,82,83)*. Two were complicated by thrombotic events *(23,37)*.

A practical dilemma confronting the practitioner, that might be illuminated by the literature review, is the necessity to set up monitoring and a patient-contact program that would prevent a metabolic emergency during glucocorticoid therapy of ambulatory patients. Short-term therapy *(25,32)* and intra-articular injection *(40,42,43)* generally carry low risk to patient safety. However, the literature review on metabolic emergency shows that the fractions of cases occurring in the ambulatory setting were ≥12/21 ketoacidosis or 57% and ≥22/44 HHS or 50%. The fractions of cases occurring during glucocorticoid treatment of <2 wk duration were ≥3/21 ketoacidosis or 14 %, and ≥9/44 HHS or 20 % (*see* Table 2). Some cases occurred during tapering of the glucocorticoid regimen *(27,34,45,52)* or during alternate-day therapy *(47)*. At least three of the fatalities in the HHS group occurred during ambulatory glucocorticoid therapy that had been of less than 2-wk duration *(31,45)*. Thus, the literature review showed that even though a majority or plurality of cases of diabetic ketoacidosis (DKA) or HHS respectively occurred later than 2 wk after the initiation of glucocorticoid therapy, there was no apparent early window of safety during which education and monitoring might safely be neglected.

Many of the foregoing cases occurred before monitoring of capillary blood glucose had gained widespread acceptance. Although this historical review may not represent

Table 2
Metabolic Emergencies During Glucocorticoid Therapy

	Setting			Duration of glucocorticoid therapy			
Metabolic emergencies and no. of cases	Amb	Hosp	Unkn, other	≥2 wk	<2 wk	Unkn, other	Fatal
Ketoalkalosis							
1 1957 Simpson (15)	1			1			
Hypoglycemia							
1 1969 Arai et al. (123)	1			1			1
Ketoacidosis							
1 1956 Berg (13)	1					1	
2 1957 Ranney and Gellham (14)			2			2	
1 1962 Gregory and Sayle (18)	1			1			
1 1964 Blereau and Weingarten (19)	1			1			
2 1967 Zangel and Mazzi, cases 1–2 (29)			2	2			
1 1969 Spenney et al., case 3 (34)		1			1		
4 1971 Alavi et al., cases 1–4 (35)	4			4			
1 1973 Ruiz et al., case 1 (81)	1			1			
1 1974 Hill et al. (82)			1			1	
2 1982 Perlman and Erlich (113)	2			2			
1 1984 Ivanova et al. (46)		1		1			1
2 1995 Haggerty et al. (58)	2			2			1
2 2000 Bouhanick et al. (116)		2			2		
21 Totals for ketoacidosis	12	4	5	14	3	4	2
Hyperglycemic hyperosmolar state							
1 1963 Mach and Sousa (20)	1			1			
1 1965 Brocard et al. (23)		1		1			
1 1965 Schwartz and Apfelbaum (24)	1			1			
3 1967 Boyer (27)	3			2	1		1
1 1967 Planchu et al. (28)	1				1		
2 1968 Kumar (30)	1	1		1	1		1
2 1968 Pyörälä et al. (31)	1	1		1	1		1
2 1969 Spenney et al., cases 1–2 (34)	2			2			
1 1971 Corcoran et al. (37)	1			1			1
1 1971 Limas et al. (36)	1			1			
1 1971 Szewczyk et al. (112)		1		1			1
1 1972 Daouk et al. (80)	1			1			
1 1973 Ruiz et al., case 10 (81)	1			1			
1 1974 Hill et al. (82)			1			1	
3 1975 Woods et al., cases 3, 5, 11 (83)		1	2	2	1		
3 1983 Fujikawa et al. (45)	2	1			3		2
1 1984 Lohr et al. (47)	1			1			
2 1987 Thomas et al., cases WH, TG (52)			2	2			
10 1987 Wachtel et al. (51)			10			10	
1 1989 Black and Filak (53)	1				1		
4 1989 Shi and Zhang (55)	4					4	1
1 1997 Kirkman et al. (97)			1	1			
44 Totals for hyperglycemic hyperosmolar state	22	6	16	20	9	15	8
67 **Overall totals**	**37**	**10**	**20**	**36**	**12**	**19**	**11**

present-day risk, unreported cases of metabolic emergency during glucocorticoid therapy continue to occur. The historical data underscore the importance of detecting diabetes and taking active preventive measures against the development of a metabolic emergency once diabetes is recognized. The data suggest that appropriate patient education must be in place from the very beginning.

DIAGNOSIS, PATIENT EDUCATION, AND MONITORING

When glucocorticoid therapy is contemplated, the question of whether diabetes is present should be addressed (7). For patients not known to have diabetes, the physician conducting glucocorticoid therapy should determine a casual or fasting plasma venous glucose concentration before initiation of glucocorticoid therapy (see Fig. 1).

Education and Monitoring of Previously Nondiabetic Patients

The nondiabetic patient should receive education on the possibility that diabetes mellitus could occur. For ambulatory patients without known diabetes, urine testing should be cost-effective and sufficient for detection of impending hyperglycemic crisis if performed twice daily at the initiation of therapy and three times weekly during long-term therapy. In addition, the provider should monitor fasting plasma venous glucose (FPVG) or casual plasma venous glucose at periodic intervals for hospitalized patients and, initially at 1- to 2-wk intervals for ambulatory patients.

Detection of Steroid Diabetes

If glycosuria or hyperglycemia appears, confirm the diagnosis of steroid diabetes by measurement of FPVG (7). For patients with new-onset steroid diabetes, educate them on self-monitoring of blood glucose (SMBG).

Education and Monitoring for Diabetic Patients

Patients with diabetes recognized prior to glucocorticoid therapy and not yet taking insulin should perform SMBG at least twice a day during initiation of glucocorticoid therapy and should be educated on the possibility that destabilization of glycemic control could occur. Those who are poorly controlled when first starting glucocorticoids, who are extremely insulin resistant, and/or who have any of the usual risk factors for HHS should be followed with special vigilance. It has been observed by diabetes educators that diabetes often is not the primary focus of care for these patients, that their medical care may be fragmented among specialists, and that the need to provide flexible instructions about diabetes may be a difficult challenge to the educator, requiring individualized attention to details of their glucocorticoid treatment plan (57,71).

Alert Parameters for Diabetic Patients

Special educational emphasis on the risk of metabolic decompensation is necessary for the elderly and their caregivers, for patients at risk of dehydration, for other patients at high risk for HHS, and for those receiving high-dose glucocorticoid therapy or intermediate- to long-term therapy (longer than 2–4 wk). The provider should be contacted for a premeal glucose >300 mg for two tests in a row or a premeal blood glucose >140 mg/dL for 3 d in a row. Patients receiving antihyperglycemic drugs should call for blood glucose <120 mg/d during glucocorticoid tapering and for blood glucose <80 mg/dL or symptoms of hypoglycemia during stable glucocorticoid therapy.

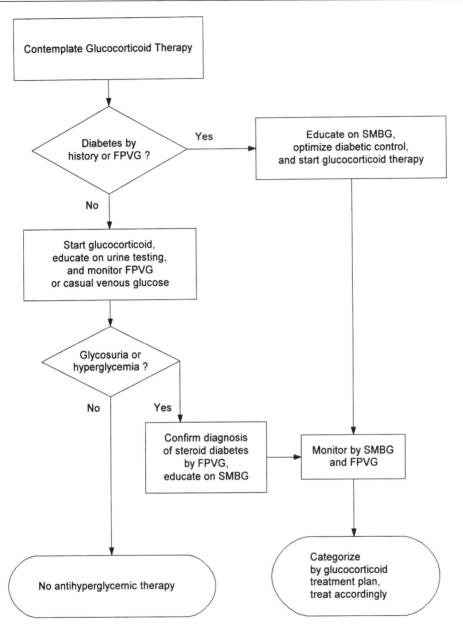

Fig. 1. Detection and monitoring of diabetes during glucocorticoid therapy. FVPG, fasting venous plasma glucose; SMBG, self-monitoring of blood glucose.

MANAGEMENT OF STEROID DIABETES
AND GLUCOCORTICOID-INDUCED EXACERBATION
OF PREEXISTING DIABETES

Unless otherwise specified, the following management plans are appropriate for ambulatory patients or inpatients. Initiation of therapy refers to the first exposure of patients to glucocorticoid therapy in doses equivalent to at least 30–60 mg of prednisone daily. Tapering refers to decrements from pharmacologic to physiologic doses of glucocorticoids, or rapid discontinuation of short-term therapy.

Whenever possible, diabetic patients should be rendered normoglycemic before starting glucocorticoid therapy.

Categorization of Glucocorticoid Treatment Plan at Initiation of Therapy, Target Range Blood Glucose Levels, and Indications for Antihyperglycemic Therapy

At initiation of glucocorticoid therapy, after classifying patients as diabetic or non-diabetic, the provider should further individualize management according to the anticipated glucocorticoid treatment plan *(61,64)*. Not every patient who newly develops hyperglycemia will require therapy with antihyperglycemic drugs, and not every patient with known diabetes will require revision of antihyperglycemic therapy during glucocorticoid treatment *(39)*.

CATEGORY 1. SINGLE INJECTIONS OF GLUCOCORTICOID; OR GLUCOCORTICOID THERAPY THAT WILL BE RAPIDLY TAPERED AND DISCONTINUED OVER THE SHORT TERM (<2 WK)

The target range premeal glucose is 80–200 mg/dL during short-term rapidly tapering glucocorticoid therapy for those receiving no insulin or insulin secretogogue therapy, or 120–200 mg/dL for those receiving insulin or insulin secretogogue therapy. Because of the time course for dissipation of glucocorticoid effect, intra-articular glucocorticoid therapy is classified as an example of short-term rapidly tapering therapy *(40,42,43)*.

Some patients with blood glucose levels above target become candidates for supplemental premeal regular insulin because they present special risk factors for HHS, because monitoring suggests impending metabolic emergency, or because they will require repeated courses of glucocorticoids. Patients already using insulin should employ compensatory dosing with short-acting insulin (*see* below). For many other patients observed during short-term rapidly tapering glucocorticoid therapy, hyperglycemia above target may occur but need not be treated (*see* Fig. 2).

CATEGORY 2. FIXED-DOSE, SHORT-TERM GLUCOCORTICOID THERAPY (<2 WK); OR INTERMEDIATE-TERM GLUCOCORTICOID THERAPY (2–4 WK)

The target range premeal glucose is 80–200 mg/dL for patients receiving fixed-dose, short-term therapy (<2 wk) or intermediate-term glucocorticoid therapy (2–4 wk).

Because of the risk of rapid deterioration of glycemic control, for any patient having premeal glucose >200 mg/dL and for many others having premeal glucose 140–200 mg/dL in the setting of fixed-dose short-term therapy or intermediate-term glucocorticoid therapy, split-mixed insulin should be initiated (*see* later subsection). For some previously diabetic patients, a temporary conversion from dietary therapy or oral agents to insulin or adjustment of daily insulin dose will be necessary (*see* Fig. 3).

CATEGORY 3. LONG-TERM GLUCOCORTICOID THERAPY (>4 WK)

The target ranges for glucose for patients who receive long-term glucocorticoid therapy are 80–130 mg/dL before meals and 100–150 mg/dL at bedtime, the same as for other patients having diabetes *(8)*. Additionally, the hemoglobin A_{1c} should be <7.0%. If patients receive pulse-dose augmentation of their long-term glucocorticoid therapy, the target blood glucose range may be temporarily increased to 120–200 mg/dL.

Sometimes, the A_{1c} exceeds target despite premeal normoglycemia. In such cases, postprandial testing should be performed. If the increase of postprandial blood glucose

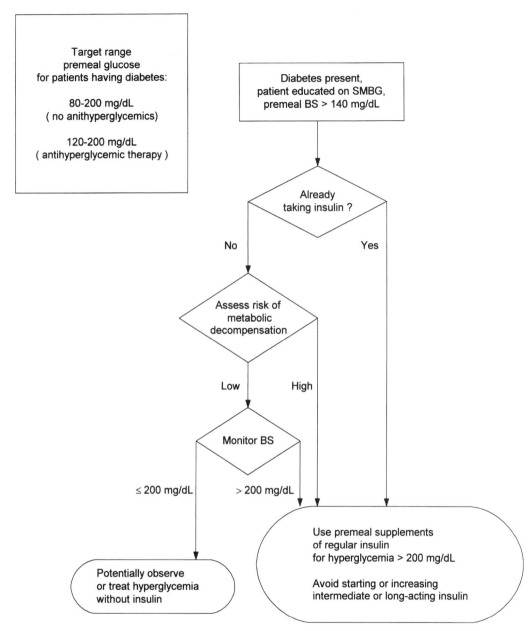

Fig. 2. Single injections of glucocorticoid, or glucocorticoid therapy that will be rapidly tapered and discontinued over the short term (<2 wk).

above premeal values exceeds 20–50 mg/dL, therapy for postprandial hyperglycemia may be indicated. For patients on long-term glucocorticoid therapy who experience mild deterioration of glycemic control during pulse dosing but who otherwise do not require antihyperglycemic treatment, repaglinide may be useful. For most patients with fasting blood glucose >140 mg/dL during long-term glucocorticoid therapy, insulin therapy is appropriate. For previously nondiabetic patients split-mixed insulin should be initiated

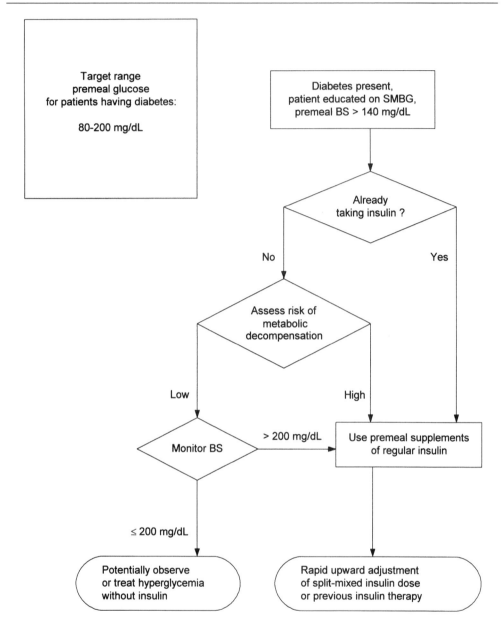

Fig. 3. Fixed-dose, short-term glucocorticoid therapy (<2 wk), or intermediate-term glucocorticoid therapy (2–4 wk).

(*see* later subsection), and for previously diabetic patients conversion to insulin or adjustment of daily insulin dose should be undertaken (*see* Fig. 4).

Compensatory Dosing with Short-Acting Insulin

Compensatory dosing for hyperglycemia with short-acting insulin is appropriate for any insulin user and also for any patient formerly naïve to insulin who is newly started on insulin during glucocorticoid therapy. Objective studies have not been undertaken

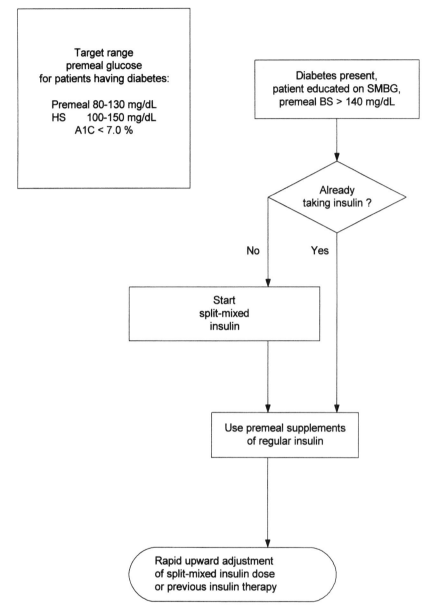

Fig. 4. Long-term glucocorticoid therapy (>4 wk).

that would establish preference among particular short-acting species of insulin during concomitant use of glucocorticoids. For patients having fasting or premeal hyperglycemia >140 mg/dL, the subcutaneous use of rapidly absorbed short-acting insulins such as lispro or aspart may fail to provide adequate "holding power" to prevent recurring premeal hyperglycemia. Therefore, because most patients with steroid diabetes either do not take basal insulin or do not complement their basal insulin with short-acting insulin at all three meals (lunch, breakfast, and supper), for these patients during glucocorticoid therapy the author prefers regular insulin to lispro or aspart.

For patients previously not taking insulin, a starting dose might be 4 U of regular insulin for premeal blood glucose of 140–239 mg/dL and 8 U for blood glucose ≥240 mg/dL. Insulin-treated patients who are knowledgeable about compensatory dosing might use their usual sick-day management plans to supplement with extra short-acting insulin (regular, lispro, or aspart). Insulin-treated patients who do not have a sick-day plan may employ a simple rule of taking a supplement of premeal regular insulin consisting of 10% of the total daily insulin dose or 4 U, whichever is larger, for a premeal glucose of 140–239 mg/dL, and 20% of the total daily insulin dose or 8 U, whichever is larger, for a premeal glucose ≥240 mg/dL. If hypoglycemia occurs, the supplement of regular insulin should be reduced to perhaps 4 U or 10% for a blood glucose over 240 mg/dL, and timing should be considered as a possible factor. In treating hospitalized patients, the physician may recommend algorithms for premeal supplementation that are more complex.

Although compensatory dosing normally is used only at mealtime, patients with severe premeal hyperglycemia may need subcutaneous short-acting insulin supplements in high dosage around the clock to gain initial control, combined with rapid adjustment of the daily dose of insulin. If the premeal blood glucose exceeds 300 mg/dL, the compensatory supplement of regular insulin should be repeated every 3–4 h with a snack, or lispro or aspart every 2 h, and if the response is unsatisfactory, higher doses of supplemental regular insulin or insulin drip therapy should be considered.

Initiation of Split-Mixed Insulin and a Rapid Insulin Adjustment Subroutine

The algorithm to follow focuses on the needs of patients not yet treated with insulin or type 2 diabetes patients who do not use intensive insulin management plans. When such patients do require treatment, a common regimen is the so-called "split-mixed" neutral protamine Hagedorn (NPH) and regular insulin treatment plan in which a mixture of NPH and regular insulin is given before breakfast and supper. Use of the algorithm should be complemented by individualization of therapy when glycemic targets are not met. Patients who have had previous glucocorticoid therapy, when rechallenged under similar conditions of health with similar glucocorticoid dose, may benefit from antihyperglycemic therapy that worked the previous time (71).

Decisions to initiate or increase the doses of intermediate- or long-acting insulins are influenced by the intended duration of glucocorticoid treatment and patient-related risks. Split-mixed insulin therapy usually is not employed for hyperglycemia complicating single injections of glucocorticoid or short-term rapidly tapering therapy. Split-mixed insulin sometimes is appropriate for high-risk patients experiencing hyperglycemia during fixed-dose, short-term therapy or intermediate-term therapy with glucocorticoids. "Split-mixed" insulin is employed routinely for patients newly requiring insulin during long-term glucocorticoid therapy.

A simple regimen by which the physician may initiate split-mixed insulin therapy is to use at least 8–10 U of premixed 70/30 NPH/regular insulin before breakfast and 4–5 U of premixed 50/50 or 70/30 insulin before supper. For patients already taking insulin, the needed adjustment of daily insulin requirement during glucocorticoid therapy is unpredictable but may exceed a 50% increase over the pretreatment requirement (49,89). If premeal glucose readings are 140–240 mg/dL, the increments usually are 10% of the daily dose of insulin, made every third day.

Patients whose premeal glucose exceeds 240 mg/dL during glucocorticoid therapy and who are selected for split-mixed insulin therapy are appropriate candidates for the "rapid insulin adjustment subroutine." The goal of rapid insulin adjustment is to provide a safe method of working up the daily dose of split-mixed insulin over several days, preventing metabolic emergency, but also avoiding hypoglycemia (*see* Figs. 5 and 6). In brief, this is the method:

> *The daily dose of insulin is administered as split-mixed NPH and regular insulin before breakfast and supper (or NPH insulin before breakfast and bedtime). In addition, premeal supplements of compensatory regular insulin are taken before breakfast, lunch, or supper. Each day, an increase of the daily dose of premixed or NPH insulin is made, in an amount equal to two-thirds of the number of units given as supplemental regular insulin the previous day.*

The routine is easily applied by house officers or, in frequent telephone consultation, by patients at home. Concern about hypoglycemia may be raised by the physicians, nursing staff, or patients because the peak actions of supplements of regular insulin will overlap the peak actions of split-mixed insulin as recommended under the rapid insulin adjustment subroutine (*see* Fig. 4). In response to those concerns, it should be noted first that the risk of hypoglycemia is reduced during high-dose glucocorticoid therapy because of insulin resistance; adequacy of the total daily insulin dose may be a more important consideration. Second, peak effects of insulin cannot be assumed to occur at the anticipated times when large doses are injected *(3)*; the actions of both regular and NPH insulin potentially are prolonged. Nevertheless, to address possible concerns about overlapping peak actions of the components of insulin therapy, an alternative plan is outlined under which the daily dose may be converted temporarily to split-dose NPH insulin rather than split-mixed NPH/regular insulin (*see* Fig. 5). This alternative plan of converting to split-dose NPH is especially appropriate for patients undergoing upward insulin dose titration whose daily dose exceeds 80 U or who have shown a propensity to hypoglycemia dependent on timing of peak insulin action.

Premeal supplementation with regular insulin should be discontinued once premeal glucose readings are under 240 mg/dL, and at that point upward adjustments of the daily dose of insulin should be made only every third day. Those patients who have been receiving the daily dose as NPH should be converted to a split-mixed regimen, distributed two-thirds before breakfast as 70/30 insulin and one-third before supper as 50/50 or 70/30 insulin, in amounts equal to the total previously given as a daily NPH dose. If premeal blood glucose levels have exceeded 140 mg/dL and the patient has been free of hypoglycemia for 3 d, a 10% increase of the daily dose of insulin may be made. The physician also should be alert to the possibility of late "snowballing" of effect of large doses of subcutaneous insulin; hypoglycemia may occur after supplementation of regular insulin has been discontinued, necessitating a reduction of daily dosage.

Individualization of therapy is especially important as the patient begins to approach good control. Some patients taking a mixture of NPH/regular insulin at supper will have poor control at bedtime but hypoglycemia in the early morning. They are the ones who may fare better with a 50/50 than 70/30 mixture of NPH/regular insulin at supper or may do best without any intermediate-acting insulin at night, taking only presupper regular insulin. Some patients will need to convert from premixed to self-mixed insulin in order to achieve pattern adjustment. Those patients using a small dose of prednisone taken only in the morning sometimes may need no evening dose of insulin at all.

Patients with type 1 diabetes or patients who already are proficient at insulin self-management, including type 2 diabetes patients who use multiple daily injections, may benefit from algorithms more complex than the above-described.

Starting daily doses of premixed insulin:

Premixed _70/30_ insulin before breakfast: __8__ units.

Premixed _70/30_ insulin before supper: __4__ units.

Supplements of regular insulin:

If premeal blood sugar is over 240 mg/dL before breakfast, lunch or supper, take

__8__ units of regular insulin.

Adjustment of daily doses of premixed insulin:

If yesterday's supplements of regular insulin added up to:	then please increase today's doses of premixed insulin by:
__8__ units	__4__ units before breakfast and
	__2__ units before supper.
__16__ units	__8__ units before breakfast and
	__4__ units before supper.
__24__ units	__12__ units before breakfast and
	__6__ units before supper.

- Test blood glucose before each meal and before the bedtime snack.
- If the premeal glucose exceeds 300 mg/dL twice in a row, call me.
- If you have a hypoglycemic insulin reaction or premeal glucose under 80 mg/dL, call me and do not make any upward adjustment of the premixed insulin.
- This is a **temporary** plan for rapid insulin adjustment.
- Call me every three days at (GET)FBS-GOOD.

Fig. 5. A typical plan is shown for a newly diabetic person or a person with known type 2 diabetes whose treatment is being converted from oral agents to insulin at the time of initiation of glucocorticoid therapy. For simplicity, the daily dose initially may consist of premixed insulin, administered two-thirds before breakfast and one-third before supper, using 70/30 NPH/regular insulin before breakfast and 50/50 or 70/30 NPH/regular before supper. The premeal supplements initially are about 8 U, and later 8 U or one-fifth of the daily dose, whichever is greater, given as regular insulin for premeal glucose exceeding 240 mg/dL. Each day's daily dose may be increased by two-thirds the number of units given as regular insulin the previous day. As control improves, supplementation with regular insulin will be discontinued; for premeal blood glucose levels consistently between 140 and 240 mg/dL, upward adjustments of the split-mixed NPH/regular insulin doses will be made only every third day, and individualization of the treatment plan will occur.

Rapid Upward Insulin Adjustment

New daily doses of NPH insulin:

NPH insulin before breakfast: _72_ units.

NPH insulin before bedtime snack: _36_ units.

Supplements of regular insulin:

If premeal blood sugar is over 240 mg/dL before breakfast, lunch or supper, take

   _22_ units of regular insulin.

Adjustment of daily doses of NPH insulin:

If yesterday's supplements of regular insulin added up to:	then please increase today's doses of NPH insulin by:
_22_ units	_10_ units before breakfast and
	_5_ units before bedtime snack.
_44_ units	_20_ units before breakfast and
	_10_ units before bedtime snack.
_66_ units	_30_ units before breakfast and
	_15_ units before bedtime snack.

- Test blood glucose before each meal and before the bedtime snack.
- If the premeal glucose exceeds 300 mg/dL twice in a row, call me.
- If you have a hypoglycemic insulin reaction or premeal glucose under 80 mg/dL, call me and do not make any upward adjustment of the NPH insulin.
- This is a **temporary** plan for rapid insulin adjustment.
- Call me every three days at (GET)FBS-GOOD.

Fig. 6. A typical plan is shown for a person with known type 2 diabetes who had satisfactory control on 108 U of daily split-mixed insulin at the time of initiation of long-term glucocorticoid therapy. The example demonstrates the option of temporary conversion of the daily dose to NPH insulin, administered before breakfast and bedtime, with two-thirds of the daily dose before breakfast and one-third before the bedtime snack. Supplementation with premeal regular insulin is calculated as in Fig 5. As control improves, the total daily dose will be converted from NPH insulin to an individualized split-mixed NPH/regular regimen administered before breakfast and supper, and for premeal blood glucose levels consistently between 140 and 240 mg/dL, upward adjustments of insulin dose will be made only every third day.

Treatment of Type 1 Diabetes During Glucocorticoid Therapy

For patients with type 1 diabetes, the caregiver is obligated to provide adequate basal insulin coverage in some form, either as intermediate insulin administered twice daily (NPH or lente), as long-acting insulin (glargine or ultralente), or as continuous subcutaneous insulin infusion of short-acting insulin. For patients with insulin-dependent diabetes, the basal rate of hepatic glucose production and fasting plasma glucose levels are increased among steroid-treated patients, compared to untreated patients *(89)*. The basal doses may need to be increased during glucocorticoid therapy. Because many glucocorticoid-treated patients receive a single morning dose of glucocorticoid and demonstrate greater daytime than nocturnal or predawn insulin resistance *(71)*, NPH may be preferred to a single daily injection of glargine. In order to use glargine effectively during glucocorticoid therapy, the glargine component may constitute less than 50% of the daily insulin dose, and the balance of the daily dose is provided as mealtime short-acting or rapid-acting insulin administered at all three meals.

Oral Antihyperglycemic Agents in Steroid Diabetes

The oral antihyperglycemic drugs marketed in the United States have been meticulously evaluated for efficacy in the treatment of type 2 diabetes by preclinical trials that usually excluded users of glucocorticoids from enrollment. The efficacy of oral agents in steroid diabetes has not been established, and predictors of response are not known. Because of the risk of rapid deterioration of diabetic control among glucocorticoid-treated patients, it is an obstacle to oral therapy, thus, that for most agents, gradual dose titration is recommended.

A majority of patients having steroid-induced abnormalities of carbohydrate metabolism demonstrate dominantly postprandial hyperglycemia *(86)*. Whether treating postprandial hyperglycemia in this setting can prevent further deterioration of glycemic control is unknown. If therapy is selected to target postprandial hyperglycemia, available oral agents include α-glucosidase inhibitors *(63)*, repaglinide, and nateglinide, but their efficacy in steroid diabetes has not been specifically reported. The oral agents most commonly cited in older literature on steroid diabetes are sulfonylureas. Biguanides occasionally have been used to treat steroid diabetes *(22,39)*, but there are no controlled studies on safety or efficacy. Some of the conditions for which glucocorticoid are prescribed constitute a contraindication to the use of metformin because of the increased risk of lactic acidosis. Although use of insulin sensitizers of the thiazolidinedione class for steroid diabetes seems logical, it is not clear that the mechanism of action of thiazolidinediones bypasses those specific defects resulting in insulin resistance that may be induced by glucocorticoids, and efficacy is not predictably strong *(62,67,70,76)*. Thiazolidinedione therapy was superior to sulfonylurea treatment in one reported case, but the corticosteroid dose was low—7.5 mg prednisolone daily *(67)*.

Some authorities argue for a trial of oral agents for mild hyperglycemia (e.g., patients having fasting blood glucose <200 mg/dL) *(60,66,69)*. In practice, it is the experience of this author that if patients persistently have a first-morning fasting blood glucose >140 mg/dL during glucocorticoid and oral antihyperglycemic therapy, generally their diabetic control will remain unsatisfactory or deteriorate over weeks or months, unless tapering of glucocorticoid occurs at the same time *(65)*. The risk of deterioration probably is greatest if intrinsic β-cell dysfunction is present or if drug-induced β-cell dysfunction occurs, as during cyclosporin or tacrolimus therapy.

If tapering of glucocorticoids is expected to occur, patients with first-morning fasting blood glucose ≤140 mg/dL but with other premeal glucose values between 140 and 200 mg/dL may be offered a trial of an insulin secretogogue. In order to provide postprandial coverage and to reduce the risk of nocturnal hypoglycemia sometimes observed during sulfonylurea therapy *(71)*, it is especially useful to choose a short-acting drug such as repaglinide.

Insulin Drip Therapy

If ambulatory therapy fails, for dehydration or impending HHS the patient may require hospitalization. In the dehydrated individual, intravenous regular infusion is the best route to ensure absorption of insulin.

For already hospitalized diabetic patients with poor control or perioperative patients having extreme insulin resistance because of high-dose glucocorticoid therapy, again intravenous insulin infusion may be the preferred therapy. The starting rate of insulin infusion for euglycemic patients with glucocorticoid-induced insulin resistance may be 2 U/h. An initial priming bolus of intravenous regular insulin is needed. An algorithm, evaluated in postoperative heart patients, includes a provision for those treated with glucocorticoids and works well among other patients who require insulin drip therapy *(11)*.

Subcutaneous short-acting and intermediate-acting insulin should be given 2 h before drip discontinuation. The rate of insulin infusion can be used to predict insulin requirement at the time of drip discontinuation *(4)*. If all else is stable and if the insulin infusion rate has been consistent, the new daily subcutaneous insulin dose may be prescribed as split-mixed insulin at approx 80% of the dose given as intravenous insulin used during the preceding 24 h.

Tapering of Glucocorticoid and Antihyperglycemic Therapy

The target range premeal glucose is 120–200 mg/dL for patients whose glucocorticoid dose has been reduced within the past 10 d.

During glucocorticoid-tapering regimens, because severe hypoglycemia is judged a greater risk than moderate short-term hyperglycemia, there should be anticipatory reductions of the daily insulin dose. A special risk of hypoglycemia occurs when here is a changeover of caregivers during glucocorticoid tapering, as may happen at the time of hospital discharge. The outpatient physicians should be involved in discharge planning. However, the best safety net is patient knowledgeability on target blood glucose levels and self-adjustment of insulin.

It is expected that in most cases of new-onset steroid diabetes, resolution of the diabetic state will occur after discontinuation of glucocorticoid therapy *(12,57,90)*. If insulin has been newly started because of the glucocorticoids, there is a good chance of insulin discontinuation by the time the glucocorticoid dosage reaches physiologic levels. If oral agents had been required for diabetic control prior to glucocorticoid therapy, they often might be resumed after discontinuation. Patients who required insulin prior to glucocorticoid therapy are likely to continue to require insulin. In order to anticipate the reduction of their daily insulin dose during glucocorticoid tapering, it is useful to review the augmentation of daily dose that occurred during glucocorticoid initiation.

Whenever a decrement in glucocorticoid dose is planned or has just occurred, if the blood glucose has been <140 mg/dL before meals or <160 mg/dL at bedtime during the preceding 3 d, part of the anticipated reduction of the insulin dose should be made, often by about 15–20% of the daily dose. When the daily insulin dose is less than 12–20 U, conversion to oral agents or replacement of insulin therapy with dietary therapy may be considered.

Alternate-Day Glucocorticoid Treatment Plans

Alternate-day glucocorticoid therapy can result in marked differences of glycemic control between the "on" day and the "off" day *(50,71)*. Some patients report greater daily variability than others. Because some patients require alternate-day insulin plans, individualization is necessary.

CONCLUSION

Beneficial glucocorticoid therapy should not be denied to patients having preexisting diabetes or developing steroid diabetes. At the initiation of glucocorticoid therapy, after classifying patients as diabetic or nondiabetic, the provider should individualize management according to the anticipated glucocorticoid treatment plan. The question is raised of whether undertreatment of transplant diabetes, or avoidance of insulin therapy specifically, is partly responsible for the observed increase of infectious complications among diabetic transplant recipients. A metabolic emergency can occur early in relation to ambulatory initiation of glucocorticoid therapy. Therefore, appropriate patient education must be in place from the very beginning and must be followed by effective treatment once hyperglycemic supervenes.

REFERENCES

1. Lim KC, Walsh CH. Diabetic ketoalkalosis: a readily misdiagnosed entity. Br Med J 1976;2:19.
2. Sanders G, Boyle G, Hunter S, Poffenbarger PL. Mixed acid-base abnormalities in diabetes. Diabetes Care 1978;1:362–364.
3. Zinman B. The physiologic replacement of insulin: an elusive goal. N Engl J Med 1989;321(6):363–370.
4. Hawkins JB, Jr, Morales CM, Shipp JC. Insulin requirement in 242 patients with type II diabetes mellitus. Endocrine Prac 1995;1(6):385–389.
5. Hirsch IB, Paauw DS. Inpatient management of adults with diabetes. Diabetes Care 1995;18(6):870–878.
6. Pomposelli JJ, Baxter JK, Babineau TJ, et al. Early postoperative glucose control predicts nosocomial infection rate in diabetic patients. J Parent Enteral Nutr 1998;22(2):77–81.
7. Anonymous ADA. Report of the expert committee on the diagnosis and classification of diabetes mellitus. Diabetes Care 2001;24:S5–S20.
8. Anonymous ADA. Standards of medical care for patients with diabetes mellitus. Diabetes Care 2001;24:S33–S43.
9. Kitabchi AE, Umpierrez GE, Murphy MB, et al. Management of hyperglycemic crises in patients with diabetes. Diabetes Care 2001;24(1):131–153.
10. Van den Berghe G, Wouters P, Weekers F, Other ea. Intensive insulin therapy in critically ill patients. New Engl J Med 2001;19:1359–1367.
11. Markovitz L, Wiechmann R, Harris N, et al. Description and evaluation of a glycemic management protocol for diabetic patients undergoing heart surgery. Endocrine Prac 2002;8(1):10–18.
12. Bookman JJ, Drachman SR, Schaefer LE, Adlersberg D. Steroid diabetes in man. Diabetes 1953;2(2):100–111.
13. Berg E-G. Nil nocere!: Über Schäden und Nebenwirkungen bei der therapeutischen Verwendung von Cortison und ähnlichen Steroidhormonen. Münchener Medizinische Wochenschrift 1956;98:1614–1622.
14. Ranney HM, Gellhorn A. The effect of massive prednisone and prednisolone therapy on acute leukemia and malignant lymphomas. Am J Med 1957;22:405–413.
15. Simpson JR. Steroid diabetes—case report. Harper Hospital Bull 1957;15:43–51.
16. Grilliat J-P, Koenig E, Vaillant G. Diabéte survenant au cours de cirrhoses traitées par delat-cortisone. Revue Médicale de Nancy 1959;84:720–727.
17. Baldwin HS, Dworetzky M, Isaacs NJ. Evaluation of the steroid treatment of asthma since 1950. J Allergy 1961;32:109–118.
18. Gregory RL, Sayle BA. Steroid diabetes. TX St J Med 1962;58:788–793.
19. Blereau RP, Weingartern CM. Diabetic acidosis secondary to steroid therapy. N Engl J Med 1964;271:836.
20. Mach RS, de Sousa RC. Coma avec hyperosmolalité et déshydratation chez des malades hyperglycémiques sans acidocétose. Schweizerishce Medizinische Wochenschrift 1963;36:1256–1263.
21. Keeney EL. The condition of asthmatic patients after daily long-term corticosteroid treatment. AZ Med 1964;21:463–469.

22. Miller SEP, Neilson Jm. Clinical features of the diabetic syndrome appearing after steroid therapy. Postgrad Medical J 1964;40:660–669.

23. Brocard H, Akoun G, Grand A. Diabète stéroïde compliqué d'un coma de type hyperosmolaire. Bulletins et Mémoires de la Société Médicale des Hôpitaux de Paris 1965;116:353–363.

24. Schwartz TB, Apfelbaum RI. Nonketotic diabetic coma. In: Schwartz TB, ed. Year Book of Endocrinology (1965–1966 Year Book Series). Year Book Publishers, Chicago, IL, 1965–1966, pp. 165–181.

25. Coles RS. Steroid therapy in uveitis. International Ophthalmology Clinics 1966;6(4):869–901.

26. Walsh SD, Grant IWB. Corticosteroids in treatment of chronic asthma. Br Med J 1966;2:796–802.

27. Boyer MH. Hyperosmolar anacidotic coma in association with glucocorticoid therapy. JAMA 1967;202:95–1009.

28. Plauchu M, Paliard P, Malluret J, Noel P, de Montgolfier R. Un nouveau cas d'état d'hyperosmolarité plasmatique ou de coma hyperosmolaire déclenché par les corticoïdes chez un diabétique latent, porteur d'une lymphose. Lyons Med 1967;217(26):1921–1932.

29. Zangel V, Masszi J. Ketozisba átmenő steroid-diabetes három esete. Orvosi Hetilap 1967;108:395,396.

30. Kumar RS. Hyperosmolar non-ketotic coma. Lancet 1968;1:48,49.

31. Pyörälä K, Suhonen O, Pentikäinen P. Steroid therapy and hyperosmolar non-ketotic coma. Lancet 1968;1:596–597.

32. Smyllie HC, Connolly CK. Incidence of serious complications of corticosteroid therapy in respiratory disease. Thorax 1968;23:571–581.

33. Williams ER. Systemic lupus erythematosus and diabetes mellitus. Br J Clin Prac 1968;22:461–463.

34. Spenney JG, Eure CA, Kreisberg RA. Hyperglycemic, hyperosmolar, nonketoacidotic diabetes: a complication of steroid and immunosuppressive therapy. Diabetes 1969;18:107–110.

35. Alavi IA, Sharma BK, Pillay VKG. Steroid-induced diabetic ketoacidosis. Am J Med Sci 1971;262(1):1971.

36. Limas CJ, Samad A, Seff D. Hyperglycemic nonketotic coma as complication of steroid therapy. NY St J Med 1971;71:1542,1543.

37. Corcoran FH, Granatir RF, Schlang HA. Hyperglycemic hyperosmolar nonketotic coma associated with corticosteroid therapy. J FL Med Assoc 1971;58:38–39.

38. Lieberman P, Patterson R, Kunske R. Complications of long-term steroid therapy for asthma. J Allergy Clin Immunol 1972;49:329–336.

39. Klein W. Behandlung mit Glukokortikoiden bei Diabetikern. Zeitschrigft für Allgemeinmedizin 1974;25:1101–1105.

40. Koehler BE, Urowitz MB, Killinger DW. The systemic effects of intra-articular corticosteroid. J Rheumatol 1974;1:117–125.

41. David DS, Cheigh JS, Braun DW, Fotino M, Stenzel KH, Rubin AL. HLA-A28 and steroid-induced diabetes in renal transplant patients. JAMA 1980;243(6):532,533.

42. Gottlieb NL, Riskin WG. Complications of local corticosteroid injections. JAMA 1980;243:1547,1548.

43. Armstrong RD, English J, Gibson T, Chakroborty J, Marks V. Serum methylprednisolone levels following intra-articular injection of methylprednisolone acetate. Ann Rheum Dis 1981;40:571–574.

44. Pagano G, Cavallo-Perin P, Cassader M, Bruno A, Ozzello A, Masciola P. An in vivo and in vitro study of the mechanism of prednisone-induced insulin resistance in healthy subjects. J Clin Invest 1983;72:1814–1820.

45. Fujikawa LS, Meisler DM, Nozik RA. Hyperosmolar hyperglycemic nonketotic coma. Ophthalmology 1983;90:1239–1242.

46. Ivanova II, Vasiutkova LA, Ivanov VA. Hyperglycemic coma after corticosteroid therapy. Sovetskaia Meditsina 1984;10:112,113.

47. Lohr KM. Precipitation of hyperosmolar nonketotic diabetes on alternate-day corticosteroid therapy. JAMA 1984;252(5):628.

48. Ferguson RP. A comparison of steroid and thiazide diabetes. CT Med 1986;50:506–509.

49. Bruno A, Cavallo-Perin P, Cassader M, Pagano G. Deflazacort vs prednisone: effect on blood glucose control in insulin-treated diabetes. Arch intern Med 1987;147:679,680.

50. Greenstone MA, Shaw AB. Alternate day corticosteroid causes alternate day hyperglycemia. Postgrad Med J 1987;63(743):761–764.

51. Wachtel TJ, Silliman RA, Lamberton P. Predisposing factors for the diabetic hyperosmolar state. Arch Intern Med 1987;147:499–501.

52. Thomas JW, Vertkin A, Nell LJ. Antiinsulin antibodies and clinical characteristics of patients with systemic lupus erythematosus and other connective tissue diseases with steroid induced diabetes. J Rheumatol 1987;14(4):732–735.

53. Black DM, Filak AT. Hyperglycemia with non-insulin dependent diabetes following intraarticular steroid injection. J Fam Prac 1989;28(4):462,463.

54. Pagano G, Bruno A, Cavallo-Perin P, Cesco L. Glucose intolerance after short-term administration of corticosteroids in healthy subjects. Arch Intern Med 1989;149:1093–1101.

55. Shi M-z, Zhang S-f. Steroid diabetes: an analysis of 28 cases. Chin J Int Med 1989;28(3):139–141;185.

56. Gurwitz JH, Bohn RL, Glynn RJ, Monane M, Mogun H, Avorn J. Glucocorticoids and the risk for initiation of hypoglycemic therapy. Arch Intern Med 1994;154:97–101.

57. Siminerio LM, Carroll PB. Educating secondary diabetes patients. Diabetes Spectrum 1994;7(1):8–14.

58. Haggerty RD, Bergsman K, Edelson GW. Steroid-induced diabetic ketoacidosis. Prac Diabetol 1995;14(2):24–25.

59. Braithwaite SS, Barr WG, Thomas JD. Diabetes management during glucocorticoid therapy of nonendocrine disease. Endocrine Prac 1996;2:320–325.

60. Hirsch IB, Paauw DS. Diabetes management in special situations. Endocrinol Metab Clin N Am 1997;26(3):631–645.

61. Braithwaite SS, Barr WG, Rahman A, Quddusi S. Managing diabetes during glucocorticoid therapy. Postgrad Med 1998;104(5):163–166,171,175,176.

62. Okumura S, Takeda N, Takami K, et al. Effects of troglitazone on dexamethasone-induced insulin resistance in rats. Metabolism 1998;47(3):351–354.

63. Tanaka M, Endo K, Suzuki T, Maruyama Y, Kondo A. Treatment for steroid-induced diabetes with alpha-glucosidase inhibitor, voglibose. Eur J Neurol 1998;5(3):315.

64. Braithwaite SS, Barr WG, Rahman A, Quddusi S. An algorithm for diabetes management during glucocorticoid therapy of nonendocrine disease. In: Meikle AW, ed. Hormone Replacement Therapy. 1st ed. Humana Press, Totowa, NJ, 1999, pp. 191–207.

65. Carolan J. Insulin versus oral agents for 'steroid-induced' diabetes [letter; comment]. Postgrad Med 1999;105(5):36.

66. Hoogwerf B, Danese RD. Drug selection and the management of corticosteroid-related diabetes mellitus. Rheum Dis Clin N Am 1999;25(3):489–505.

67. Fujibayashi K, Nagasaka S, Itabashi N, et al. Troglitazone efficacy in a subject with glucocorticoid-induced diabetes. Diabetes Care 1999;22(12):2088,2089.

68. Niewoehner DE, Erbland ML, Deupree RH, et al. Effect of systemic glucocorticoids on exacerbations of chronic obstructive pulmonary disease. N Engl J Med 1999;340:1941–1947.

69. Pauw DS. Case study: a 60-year-old woman with type 2 diabetes and COPD: worsening hyperglycemia due to prednisone. Clin Diabetes 2000;18(2):89,90.

70. Morita H, Oki Y, Ito T, Ohishi H, Suzuki S, Nakamura H. Administration of troglitazone, but not pioglitazone, reduces insulin resistance caused by short-term dexamethasone (DXM) treatment by accelerating the metabolism of DXM. Diabetes Care 2001;24(4):788,789.

71. Volgi J, Baldwin DJ. Glucocorticoid therapy and diabetes management. Nurs Clin N Am 2001;36(2):333–339.

72. Long CNH, Katzin B, Fry EG. The adrenal cortex and carbohydrate metabolism. Endocrinology 1940;26:309–344.

73. Ingle DJ, Sheppard R, Evans JS, Kuizenga MH. A comparison of adrenal steroid diabetes and pancreatic diabetes in the rat. Endocrinology 1945;37:341–356.

74. Owen OE, Cahill GF. Metabolic effects of exogenous glucocorticoids in fasted man. J Clin Invest 1973;52:2596–2605.

75. Rizza RA, Mandarino LJ, Gerich JE. Cortisol-induced insulin resistance in man: impaired suppression of glucose production and stimulation of glucose utilization due to a postreceptor defect of insulin action. J Clin Endocrinol Metab 1982;54:131–138.

76. Weinstein ST, Holand A, O'Boyle E, Haber RS. Effects of thiazolidinediones on glucocorticoid-induced insulin resistance and GLUT4 glucose transporter expression in rat skeletal muscle. Metabolism 1993;42(10):1365–1369.

77. Tappy L, Randin D, Vollenweider P, et al. Mechanisms of dexamethasone-induced insulin resistance in healthy humans. J Clin Endocrinol Metab.1994;79(4):1063–1069.

78. Matsumoto K, Yamasaki H, Akazawa S, et al. High-dose but not low-dose dexamethasone impairs glucose tolerance by inducing compensatory failure of pancreatic beta-cells in normal men. J Clin Endocrinol Metab 1996;81(7):2621–2626.

79. Henriksen JE, Alford F, Ward GM, Beck-Nielsen H. Risk and mechanism of dexamethasone-induced deterioration of glucose tolerance in non-diabetic first-degree relatives of NIDDM patients. Diabetologia 1997;40:1439–1448.

80. Daouk AA, Malek GH, Kauffman HM, Kisken WA. Hyperosmolar non-ketotic coma in a kidney transplant recipient. J Urol 1972;108:524,525.
81. Ruiz JO, Simmons RL, Callender CO, Kjellstrand CM, Buselmeier TJ, Najarian JS. Steroid diabetes in renal transplant recipients: pathogenetic factors and prognosis. Surgery 1973;73(5):759–765.
82. Hill CM, Douglas JF, Rajkumar KV, McEvoy J, McGeown MG. Glycosuria and hyperglycaemia after kidney transplantation. Lancet 1974;2:490–542.
83. Woods JE, Zincke H, Palumbo PJ, et al. Hyperosmolar nonketotic syndrome and steroid diabetes. JAMA 1975;231:1261–1263.
84. Gunnarsson R, Arner P, Lundgren G, Magnusson G, Östman J, Groth CG. Steroid diabetes after renal transplantation—a preliminary report. Scand J Urol Nephrol 1977;42:191–194.
85. Gunnarsson R, Lundgren G, Magnusson G, Ost L, Groth CG. Steroid diabetes—a sign of overtreatment with steroids in the renal graft recipient? Scand J Urol Nephrol 1980;54:135–138.
86. Pagano G, Lombardi A, Ferraris GM, Imbimbo B, Perin PC. Acute effect of prednisone and deflazacort on glucose tolerance in prediabetic subjects. Eur J Clin Pharmacol 1982;22:469–471.
87. Arner P, Gunnarsson R, Blomdahl S, Carl-Gustav G. Some characteristics of steroid diabetes: a study in renal-transplant recipients receiving high-dose corticosteroid therapy. Diabetes Care 1983;6(1):23–25.
88. Roth D, Milgrom M, Esquenazi V, Fuller L, Burke G, Miller J. Posttransplant hyperglycemia. Increased incidence in cyclosporine-treated renal allograft recipients. Transplantation 1989;47(2):278–281.
89. Ekstrand AV. Effect of steroid-therapy on insulin sensitivity in insulin-dependent diabetic patients after kidney transplantation. J Diabetic Complic 1991;5(4):244–248.
90. Hricik DE, Bartucci MR, Moir EJ, Mayes JT, Schulak JA. Effects of steroid withdrawal on posttransplant diabetes mellitus in cyclosporine-treated renal transplant recipients. Transplantation 1991;51(2):374–377.
91. Sumrani NB, Delaney V, Ding ZK, et al. Diabetes mellitus after renal transplantation in the cyclosporin era—an analysis of risk factors. Transplantation 1991;51(2):343–347.
92. Sumrani NB, Delaney V, Daskalakis P, et al. Retrospective analysis of posttransplantation diabetes mellitus in black renal allograft recipients. Diabetes Care 1991;14(8):760–762.
93. Vesco L, Busson M, Lang P. Characteristics of postrenal transplant diabetes mellitus. Transplant Proc 1995;27(4):2465,2466.
94. Ekstrand A, Schalin-Jäntti C, Löfman M, et al. The effect of (steroid) immunosuppression on skeletal muscle glycogen metabolism in patients after kidney transplantation. Transplantation 1996;61(6):889–893.
95. Vesco L, Busson M, Bedrossian J, Bitker M, Hiesse C, Lang P. Diabetes mellitus after renal transplantation: characteristics, outcome, and risk factors. Transplantation 1996;61(10):1475–1478.
96. Hjelmesaeth J, Hartmann A, Kofstad J, et al. Glucose intolerance after renal transplantation depends upon prednisolone dose and recipient age. Transplantation 1997;64(7):979–983.
97. Kirkman MS, Wittle B, Benzing M, Johnson P. Hyperosmolar non-ketotic state as first manifestation of diabetes mellitus. Diabetes Spec 1997;10(3):175,176.
98. Veenstra DL. Incidence and long-term cost of steroid-related side effects after renal transplantation. Am J Kidney Dis 1999;33(5):829–839.
99. Weir MR, Fink JC. Risk for posttransplant diabetes mellitus with current immunosuppressive medications. Am J Kidney Dis 1999;34(1):1–13.
100. Depczynski B, Daly B, Campbell LV, Chisholm DJ, Keogh A. Predicting the occurrence of diabetes mellitus in recipients of heart transplants. 2000;17(1):15–19.
101. Jindahl RM. Impact and management of posttransplant diabetes mellitus. Transplantation 2000;70:ss58–63.
102. Tenderich G, Schulte-Eistrup S, Petzoldt R, Koerfer R. Cardiac transplantation in patients with insulin-treated diabetes mellitus. 2000.
103. Blanco JJ, Herrero JI, Quiroga J, et al. Liver transplantation in cirrhotic patients with diabetes mellitus: midterm results, survival, and adverse events. Liver Transplantation 2001;7(3):234–237.
104. Duijnhoven EM, Boots JM, Christiaans MH, Wolffenbuttel BH, Van Hooff JP. Influence of tacrolimus on glucose metabolism before and after renal transplantation: a prospective study. J Am Soc Nephrol 2001;12(3):583–588.
105. Hjelmesaeth J, Hartmann A, Midtvedt K, et al. Metabolic cardiovascular syndrome after renal transplantation. Nephrol, Dial Transplant 2001;16(5):1047–1052.
106. Hjelmesaeth J, Hartmann A, Kofstad J, Egeland T, Stenstrøm J, Fauchald P. Tapering off prednisolone and cyclosporin the first year after renal transplantation: the effect on glucose tolerance. Nephrol, Dial Transplant 2001;16(4):829–835.

107. Nam JH, Mun JI, Kim SI, et al. Beta-cell dysfunction rather than insulin resistance is the main contributing factor for the development of postrenal transplantation diabetes mellitus. Transplantation 2001;71(10):1417–1423.
108. Nieuwenhuis MG, Kirkels JH. Predictability and other aspects of post-transplant diabetes mellitus in heart transplant recipients. J Heart Lung Transplant 2001;20(7):703–708.
109. Paolillo JA, Boyle GJ, Law YM, et al. Posttransplant diabetes mellitus in pediatric thoracic organ recipients receiving tacrolimus-based immunosuppression. Transplantation 2001;71(2):252–256.
110. Steinmuller T, Stockmann M, Jonas S, et al. The impact of liver transplantation on diabetes mellitus. Transplant Proc 2001;33(1–2):1393.
111. Sutherland DER, Gruessner RWG, Dunn DL, et al. Lessons learned from more than 1000 pancreas transplants at a single institution. Ann Surg 2001;233(4):463–501.
112. Szewczyk Z, Ratajczyk T, Rabczynski J. Hyperosmotic coma in steroid-induced diabetes complicating subacute glomerulonephritis in a 16-year-old boy. Polski Tygodnik Lekarski 1971;26:1988–1990.
113. Perlman K, Ehrlich RM. Steroid diabetes in childhood. Am J Dis Child 1982;136:64–68.
114. Robert JJ, Tete MJ, Crosnier H, Broyer M. Diabète sucré aprés transplantation rénale chez l'enfant. Ann Pédiatr (Paris) 1993;40(2):112–118.
115. Covar RA, Leung DYM, Mc Cormick D, Steelman J, Zeitler P, Spahn JD. Risk factors associated with glucocorticoid-induced adverse effects in children with severe asthma. J Allergy Clin Immunol 2000;106(4):651–659.
116. Bouhanick B, Biquard F, Hadjadj S, Roques MA. Does treatment with antenatal glucocorticoids for the risk of premature delivery contribute to ketoacidosis in pregnant women with diabetes who receive continuous subcutaneous insulin infusion (CSII)? Arch Intern Med 2000;160:242,243.
117. Wiczynska-Zajac A, Bomba-Opon DA, Domanska-Janczewska E, Jozwicka E, Marianowski L. The influence of prenatal glucocorticoids on glycemic control among pregnant women with type I diabetes. Ginekologia Polska 2000;71(8):900–905.
118. Pearson DW, Thomson JA, Kennedy AC, Toner PG, Ratcliffe JG. Diabetic ketoalkalosis due to ectopic ACTH production from an oat cell carcinoma. Postgrad Med J 1981;57:455,456.
119. Kendall-Taylor P. Hyperosmolar coma in Cushing's disease. Lancet 1974;1:409.
120. Kreze A, Mikulecky M, Moravick M. Factors influencing the development of glucose intolerance in Cushing syndrome. Acta Medica Austriaca 1995;22(5):110–112.
121. Leibowitz G, Tsur A, Chayen SD, et al. Pre-clinical Cushing's syndrome: an unexpected frequent cause or poor glycemic control in obsese diabetic patients. Clin Endocrinol 1996;44:717–722.
122. Mann M, Koller E, Murgo A, Malozowski S, Bacsanyi J, Leinung M. Glucocorticoidlike activity of megestrol. Arch Intern Med 1997;157:1651–1656.
123. Arai J, Miyakawa Y, Kataoka K, Matsuki S, Asano S. Case of fatal hypoglycemic coma during sulfonylurea administration for the therapy of steroid diabetes following adrenalectomy. Saishin Igaku Recent Med 1969;1969(24):2524–2529.
124. McConnell EM, Bell PM, Hadden DR, McCance DR, Sheridan B, Atkinson AB. Prevalence of diabetes and impaired glucose tolerance in adult hypopituitarism on low dose oral hydrocortisone replacement therapy. Clin Endocrinol 2001;54(5):593–599.

15

Exercise and Managing Diabetes

Robert E. Jones, MD

INTRODUCTION

Diabetes mellitus is characterized by hyperglycemia resulting from either an absolute or relative insulin deficiency and affects more than 16 million people in the United States. Diabetes is classified into several types *(1)*, but the most frequently encountered categories are types 1 and 2 diabetes. Type 1 diabetes is secondary to pancreatic β-cell destruction, which results in an absolute insulin deficiency. On the other hand, type 2 diabetes is characterized initially by insulin resistance followed by a progressive decline in insulin secretion *(2)*.

In addition to the use of hypoglycemic agents, the management of diabetes includes both dietary planning and suggestions for regular physical exercise. Although exercise has been shown to be beneficial in the treatment of diabetes through its effects on improving insulin sensitivity *(3)* and assisting with weight control, there are significant potential dangers associated with exercise in diabetics. For example, vigorous exercise in patients treated with insulin or sulfonylureas may be associated with hypoglycemia during or following the event, and, occasionally, the micro- or macrovasular complications associated with diabetes might be aggravated by participation in an exercise program. A variety of techniques may be implemented to reduce the risk of hypoglycemia in physically active people with diabetes and careful attention to the presence of existing complications should identify those individuals who are at risk for potential exacerbation due to exercise.

From: *Endocrine Replacement Therapy in Clinical Practice*
Edited by: A. Wayne Meikle © Humana Press Inc., Totowa, NJ

METABOLIC RESPONSES TO EXERCISE

The biochemical and hormonal responses to exercise are dependent on a variety of factors. For example, the degree of prior conditioning, the intensity of exercise, and the duration of the activity all play major roles in the adaptive responses and type of substrate fluxes noted during exercise.

Energy demands during exercise are met through the oxidation of fatty acids and glucose, and the synthesis and storage of these depot fuels, glycogen and triglycerides, are dependent on insulin. In addition, the glucose counterregulatory hormones, cortisol, growth hormone, catecholamines, and glucagon, either actively or permissively facilitate substrate mobilization by enhancing gluconeogenesis, lipolysis, or glycogenolysis. The concerted interplay between insulin and these counterregulatory hormones allows for constancy of blood glucose levels and provides additional substrates for oxidation. During exercise in people without diabetes, insulin levels appropriately decline, which results in the mobilization of free fatty acids and the facilitation of gluconeogenesis from muscle-derived lactic acid and glycerol from adipocytes. Additionally, the decrease in insulin concentration is also associated with the cessation of glycogen synthesis in both muscle and liver while permissively allowing glycogenolysis. Following exercise, both hepatic and muscle glycogen stores are rapidly repleted (4). The biochemical effects of exercise on glucose metabolism have been recently reviewed (5).

Exercise in Type 1 Diabetes

In contrast to normal individuals, insulin levels in people with type 1 diabetes are basically unregulated because of their reliance on injected insulin. If the type 1 patient is underinsulinized, substrate production and mobilization are unrestrained because of the lack of opposition of the counterregulatory hormones. This may result in an exaggeration of preexisting hyperglycemia and may predispose to the development of ketoacidosis. If the patient is overinsulinized at the time of exercise, hypoglycemia will result because of augmentation of tissue glucose uptake and suppression of hepatic gluconeogenesis. This insulin-induced stimulation of glucose uptake in muscle clearly augments non-insulin-mediated glucose disposal that is already activated in exercising muscle (5,6). Additionally, elevated insulin levels also suppress lipolysis which results in an impaired delivery of free fatty acids to myocytes and indirectly increases the oxidation of glucose because of the glucose-sparing actions of intracellular lipids.

Exercise in Type 2 Diabetes

The effects of exercise in people with type 2 diabetes are nearly identical, but because basal insulin secretion is generally maintained in these patients, the risk of developing ketoacidosis is nonexistent. However, if the patient is poorly controlled prior to exercise, a worsening of hyperglycemia may be observed. Similar to the risk seen in people with type 1 diabetes, type 2 patients treated with either insulin or sulfonylureas may experience hypoglycemia during exercise. On the other hand, hypoglycemia is extremely rare in people taking metformin (7) and has not been described with the use of either α-glucosidase inhibitors or thiazolidinediones.

AVOIDANCE OF HYPOGLYCEMIA

Fatigue may be the only manifestation of a mild hypoglycemic reaction. As the degree of hypoglycemia increases, the sympathetic nervous system is activated, and if corrective measures are not taken, neuroglycopenia may occur. The hypoglycemic effects of exercise may persist for many hours after completion of the event as a result of delays in replenishment of hepatic or muscle glycogen and of the effect of exercise on enhancing insulin sensitivity. Postexercise late-onset hypoglycemia has been observed in young people with type 1 diabetes and may occur up to 24 h following strenuous exercise (8).

Nutritional Supplements

Either adding nutritionally supplements prior to exercise or reducing the insulin dosage is the mainstay of therapeutic approaches to prevent exercise-induced hypoglycemia (9). Depending on specific circumstances, they can be used together or individually, but there can be no substitution for meticulous monitoring of capillary blood glucose before, during, and after exercise in order to assess the regimen or to prevent hypoglycemia. Ideally, exercise should be planned when blood glucose levels are highest, which is generally 1–3 h following a meal. Prior to exercise, blood glucose levels should be between 100 and 200 mg/dL (5.5–11.1 mM). If the patient is severely hyperglycemic (glucose in excess of 300 mg/dL or 16.7 mM), activity should be delayed in order to prevent an exacerbation of diabetic control. Relative pre-exercise hypoglycemia (glucose less than 80 mg/dL or 4.4 mM) should be treated by supplemental carbohydrate. Consumption of 15–20 g of readily absorbable carbohydrate is generally sufficient to prevent hypoglycemia during exercise (see Table 1).

Supplemental calories should be consumed immediately before and every 30–60 min during exercise. Simple carbohydrates, up to 40 g for adults and 25 g for children may be used; however, this approach may occasionally be associated with an excessive glycemic excursion and may exacerbate fluid losses that normally occur during exercise. Dietary supplements containing a balanced mixture of complex carbohydrates, protein, and fat such as whole milk (10) may provide a more prolonged, even absorption of glucose, thereby providing longer protection against hypoglycemia without tending to dramatically elevate blood glucose levels. Dietary supplementation is usually all that is required to prevent hypoglycemia during less strenuous exercise of modest duration (less than 45 min).

Alterations in Medical Regimen

Alterations in insulin dosage are often necessary prior to more intense or extended periods of exercise. Lowering the amount of insulin projected to peak during the event by 25–75% is generally adequate to prevent exercise-induced hypoglycemia (11). Elite athletes may reduce their total insulin dosage up to 40% prior to engaging in exhaustive competitions (12). All adjustments in insulin dosage are dependent on the types of insulin employed, the schedule of injections, and the time of day the exercise period is planned. For example, an exercise session that is planned prior to noon may necessitate a reduction in the dose of rapid-acting administered in the morning. If a mid-afternoon event is scheduled, lowering the amount of intermediate-acting insulin may be needed. The unusual patient who is managed with a single daily injection of intermediate-acting insulin may display a deterioration in control of fasting glucose levels if their dosage of insulin is decreased in order to accommodate an exercise session. In order to avoid this problem, the patient should be placed on twice-daily injections of insulin, and specific adjustments in dosage can be made on the timing of the exercise period. Patients managed using intensive conventional insulin therapy based on a regimen of ultralente and

Table 1
Carbohydrate Sources (Equal to 15 g)

- 1/2 cup of regular soda
- 1/2 cup of orange, apple, grapefruit juice
- 2 tbs of sucrose dissolved in water
- 1 tube (15 g) of Glutose 15®
- 2 tbs of raisins
- 3 glucose tablets (5 g)
- 7–8 oz of milk
- 8–10 hard candies
- 1 cup Gatorade®

preprandial injections of a rapid-acting insulin such as regular, insulin lispro, or insulin aspart frequently do not require an alteration in their dose of ultralente but should not use their rapid-acting insulin prior to the event. Insulin glargine, a bioengineered basal insulin, deserves special comment. Because of its lower isoelectric point, glargine forms a microprecipitate at the site of injection (13) and is slowly absorbed over a 24-h period with a relatively peakless activity profile (14). If glargine is injected intravenously, it is comparable to native human insulin (15). Therefore, it is reasonable to conclude that the risk of prolonged hypoglycemia during exercise is no greater with glargine than with any other type of insulin, and until greater experience is gained, dosage adjustments for exercise should be individualized. A similar strategy can be taken for patients using an insulin pump. Generally, the basal rate does not need to be lowered for short-duration exercise; however, many elite athletes will temporarily lower their basal rate up to 50% for sustained, intensive exercise. However, whereas lowering their basal may eliminate the risk of hypoglycemia, they may develop paradoxical hyperglycemia during their workout. As with multiple daily insulin injection regimens, insulin boluses should be avoided prior to exercise. If the patient on an insulin pump is participating in either a water or contact sport, the pump should be disconnected and the tubing capped prior to the event. Once the insulin pump has been discontinued and insulin delivery has ceased, the patient is at an increased risk for developing ketosis because of the decline in insulin and the concurrent increase in counterregulatory hormones induced by exercise. Therefore, the patient should be monitored closely, and the time off the pump should be kept to a minimum. Lispro and aspart have become the standard type of insulin employed in subcutaneous insulin infusion devices; and, because of their extremely short half-lives, patients using these insulins in their pumps should be advised to limit their time off the pump to less than 3 h (16,17). If the patient is using regular insulin in their pump, the time off the pump is longer and may be prolonged up to 4 h.

Other factors influencing the kinetics of insulin absorption must be considered when advising patients about avoiding exercise-related hypoglycemia. Local factors such as increased blood flow can enhance the absorption of insulin from the injection site (18), and patients should be advised to refrain from administering insulin into an extremity that will be exercised. Instead, a consistent injection site (such as their abdomen) should be suggested. Increased insulin sensitivity is one of the benefits derived from exercise, and physically active patients may develop lower insulin requirements as a consequence. Indeed, it is common to see reductions in insulin requirements ranging between 20 and 50% as patients improve their conditioning levels.

Table 2
Symptoms and Management of Hypoglycemia

Degree of hypoglycemia	Symptoms	Treatment	Return to activity
Mild	Fatigue, weakness, nausea, anxiety, tremor, palpitations	10–15 g of readily absorbable carbohydrate	15 min following improvement in symptoms
Moderate	Tachycardia, diaphoresis, headache, mood and personality changes	10–20 g of readily absorbable carbohydrate	15 min following complete resolution of symptoms
	Stupor, somulence, apathy	Observe patient closely following initial therapy; retreat for recurrent symptoms	Consider termination of activity
Severe	Loss of consciousness or seizures	Administer glucagon 1 mg im or sc or give 50% dextrose iv	Medical re-evaluation before exercising

Source: Modified from ref. 20.

The phenomenon of postexercise late-onset hypoglycemia can result in severe episodes of nocturnal neuroglycopenia and can be avoided by counseling the patient to increase their evening caloric intake and closely monitor capillary blood glucose levels. If the patient is just beginning an exercise program or is unaccustomed to an increased degree of physical activity, it may be prudent to prophylactically reduce the amount of insulin taken in the evening following exercise (8).

There are a paucity of data concerning the use of oral hypoglycemics in patients participating in athletics. Sulfonylureas have been associated with prolonged or recurrent events of hypoglycemia, and it may be prudent to avoid the use of these agents in the management of patients who are participating in an intensive conditioning program or engaging in competitive sports. In contrast to the sulfonylureas, the meglitinides, nateglinide and repaglinide have a shorter duration of action and do not enhance insulin secretion unless there is glucose stimulation of the islets. They may have great potential for use in association with exercise in people having difficulty controlling postprandial hyperglycemia, but, unfortunately, there are no data on the meglitinides and exercise, and hypoglycemia has been observed with the drugs in this class (19). As an alternative, the patient may be placed on insulin or changed to another oral agent not associated with hypoglycemia, such as a thiazolidinedione or an α-glucosidase inhibitor. Using metformin in this circumstance may be inadvisable because of possible development of lactic acidosis secondary to exercise-induced hypoxemia or acidosis (7).

Treatment and preventative measures against hypoglycemia are reviewed in Tables 2 and 3.

EFFECTS OF EXERCISE ON GLYCEMIC CONTROL AND DIABETIC COMPLICATIONS

It is clear that exercise has beneficial effects on both glucose homeostasis and insulin sensitivity, but several studies (21–23) have failed to document an improvement in long-

Table 3
Recommendations for Pre-Exercise Planning

- Schedule exercise 1– 3 h after eating.
- Pre-exercise blood glucose should be between 100 and 200 mg/dL.
- If glucose prior to exercise is <80 mg/dL, consume 15–20 g carbohydrate.
- If glucose prior to exercise is >300 mg/dL or urine if ketones are positive, delay activity.
- Consume carbohydrate immediately prior to and every 30–60 minutes during exercise.
- Reduce insulin dose anticipated to peak during exercise by 25–75%.

Adapted from refs. *9* and *11*.

term glycemic control in patients engaging in regular exercise or sports; however, short-term improvements in glycemic control have been noted *(24,25)*. The explanations underlying these observations are unclear but may be related to pre-exercise carbohydrate loading *(12)*, which may result in hyperglycemia at the onset and during the event, or to overcorrection of hypoglycemia *(21)* either during or following exercise, or to physiologic barriers *(26–28)* described in subjects with type 2 diabetes. In addition to the immediate effects of exercise on diabetic control, it has been shown that the benefits of exercise in type 1 diabetes, at least, may persist long after participation in sports and are manifest as a reduction in the risk of macrovascular complications *(29)* without increasing the risk for microvascular complications such as retinopathy *(30)*. Short-term aerobic exercise has been shown to dramatically improve endothelial function in people with type 2 diabetes *(31)*.

ASSESSMENT GUIDELINES

The recommendations for evaluating a patient prior to participation in sports activities or a general conditioning program are based on the age of the patient, the type of diabetes, and the length of time the patient has had diabetes. Because insulin resistance and asymptomatic hyperglycemia typically antedate the diagnosis of type 2 diabetes by several years, duration of illness is less critical in the assessment of these patients.

General Assessment

The initial evaluation of the patient should include a general assessment of health. Any symptoms suggesting vascular disease or preexisting conditions that could be aggravated by participation in an exercise program should be investigated prior to granting medical clearance. Specific information crucial in assessing the patient with diabetes includes a review of the patient's short- and long-term glycemic control, an evaluation of the frequency and duration of hypoglycemic episodes, and a systematic investigation to diagnose any complication resulting from diabetes that could be aggravated by participation in sports *(32)*.

Glycemic Control

Measuring a hemoglobin A_{1c} is indispensable in determining long-term metabolic control, and a careful review of the results of self-monitoring of capillary blood glucose will give an appraisal of short-term or day-to-day control. If the mean blood glucose is under 150 mg/dL (8.3 m*M*) and the hemoglobin A_{1c} is 7.0% or less, the patient is under acceptable control *(33)*. On the other hand, a hemoglobin A_{1c} greater than 9.5% is consistent with poor control, and the patient should be counseled to avoid participation in competitive events, but enrollment in a conditioning program may benefit the overall control. In addition, symptoms of hyperglycemia or changes in weight should be obtained.

Hypoglycemia and Hypoglycemia Unawareness

A careful history of the frequency, duration, and presence of prodromal symptoms of hypoglycemia is also vital. The lack of an adrenergic prodrome to signal hypoglycemia is termed "hypoglycemia unawareness" and is typically manifest as recurrent, severe episodes of neuroglycopenia. Frequently, these patients also have difficulty in the effective counterregulation of blood glucose that results in prolonged episodes of hypoglycemia that generally require medical assistance to facilitate recovery. Obviously, these patients should be precluded from participation in sporting events, such as swimming, scuba diving, or climbing, in which a sudden alteration in mental alertness could have drastic consequences. These patients should be encouraged to participate in activities where close supervision is possible. Because both alterations in the insulin regimen or supplemental feedings are used to prevent hypoglycemia during exercise, the history should also be directed to determine if the patient has unusual insulin absorption kinetics or may have delayed gastric emptying.

Exercise-Induced Hypertension

Exercise-induced hypertension can be diagnosed by obtaining vital signs before and after moderate exercise *(34)*. This condition is defined as a peak systolic blood pressure greater than 210 mm Hg in men and 190 mm Hg in women *(35)*, and has been associated with cardiovascular disease. If the response to exercise is normal, periodic re-evaluation to exclude exercise-induced hypertension should be undertaken. Although there is no consensus concerning management of these patients, it would be prudent to advise against participation in high-intensity events, and the patient should be directed to sports with low static demands.

Retinopathy

Patients with proliferative retinopathy should be excluded from contact sports or events like weight lifting because of the risk of vitreous hemorrhage or retinal detachment possibly resulting in blindness. Routine office funduscopy is usually inadequate to detect peripheral retinal lesions, and consultation with an ophthalmologist or retinal photographs are necessary to exclude retinopathy. It is not necessary to restrict activities of patients with mild background retinopathy or no retinal findings.

Nephropathy

The earliest manifestation of diabetic nephropathy is the presence of albuminuria or proteinuria *(36,37)*. The most sensitive screening test to detect this complication is the measurement of the microalbumin excretion rate. Although there is no evidence that exercise exacerbates fixed diabetic nephropathy, it may transiently increase the urinary excretion of albumin and protein *(38)*. Exercising patients with incipient nephropathy should be monitored closely with periodic measurements of both creatinine clearance and protein excretion rates in order to ensure stability of renal function. Because of the close linkage between diabetic nephropathy and retinopathy, the renal–retinal syndrome *(39)*, patients with either component should be observed closely for the possible development of either complication.

Table 4
Medical Conditions Potentially Limiting
Strenuous Exercise

- Hypoglycemia unawareness
- Proliferative diabetic retinopathy
- Persistent hyperglycemia
- Uncontrolled hypertension
- Significant peripheral sensory neuropathy
- Autonomic insufficiency
- Coronary artery disease
- Peripheral vascular disease
- Persistent albuminuria/proteinuria
- Nephropathy
- Nonadherence to medical regimen

Adapted from ref. 20.

Neuropathies

Peripheral sensory neuropathies are the most common neurologic complication of diabetes and can predispose to injury because of the risk of overusage because of an increased pain threshold or because of joint laxity resulting from impaired proprioception. If a patient has normal vibratory and position sense on examination, it is very unlikely they have any significant sensory neuropathy. Dysfunction of the motor nerves is associated with weakness and atrophy that serve to limit participation in a variety of different activities. Because these symptoms are the result of deinnervation, attempts to improve strength and bulk of the affected muscles are essentially fruitless.

The easiest diagnostic maneuvers to assess for the presence of autonomic neuropathy are the determinations of the blood pressure and pulse response to orthostatic and Valsalva maneuvers. If these are normal, autonomic dysfunction is doubtful. The major clinical complications associated with autonomic neuropathies are diabetic gastroparesis with delayed gastric emptying and striking fluctuations in blood pressure.

Atherosclerosis

Monitored exercise tolerance testing should be considered in all people with type 2 diabetes who are over the age of 40 or those who have had the condition for more than 10 yr. Those with type 1 diabetes who have a greater than a 15-yr history of diabetes should similarly be considered for screening. As an alternative to standard exercise tolerance testing, newer paradigms for screening with exercise echocardiography have been suggested (40). In addition to an increased risk for coronary artery disease and diastolic dysfunction (41), people with diabetes have a several-fold higher chance of developing peripheral vascular disease. Diminished pulses, vascular bruits, and delayed capillary refill times should prompt further evaluation of possible vascular insufficiency.

Conditions prompting limitations in sporting activities or conditioning programs are listed in Table 4.

CONCLUSIONS

If patients are carefully screened and counseled prior to participation in sports or a conditioning program, exercise appears beneficial in the management of diabetes and seems not to be associated with precipitating diabetic complications. The major exercise-related difficulty in diabetics is the occurrence of hypoglycemia, which can be immediate or appear hours following exercise. The judicious use of nutritional supplements prior to and during exercise coupled with carefully designed alterations in the patient's medical regimen is generally adequate to avoid this problem. Periodic reassessment of the patient and a critical review of both short- and long-term glycemic control are crucial in evaluating the efficacy of any therapeutic modifications made to accommodate an exercise program.

REFERENCES

1. Expert Committee on the Diagnosis and Classification of Diabetes Mellitus. Report of the expert committee on the diagnosis and classification of diabetes mellitus. Diabetes Care 1997;20:1183.
2. Seely BL, Olefsky JM. Potential cellular and genetic mechanisms for insulin resistance in the common disorders of diabetes and obesity. In: Moller DE, ed. Insulin Resistance. John Wiley, West Sussex, UK, 1993, pp. 187=252.
3. Krotkiewski M, Lonnroth P, Mandroukas K, et al. The effects of physical training on insulin secretion and effectiveness and on glucose metabolism in obesity and type 2 (non-insulin dependent) diabetes mellitus. Diabetologia 1985;28:881.
4. Yeaman SJ, Armstrong JL, Bonavaud BD, et al. Regulation of glycogen synthesis in human muscle cells. Biochem Soc Trans 2001;29:537.
5. Ryder JW, Chibalin AV, Zierath JR. Intracellular mechanisms underlying increases in glucose uptake in response to insulin or exercise in skeletal muscle. Acta Physiol Scand 2001;171:249.
6. Ploug T, Galbo H, Richter EA. Increase muscle glucose uptake during contractions: no need for insulin. Am J Physiol 1984;247:E726.
7. Bailey CJ, Turner RC. Metformin. N Engl J Med 1996;334:574.
8. MacDonald MJ. Postexercise late-onset hypoglycemia in insulin dependent diabetic patients. Diabetes Care 1987;10:584.
9. Horton ES. Role and management of exercise in diabetes mellitus. Diabetes Care 1988;11:201.
10. Nathan DM, Madnek SF, Delahanty L. Programming pre-exercise snacks to prevent post-exercise hypoglycemia in intensively treated insulin dependent diabetics. Ann Int Med 1985;102:483.
11. Rabasa-Lhoret R, Bourque J, Ducros F, Chiasson JL. Guidelines for premeal insulin dose reduction for postprandial exercise for different intensities and durations in type 1 diabetic subjects treated intensively with a basal-bolus insulin regimen (ultralente-lispro). Diabetes Care 2001;24:625.
12. Koivisto VA, Sane T, Ehyrquist F, Pelkonen R. Fuel and fluid homeostasis during long- term exercise in healthy subjects and type I diabetic patients. Diabetes Care 1992;15:1736.
13. Gillies PS, Figgitt DP, Lamb HM. Insulin glargine. Drugs 2000;59:253.
14. Lepore M, Pampanelli S, Fanelli C, et al. Pharmacokinetics and pharmacodynamics of subcutaneous injection of long-acting human insulin analog glargine, NPH insulin, and ultralente human insulin and continuous subcutaneous infusion of insulin lispro. Diabetes 2000;49:2142.
15. Dagogo-Jack S, Askari H, Morrill B, et al. Physiological responses during hypoglycemia induced by regular human insulin or a novel human analog, insulin glargine. Diabetes Obes Metab 2000;2:373.
16. HollemanF, Hoekstra JBL. Insulin lispro. N Engl J Med 1997;337:176.
17. Hedman CA, Lindstrom T, Arnqvist HJ. Direct comparison of insulin lispro and aspart shows small differences in plasma insulin profiles after subcutaneous injection in type 1 diabetes. Diabetes Care 2001;24:1120.
18. Koivisto V, Felig P. Effects of acute exercise on insulin absorption in diabetic patients. N Engl J Med 1978;298:79.
19. Dunn CJ, Foulds D. Nateglinide. Drugs 2000;60:607.
20. Jones RE. The diabetic athlete. In: Lillegard W, Butcher JD, Rucker KS, eds. Handbook of Sports Medicine: A Symptom-Oriented Approach. 2nd ed. Butterworth Heinmann, Newton, MA, 1999, p. 345.
21. Weiliczko MC, Gobert M, Mallet E. The participation in sports of diabetic children. A survey in the Rouen region. Ann Pediatr Paris 1991;38:84.
22. Selam JL, Casassus P, Bruzzo F, et al. Exercise is not associated with better diabetes control in type 1 and type 2 diabetic subjects. Acta Diabetol 1992;29:11.

23. Sackey AH, Jefferson IG. Physical activity and glycemic control in children with diabetes mellitus. Diabet Med 1996;13:789.
24. Stratton R, Wilson DP, Endres RK, Goldstein DE. Improved glycemic control after a supervised eight week exercise program in insulin-dependent diabetic adolescents. Diabetes Care 1987;10:589.
25. Boule NG, Haddad E, Kenny GP, et al. Effects of exercise on glycemic control and body mass in type 2 diabetes mellitus: a meta-analysis of controlled clinical trials. JAMA 2001;286:1218.
26. Regensteiner JG, Sippel J, McFarling ET, et al. Effects of non-insulin dependent diabetes on oxygen consumption during treadmill exercise. Med Sci Sports Exerc 1995;27:875.
27. Joseph LJ, Trappe TA, Farrell PA, et al. Short-term moderate weight loss and resistance training do not affect insulin-stimulated glucose disposal in postmenopausal women. Diabetes Care 2001;24:1863.
28. Blaak EE, Wolffenbuttel BH, Saris WH, et al. Weight reduction and the impaired plasma- derived free fatty acid oxidation in type 2 diabetic subjects. J Endocrinol Metab 2001;86:1638.
29. LaPorte RE, Dorman JS, Tajima N, et al. Pittsburgh insulin-dependent diabetes mellitus morbidity and mortality study: physical activity and diabetic complications. Pediatrics 1986;78:1027.
30. Cruickshanks KJ, Moss SE, Klein R, Klein BE. Physical activity and proliferative retinopathy in people diagnosed with diabetes before age 30 years. Diabetes Care 1992;15:1267.
31. Maiorana V, O'Driscoll G, Cheetham C, et al. The effect of combined aerobic and resistance exercise training on vascular function in type 2 diabetics. J Am Coll Cardiol 2001;38:860.
32. Chipkin SR, Klugh SA, Chasan-Taber L. Exercise and diabetes. Cardiol Clin 2001;19:489.
33. American Diabetes Association. Standards of medical care for patients with diabetes mellitus. Diabetes Care 2001;24(suppl 1):S33.
34. Blake GA, Levin SR, Koyal SN. Exercise-induced hypertension in normotensive patients with NIDDM. Diabetes Care 1990;7:799.
35. Lauer MS, Levy D, Anderson KM, Plehn JF. Is there a relationship between exercise systolic blood pressure and left venticular mass? Ann Int Med 1992;116:203.
36. Mogensen CE, Christensen CK. Predicting diabetic nephropathy in insulin-dependent patients. N Engl J Med 1984;311:89.
37. Mogensen CE. Microalbuminuria predicts clinical proteinuria and early mortality in maturity-onset diabetes. N Engl J Med 1984;310:356.
38. Agarwal RP, Thanvi I, Vachhani G, et al. Exercise induced proteinuria as an early indicator of diabetic nephropathy. J Assoc Physicians India 1998;46:772.
39. Lloyd CE, Orchard TJ. Diabetes complications: the renal-retinal link. An epidemiological perspective. Diabetes Care 1995;18:1034.
40. Elhendy A, Arruda AM, Mahoney DW, Pellikka PA. Prognostic stratification of diabetic patients by exercise echocardiography. J Am Coll Cardiol 2001;37:1551.
41. Zabalgoitia M, Ismaeil MF, Anderson L, Maklady FA. Prevalence of diastolic dysfunction in normo- tensive, asymptomatic patients with well-controlled type 2 diabetes mellitus. Am J Cardiol 2001;87:320.

V ADRENAL

16

Glucocorticoid Treatment
in Prenatal and Postnatal Life

Lynnette K. Nieman, MD
and Kristina I. Rother, MD

INTRODUCTION

Untreated, complete glucocorticoid insufficiency leads to circulatory collapse and death. Although uncommon, the possibility of this endocrine emergency engenders vigilance, both for a new diagnosis of adrenal insufficiency as well as for exacerbation of a chronic, known condition. Conversely, overtreatment of adrenal insufficiency with excessive glucocorticoid carries the morbidity associated with iatrogenic Cushing's syndrome. Thus, glucocorticoid insufficiency presents two major challenges for clinicians: timely diagnosis and appropriate treatment.

CAUSES OF ADRENAL INSUFFICIENCY

The causes of glucocorticoid insufficiency can be subdivided according to the anatomic site of the defect. Primary adrenal insufficiency reflects an inability of the adrenal glands to synthesize steroids, whereas secondary adrenal insufficiency reflects an inability of the hypothalamic–pituitary unit to deliver CRH and/or adrenocorticotropin

From: *Endocrine Replacement Therapy in Clinical Practice*
Edited by: A. Wayne Meikle © Humana Press Inc., Totowa, NJ

(ACTH), thus reducing trophic support to otherwise normal adrenal glands. This anatomic distinction results in an important clinical difference: Patients with primary adrenal disease tend to have destruction of all layers of the adrenal cortex, so that mineralocorticoid as well as glucocorticoid function is lost. In contrast, the diminished ACTH levels in patients with secondary adrenal insufficiency markedly decrease cortisol production, but does not affect mineralocorticoid production, so that mineralocorticoid activity is intact.

PRIMARY ADRENAL INSUFFICIENCY

Primary adrenal insufficiency may be caused by a number of conditions. Autoimmune destruction of the gland is the most common etiology in the United States (more than 80%) and may occur alone or in association with other endocrinopathies. These latter autoimmune polyglandular syndromes tend to present either in childhood (type 1), in association with hypoparathyroidism and mucocutaneous candidiasis (1), or in adulthood, in association with insulin-dependent diabetes mellitus, autoimmune thyroid disease, alopecia areata, and vitiligo (2). Radiographically, these adrenal glands are small.

Infections cause about 15% of primary adrenal insufficiency and typically include tuberculosis, systemic fungal diseases (histoplasmosis, coccidiomycosis, blastomycosis), and acquired immunodeficiency syndrome (AIDS)-associated opportunistic infections such as cytomegalovirus (CMV) (3). These adrenal glands tend to be large on computed tomography (CT) scan.

Adrenal tissue may be replaced by bilateral metastases (most commonly primary carcinoma of the lung, breast, kidney, or gut, or primary lymphoma) (4) or by hemorrhage, leading to insufficient steroidogenesis (5). Obviously, bilateral adrenalectomy removes all steroidogenic tissue, leaving a life-long deficit.

Medications that inhibit specific enzymatic steps of steroidogenesis, including ketoconazole, mitotane, aminoglutethimide, trilostane, and metyrapone, can cause primary adrenal failure. These medications are usually prescribed in the setting of hypercortisolism, to exploit this ability and reduce glucocorticoid production (6). However, this side effect of the imidazole derivatives may not be anticipated in patients treated for fungal disease.

A number of rare genetic disorders may cause adrenal insufficiency in childhood, including congenital lipoid adrenal hyperplasia (7), adrenoleukodystrophy (8) and the congenital adrenal hyperplasias.

Mutations of genes required for adrenal development *in utero* may lead to adrenal dysplasia and congenital adrenal insufficiency (9). Defects in the transcription factors SF-1 and DAX-1 or in the ACTH receptor result in syndromes that include adrenal abnormalities as well as other clinical features at birth.

Adrenaleukodystrophy, a rare (1/25,000) X-linked condition, is characterized by deficiency of peroxisomal membrane adrenoleukodystrophy protein, which transports activated acyl-CoA derivatives into the peroxisomes, where they are shortened by β-oxidation. This deficiency results in accumulation of very long-chain fatty acids (VLCFAs) in the central nervous system and other tissues, as well as increased circulating levels that can be detected as an increase in plasma C26:0 fatty acids. Incomplete penetrance of the genetic defect and variable accumulation of VLCFAs in the adrenal gland, brain, testis, and liver account for the clinical phenotypes, which differ by age and presentation. Cerebral adrenaleukodystrophy, presenting in childhood, is characterized by cognitive and gait disturbances, whereas the adult form, adrenomyeloneuropathy, is characterized by spinal cord and peripheral nerve demyelination. In both forms, accumulation of VLCFAs in the adrenal cortex alters membrane function and inhibits signal transduction by ACTH. Because a substantial minority of patients in both groups present first with adrenal insufficiency, boys and young men with adrenal insufficiency should be screened for adrenaleukodystrophy.

The congenital adrenal hyperplasias (CAHs) are a disparate group of diseases that reflect deficiency of one of the enzymes needed for adrenal steroidogenesis (10). Patients with nearly complete deficiency of an enzyme required for cortisol synthesis present in childhood with adrenal insufficiency and salt-wasting crisis. Deficiency of 21-hydroxylase (CYP21 gene) accounts for 90% of CAH cases. The increase in ACTH levels caused by cortisol deficiency drives the intact steroidogenic pathways so that there is excessive production of the steroids just proximal to the enzymatic block, 17-hydroxyprogesterone and 11-deoxycortisol in 21-hydroxylase and 11β-hydroxylase deficiency, respectively. Because of the increased levels of precursor steroids, adrenal androgen levels increase. As a result, severely affected girls may be virilized *in utero*, and less affected girls and women become hirsute after puberty (11).

Similarly, abnormalities in cholesterol production or delivery to cells, such as the abnormality in Smith–Lemli–Opitz syndrome, cause defective steroidogenesis (12).

The initial presentation of patients with primary adrenal insufficiency is either acute or chronic. The characteristic features of acute adrenal insufficiency include orthostatic hypotension, circulatory collapse, fever, hyperkalemia, hyponatremia, and hypoglycemia. These patients often have hemorrhage, metastasis, or acute infection and lack the typical history and clinical findings of patients with chronic primary adrenal insufficiency. The latter individuals present with a longer history of malaise, fatigue, anorexia, weight loss, joint and back pain, and darkening of the skin. Although hyperpigmentation is dramatic in sun-exposed areas, it is present in other areas also and should be sought in the creases of the hands, extensor surfaces, recent scars, buccal and vaginal mucosa, and nipples. Associated biochemical features include hyponatremia, hypoglycemia, and hyperkalemia.

SECONDARY ADRENAL INSUFFICIENCY

Suppression of the hypothalamic–pituitary–adrenal axis by exogenous or endogenous glucocorticoids is the most common cause of secondary adrenal insufficiency. It is important to recognize that this axis may not recover full function for up to 18 mo after cure of Cushing's syndrome (13) or discontinuation of medication (14), during which time the patient should receive supplemental steroids during severe physiologic stress (*see* section on Treatment of Glucocorticoid Insufficiency). Secondary adrenal insufficiency also may result from structural lesions of the hypothalamus or pituitary gland that interfere with CRH production or transport or with corticotrope function. This includes tumors, destruction by infiltrating disorders, X-irradiation, and lymphocytic hypophysitis. Although the loss of ACTH function is usually accompanied by other pituitary deficiencies, isolated ACTH deficiency may occur, although rarely (15).

DIAGNOSIS OF ADRENAL INSUFFICIENCY

The diagnosis of adrenal insufficiency rests on biochemical testing. In a patient without a known diagnosis of adrenal insufficiency, blood is obtained for measurement of cortisol when the intravenous line is inserted. In patients with adrenal insufficiency, the cortisol value generally will return in the normal or subnormal range. Such a value is inappropriately low for the physiologic state of hypotension, in which cortisol values are usually well above 18 μg/dL.

In a nonemergent presentation, the cortisol response to administration of ACTH, 250 μg, is the gold standard test of adrenal steroidogenic ability *(16,17)*. Other tests, such as metyrapone stimulation test, insulin-induced hypoglycemia and lower doses of the ACTH stimulation test *(18)*, may have merit in specific circumstances, but cannot be advocated as the appropriate initial screening test *(17)*. Both insulin and metyrapone carry significant risks in individuals who lack appropriate counter-regulatory processes.

In the classic test, 250 μg of ACTH (1-24, cosyntropin) is given either intravenously or intramuscularly, at any time of the day. This supraphysiologic dose of ACTH delivers a maximal stimulus to the adrenal gland so that the peak cortisol response measured 30–60 min later is greater than 18 μg/dL. The actual plasma cortisol value at 30 min is the most consistent measure and does not change in relationship to the basal cortisol level. Although the absolute increase in cortisol is usually greater than 7 μg/dL, this criterion alone cannot be used to determine adequacy of the response. In particular, critically ill patients with a high basal cortisol level may not show a further increase after ACTH administration. The increased basal value reflects a normal adrenal response to the stressful condition.

In theory, the 250-μg ACTH test evaluates the integrity of the entire hypothalamic–pituitary–adrenal axis, because lack of ACTH leads to atrophy of the adrenal glands and an inability to respond to exogenous ACTH. However, it is important to recognize that a normal response to ACTH, 250 μg, may occur in the setting of mild hypothalamic–pituitary disease, particularly of recent onset *(19)*. In this setting, ACTH levels are reduced, but are adequate to sustain some adrenal steroidogenesis, so that cortisol secretion is apparently normal when a pharmacologic dose of ACTH is given.

The lower-dose ACTH tests have not yet been fully validated, but hold promise. Proponents of the 1-μg test indicate that it is more sensitive than the 250-μg ACTH test *(18,20)*. A number of small series report that patients with secondary adrenal insufficiency may respond normally to the standard ACTH test but subnormally to the insulin, metyrapone, or the low-dose ACTH test(s) *(18,20–24)*. However, in the absence of clinical features of adrenal insufficiency, others argue that the normal response to the standard ACTH test correctly reflects a lack of disease *(25)*. An additional problem is the lack of consensus on the optimal cutpoint for interpretation of the cortisol response to the low-dose ACTH test.

Other issues surrounding the low-dose ACTH test relate to the formulation of the dose and the method of administration. Because there is no commercial formulation of ACTH for the low-dose test, the product must be diluted and delivered on site, leading to concerns about the accuracy of the administered dose.

Primary and secondary adrenal insufficiency may be distinguished by biochemical tests. The basal plasma ACTH in currently available commercial assays is generally above the normal range in primary adrenal insufficiency and may exceed the normal range before the cortisol response to ACTH stimulation is subnormal. Measurement of basal ACTH works as well as the CRH-stimulated ACTH value for discriminating primary and secondary adrenal insufficiency (26). Primary adrenal insufficiency may also be identified by failure of plasma aldosterone to reach 16 ng/dL at 30 min after cortrosyn (250 μg), as normal individuals and those with secondary adrenal insufficiency exceed this value (27).

Individuals suspected of having congenital adrenal hyperplasia should undergo additional measurement of precursor and product hormones to delineate the site of enzymatic deficiency, as detailed elsewhere (11,28). When a family has an affected infant, subsequent prenatal diagnosis for 21-hydroxylase deficiency using molecular probes of the CYP21 gene (28–31), or human leukocyte antigen (HLA) (32) genes, and material obtained from chorionic villous sampling at 8–10 wk gestation is now available, albeit primarily in a research setting. The CYP21 gene is closely linked to the HLA major histocompatibility complex (MHC) on chromosome 6, so that affected siblings usually share the identical HLA type. Because patients with 21-hydroxylase deficiency may carry many different mutations, molecular diagnosis is not a straightforward commercially available test. These molecular techniques have supplanted diagnostic measurement of 17-hydroxyprogesterone and testosterone in amniotic fluid at 16–18 wk, because they allow for earlier discontinuation of dexamethasone treatment of an unaffected fetus.

TREATMENT OF GLUCOCORTICOID INSUFFICIENCY

Chronic therapy of glucocorticoid insufficiency is designed to provide a physiologic amount of glucocorticoid. This is best done by administering 12–15 mg/m^2 of hydrocortisone daily in one or two oral doses. Ideally, the morning dose is given as soon after waking as possible; for individuals who feel extremely fatigued in the morning, a strategy of taking the medication 30 min before arising may be helpful. Although many patients do well on a single morning dose, others complain of pronounced fatigue in the afternoon and evening. For these individuals, a split dose of hydrocortisone, in which about one-third of the daily dose is given around 4 PM, may be useful. Many adults complain of insomnia and overly vivid dreams if glucocorticoid is given later in the evening, so that this timing is best avoided.

Other glucocorticoids may be used for daily replacement therapy, according to their relative potency to hydrocortisone (see Table 1). Prednisone and dexamethasone offer longer biologic half-lives, which may be advantageous for individuals with pronounced afternoon and evening symptoms. However, hydrocortisone, although shorter acting, offers the advantage of multiple-dose tablets, which allows for fine adjustment and splitting of the daily dose.

Patients with primary adrenal insufficiency should also receive mineralocorticoid (see Chapter 17). When mineralocorticoid is not given as part of the chronic therapy of primary adrenal insufficiency, often the dose of hydrocortisone or another steroid with mineralocorticoid activity is increased to ameliorate hyperkalemia or salt-craving. The problem with this approach is that the amount of administered glucocorticoid activity also increases, beyond the level of physiologic replacement, so that the patient becomes Cushingoid.

In suspected acute adrenal insufficiency, hydrocortisone is the treatment of choice because it has both glucocorticoid and mineralocorticoid activity. Treatment with intra-

Table 1
Comparison of Commonly Used Glucocorticoids

Agent	Biologic half-life (h)	Equivalent dose (mg)	Relative mineralocorticoid activity
Cortisone	8–12	25	0.8
Cortisol (hydrocortisone)	8–12	20	1
Prednisone	12–36	5	0.8
Dexamethasone	36–72	0.3	0
Fludrocortisone			250

venous saline for volume expansion, glucose for hypoglycemia, and intravenous hydrocortisone, 100 mg, should be started immediately after placement of an intravenous line and withdrawal of blood for documentation of the cortisol value. Patients with adrenal insufficiency will recover blood pressure and normalize symptoms rapidly, usually within 1 h. Persistent symptoms should provoke evaluation of other disorders.

ADJUSTMENT OF GLUCOCORTICOID DOSE

All patients receiving chronic glucocorticoid replacement therapy should be instructed that they are "dependent" on taking glucocorticoids as prescribed and that failure to take or absorb the medication will lead to adrenal crisis and possibly death. They should also obtain a medical information bracelet or necklace that identifies this requirement (Medic Alert Foundation, 2323 Colorado Ave., Turlock, CA 95382; telephone 1-888-633-4298; www.medicalert.org). Caregivers must educate these patients and their families about how to adjust their medication dose for mild physiologic stress conditions and how to respond to more severe situations, including administration of intramuscular glucocorticoid.

Conventional wisdom recommends that the daily oral glucocorticoid dose be doubled for "stressful" physiologic conditions such as fever, nausea, and diarrhea. Apart from reduced absorption because of vomiting or diarrhea, there are relatively little data in the medical literature to support this requirement. Additionally, this practice may lead to chronic overmedication by the patient because of a liberal interpretation of what constitutes physical stress. Thus, education of when and how to change the dose of steroid should be reinforced periodically, preferably with written material, and the dangers of excessive steroid use should be emphasized.

In predictable stressful conditions, such as surgery, glucocorticoid doses are increased in proportion to the amount of stress. Thus, during maximally stressful situations (e.g., in the setting of adrenal crisis, major surgery, trauma, or labor and delivery), the daily hydrocortisone dose will be 100–300 mg. (Although there are few data to support the need use of a 10-fold increase over the physiologic replacement dose, as opposed to mere replacement, the safety of not following this practice has not been established.) For more moderate stress, such as that of cholescystectomy, the dose is reduced to 75–100 mg hydrocortisone on the day of surgery, and the dose is tapered more rapidly. Patients undergoing minimal stress such as tooth extraction or short operative orthopedic procedures may not require any additional supplementation (33).

However, as not all stressful conditions are scheduled, the patient or a family member should be taught how to administer intramuscular injections and should be given an emergency kit containing prefilled syringes with injectable steroid (5 mg dexamethasone or 100 mg hydrocortisone). If the patient experiences trauma, vomiting, or is found unconscious, the medication should be administered, and the patient transported to the hospital. In the hospital, from 100 to 300 mg of hydrocortisone should be given by vein each day, in split doses every 6 to 8 h. These increases in oral or parenteral glucocorticoid doses should be continued only for a few days, until the acute event has resolved, and are then tapered by 50% each day until the usual oral dose is resumed. For acute gastrointestinal illnesses or less severe systemic illness, patients should double their usual oral dose and seek advice from a physician.

Glucocorticoid therapy may require adjustment in conditions where the metabolism of the agent might be altered. In particular, hyperthyroidism increases and hypothyroidism decreases the metabolism of glucocorticoids so that the administered dose of medication may need to be adjusted dramatically. Drugs such as rifampin, phenobarbital, and phenytoin, which induce hepatic microsomal enzymes that catabolize steroids, reduce the bioavailability of these agents.

EVALUATION OF THERAPEUTIC EFFICACY

In the setting of chronic adrenal insufficiency, clinical assessment is the best way to judge whether the glucocorticoid dose is correct. Symptoms of adrenal insufficiency, such as nausea, anorexia, and diarrhea, ameliorate quickly with the initiation of therapy, and the patient gains lost weight. Joint aches and pains may resolve more slowly. With appropriate additional mineralocorticoid replacement in the setting of primary adrenal insufficiency, salt-craving decreases.

Although biochemical abnormalities also normalize, these should not be used as the only index of appropriate therapy. When glucocorticoid and mineralocorticoid replacement of patients with primary adrenal insufficiency is adequate, plasma ACTH levels decrease, but still remain elevated in the range of 100–200 pg/mL. Renin values, however, normalize completely and may be used to judge the adequacy of mineralocorticoid replacement. Increases in ACTH alone above 200 pg/mL suggest inadequate glucocorticoid replacement; if both ACTH and renin are increased, the mineralocorticoid dose should be increased before the glucocorticoid dose is adjusted, to prevent iatrogenic Cushing's syndrome. Although hydrocortisone is metabolized to cortisol, plasma cortisol values should not be used to monitor therapy, as clearance from the bloodstream is rapid and circulating values are low for most of the day. Other steroids such as dexamethasone or prednisone do not crossreact fully in the cortisol assays; thus, measurement of plasma cortisol does not provide a good measure of adequate replacement if these agents are used.

Clinical features are also an excellent way to monitor for glucocorticoid excess. The development of a Cushingoid habitus, weight gain, and in children, decreased linear growth are worrisome and suggest that the glucocorticoid dose should be decreased. The development of osteopenia is possible with subtler overreplacement. If the patient is receiving hydrocortisone, increased urine free cortisol provides additional evidence that the dose is too high.

Pediatric patients receiving hydrocortisone for classical salt-wasting congenital adrenal insufficiency are monitored using these clinical criteria and by measuring the steroid immediately proximate to the enzymatic block. Thus, in 21-hydroxylase deficiency, measurement of 17-hydroxyprogesterone provides an indirect index of the ability of administered glucocorticoid to inhibit ACTH secretion. With adequate treatment, morning levels of these steroids should be reduced but not fully normalized. Overtreatment, leading to ultimate short stature from glucocorticoid excess, may be avoided by splitting the hydrocortisone dose into three evenly spaced intervals and by adequate administration of fludrocortisone. Undertreatment is often signaled by continued excessive linear growth and the development of precocious puberty *(34)*.

PRENATAL TREATMENT OF CONGENITAL ADRENAL HYPERPLASIA WITH DEXAMETHASONE

Though defects in several steroidogenic enzymes (21-hydroxylase, 11β-hydroxylase, and 3β-hydroxysteroid dehydrogenase) may result in overproduction of adrenal androgens and, subsequently, in virilization of affected female fetuses, credible experience with prenatal treatment exists only for 21-hydroxylase deficiency. In 1984, David and Forest were the first to report amelioration of virilization by administration of hydrocortisone or dexamethasone during pregnancy *(35)*. After an affected child is born to a couple, it is now recommended for subsequent pregnancies to begin hormonal treatment of the fetus—blind to its affected status and sex—by administering dexamethasone orally to the mother immediately after confirmation of pregnancy.

This strategy is based on the fact that dexamethasone, when administered to a pregnant woman, is not bound to corticosteroid-binding globulin, crosses the placental barrier, and suppresses fetal ACTH levels, which stimulate adrenal androgen production. Dexamethasone is the agent of choice because as a synthetic fluorinated steroid, it is not a ready substrate for 11β-hydroxysteroid dehydrogenase type 2 (11β-HSD-2). In contrast, only a small portion of maternally administered cortisol and prednisolone reaches the fetus in an active form because, at least during the last trimester, both placental and fetal 11β-HSD-2 rapidly converts these active 11-hydroxysteroids to inert 11-keto forms (cortisone, prednisone).

The recommended dexamethasone dose, 20 μg/kg pre-pregnancy body weight per day in two or three divided doses *(36,37)*, should be started as early as 4–5 wk gestation to prevent virilization of an affected female fetus. Chorionic villous sampling is performed at 9–11 wk; if the karyotype analysis reveals that the fetus is male, treatment is stopped. If the fetus is female, treatment is continued until the results of the DNA analysis of the affected gene or HLA type are available, when dexamethasone treatment is either discontinued, or, in the case of an affected female, continued to term.

EFFECTIVENESS OF TREATMENT

Most recently, New et al. reported that dexamethasone administered at or before 9 wk gestation prevented genital masculinization in 11 of 25 affected females; another 11 infants had only mild virilization (Prader stages 1 and 2) *(38)*. Treatment with a suboptimal dose or later onset resulted in normal external genitalia in only 1 of 24 newborns. Similarly, the Scandinavian experience confirmed the need for timely onset of treatment: virilization was completely prevented if treatment was begun before the seventh week of gestation and continued without interruption until term *(39)*. Apart from the reduction in surgery, the additional psychological benefits of ameliorating the genital masculinization are difficult to quantitate in affected patients and their families, but are likely to be substantial.

The relationship between increased fetal androgens and lower frequency of marriage and fewer children *(40)*, an increased incidence of lesbian behavior *(40,41)*, or less interest in sexual activity and a more negative body image *(42)* reported in affected untreated females, is not well understood. The contribution of fetal androgenization as opposed to the contributions of possible psychological trauma of genital surgery or parental uncertainty about the sex assignment has not been distinguished. However, the potential contribution of fetal androgens to "masculinization" of the brain represented by these alterations from the female "norm" has been invoked as an additional reason to initiate early prenatal therapy.

SIDE EFFECTS AND PITFALLS OF TREATMENT

Few clear-cut adverse effects have been reported in neonates or children who received prenatal treatment with dexamethasone, but the numbers of studies and subjects are small. No teratogenic effects have been noted. Most treated newborns have normal weight and length. However, anecdotal reports have suggested an increased risk of fetal death after acute withdrawal of glucocorticoid therapy (in unaffected pregnancies) and a possibly increased incidence of adverse events in children born after short- or long-term prenatal treatment *(29,39,43)*.

The potential for creating iatrogenic maternal Cushing's syndrome, with its known deleterious effects on fetal and maternal morbidity *(44)*, is a concern. Except for rapid weight gain, the incidence of significant maternal side effects is low in the first to early second trimester, but increases to between 10 and 50% of treated mothers when dexamethasone is continued until term *(39,43–48)*. These adverse effects include Cushingoid features, excessive weight gain, severe cutaneous striae, hypertension, abnormal glucose tolerance, proteinuria, acne, hirsutism, edema, and emotional irritability.

Seckl and Miller have recently summarized the most important current concerns regarding long-term fetal treatment *(50)*. These include unnecessary treatment of unaffected fetuses, the known adverse effects on the mother, and potential adverse effects on the child. If a couple has a child with CAH, only one in four subsequent pregnancies will be affected, and only one in eight will be an affected female; thus, seven out of eight fetuses are treated unnecessarily during the early stages of pregnancy. Although the recommended treatment, 20 µg/kg/d of dexamethasone, is a supraphysiological dose for the mother, it does not consistently prevent virilization of an affected fetus. Other concerns, based in part on animal studies, include the possibility that prenatal glucocorticoid exposure may lead to an increased risk of hypertension and cardiovascular disease, to hippocampal damage *(51)*, or to abnormalities in social play, reproductive behavior, avoidance, and spatial learning. Regarding the latter point, increased avoidance, shyness, emotionality, and internalizing problems have been reported in children exposed to dexamethasone prenatally *(52)*.

CONCLUSION

Prenatal treatment (initiated early and continued until term) of affected females with 21-hydroxylase deficiency is effective in preventing or at least ameliorating the genital malformations caused by increased androgen concentrations. However, many questions regarding long-term consequences of this treatment remain unanswered. We, therefore, support the view that prenatal treatment with dexamethasone should be recommended and patients should be closely supervised for long periods, optimally with inclusion in institutional review board-approved study protocols.

REFERENCES

1. Ahonen P, Myllarnieini S, Sipila I, et al. Clinical variation of autoimmune polyendocrinopathy-candidiasis-ectodermal dystrophy (APECED) in a series of 68 patients. N Engl J Med 1990;322:1829–1836.
2. Betterle C, Volpato M, Greggio AN, et al. Type 2 polyglandular autoimmune disease (Schmidt's syndrome). J Pediatr Endocrinol Metab 1996;9:113–123.
3. Piedrola G, Casado JL, Lopez E, et al. Clinical features of adrenal insufficiency in patients with acquired immunodeficiency syndrome. Clin Endocrinol (Oxf) 1996;45:97–101.
4. Ihde JK, Turnbull AD, Bajourunas DR. Adrenal insufficiency in the cancer patient: implications for the surgeon. Br J Surg 1990;77:1335–1337.
5. Rao RH, Vagnucci AH, Amico JA. Bilateral massive adrenal hemorrhage: early recognition and treatment. Ann Intern Med 1989;110:227–235.
6. Nieman LK. Cushing's syndrome treatment. In: C. Wayne Bardin, ed., Current Therapy of Endocrinology and Metabolism. Saunders, Philadephia, 1996, pp. 609–614.
7. Seminara SB, Achermann JC, Genel M, et al. X-linked adrenal hypoplasia congenita: a mutation in DAX1 expands the phenotypic spectrum in males and females. J Clin Endocrinol Metab 1999;84:4501–4509.
8. Rizzo WB. X-linked adrenoleukodystrophy: a cause of primary adrenal insufficeincy in males. The Endocrinologist. 1992;2:177–183.
9. Ten S, New M, Maclaren N. Clinical review 130: Addison's disease 2001. J Clin Endocrinol Metab. 2001;86:2909–2922.
10. Merke DP, Camacho CA. Novel basic and clinical aspects of congenital adrenal hyperplasia. Rev Endocr Metab Disord 2001;2:289–296.
11. White PC. Congenital adrenal hyperplasias. Best Pract Res Clin Endocrinol Metab. 2001;15:17–41.
12. Porter FD. RSH/Smith-Lemli-Opitz syndrome: a multiple congenital anomaly/mental retardation syndrome due to an inborn error of cholesterol biosynthesis. Mol Genet Metab 2000;71:163–174.
13. Avgerinos PC, Chrousos GP, Nieman LK, et al. The corticotropin-releasing hormone test in the postoperative evaluation of patients with Cushing's syndrome. J Clin Endocrinol Metab 1987;65:906–913.
14. Graber AL, Ney RL, Nicholson WE, et al. Natural history of pituitary-adrenal recovery following long-term suppression with corticosteroid. J Clin Endocrinol Metab 1965;25:11–16.
15. Yamamoto T, Fukuyama J, Haasegawa K, et al. Isolated corticotropin deficiency in adults. Report of 10 cases and reveiw of the literature. Arch Intern Med 1992;152:1705–1712.
16. Oelkers H, Diederich S, Bahr V. Diagnosis and therapy surveillance in Addison's disease: rapid adrenocorticotropin (ACTH) test and measurement of plasma ACTH, renin activity, and aldosterone. J Clin Endocrinol Metab 1992;75:259–264.
17. Grinspoon SK, Biller BM. Clinical review 62: laboratory assessment of adrenal insufficiency. J Clin Endocrinol Metab 1994;79:923–931.
18. Dickstein G, Schechner C. Low dose ACTH test - a word of caution to the word of caution: when and how to use it. J Clin Endocrinol Metab 1997;82:322.
19. Borst GC, Michenfelder HJ, O'Brian JT. Discordant cortisol responses to exogeneous ACTH and insulin-induced hypoglycemia in patients with pituitary diseases. N Engl J Med 1982;302:1462–1464.
20. Tordjman K, Jaffe A, Trostanetsky Y, et al. Low-dose (1 mcg) adrenocorticotrophin (ACTH) stimulation as a screening test for impaired hypothalamo-pituitary-adrenal axis function: sensitivity, specificity and accuracy in comparison with the high-dose (250 mcg) test. Clin Endocrinol (Oxf) 2000;52:633–640.
21. Ammari F, Issa BG, Millward E, Scanion MF. A comparison between short ACTH and insulin stress tests for assessing hypothalamo-pituitary-adrenal function. Clin Endocrinol (Oxf) 1996;44:473–476.
22. Soule SG, Fahie-Wilson M, Tomlinson S. Failure of the short ACTH test to unequivocally diagnose long-standing symptomatic secondary hypoadrenalism. Clin Endocrinol (Oxf) 1996;44:137–140.
23. Rasmuson S, Olsson T, Hagg E. A low dose ACTH test to assess the function of the hypothalamic-pituitary-adrenal axis. Clin Endocrinol (Oxf) 1996;44:151–156.
24. Cunningham SK, Moore A, McKenna TJ. Normal cortisol response to corticotropin in patients with secondary adrenal failure. Arch Intern Med 1983;143:2276–2279.

25. Clayton RN. Short Synacthen test versus insulin stress test for assessment of the hypothalamo-pitu-itary—adrenal axis: controversy revisited. Clin Endocrinol (Oxf) 1996;44:147–149.

26. Schulte HM, Chrousos GP, Avgerinos P, et al. The corticotropin-releasing hormone stimulation test: a possible aid in the evaluation of patients with adrenal insufficiency. J Clin Endocrinol Metab 1984;58:1064–1067.

27. Dluhy RG, Himathongkam T, Greenfield M. Rapid ACTH test with plasma aldosterone levels. Ann Intern Med 1974;80:693–696.

28. New MI. Minireview: 21-hydroxylase deficiency congenital adrenal hyperplasia. J Steroid Biochem Molec Biol 1994;48:15–22.

29. Miller WL. Genetics, diagnosis, and management of 21-hydroxylase deficiency. J Clin Endocrinol Metab 1994;78:241–246.

30. Speiser PW, White PC, Dupont J, et al. Molecular genetic prenatal diagnosis of congenital adrenal hyperplasia due to 21-hydroxylase deficiency by allele-specific hybridization. Recent Prog Horm Res 1994;49:367–371.

31. Barbat B, Bogyo A, Raux-Dermay MC, et al. Screening of CYP21 gene mutations in 120 French patients affected by steroid 21-hydroxylase deficiency. Hum Mutat 1995;5:126–130.

32. Couillin P, Nicolas H, Boue J, et al. HLA typing of amniotic-fluid cells applied to prenatal diagnosis of congenital adrenal hyperplasia. Lancet 1979;1:1076.

33. Coursin DB, Wood KE. Corticosteroid supplementation for adrenal insufficiency. JAMA. 2002;287:236–240.

34. Merke DP, Cutler GB. New ideas for medical treatment of congenital adrenal hyperplasia. Endocrinol Metab Clin North Am 2001;30:121–135.

35. David M, Forest MG. Prenatal treatment of congenital adrenal hyperplasia resulting from 21-hydroxy-lase deficiency. J Pediatr 1984;105:799–803.

36. Speiser PW. First trimester prenatal treatment and molecular genetic diagnosis of congenital adrenal hyperplasia (21-hydroxylase deficiency). J Clin Endocrinol Metab. 1990;70:838–848.

37. Speiser PW, New MI. Prenatal diagnosis and treatment of congenital adrenal hyperplasia. J Ped Endocrinol 1994;7:183–191.

38. New MI, Carlson A, Obeid J, et al. Prenatal diagnosis for congenital adrenal hyperplasia in 532 pregnancies. J Clin Endocrinol Metab. 2001;86:5651–5657

39. Lajic S, Wedell A, Bui TH, et al. Long-term somatic follow-up of prenatally treated children with congenital adrenal hyperplasia. J Clin Endocrinol Metab. 1998;83:3872–3880.

40. Mulaikal RM, Migeon CJ, Rock JA. Fertility rates in female patients with congenital adrenal hyper-plasia due to 21-hydroxylase deficiency. N Engl J Med 1987;316:178–188.

41. Dittmann RW, Kappes ME, Kappes MH. Sexual behavior in adolescent and adult females with con-genital adrenal hyperplasia. Psychoneuroendocrinology 1992;17:153–170.

42. Kuhnle U, Bollinger M, Schwarz HP, et al. Partnership and sexuality in adult female patients with congenital adrenal hyperplasia: first results of a cross-sectional qualtiy-of-life evaluation. J Steroid Biochem Mol Biol 1993;45:123–126.

43. Lajic S, Wedell A, Ritzen EM, et al. Scandinavian experience of prenatal treatment of congenital adrenal hyperplasia. Horm Res 1997;48:22.

44. Buescher MA, McClamrock HD, Adashi EY. Cushing's syndrome in pregnancy. Obstet Gynecol 1992;79:130–137.

45. Forest MG, Betuel H, David M. Prenatal treatment in congenital adrenal hyperplasia due to 21-hydroxylase deficiency: update 88 of the French multicentric study. Endocr Res 1989;15:277–301.

46. Dorr HG, Sippell WG, Willig RP. Praenatale Diagnostik und Therapie des Adrenogenitalen Syndroms (AGS) mit 21-Hydroxylase Defekt. Monatsschr Kinderheilkd 1992;140:661–663.

47. Forest MG, David M, Morel Y. Prenatal diagnosis and treatment of 21-hydroxylase deficiency. J Steroid Biochem Mol Biol 1993;45:75–82.

48. Pang S, Clark AT, Freeman LC, et al. Maternal side-effects of prenatal dexamethasone therapy for fetal congenital adrenal hyperplasia. J Clin Endocrinol Metab 1992;75:249–253.

49. Mercado AB, Wilson RC, Cheng KC, et al. Prenatal treatment and diagnosis of congenital adrenal hyperplasia owing to 21-hydroxylase deficiency. J Clin Endocrinol Metab1995;80:2014–2020.

50. Seckl JR, Miller WL. Commentary: how safe is long-term prenatal glucocorticoid treatment? J Am Med Assoc 1997;277:1077–1079.

51. Uno H, Lohmiller L, Thieme C, et al. Brain damage induced by prenatal exposure to dexamethasone in fetal rhesus macaques. I. Hippocampus. Brain Res Dev 1990;53:157–167.

52. Trautman PD, Meyer-Bahlburg HFL, Postelnek J, New MI. Effects of early prenatal dexamethasone on the cognitive and behavioral development of young children: results of a pilot study. Psychoneuro-endocrinology 1995;20:439–449.

17

Mineralocorticoid Deficiency Syndromes

Robert G. Dluhy, MD

MINERALOCORTICOID PHYSIOLOGY

Aldosterone, the most important mineralocorticoid in humans, is produced in the zona glomerulosa of the adrenal cortex. It acts on the principal cells of the distal convoluted tubule of the kidney, intestine, and salivary gland to stimulate sodium absorption and potassium excretion. The adrenocortical steroidogenic cells of the zona glomerulosa are unique in that they express aldosterone synthase (18-hydroxylase) activity, which converts corticosterone to aldosterone. On the other hand, these cells lack 17α-hydroxylase activity, which is present in the cortisol-producing zona fasciculata.

Although the control of cortisol secretion is primarily regulated by adrenocorticotropin (ACTH), the control of aldosterone secretion is more complex. There are two major secretagogues of aldosterone secretion: potassium and angiotensin II. Minor regulators that either stimulate or inhibit aldosterone secretion include ACTH, vasopressin, dopamine, atrial natriuretic peptide, serotonin, somatostatin, and β-adrenergic agents.

Potassium depolarizes voltage-sensitive calcium channels on the plasma membrane of cells of the zona glomerulosa, resulting in an influx of calcium. This increase in cytosolic calcium activates a cascade of second messengers that result in aldosterone synthesis and release from the cell.

The renin–angiotensin system is the other major regulator of aldosterone secretion. The juxtaglomerular apparatus, a baroreceptor located in the afferent arteriole, and the macula densa in the distal convoluted tubule of the kidney, regulate renin release in response to stretch and the ion content of the luminal tubular fluid, respectively. The

From: *Endocrine Replacement Therapy in Clinical Practice*
Edited by: A. Wayne Meikle © Humana Press Inc., Totowa, NJ

enzyme renin is the rate-limiting step in the production of angiotensin II (Ang II). An increase in the release of renin results in action on angiotensinogen to produce the decapeptide Ang I. Angiotensin-converting enzyme (ACE) converts this inactive peptide into the biologically active octapeptide angiotensin II (Ang II), a potent vasoconstrictor as well as a secretagogue of aldosterone. Ang II can be further metabolized to angiotensin III, which is equipotent in its effects on aldosterone secretion but lacks the vasoconstrictive properties of Ang II.

The renin–angiotensin system was previously viewed as a classic circulating hormonal system; recent studies have shown that all components of this system are also present in the kidney, heart, and peripheral vasculature, allowing for the local (paracrine) regulation of function by tissue Ang II.

Adrenocoticotropin can transiently increase aldosterone levels, particularly during stress. However, in ACTH-deficient patients, such as steroid-suppressed subjects, aldosterone secretion is still normally regulated by potassium and the renin–angiotensin system.

ALDOSTERONE-DEFICIENCY SYNDROMES

Although the causes of aldosterone deficiency are numerous (*see* Table 1), the clinical presentation is often similar with the severity of the syndrome related to the degree of the hormonal-deficiency state. A useful approach for organizing the diagnosis of these conditions (*see* Fig. 1) is based on the renin status of the patient; aldosterone deficiency can therefore be classified as hyporeninemic (secondary) or hyperreninemic (primary). Thus, hypoaldosteronism can arise from a deficiency of aldosterone secretagogues (primarily renin) or as a result of adrenocortical failure. In the latter circumstance as well as in aldosterone resistant states, the renin levels will be elevated. Drugs can produce mineralocorticoid deficiency by a variety of mechanisms including renin–angiotensin lowering actions, effects on adrenocortical steroidogenesis, or antagonizing the actions of aldosterone (*see* Table 2).

Hyporeninemic Hypoaldosteronism

ACQUIRED

Hyporeninemic hypoaldosteronism (HH) accounts for approx 10% of all cases of hyperkalemia and up to 50% of previously unexplained hyperkalemia (*1*). It is a heterogeneous syndrome in which isolated aldosterone deficiency results from decreased renin release from the kidney. Acute provocative maneuvers, such as sodium restriction, volume depletion with diuretics, and upright posture, fail to simulate renin release. Aldosterone responsiveness to Ang II and ACTH is variable, and patients also fail to exhibit normal potassium-stimulated aldosterone production (*2*).

This syndrome has multiple etiologies and occurs most commonly in the seventh decade of life. Most patients have mild to moderate renal insufficiency. However, creatinine clearance exceeds the levels that usually are associated with hyperkalemia (<10 mL/min). Diabetes mellitus is the most common disease associated with HH, but other concurrent illnesses such as multiple myeloma, systemic lupus erythematosis, amyloidosis, cirrhosis, acquired immunodeficiency syndrome (AIDS) or sickle cell disease have also been reported. It has been hypothesized that autonomic insufficiency (often seen in long-standing diabetes mellitus) and/or renal prostaglandin deficiency

Table 1
Etiologies of Aldosterone-Deficiency/Resistance States

Secretagogue deficiency
    Hyporeninemia
    Diabetes mellitus
    Drugs (β-blockers, prostaglandin inhibitors)
    Angiotensin II deficiency (ACE inhibitors) or blockade (AT1 receptor antagonists)
    Hypokalemia
Adrenocortical dysfunction
    Autoimmune destruction (idiopathic Addison's disease)
    Adrenal hemorrhage
    Infectious/infiltrative diseases (e.g., cytomegalovirus in AIDS patients)
    Steroidogenic defects (CMO deficiency)
    Drugs (heparin)
Intrinsic renal abnormalities
    Mineralocorticoid receptor
        Mutation (autosomal dominant pseudohypoaldosteronism type I [PHA I])
        Drugs (spironolactone, eplerenone)
    Epithelial sodium channel
        Mutation (autosomal recessive PHA I)
        Drugs (amiloride, trimethoprim, triamterene)

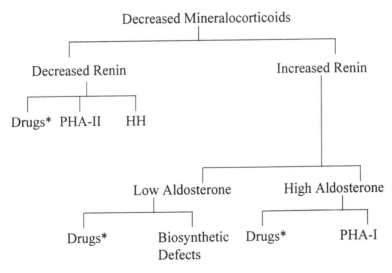

Fig. 1. Diagnostic algorithm for the mineralocorticoid-deficient patient. *See* Table 2. PHA, pseudohypoaldosteronism; HH, hyporeninemic hypoaldosteronism.

(including nonsteroidal anti-inflammatory medications) are alternative mechanisms that underlie the hyporeninemic state. Additionally, some patients with renal insufficiency are volume expanded, and this may contribute to the suppressed renin levels.

The diagnosis of HH is established by demonstrating subnormal stimulation of renin and aldosterone levels following stimulation maneuvers such as upright posture and a low-sodium diet (or acute volume depletion with a diuretic such as furosemide). Cortisol

Table 2
Drug-Induced Hyperkalemia

Hypoaldosteronism
    Prostaglandin Inhibitors (inhibit renin release and aldosterone synthesis)
    β-blockers (inhibit renin release)
    ACE inhibitors (inhibit angiotensin II generation)
    Heparin (inhibits aldosterone synthesis)
    Angiotensin II receptors blockers (inhibit angiotensin II action)
Decreased renal kaliuresis
    Potassium-sparing diuretics (spironolactone, amiloride, triamterene)
    Cyclosporine
    Lithium
    Digitalis
    Trimethoprim
    Pentamidine
Altered potassium distribution
    β-blockers
    α-blockers
    Hypertonic solutions (glucose, mannitol, saline)
    Digitalis
    Succinylcholine
    Insulin antagonists (somatostatin, diazoxide) or deficiency (diabetes mellitus)

Source: Adapted from ref. *2a*.

levels, by definition, are normal and show normal responsiveness to cosyntropin. Serum potassium is consistently elevated, although symptomatic hyperkalemia is unusual. At least half of such patients also demonstrate hyperchloremic metabolic acidosis.

Treatment of the hyperkalemic HH is at the outset to limit potassium intake (40–60 mmol/d). Potassium-binding resins (Kayexalate®) and loop diuretics (furosemide) can also be used. Mineralocorticoid treatment with fludrocortisone (Florinef®) in doses of 0.05 to 0.2 mg daily in conjunction with a high sodium (150–200 mmol/d) diet is also effective. However patients with renal and/or cardiac disease may not tolerate this volume-expanding regimen.

GENETIC PSEUDOHYPOALDOSTERONISM TYPE II

Pseudohypoaldosteronism type II (PHA II), or Gordon's syndrome *(3)*, is inherited in an autosomal dominant fashion *(4)*. The phenotype of PHA II includes hypertension, suppressed plasma renin activity, metabolic acidosis, and hyperkalemia. Patients have normal renal function, which serves to distinguish them from patients with HH.

Pseudohypoaldosteronism type II is thought to arise from enhanced absorption of chloride ions in the early portions of the distal tubule, causing proximal sodium reabsorption. This increased absorption of sodium chloride causes volume expansion and suppression of the renin–angiotensin system. Low luminal sodium concentrations may impair distal tubular potassium secretion, resulting in hyperkalemia (which increases aldosterone levels to a variable degree through potassium-stimulated aldosterone production *[5]*). There also may be a primary defect in distal tubule potassium secretion. Mutations in gene encoding the WNK family of serine–threonine kinases in the distal nephron cause PHA II.

Hyperreninemic Hypoaldosteronism

PRIMARY ADRENAL FAILURE

Primary adrenal failure usually does not cause isolated mineralocorticoid deficiency, but rather combined glucocorticoid and mineralocorticoid deficiencies (6). Rarely, however, isolated mineralocorticoid deficiency may be seen (7). Most cases result from autoimmune adrenal destruction but primary adrenal failure can also be seen as a result of bilateral adrenal hemorrhage (8), tumor infiltration of the adrenal glands, some infections (AIDS [7], histoplasmosis, mycobacterial infections, cytomegalovirus) or infiltrative diseases (amyloidosis [9], hemochromatosis).

Treatment should focus on correcting the underlying illness, as some patients will have restoration of adrenocortical function after appropriate therapy. Usually, combined glucocorticoid and mineralocorticoid replacement therapies are needed.

ACUTE, SEVERE ILLNESS

Critically ill patients can show selective hypoaldosteronism with elevated plasma renin activity (PRA) (10), but these patients are not characteristically hyperkalemic. The fact that plasma cortisol levels are normal or high in these subjects, indicates that there is selective adrenal deficiency of the zona glomerulosa. When ACTH is administered to these subjects cortisol responses are normal, but aldosterone shows a minimal response. There may be diminished aldosterone responsiveness to the infusion of Ang II in some of these patients as well (10).

The etiology of this syndrome is not understood. A number of possibilities for the selective hypoaldosteronism exist, but the most likely explanation relates to the chronic, stress-related elevation of ACTH leading to altered steroidogenesis, favoring normal cortisol production but diminished production of mineralocorticoids such as aldosterone, corticosterone and 18-hydroxycorticosterone (11,12). Chronic hypoxia, as is seen with exposure to high altitudes, has been shown to result in hyperreninemic hypoaldosteronism with preserved cortisol biosynthesis (13). Because many critically ill patients experience hypoxemia over the course of their illness, this may contribute to their hypoaldosteronism as well. Finally, hypokalemia, another common occurrence in the critically ill patient, may also contribute to the selective hypoaldosteronism.

BIOSYNTHETIC DEFECTS

Congenital hypoaldosteronism is a rare genetic disorder with an autosomal recessive pattern of inheritance. It is caused by deficiency of corticosterone 18-methyl oxidase (CMO, or P450c11Aldo), the enzyme that catalyzes the conversion of corticosterone to aldosterone (see Fig. 2). Mutations in the gene coding for P450c11Aldo (CYP11B2) have been described that affect both CMO I (14–16) and CMO II (17) isoenzymes, but CMO I deficiency is less common. Patients present with signs of hypoaldosteronism such as sodium wasting, hyponatremia, hyperkalemia, metabolic acidosis, and hypotension. During infancy, CMO deficiency can also cause growth retardation. Hyper–reninemia in infancy is marked but lacks diagnostic specificity because elevated renin levels are also seen in primary adrenal failure (Addison's disease) as well as in the aldosterone-resistance syndromes (see the following section). Symptoms are most pronounced early in life and tend to improve gradually as the child ages.

Both CMO I and CMO II deficiency can be difficult to differentiate clinically or in severity of symptoms (18). However, the syndromes are easily differentiated biochemically. CMO II is characterized by extremely high 18-hydroxycorticosterone levels, with

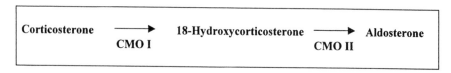

Fig. 2. Biosynthetic pathway of aldosterone production from its precursor corticosterone. Congenital hypoaldosteronism results from a deficiency in corticosterone 18-methyl oxidase (CMO). CMO I and II deficiencies have similar clinical presentations but can be biochemically differentiated by the elevation of 18-hydroxycorticosterone levels in CMO II deficiency; in contrast, levels of this compound are subnormal in CMO I deficiency.

a ratio of 18-hydroxycorticosterone to aldosterone exceeding *(5)*. In contrast, subnormal levels of 18-hydroxycorticosterone are seen in CMO I deficiency. Treatment is similar for both syndromes and involves mineralocorticoid replacement with fludrocortisone *(19)*.

Aldosterone-Resistance Syndromes

PSEUDOHYPOALDOSTERONISM TYPE I

There are both autosomal dominant and recessive forms of pseudohypoaldosteronism type I (PHA I). PHA I features include renal salt wasting, hyperkalemia, and metabolic acidosis in presence of markedly elevated aldosterone levels (so-called pseudo-hypoaldosteronism) *(20)*.

The rare, autosomal recessive disorder results from mutations of the aldosterone-regulated amiloride-sensitive epithelial sodium channel (ENaC), resulting in loss of ENaC function *(21)*. Infants with this syndrome show phenotypic features of hypoaldosteronism, including renal salt wasting, hypotension, hyperkalemia, and hyperchloremic metabolic acidosis. Affected individuals also exhibit marked elevation of plasma renin activity and plasma aldosterone levels. Treatment with exogenous mineralocorticoids logically does not correct the hyperkalemia because of the renal resistant state *(22)*. Therapy includes administration of potassium-binding resins, potassium-wasting diuretics, and high sodium intake to maintain extracellular and intravascular volume. The syndrome is often self-limited, and salt supplementation can often be discontinued after several years.

The autosomal dominant form of PHA I results from heterozygous loss-of-function mutations in the mineralocorticoid receptor (MR). This loss of MR function results in reduced EnaC activity and phenotypic features early in life similar to the recessive PHA I disorder. Characteristically, these patients become asymptomatic later in life.

PSEUDOHYPOALDOSTERONISM TYPE III

Pseudohypoaldosteronism type III (PHA III) is most commonly diagnosed in normotensive adults with hyperkalemia. Plasma aldosterone are elevated and there is impaired renal potassium excretory capacity which is refractory to exogenous mineralocorticoids. Most patients have tubulointerstitial renal disease (Fanconi syndrome, multiple myeloma, etc.). Treatment involves use of kaliuretic diuretics, potassium-binding resins, and sodium chloride supplementation to maintain intravascular volume.

DRUG-INDUCED HYPERKALEMIC STATES

Aldosterone Deficiency

INHIBITORS OF RENIN RELEASE

Inhibitors of the cyclooxygenase pathway of prostaglandin synthesis have been shown to reversibly inhibit renin release independent of the precipitation of renal insufficiency resulting from the reduction of renal blood flow (23,24). However, patients with under-lying renal insufficiency (particularly diabetes mellitus—*see* section on Hyporeninemic Hypoaldosteronism) are at higher risk for clinically significant hypoaldosteronism and resultant hyperkalemia when treated with these medications. Because another important determinant of renin release is the sympathetic nervous system (25,26), interruption of the adrenergic system with β-blockers can inhibit renin release, thereby secondarily decreasing the production of Ang II and aldosterone. However, precipitation of hyper-kalemia with β-blockers alone is rare, usually occurring in patients with preexisting chronic renal insufficiency and/or diabetes mellitus.

INHIBITORS OF ANG II PRODUCTION OR ACTION

In normal subjects ACE inhibitors modestly reduce aldosterone levels by inhibiting Ang II formation. They can precipitate hyperkalemia, but usually this occurs only in the setting of underlying renal insufficiency or bilateral renal artery stenosis. This is particu-larly important in diabetic patients where ACE inhibitors are the agents of choice to reduce protein excretion and preserve renal function. Angiotensin type I receptor an-tagonists (e.g., losartan, valsartan) block the actions of Ang II in target tissues, resulting also in a reduction of aldosterone levels. However, hyperkalemia is uncommonly seen with these agents, but it would be anticipated in patients with renal insufficiency.

INHIBITORS OF ALDOSTERONE SECRETION OR ACTION

Heparin, even in low doses, has been shown to cause hypoaldosteronism and hyper-kalemia (27–29). A number of mechanisms have been proposed. Chlorbutal, a preser-vative additive to commercial heparin preparations, has been shown to inhibit both the early and late biosynthetic phases of aldosterone production (30). Heparin decreases Ang II-mediated aldosterone production by decreasing receptor number and binding affinity on adrenal glomerulosa cells (31). Higher doses of heparin can also impair ACTH and potassium-stimulated aldosterone production (30). These effects may be seen as early as 4 d after initiation of therapy. Although aldosterone levels may be reduced to some extent in all patients on heparin therapy, most subjects do not show overt hypoaldosteronism because they are able to compensate by increasing renin release from the kidney. Individuals with diabetes mellitus, renal insufficiency, or critical illness may exhibit impaired compensation and are therefore at higher risk of developing heparin-induced hypoaldosteronism. A high index of suspicion must be maintained when such patients are given heparin so that hypoaldosteronism can be recognized early and severe hyperkalemia avoided.

In addition to inhibiting renin release, prostaglandin synthase inhibitors have also been shown to inhibit aldosterone secretion directly (23). Spironolactone can cause "functional" hypoaldosteronism by antagonizing the actions of aldosterone at the min-eralocorticoid receptor. Amiloride, triamterene, and trimethoprim therapy can all result in hyperkalemia; the mechanism of action is independent of aldosterone and involves a direct effect of the drug on blocking the aldosterone-regulated ENaC. This results in reduction of the transepithelial voltage in the renal tubule thus inhibiting kaliuresis *(32)*.

TREATMENT OF MINERALOCORTICOID DEFICIENCY

General Principles

There are several goals of therapy in mineralocorticoid deficient patients. The first is to assess the severity of the hyperkalemia and institute immediate treatment if required.

Hyperkalemia may require emergency treatment when it is severe and especially if it occurs rapidly. Electrocardiographic features of life-threatening hyperkalemia (peaked T-waves, shortening of QTc, widening of QRS) mandate immediate emergency treatment 33. Intravenous calcium gluconate (two to four ampules of 10% calcium gluconate) or calcium chloride (10 mL of 10% calcium chloride over 2–5 min) will acutely raise the threshold potential of cell membranes and lower excitability. Extracellular potassium can also be temporarily shifted into the intracellular compartment by intravenous administration of insulin (5 U Regular insulin with 50 mL of 50% dextrose to prevent hypoglycemia) or sodium bicarbonate (50–150 meq sodium bicarbonate) and by nebulized albuterol. However, maneuvers to shift potassium into the intracellular compartment are only temporizing measures, lasting 20–30 min. Additional long-term therapies should be simultaneously initiated and directed at the etiology of the hyperkalemic state.

Acidosis should be corrected with intravenous sodium bicarbonate administration. Hemodialysis can rapidly lower blood potassium levels and may be needed in some emergency cases. Additional therapies to lower potassium, such as potassium-binding resins (15–20 g po q2h Kayexelate®; 50 g po/pr q4-6h Resonium®) are useful in chronic hyperkalemic states, such as renal insufficiency (1 g of Kayexelate, has an in vitro exchange capacity of about 3 meq of potassium). Potassium-binding resins should be complimented by a low-potassium diet and, if needed, potassium-wasting diuretics (primarily furosemide). Some of these therapies, especially diuretics, are useful in treating elderly patients with hypoaldosteronism who are prone to volume overload as a result of renal insufficiency and/or congestive heart failure. In the aldosterone-insufficient subject, correction of the deficiency will ultimately restore potassium homeostasis by promoting kaliuresis. Finally, it is necessary to identify possible medications that may have precipitated or worsened the hyperkalemic state (*see* Table 2). Medications such as ACE inhibitors should be discontinued and judiciously reinstated later if they are felt to be absolutely necessary for the management of the patient.

A second major goal of therapy is to simultaneously correct the volume depletion and hypotension that may occur in some mineralocorticoid-deficient patients. Patients should be given intravenous isotonic saline or be maintained on a high-salt diet; sodium chloride tablets (10–12 g/d) may be useful in some patients. However, caution should be exercised not to overhydrate hyperkalemic patients who may also be concomitantly volume expanded (such as patients with renal insufficiency).

Mineralocorticoid Replacement

Along with a normal sodium intake (100–150 mmol/d), fludrocortisone (Florinef®), a synthetic mineralocorticoid, is the cornerstone of maintenance therapy of the aldosterone-deficient patient. Most patients with aldosterone insufficiency require a daily dose of 0.1 mg/d (dose range: 0.05–0.2 mg/d). Larger doses may be needed in selected patients, such as subjects with HH and PHA III. Fludrocortisone can be administered in a single daily dose, although patients who require larger doses may benefit from twice-a-day dosing. Therapy should be initiated at low doses, especially in the elderly or in patients with a history of congestive heart failure. When increasing the dose of fludrocortisone, patients should have their dosage increased gradually over days to prevent excessive sodium retention or rapid volume expansion. Ambulatory patients can monitor adequacy of treatment by recording accurate daily weights as a sensitive measure of salt and water retention.

Mineralocorticoid treatment is usually not necessary in the hospitalized patient with acute primary adrenal insufficiency. In such patients, the pharmacological doses of parenteral glucocorticoids that are commonly used to prevent adrenal crisis (bolus hydrocortisone, 100 mg iv q8h or continuous hydrocortisone infusion, 10 mg/h) exert sufficient mineralocorticoid action to obviate the need for mineralocorticoid treatment. In addition, there are no parenteral mineralocorticoid formulations available to treat patients whose oral intake has been curtailed. Another cornerstone of management in acutely ill patients who are mineralocorticoid deficient is adequate sodium repletion, primarily with isotonic saline. It is emphasized that mineralocorticoid treatment alone can never replete extracellular volume in a mineralocorticoid and volume-depleted subject without providing adequate substrate (sodium). Careful attention should also be given to maintenance of blood pressure and renal function (such as the BUN/creatinine ratio and adequate urine output).

REFERENCES

1. Tan SY, Burton M. Hyporeninemic hypoaldosteronism. An overlooked cause of hyperkalemia. Arch Intern Med 1981;141:30–33.
2. Schambelan M, Stockigt JR, Biglieri EG. Isolated hypoaldosteronism in adults: a renin-deficiency syndrome. N Engl J Med 1972;287:573.
2a. DeFronzo RA, Bia M, Smith D. Clinical disorders of hyperkalemia. Annu Rev Med 1982;33:521–554.
3. Gordon RD. Syndrome of hypertension and hyperkalemia with normal glomerular filtration rate. Hypertension 1986;8:93.
4. Mansfield TA, Simon DB, Farfel Z, Bia M, Tucci JR, Lebel M, et al. Multilocus linkage of familial hyperkalaemia and hypertension, pseudohypoaldosteronism type II, to chromosomes 1q31-42 and 7p11-q21. Nat Genet 1997;16(2):202-205.
5. Schambelan M, et al. Mineralocorticoid-resistant renal hyperkalemia without salt-wasting (type II pseudohypoaldosteronism): Role of increased renal chloride reabsorption. Kidney Int 1981;19:716.
6. Oelkers W. Adrenal insufficiency. N Engl J Med 1996;335:1206–1212.
7. Guy RJ, Turberg Y, Davidson RN, et al. Mineralocorticoid deficiency in HIV infection . Br Med J 1989;298:496–497.
8. Dahlberg PJ, Goellner MH, Pehling GB. Adrenal insufficiency secondary to adrenal hemorrhage. Two case reports and a review of cases confirmed by computed tomography. Arch Intern Med 1990;150:905–909.
9. Agmon D, Green J, Platau E, et al. Isolated adrenal mineralocorticoid deficiency due to amyloidosis associated with familial Mediterranean fever. Am J Med Sci 1984;288:40–43.
10. Zipser RD, Davenport MW, Martin KL, et al. Hyperreninemic hypoaldosteronism in the critically ill: a new entity. J Clin Endocrinol Metab 1981;53:867–873.
11. Biglieri EG, Schambelan M, Slaton Jr. PE. Effect of adrenocorticotropin on desoxycorticosterone, corticosterone and aldosterone excretion. J Clin Endocrinol Metab 1969;29:1091.
12. Kraiem Z, Rosenthal T, Rotzak R, et al. Angiotensin II and K challenge followed by prolonged ACTH administration in normal subjects. ACTA Endocrinol (Copenh) 1979;91:657.
13. Slater JDH, Tuffley RE, Williams ES, et al. Control of aldosterone secretion during acclimatization to hypoxia in man. Clin Sci 1969;37:237.
14. Nomoto S, Massa G, Mitani F, et al. CMO I deficiency caused by a point mutation in exon 8 of the human CYP11B2 gene encoding steroid 18-hydroxylase (P450C18). Biochem Biophys Res Commun 1997;234(2:)382–385.

15. Mitsuuchi Y, Kawamoto T, Miyahara K, et al. Congenitally defective aldosterone biosynthesis in humans: inactivation of the P-450C18 gene (CYP11B2) due to nucleotide deletion in CMO I deficient patients. Biochem Biophys Res Commun 1993;190:(3)864–869.

16. Peter M, Fawaz L, Drop SLS, et al. A prismatic case. Hereditary defect in biosynthesis of aldosterone: aldosterone synthase deficiency 1964–1997. J Clin Endocrinol Metab 1997;82(11):3525–3528.

17. Mitsuuchi Y, Kawamoto T, Naiki Y, et al. Congenitally defective aldosterone biosynthesis in humans: the involvement of point mutations of the P-450C18 gene (CYP11B2) in CMO II deficient patients. Biochem Biophys Res Commun 1992;182(2):974–979.

18. Peter M, Sippel WG. Congenital hypoaldosteronism: the Visser-Cost-Syndrome revisited. Pediatr Res 1996;39:554–560.

19. Yong AB, Montalto J, Pitt J, et al. Corticosterone methyl oxidase type II (CMO II) deficiency: biochemical approach to diagnosis. Clin Biochem 1994;27:(6)491–494.

20. Cheek DB, Perry JW. A salt-wasting syndrome in infancy. Arch Dis Child 1958;33:252.

21. Chang SS, Grunder S, Hanukoglu A, et al. Mutations in subunits of the epithelial sodium channel cause salt wasting with hyperkalaemic acidosis, pseudohypoaldosteronism type 1. Nat Genet 1996;12:(3)248–253.

22. Oberfield SE, et al. Pseudohypoaldosteronism: multiple target organ unresponsiveness to mineralocorticoid hormones. J Clin Endocrinol Metab 1979;48:228.

23. Saruta T, Kaplan NM. Adrenocortical steroidogenesis: the effects of prostaglandins. J Clin Invest 1972;51:2246.

24. Franco-Saenz R, et al. Prostaglandins and renin production: a review. Prostaglandins 1980;20:1131.

25. Holdaas H, Dibona GF, Kiil F. Effect of low-level renal nerve stimulation on renin release from non-filtering kidneys. Am J Physiol 1981;241:F156–F161.

26. Gross R, Hackenberg HM, Hackenthal E, et al. Interaction between perfusion pressure and sympathetic nerves in renin release by carotid baroreflex in conscious dogs. J Physiol 1981;313:237–250.

27. Oster JR, Singer I, Fishman LM. Heparin-induced hypoaldosteronism and hyperkalemia. Am J Med 1995;98(6):575–586.

28. Aull L, Chao H, Coy K. Heparin-induced hyperkalemia. DICP 1990;24:244–246.

29. Levesque H, Verdier S, Cailleux N, et al. Low molecular weight heparins and hypoaldosteronism. Br Med J 1990;300:1437–1438.

30. Sequeira SJ, McKenna TJ. Chlorbutal, a new inhibitor of aldosterone biosynthesis identified during examination of heparin effect on aldosterone production. J Clin Endocrinol Metab 1986;63(6):780–784.

31. Azukizawa S, Iwasaki I, Kigoshi T, et al. Effects of heparin treatments in vivo and in vitro on adrenal angiotensin II receptors and angiotensin II-induced aldosterone production in rats. ACTA Endocrinol (Copenh) 1988;119(3):367–372.

32. Velazquez H, Perazella MA, Wright FS, et al. Renal mechanism of trimethoprim-induced hyperkalemia. Ann Intern Med 1993;119(4):296–301.

33. Clark BA, Brown RS. Potassium homeostasis and hyperkalemic syndromes. Endocrinol Clin N Am 1995;24(3):573–591.

18 Dehydroepiandrosterone and Pregnenolone

Syed H Tariq, MD, Hosam Kamel, MD, and John E. Morley, MB, BCh

CONTENTS

INTRODUCTION
DHEA
PREGNENOLONE
CONCLUSIONS
REFERENCES

INTRODUCTION

Steroid hormones play a multifactorial role in human physiology. They facilitate coordinative processes that enable neural, endocrine, immune, and metabolic systems separately or collectively, to operate in solving problems of survival and reproduction. Both pregnenolone and dehydroepiandrosterone (DHEA) are key hormones early in the pathway of steroid hormones biosynthesis (see Fig. 1). Pregnenolone is the precursor of all the known steroid hormones, and its formation from cholesterol via the action of cytochrome P450scc, is the rate-limiting step in steroid hormone formation. DHEA and its sulfated conjugate, dehydroepiandrosterone sulfate (DHEAS), on the other hand, serve as precursors for both androgenic and estrogenic steroids and are the most abundant steroid hormones in the human body. Furthermore, based on multiple animal and human studies, there is now accumulating evidence to suggest a potential role for both of these hormones in the prevention of multiple morbidities associated with aging process. This chapter reviews the biological roles of DHEA and pregnenolone with aging process and draws implications for their possible role as antiaging agents.

DHEA

Dehydroepiandrosterone and its sulfated conjugate, DHEAS, are the most abundant steroid hormones in the human body (1). Despite this, very little is known about their physiological role.

From: *Endocrine Replacement Therapy in Clinical Practice*
Edited by: A. Wayne Meikle © Humana Press Inc., Totowa, NJ

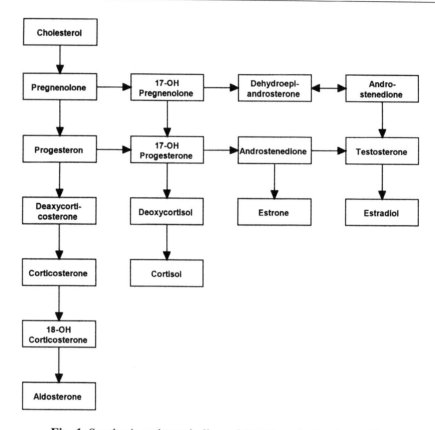

Fig. 1. Synthesis and metabolism of DHEA and related steroids.

For many years, DHEA has enjoyed the reputation that it is the fountain of youth even though evidence for its beneficial effects in humans was virtually nonexistent. Over the past decade, however, this situation has changed. Two observations renewed interest among aging researchers in DHEA and DHEAS. First, there is a decline in circulating levels of these hormones with aging. Second, animal studies have demonstrated the beneficial effects of DHEA administration in preventing obesity, diabetes, cancer, and heart disease, and in enhancing the immune system. Collectively, these observations have led investigators to question whether DHEA administration can reverse some of the degenerative changes associated with human aging. This resulted in several human studies being conducted that tested the effects of DHEA administration on various organ systems. In this chapter, we discuss the biological role of DHEA and review its antiaging effects as demonstrated by both animal and human studies, with special emphasis on the latter (*see* Appendix for an overview of human DHEA studies).

DHEA: Synthesis and Biological Role

Dehydroepiandrosterone is a C-19 steroid first isolated in 1934 from urine by Butenandt and Dannenbaum *(2)*. Most DHEA is produced in the adrenal cortex from cholesterol and another 5% is produced by the testes and ovaries *(3)*. Ninety-nine percent of circulating DHEA is the water-soluble sulfate conjugate DHEAS. Baulieu et al. have shown that free DHEA and DHEAS as metabolically active interconvertible by phosphoadenosine–phosposulfate-dependent sulfotransferase *(4,5)*. DHEA(S) circulates in the blood in a free form as well as bound to albumin and sex-hormone-binding globulin (SHBG) *(6)*.

How DHEA exerts its biologic actions remains a mystery. DHEA may act by influencing several key metabolic enzymes, such as glucose-6-phosphate dehydrogenase or glycerol-3-phosphate dehydrogenase, by altering physicochemical parameters via interpolation into cellular membranes, or by conversion to androgens, estrogens, or other metabolites. A putative binding site for DHEA has been demonstrated on hepatocytes and human leukocytes, but a specific DHEA receptor has not yet been characterized *(1)*.

DHEA and Aging

Both cross-sectional *(7)* and longitudinal studies *(8)* have demonstrated the decline of DHEA and DHEAS levels with advancing age. Liu et al. *(9)* reported that there is progressive decline in DHEA and DHEAS with aging, reflecting a relative deficiency of 17,20-desmolase occurs in both men and women. Both 17α-hydroxylase and 17,20-desmolase are P450 enzymes encoded by a single gene *(10)*. There is a decrease in 17,20-desmolase activity, and 17α-hydroxylase activity is unchanged in older adults, suggesting a functional shift with aging opposite that is seen in puberty/adrenarche. Also, there is progressive blunting of adrenocorticotropin (ACTH)-mediated pulsatile activity of DHEA with advancing age *(11)*.

It has been shown that, with age, levels of DHEA and DHEAS in both sexes decrease at a relatively constant rate: 2.3% per year for men and 3.9% per year for women *(12)*. Hence, at age 80, levels are only about 20% of those at age 25 *(13)*. Most studies report 10–30% higher levels of DHEAS in young men than young women. This gender difference, however, largely disappears after age 50. Moreover, important genetic differences appear to exist, for example, Japanese men have significantly lower levels than American white men *(14)*.

The decline in DHEA serum levels with age is parallel to the development of decreased immunity, physical frailty, decreased muscle mass, increased fat mass, decreased ability to cope, disrupted sleep patterns, and increased incidents of disease *(see* Fig. 2). Thus, DHEA can be viewed as a marker of aging in humans *(13)*. Low serum levels of DHEAS have been related to increased all-cause and cardiovascular mortality in men over the age of 50 *(15)*. Recently, Baulieu et al. *(12)* reported in a prospective study with an 8-yr follow-up that no association was found among DHEA levels, mortality, and women, whereas in men, the lower the DHEA, the higher the risk of mortality under the age of 70 yr. In this study, the risk of death was higher in male smokers, suggesting that DHEA levels is a reliable predictor of death in male smokers.

DHEA: Antiaging Effects

Although numerous animal studies have demonstrated that DHEA has multiple antiaging effects, it should be kept in mind that most of these animal studies were conducted in rodents, which have little, if any, circulating DHEA. Hence, a major question is whether any of these beneficial consequences of DHEA administration demonstrated in animal models can be shown to be relevant in human beings. This led several investigators to administer DHEA to human studies. In the following sections, we explore the various effects of DHEA as demonstrated by both animal and human studies.

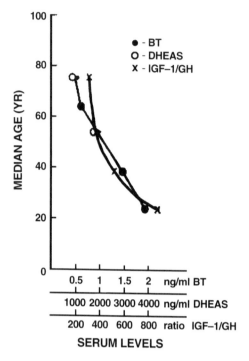

Fig. 2. Age-related decline in dehyroepiandrosterone sulfate in humans. (From ref. *140.*)

DHEA and Cardiovascular Disease

Lower levels of DHEA(S) and its urinary metabolites, 17 keto-steroids were found in men with artherosclerotic disease *(16–18)*. This led to the assumption that DHEA(S) might protect against cardiovascular disease *(19)*. Barrett-Connor et al. examined this hypothesis in a large 12-yr longitudinal study *(10)* and reported that DHEA(S) levels were inversely related to the cardiovascular mortality in men. However, this inverse association between DHEAS levels and cardiovascular disease has not been consistently found in subsequent studies in women *(20)* or in other cohorts *(21–23)*.

The association between DHEAS and cardiovascular disease in this epidemiologic data could be merely an epiphenomenon; that is, because the incidence of atherosclerosis is related to age, the decline in plasma DHEAS with aging may be coincidental and not casual *(24)*. The hypothesis that DHEA protect against cardiovascular diseases was tested in animal models. These studies showed that oral administration of DHEA has a great protective effect against atherosclerosis in cholesterol-fed animals *(25–27)*. Epidemiologic studies in human have shown conflicting reports with the effect limited to men. Zumoff et al. reported that men with abnormal coronary angiogram had lower levels of DHEAS than in men with no abnormality *(28)*. In another study, men with 50% or greater stenosis has significant lower DHEAS than with men without stenosis *(28a)*. In the Honolulu heart study, 82 men died during follow-up; after their autopsy, there was no significant association between baseline DHEAS levels and the extent of atherosclerosis *(21)*. In one study, women with definite diagnosis of coronary artery disease on angiography had lower levels of DHEAS than in women with angina but no definite lesions on angiography *(29)*. In a longitudinal study, the Massachusetts Women Health

Study reported that women with higher DHEA(S) levels might have greater risks factors for cardiovascular disease.

The association between DHEA(S) and total cholesterol varies *(30–32)*. Most of the studies failed to show any significant association between DHEA(S) and hugh-density lipoprotein (HDL)-cholesterol; one study reported a positive correlation *(31–33)*. Similarly, some have reported a positive correlation between low-density lipoprotein (LDL)-cholesterol and DHEAS; others have reported a negative association *(32,33)*.

Dehydroepiandrosterone possibly interferes with the atherogenic process by inhibiting glucose 6-phospahte dehydrogenase, which is the entry point into the pentose phosphate pathway *(34)*. Both in vitro and in vivo studies showed that DHEA and DHEAS have inhibitory effects on platelet activation. When DHEAS was added to pooled platelet-rich plasma before the addition of the agonist arachidonate, the platelet aggregation was inhibited. Inhibition of platelet aggregation by DHEA was both dose and time dependent. Inhibition of platelet aggregation by DHEA was accompanied by reduced platelet thromboxane B_2 production. The effect of DHEA on platelet function was also tested in vivo. In a randomized double-blinds study by Jesse et al. *(24)*, 10 normal men received either DHEA 300 mg ($n = 5$) or placebo capsule ($n = 5$) orally three times per day for 14 d. Platelet aggregation was either slowed or completely inhibited in the DHEA group.

Dehydroepiandrosterone administration has also been shown to enhance nitric oxide activity in human studies. Nitric oxide is a potent vasodilator; thus, vasodilation resulting from increased nitric oxide production is a mechanism that may be involved in the protective action of DHEA against coronary artery disease *(35)*. Finally, Beer et al., in a double-blind, placebo-controlled, study demonstrated that the administration of DHEA to human subjects caused a decrease in both plasma plasminogen activator inhibitor type 1 (PAI-1) and tissue plasminogen activator (tPA) antigens *(36)*. Both PAI-1 and tPA antigens are circulating markers of fibrinolytic potential, and their elevation is a risk factor for heart disease in men.

DHEA and Cancer

Animal studies have repeatedly shown that DHEA supplementation slows the development of several cancers such as testicular cancer *(37)*, skin cancer *(38)*, pancreatic cancer *(39)*, and colorectal cancer *(40)*. Epidemiological studies have shown low DHEA levels to be associated with premenopausal breast cancer *(41)*, gastric cancer *(42)*, lung cancer *(43)*, bladder cancer *(44)*, and hairy cell leukemia *(45)*.

The association between breast cancer and DHEAS is controversial. Helzlsouer et al. *(41)*, with a mean age of 40 yr, suggested that DHEAS levels were 10% lower in the subjects who developed breast cancer compared to control, but there was no difference in DHEA and DHEAS between the cases and controls. The odd ratio of developing premenopausal breast cancer for the upper tertile DHEAS is 0.4, for the middle tertile, it is 0.76 and for the lower tertile, it is 1, suggesting a dose-response relationship. Similarly, others have reported the same—that there is an increasing protective association between DHEAS and breast cancer *(18,46)*. There are reports suggesting that there is a difference in association between breast cancer and menopausal status. Barrett-Conner et al. *(47)* reported, in women aged 59–79 yr that after adjusting for age, body mass index, estrogen use, and smoking use there was no association between risk of breast cancer and DHEAS. They further concluded that DHEAS has no protective role in the development of postmenopausal breast cancer. In another prospective study of postmenopausal breast cancer, higher levels of DHEAS were associated with development of breast cancer compared to controls *(48)*. Hankinson et al. *(49)* reported in the Nurses Health Study that persons with elevated plasma estradiol, testosterone, and DHEAS were at significantly increasing risk when the relationship of each hormone was analyzed separately.

Dietary supplementation with DHEAS is taken to stop the aging process. In a recent review, Stoll et al. (50), suggested that prolonged intake of DHEA may stimulate postmenopausal breast cancer. This is particularly very important in women with postmenopausal obesity.

In vitro, DHEA has been shown to have paradoxical effects, slowing the growth of human breast cancer cells in some studies *(51,52)*, but not in others *(53)*. This was attributed to the activation of androgen receptors in a human breast cancer cell line *(52)*. Prospective human studies are required before definitive statements can be made concerning the role of DHEA supplementation in cancer prevention in humans.

DHEA and Immunomodualtion

Dehydroepiandrosterone improves the age-related decline in the immune system in older animals *(54)* and those with thermal injury *(55)*, and it reverses immune suppression by antigens used in higher doses *(56)*. In elderly individuals, there is decreased production of antibodies *(57)*, as a response to influenza, pneumococcal, and hepatitis B vaccines *(58)*. Primary immune response is markedly impaired *(59,60)*, but the response to recall antigen remains intact with aging *(61)*. When DHEA is administer to the elderly as an adjuvant to vaccines such as influenza, there was no improvement in immune response *(62)*; others reported that DHEA does not alter the immune system *(63,64)*.

Sepsis is associated with decreased cellular immune function, whereas DHEA is considered to have immunoenhancing properties. Male mice with sepsis when treated with DHEA have shown improvement in T-cell immunity and reduction in tumor necrosis factor (TNF)-α serum concentration, resulting in improved survival and a possible beneficial role in systemic inflammation (65). Rasmussen et al. has reported that higher doses of DHEA are required to protect the immune system of mice suppressed by both dexamethasone and infection *(66)* and to reduce mortality in mice infected with lethal injection *(67)*.

Dehydroepiandrosterone in a 3-mo randomized double-blind trial of 28 female patients with systemic lupus erythematosus (SLE) produced improvement in disease parameters tested using a scoring system and visual analog scale *(68)*. In another trial, there was no significant difference in patients with severe SLE in the control and treatment groups at 6 mo duration *(69)*. DHEA in a multicenter, randomized, placebo-controlled trial, produced a decrease in the use of corticosteroids in the treatment group compared to placebo *(70)*. The most frequent side effects were mild acneiform dermatitis and lowering of HDL-cholesterol long term.

Recently, there has been growing interest in DHEA in relation to the acquired immunodeficiency syndrome (AIDS). Changes in cytokine production in patients with AIDS are very similar to those seen in aging, but less dramatic. Chatteron et al. *(71)* in an 11-yr longitudinal study demonstrated that in patients infected with the human immunodeficiency virus (HIV) virus, there is a progressive decline in serum DHEA levels that, in some cases, preceded a precipitous fall in CD4 cell count. In another study by Dyner et al. *(144)*, DHEA supplementation to patients with AIDS resulted in a 40% reduction in serum neopterine, one of the markers of HIV infection progression, but it did not have any effect on CD4 cell count. Although the role of DHEA in the treatment of AIDS has not yet been determined, the drug appears to show potential for clinical benefit that warrants evaluation in large, randomized, controlled trials.

Dehydroepiandrosterone may produce its beneficial effects on the immune system by producing changes in cytokines (72), interleukins (73), and lymphocytes viability (74). Yen et al. (11) conducted a placebo-controlled trial in which he administered DHEA 50 mg/d to nine healthy older men for 5 mo duration. DHEA resulted in enhancing T-cell mitogenesis and natural-killer cell activity, as well as increased production of growth factors. Both the lymphoid system of human (75) and murine cell lines (76) have DHEA receptors.

DHEA and Diabetes Mellitus

Insulin action appears to influence DHEA metabolism. The human adrenal glands have receptors for insulin and insulin-like growth factor-I (77), suggesting a possible role for insulin in the regulation of adrenal function. Several epidemiologic studies report that serum DHEA in men is reduced in conditions such as obesity (78), hypertension (79), and untreated type 2 diabetes mellitus (80). In addition, Nestler et al. (81) reported that, in men, infusion of insulin acutely lowers the serum DHEA(S) level. Amelioration of insulin resistance and hyperinsulinemia is associated with a rise is serum DHEA over a broad range of ages (82). Insulin increases the metabolic clearance rate of DHEA (83), and inhibits adrenal androgen production (84).

These observations led investigators to suggest that reduced serum DHEA may be an indicator of insulin sensitivity problems and that insulin resistance may be ameliorated by DHEA administration (85). Bates et al., in a placebo-controlled trial administered 50 mg of DHEA daily to 15 postmenopausal women for a 3-wk period and demonstrated a significant enhancement in insulin sensitivity index (86). Casson et al. has reported similar finding in 11 postmenopausal women who were given 50 mg of DHEA (87). With the current evidence, it is not recommended to administer DHEA to patient with diabetes. Long-term trials are needed to show the effect of DHEA on diabetes.

DHEA and Adrenal Insufficiency

Dehydroepiandrosterone and DHEAS in humans is produced in adrenal glands in larger amounts and decreases with age, which is further decreased in adrenal insufficiency. The amount of DHEA required for women with adrenal insufficiency according to one study of 3-mo duration is 50 mg of DHEA daily. This provides DHEA levels close to physiological levels in these women without any adverse effects (88). When replaced with physiologic doses of DHEA, patients with adrenal insufficiency when replaced with physiologic doses of DHEA had no significant changes on carbohydrate metabolism, body composition, or exercise capacity (89,90). In a double-blind placebo-controlled cross-over study of 4-mo duration, women with adrenal insufficiency were treated with a 50-mg dose of DHEA orally. In this particular study, DHEA improved general well being, sexual thoughts, sexual interest, and satisfaction with both physical and mental aspects of sexuality in women with adrenal insufficiency (90,91). Long-term studies are required in both men and women to further define the role of DHEA as a component of the standard replacement for adrenal insufficiency.

DHEA and Osteoporosis

Low serum levels of DHEA were postulated as a possible risk factor for the development of osteoporosis (92,93), whereas others reported no such association (16). A positive correlation between serum levels of DHEAS and bone mineral density in the lumbar spine, femoral neck, and radius mid-shaft has been demonstrated in women aged 45–69 yr (92). However, the mechanism(s) by which DHEA may offer protection against osteoporosis remains unclear. DHEA may have a nonestrogenic effect on bone, as there were no significant differences in estrogen levels among women with different bone densities (92). However, DHEA may be converted by bone osteocytes to estrogen resulting in slowing down of bone resorption. Furthermore, a metabolite of DHEA and DHEAS, 4-androstene-3β, 17-β-diol, has an affinity for estrogen receptors (94) and may act as an antiresortptive agent. In a double-blind, placebo-controlled trial, men and women 60–79 yr of age were given 50 mg of DHEA, orally for 1 yr. This study showed that in women >70 yr of age, there was improvement of bone turnover as measured by dual-energy X-ray absorptiometry (DEXA) and decrease in osteoclastic activity (95). Prospective placebo-controlled trials are needed, however, to confirm the protective effect of DHEA against osteoporosis and to define recommendations for therapeutic interventions.

DHEA and the Central Nervous System

Dehydroepiandrosterone has been shown to improve memory in young and old mice (96a). The addition of steroid sulfatase inhibitors to DHEA further increases enhancement of memory in rats (97). DHEA(S) are also produced by the brain along with the adrenal gland (98) and is aneuroprotective agent (99,100). DHEA(S) also increases the effect of glutamate and decreases the effect of GABA, an excitatory and inhibitory neurotransmitter, respectively (101).

Some studies have reported that patients with Alzheimer's disease were found to have lower levels of DHEA and DHEAS (102–105); however, others reported no difference (106,107). Rudman et al. (108) reported lower levels of DHEA in male nursing home patients compared to the community; furthermore, plasma DHEAS levels were inversely related to the presence of organic brain syndrome and to the degree of dependence in activities of daily living.

When administered to depressed patients, DHEA resulted in improvement in depressive symptoms (109), length and quality of sleep, and well being in aged men and women (11,110). Thus, it appears from the initial pilot studies that DHEA is involved in behavior. A larger-scale double-blind study failed to demonstrate any effect of DHEA on mood (111), whereas Hunt et al. (112), in a randomized control trial, reported improvement in mood and fatigue in patient with Addison's disease who were given 50 mg of DHEA orally for 12 wk and Barnhart et al. (113) showed no effect on mood in perimenopausal women.

Dehydroepiandrosterone decreases as HIV disease progresses. In a double-blind placebo-controlled trial, 32 patients with mean age of 44 ± 11 yr, 50 mg of DHEA or placebo was administered to patient with advanced HIV disease for 4 mo, with the primary end point of this study being quality of life. At the end of the study, patients in the DHEA group had improved mental functions and better quality of life than the placebo group. No significant side effects were noted in the treatment group and no worsening of CD4 counts were seen in the treatment group (114).

Currently, there is no evidence to support DHEA/S supplementation for cognitive function improvement in normal older people. There are no data available in patients with dementia and DHEA(S) replacement *(115)*.

Baulieu et al. *(97)* studied 280 healthy men and women with age ranged from 60–79 yr of age the so-called "DHEA study." These individual were given, in a double-blind, placebo-controlled fashion either 50 mg of DHEA orally or placebo for 1 yr. DHEA replacement re-established a "young" concentration of DHEA and showed a small increase in the concentration of testosterone and estradiol in women. DHEA replacement demonstrated improved bone turnover in women older than 70 yr, improvement in skin status and increased libido in older women. Replacement of DHEA at 50 mg/d showed no biochemical signs of deficiency for 1 yr, indicating that replacement of DHEA normalizes the effects of aging, but does not create " supermen/women."

Current DHEA Status

Although the results from initial human studies appear promising, they still need to be confirmed by large-scale controlled studies. At the present time, beneficial effects of chronic DHEA administration are virtually unknown. Thus, it does not seem reasonable at the present time to dispense DHEA. This status, however, is expected to change in the near future given the magnitude of current human DHEA-related research. It is expected that a therapeutic role for DHEA will be established which could take the form of hormone replacement therapy or as pharmacological therapy for specific pathologic conditions *(1)*.

PREGNENOLONE

Pregnenolone is the precursor of all of the known steroid hormones *(see* Fig. 1) and as such, possesses several typical steroid hormonal effects *(116,117)*. The formation of pregnenolone, by the conversion from cholesterol via the action of cytochrome P450scc (side-chain cleavage), is the rate-limiting step in steroid hormone formation. Pregnenolone, like DHEA, is secreted from the adrenal gland and declines with age, showing a 60% reduction at 75 yr compared to the mean value observed at 35 yr.

Effects of Pregnenolone on Physical Decline

Pregnenolone, like its derivates, may be involved in the modulation of muscle strength, osteoporosis, and immune function, which may be achieved directly or from its conversion to other steroid hormones. In a recent animal study, injection of pregnenolone prior to administration of a lysozyme antigen increased titers of antilysozyme IgG compared with controls, suggesting its role in the regulation of body's immune response *(118)*.

In the 1940s and 1950s, pregnenolone was safely used as a treatment for rheumatoid arthritis and other inflammatory conditions. Outcomes in the treatment of rheumatoid arthritis were variable, improving symptoms in majority of patients in most studies but having few effects in other studies *(119,120)*. From anecdotal evidence volunteered by our subjects in preliminary studies, pregnenolone administration mitigated "aches and pains" attributed to arthritis. The mechanism of the anti-inflammatory effects of pregnenolone is unclear, and its impact on aspects of frailty in humans has not been explored.

Pregnenolone and the Central Nervous System

In addition to serving as a precursor for the formation of different steroids, pregnenolone also appears to directly affect both GABA (A) (γ amino butyric acid A) and NMDA (N-methyl-D-aspartate) receptors in the central nervous system (CNS) *(121–123)*. Pregnenolone sulfate inhibits GABA-gated chloride channels by increasing receptor desensitization and stabilizing desensitized states *(124)*. As a neurosteroid, pregnenolone may have a role in the regulation of behavior, mood, anxiety, learning, and sleep. Within animal brains, regional alterations in the concentration of pregnenolone sulfate have been associated with different physiological states, (i.e., stress, diurnal cycles, or sexual activities) *(125)*.

During the mid-1940s, several experiments were performed examining the effects of pregnenolone on psychomotor performance in humans. In a study of nearly 300 factory workers who were given up to 70 mg of pregnenolone for up to 3 mo, pregnenolone improved production efficiency in groups deemed to be working under stressful conditions, those being paid per piece rather than paid per hour *(126,127)*. Effects of pregnenolone administration on psychomotor performance in pilots included a decrease in fatigue and an improvement in targeting scores *(128)*. In a recent study in humans, 1-mg doses of pregnenolone affected EEG patterns during sleep, improved sleep efficiency, and decreased intermittent wakefulness *(129)*.

Pregnenolone and Memory

Neurosteroids have higher concentration in the brain than in plasma and have effects on anxiety and convulsions *(130)*, influences cognitive function and the memory process. It is proposed that the hippocampal content of pregnenolone sulfate is responsible for playing a physiological role in preserving cognitive abilities in older animals, possibly by interaction with acetylcholine *(131)*. Pregnenolone induces memory enhancement in aged mice *(132)* and rats *(133)*. Systemic or intracerebral administration of pregnenolone or its sulfate amplifies memory in rodents by improving natural performance or by preventing pharmacologically induced amnesia *(96,124,133,134)*. Pregnenolone sulfate is reported to exacerbate NMDA-induced death of hippocampal neurons *(135)* and protects mouse hippocampal cells against glutamate and amyloid β-toxicity *(136)*. Our group also demonstrated that pregnenolone, when injected directly in the mouse brain, enhances posttraining memory processes *(96,123)*. The effect of pregnenolone on memory in humans has not been established.

Pregnenolone in Humans

In our preliminary study, 22 healthy men and women aged 20–88 yr were given 500 mg pregnenolone each day for a period of 12 wk. This study found no effects on strength, balance, or memory *(137)*. Early studies had suggested that pregnenolone might improve attention span and performance in humans *(138)*.

Pregnenolone: Side-Effects Profile

Problems often arise that preclude prolonged hormonal replacement. For example, in men, prostatic hypertrophy and polycythemia are risks of long-term testosterone replacement. Multiple studies in humans and animals have demonstrated no significant untoward effects owing to pregnenolone, even with long-term administration. Specifically, there have been no reported effects on glucose, weight, heart rate, blood pressure, gastrointestinal symptoms, or menstrual cycles *(119,120,139)*. One case of mild rash was reported to occur with oral pregnenolone *(140)*. The minimum of side effects noted with pregnenolone may be attributed to the maintenance of normal steroid patterns, minimizing the disruption of feedback mechanisms in steroid formation and competition of steroid for receptor binding sites. Pregnenolone alone or with small amounts of androgens, estrogens, or DHEA may avoid the side effects of large doses of these derivatives. Pregnenolone could serve as a precursor of indigenous synthesis of these hormones and may facilitate their actions through allosteric effects exerted by binding at different loci of the same receptors.

CONCLUSIONS

Because there are many tantalizing clues suggesting salutary effects of DHEA and pregnenolone on the aging process, controlled studies so far have failed to demonstrate these benefits in a convincing manner. There is a clear need for further long-term controlled studies. Our preliminary studies have questioned whether commercially available DHEA always contains the amounts of DHEA stated on the bottle. This further confuses an already complex field.

Appendix: Overview of Human DHEA Studies

Researchers/type of study	Dose and period of subjects	Age and number	Results
Yen et al. (11)	50 mg cap/oral/sublingual	8 men/8 women, age: 40–70	DHEA, A, T, DHT were similar in two routes, but there was rapid and marked elevation of DHEA for 2 h after sublingual than after oral route.
Yen et al. (11); randomized, placebo-controlled	50 mg oral cap for 6 mo	13 men/17 women, age: 40–70	Twofold increase of A, T, DHT in women with only slight increase in men. Small decrease in HDL in women, no change in other lipids. No change in SHBG E1-E2 in both women and men. No change in insulin sensitivity, body fat mass. No change in libido. Increase in perceived physical and psychological well-being (men, 67%, women 84%)
Yen et al. (11); randomized, placebo-controlled	100 mg cap for 1 yr	8 men/8 women, age: 50–65	Increase in SHBG in women with no change in men. Fivefold increase in A, T, DHT in women, but only twofold increase in men. No change in gonadotropin in both groups. Increase in lean body mass only in men. Increase in IGF-I in both groups. No change in lipids profile, apolipoprotein, insulin, glucose, metabolic rate, and bone mineral density.
Yen et al. (11); single-blind, placebo- controlled	50 mg cap: 2 wk placebo then 20	9 men	Stimulation of immune function. Increase in NK cells and IL-2.
Buster et al. (141); open-label, noncontrolled trial	Placebo or 150 or 300 mg DHEA	8 postmenopausal women not on hormone replacement	Increase in DHEA, DHEAS, T. No change in estradiol levels. Increase in LET in one of subjects. Direct assay of T overestimated it by 300%.

Researchers/type of study	Dose and period of subjects	Age and number	Results
Vollenhoven et al. (*142*); open noncontrolled trial	200 mg DHEA for 3–6 wk	10 women with SLE, average age 35.7 yr	Improved SLE activity. Decrease requirement of prednisone. Decrease in proteinuria. Improvement in well being and energy. Four subjects developed acne form dermatitis. Two subjects developed mild hirsutisms that were also on prednisone.
Arano et al. (*143*); double-blind, randomized, placebo-controlled study	(1) 50 mg oral DHEA or placebo twice daily for 4 d beginning 2 d before tetanus vaccination	(1) 66 men, age >65	No difference between DHEAS group and placebo group, no detrimental effects of DHEAS on outcome of tetanus vaccination
	(2) 50 mg oral DHEA or placebo for 2 d beginning with the day of influenza vaccination	(2) 67 elderly persons, age: ?	41.2% of DHEAS group have greater than fourfold increase in HAI titer, only 27% of placebo group have greater than fourfold increase in HAI titer. Response to N1H1 antigen was 39.9% in placebo group and 47.1% in DHEAS group. Response to influenza B was marked increase in titer in only three of placebo group and six of DHEAS group.
Dyner et al. (*144*); open-label uncontrolled trial	250–500–750 mg oral DHEA tid for 16 wk	31 homosexual men	No dose-limiting side effects. No sustained improvement in CD4. No change in P24 Ag or β-macroglobulin. Transient decrees in neopterin at 8 wk.
Jakubowicz et al. (*35*); double-blind placebo-controlled study	(1) Acute test: 300 mg of DHEA; 6 were given (L-NAME), a specific inhibitor of NO synthase. The rest of subjects were given intravenous saline.	(1) 14 men (out of 22)	Increase in IGF-1 and C-GMP in saline group. Increase in IGF-1 in DHEA–L-NAME group, which indicates that DHEA's effects are medicated via NO.
	(2) 100 mg oral DHEA qd for 1 mo	(2) 22 men, mean	Increase in plasma C-GMP and IGF-1 after 1 mo of DHEA replacement.

(continued)

Appendix: Overview of Human DHEA Studies (continued)

Researchers/type of study	Dose and period of subjects	Age and number	Results
Jesse et al. (24); randomized, double-blind, placebo-controlled trial	300 mg oral DHEA tid for 14 d	10 normal men	Platelet aggregation rates were prolonged in 4 out of 5 in DHEA group. No side effects reported.
Beer et al. (36); randomized, double blind, placebo-controlled trial	50 mg oral DHEA tid for 12 d	34 men, age: 47–75	Decrease in plasma plasminogen activator inhibitor type 1 (PAI-1) and tissue plasminogen activator (tPA). Decrease in diastolic blood pressure (BP) in DHEA group compared with slight increase in BP in placebo group. Two- to fivefold increase in serum DHEAS; no change in serum DHEA in DHEA group. 55% increase in A in DHEA group. No change in systolic BP in both groups. No change in body mass index in both groups.
Wolkowitz et al. (109)	30–90 mg of oral DHEA qd for 4 wk	3 men/3 women (major depression patients), age: 51–72	Increase in serum levels of DHEA and DHEAS. Improvement in HDRS, global depression, SCL90, BDI; improvement in automatic memory functions. Return of behavioral and cognitive measures to baseline after DHEA withdrawal.
Friess at al. (145); placebo-controlled study	Single 500 mg oral dose	Ten young healthy men, mean age: 24.9	Significant increase in REM sleep, with no change in other sleep variables. DHEA may play a role of GABAa-agonist/antagonist.

320

Researchers/type of study	Dose and period of subjects	Age and number	Results
Buffington et al. (146); case study	0.25 mg dexamethasone for 1 mo, then 0.25 mg + DHEA (150 bid)	One woman (NIDDM, primary amenorrhea), age: 15	No change in body weight, and percent of body fat. Dexamethasone treatment caused eightfold increase in serum cortisol, 28-fold decrease in DHEAS and fivefold decrease in testosterone. DHEA administration did not affect cortisol levels, but caused increase in DHEAS and testosterone. DHEA caused increase in the disappearance rate of glucose in response to intravenous insulin, suggesting enhanced peripheral tissue insulin sensitivity. DHEA caused threefold increase in the hypoglycemic response to intravenous insulin, and 30% increase in insulin binding.
Bates et al. (86); randomized, double-blind, placebo-controlled trial	50 mg oral DHEA qd for 3 wk	15 patients	Insulin sensitive index increased in the DHEA group. No change in weight body mass index.
Casson et al. (147); placebo-controlled, randomized trial	50 mg oral DHEA qd for 3 wk	11 postmenopausal women	Increase in DHEA, DHEAS, T free T Decrease in fasting triglycerides with no change in other lipid profile. Increase in insulin sensitivity. Increase in SHBG.
Usiskin et al. (148)	1600 mg DHEA/d for 28 d	6 obese men	No change in total body weight, body fat mass, tissue insulin sensitivity, serum lipids, or fat distribution.
Jones et al. (149); case report	Oral DHEA	Patient with advanced prostate cancer	Symptoms improved Cancer flared. Previously hormonally unresponsive cancer responded transiently to third-line hormonal therapy with diethylstilbestrol.

(continued)

321

Appendix: Overview of Human DHEA Studies (continued)

Researchers/type of study	Dose and period of subjects	Age and number	Results
Labrie et al. (150); non-controlled trial	10% DHEA cream for 12 mo	Fourteen 60- to 70-yr-old postmenopausal women	Stimulation of vaginal epithelium maturation. No estrogenic effect observed on endometrium. Bone mineral density at the hip significantly increased. Decreased alkaline phosphatase, and urinary/ hydroxyproline/creatine ratio. Increase in serum osteocalcin, a marker of bone formation.
Danenberg et al. (64); prospective randomized, double-blind study	Either DHEA (50 mg qd po) for 4 d or a placebo. Antibody response to the influenza vaccine was measured before and 28 d after vaccination.	71 volunteers; age: 61–89 yr	Increased DHEAS in the DHEA group. No enhancement in established immunity. Decrease in attainment of protective antibody titer against A/Texas strain in subjects with nonprotective baseline antibody titer following DHEA treatment compared with placebo.
Wolf et al. (113); double-blind, placebo-controlled trial	DHEAS 50 mg for 2 wk daily, then 2-wk wash-out period and a 2-wk placebo period	40 healthy men and women (mean age: 69 yr)	DHEA, androstenedione, and testosterone increased in both groups. No strong beneficial effects in psychological or cognitive parameter.
Evans et al. (151); randomized, double-blind trial	DHEAS 50 mg po bid for 4 d, or a placebo. Tetanus vaccine given before the fifth dose.	66 individuals; age 65 yr or older	No difference noted between groups.
Evans et al. (151); randomized, double-blind trial	DHEAS 50 mg po immediately before and 24 h after vaccination	67 individuals	Number of individuals who developed influenza protective titer was not different in the two groups. The mean log increase in the antibody response was greater in the DHEAS group.
Diamond et al. (152)	Single dailt percutaneous application of a 10% DHEA cream	15 postmenapausal women; age 60–70 yr	9.8% decrease in subcutaneous skin-fold thickness 12 mo. 11% decrease in fasting plasma glucose levels and a 17% decrease in fasting insulin levels. Overall trend toward a decrease in total cholesterol and its lipoprotein fractions. Plasma triglycerides were not affected. HDL cholesterol decreased by 8%.

Researchers/type of study	Dose and period of subjects	Age and number	Results
Baulieu et al. (98); randomized, double-blind, placebo-controlled trial	50 mg/d DHEA oral or placebo for 1 yr	280 men and women; age: 60–79 yr	No harmful effects of accumulation of DHT or other active steroids. Re-established serum levels of DHEA as of "young" concentration. Increase in concentration of T and estradiol Improved bone turnover in women >70 yr old and decrease in osteoclastic activity. Increase in libido and skin status in women. No creation of "supermen/women."

Abbreviations: A, androstenedione; T, testosterone; DHT, dehydroepiandrosterone; SHBG, sex-hormone-binding globulin; HDL, high-density lipoprotein; E1, estrone; E2, estradiol; LFT, liver function test; NK, natural-killer cells; IL, interleukin; SLE, systemic lupus erythromatosis; c-GMP, cyclic guanosine monophosphate; IGF, insulin growth factor-1; REM, rapid eye movement; HDRS, Hamilton Depression Rating Scale; BDI, Beck Depression Inventory; SCL, symptom check list; NIDDM, non-insulin-dependent diabetes mellitus.

REFERENCES

1. Nestler JE. DHEA: a coming of age. Ann NY Acad Sci 1995;774:ix–xi.
2. Butenandt A, Damembaum H. Isolierung neuen, physiologisch unwirksamen Sterindervates aus Mannerharn, Seine Verknupung mit dehdro-androsterone und Androsteron. Z Physiol Chem 1934;229:192–195.
3. Watson RR, Huls A, Araghinikaum M, et al. DHEA and disease of aging. Drugs Aging 1996;9(4):274–291.
4. Baulieu EE, Corpechot C, Dray E. An adrenal–secreted "androgen" dehydroepiandrosterone sulfate. Its metabolism and a tentative generalization on the metabolism of other steroid conjugate in men. Recent Prog Horm Res 1965;21:411–500.
5. Baulieu EE. Dehydroepiandrosterone (DHEA): a fountain of youth: J Clin Endocrinol Meytab 1996;80:3147–3151.
6. Dunn JF, Nisula BC, Rodbard D. Transport of steroid hormones: binding of 21 endogenous steroid to both testosterone-binding globulin and corticosteroid binding globulin in human plasma. J Clin Endocrinol Metab 1965;53:58–68.
7. Vermeulen A. Adrenal Androgens. Raven Press, New York, 1980, pp. 207–217.
8. Orentreich N, Brind JL, Andres R, et al. Long-term longitudanl measurements of plasma Dehydroepiandrosterone sulfate in normal men. J Clin Endocrinol Metab 1992;75:1002–1004.
9. Liu CH, Laughlin GA, et al. Marked attenuation of ultradian and circadian rhythums of DHEA in postmenopausal women: evidence of reduced 17,20-desomolase enzymatic activity. J Clin Endocrinol Metab 1990;71(4):900–906.
10. Khaw KT, Tazuke S, Barrett-Conner E. Cigarette smoking and levels of adrenal androgens in post menopausal women. N Engl J Med 1998;318:1705–1709.
11. Yen SSC, Moreles AJ, Khorram O. Replacement of DHE in aging men and women: potential remedial effects. Ann NY Acad Sci 1995;774:128–142.
12. Mazat L, Lafont S, Berr C, et al. Prospective measurements of dehydroepiandrosterone sulfate in a cohort of elderly subjects: relationship to gender, subjective health, smoking habits, and 10-yearmortality. Proc Natl Acad Sci USA.2001;98(14):8145–8150 .
13. Vermeulen A. Dehydroepiandrosterone sulfate and aging. Ann NY, Acad Sci 1995;774:121-127.
14. Roter JI, Wong L, Lifrank Et, et al. A genetic component of the variation of dehydroepiandrosterone sulfate. Metabolism 1985;34:731–736.
15. Barrett-Connor E, Khaw KT, Yen SS. A prospective study of dehydroepiandrosterone sulfate mortality, cardiovascular disease. NEJM 1986;315:1519–1524.
16. Barrett-Conner E, Kiltz- Silverstein D, Edelstein SL. A prospective study of dehydroepiandrosterone sulfate and bone mineral density in older men and women. Am J Epidemil 1993;137:201–206.
17. Marmorston J, Lewis JJ, Bernstein JL, et al. Excretion of urinary steroids by men and women with myocardial infarction. Geriatrics 1957;12:297–300.
18. Marmorston J, Griffith CC, Geller PJ, et al. Urinary steroids in the measurement of aging. J Am Geriatr Soc 1975;23:481–492.
19. Khaw KT. Dehydroepiandrosterone, dehydroepiandrosterone sulfate and cardiovascular disease. J Endocrinol 1996;150:S149–153.
20. Barret-Connor E, Edelstein SL. A prospective study of dehydroepiandrosterone sulfate and cognitive function in an older population: The Rancho Bernard Study. J Am Geriatr Soc 1994;42:420–23.
21. Lacroix AZ, Yano K, Reed DM. Dehydroepiandrosterone, incidence of myocardial infarction and extent of atherosclerosis in men. Circulation 1992;86:1529–1535.
22. Hautanen A, Mnttari M, Manninen V, et al. Adrenal androgens and testosterone as coronary risk factors in Helsinki Heart study. Arterosclerosis 1994;105:191–200.
23. Newcornewer LM, Manson JE, Barbieri RL, et al. Dehydroepiandrosterone sulfate and the risk of myocardial infarction in US male physician: a prospective study. Am J Epidemiol 1994;140:870–875.
24. Jesse RL, Loesser K, Eich DM, et al. Dehydroepiandrosterone inhibits human platelet aggregation in vitro and in vivo. Ann NY Acad Sci 1995;774:281–290.
25. Gordon GB, Bush DE, Weisiman HF. Reduction in arteriosclerosis by administration of dehydroepiandrosterone. A Study in the hypercholestrolemic New Zealand white rabbit with aortic intimal injury. J Clin Invest 1988;82:712–720.
26. Arad Y, Badimon JO, Hemmberee W, et al. Dehydroepiandrosterone feeding prevents aortic fatty streak formation and cholesterol accumulation in cholesterol-fed rabbit. Atherosclerosis 1989;9:159–166.

27. Eich DM, Nestler, Johnson DE, et al. Inhibition of accelerated coronary athreosclerosis with dehydroepiandrosterone in the hetrotropic rabbit model of cardiac transplantation. Circulation 1993;87:261–269.

28. Zumoff B, Troxler RG, O'Connor J. Abnormal hormone levels in men with coronary artery disease. Aterosclerosis 1982;2:58–67.

28a. Herrington DM, Gordon GB, Achuff SC, et al. Plasma DHEA and DHEAS in patient undergoing diagnostic coronary angiogram. J Am Coll of Cardiol 1990;16:862–870.

29. Slowinska-Srzednicka J, Makczwska B, Srzednicki M et al. Hyperinsulinaemia and decreased plasma levels of dehydroepiandrosterone in premenopausal women with coronary heart disease. J Intern Med 1995;237:465–472.

30. Barrett-Connor E, Goodman Gruen D. Dehydroepiandrosterone sulfate does not predict cardiovascular death in postmenopausal women. Circulation 1995;91:1757–1760.

31. Nafziger AN, Jenkins PL, Pearson TA. Dehydroepiandrosterone, lipids, and apoproteins: association in a free-living population. (Abstract). Circulation 1990;82:SIII-469.

32. Haffer SM, Newcomb PA, Marcus PM, et al. Relation of sex hormones and dehydroepiandrosterone sulfate to cardiovascular risk factor in postmenopausal women. Am J Epidemiol 1995;142:923–925.

33. Herrington DM, Gordon DB, Achuff SC, et al. Plasma dehydroepiandrosterone sulfate in patients undergoing diagnostic coronary angiography. J Am Coll Cardiol 1990;16:862–870.

34. Cleary MP, Zisk JF. Anti obesity effects of 2 different levels of dehydroepiandrosterone in lean and obese middle-aged femal Zucker rats. Int J Obesity 1986;10:193–204.

35. Jakubowicz D, Beer N, Rengifo R. Effects of dehydroepiandrosterone on cyclic–guanosine monophosphate and advancing age. Ann NY Acad Sci 1995;774:312–315.

36. Beer NA, Jakubowics DJ, Matt DW, et al. Dehydroepiandrosterone reduces plasma plasminogen activator antigen in men. Am J Med Sci 1996;311(5):205–210.

37. Roa MS, Subbarao V, Yeldandi AV. Inhibition of spontaneous testicular leydig cell tumor development in F-344 rats by dehydroepiandrosterone. Cancer Lett 1992;65:123–126.

38. Schwartz AG, Pashko LL. Cancer chemoprevention with the adrenalcortical steroid dehydroepiandrosterone and structure analogs. J Cell Biochem 1993;17G(Suppl):73–79.

39. Schwartz AG, Pashko LL. Cancer chemo prevention with dehydroepiandrosterone and no-androgenic structural analogs. J Cell Biochem 1995;22(suppl):210–217.

40. Klamm RC, Holbroke CT, Nyee JW. Chemotherapy of murine colorectal carcinoma with cisplatin plus 3'-deoxy 3'-azidothymidine. Anticancer Res 1992;12:781–787.

41. Helzouer KJ Gordon GB, Alberg AJ, et al. Relationship of prediagnostic serum levels of DHEA/S to the risk of developing premenopausal breast cancer. Cancer Res 1992;52:1–4.

42. Gordon GB, Helzouer KJ, Alberg AJ, et al. Serum levels of DHEA/S and the risk of developing gastric cancer. Cancer Epid Biomark Prevent 1993;2:33–35.

43. Bhatavdekar JM, Patel DD, Chikhikaar RR. Levels of circulating peptide and steroid hormones in men with lung cancer. Neoplasm 1994;41:101–103.

44. Gordon GB, Helzlsour KJ, Comstock GW. Serum levels of dehydroepiandrosterone and its sulfate and the risk of developing bladder cancer. Cancer Res 1991;51:1366–1369.

45. Magee JM, Mekenzie S, Filippa DA. Hairy cell Leukemia: durability of response to spleenectomy in 26 patients and treatment of replace with androgens in six patients. Cancer 1985;56:2557–2562.

46. Kask E. Ketosteroids and arteriosclerosis. Angioplasty 1959;10:358–368.

47. Barrett-Connor E, Friedlander NJ, Khaw KT. Dehydroepiandrosterone sulfate and breast cancer risk. Cancer Res 1990;50(20):6571–6574.

48. Gordon GB, Bush TL, Helzsour KJ. Relationship of serum levels of dehydroepiandrosterone and dehydroepiandrosterone sulfate to the risk of developing postmenopausal breast cancer. Cancer Res 1990;50:3859–3862.

49. Hankinson SE, Willett WC, Mason JE. Plasma sex steroid hormone levels and risk of breast cancer in post menopausal women. J Natl Cancer Inst 1998;90:1292–1299.

50. Stoll BA. Dietary supplements of dehydroepiandrosterone in relation to breast cancer risk. Eur J Clin Nutri 1999;53(10):771–775.

51. Liberto HM, Sonohara S, Brentant MM. Effects of androgen on proliferation and progesterone receptors levels in T47D human breast cancer cells. Tumor boil 1993;14:38–45.

52. Boccuzzi g, DiMonaco M, Brignardello E. Dehydroepiandrosterone antiestrogenic action through androgen receptor MCF-7 human breast cell line. Anticancer Res 1993;13:2267–2272.

53. Boccuzzi G, DiMonaco M, Brignardello E. Influence of dehydroepiandrosterone and 5-androster-one-3-beta-diol on the growth of MCF-7 human breast cancer cells induced by 17 beta -estradiol. Anticancer Res 1992;12:799–803.

54. Garg M, Bondada S. Reversal of age associated decline in immune response to pnu-immue vaccine by supplemantation with steroid hormone dehydroepandrosterone. Infect Immun 1993;61:2238–2241.

55. Araneo B, Daynes R. Dehydroepiandrosterone function as more than an antiglucocorticoid in preserving immunocompetence after thermal injury. Endocrinology 1995;136:393–401.

56. Kim HR, Tyu SY, Kim HS. Administration of dehydroepiandrosterone reverses the immune suppression induced by high doses antigen in mice. Immunol Invest 1995;24:583–593.

57. Beyer WE, Palache AM, Baljet M, et al. Antibody induction by influenza vaccines in the elderly: a review of the literature. Vaccine.1989;7(5):385–94.

58. Stein BE. Vaccinating elderly people. Protecting from avoidable disease. Drugs Aging 1994;5(4):242–253.

59. Miller RA. The cell biology of aging: immunological models. J Gerontol 1989;44(1):B4–8.

60. Thoman ML, Weigle WO. The cellular and sub cellular bases of immunosenescenc Adv Immunol 1989;46:221–261.

61. Sanders ME, Makgoba MW, Shaw S. Human naive and memory T cells: reinterpretation of helper-inducer and suppressor-inducer subsets. Immunol Today 1988;9(7-8):195–199.

62. Miller RA. Accumulation of hypo responsive, calcium-extruding memory T cells as a key feature of age-dependent immune dysfunction. Clin Immunol Immunopathol 1991;58(3):305–317.

63. Degelau J, Guay G, Hallgren H. The effect of DHEAS on influenza vaccination in aging adults. J Am Geriatr Soc 1997;45:747–751.

64. Dannenberg HD, Ben-Yehuda, Zakay-Rones Z. DHEA treatment in not beneficial to the immune response to influenza in elderly subjects. J Clin Endocrinol Metab 1997;82:2911–2914.

65. Oberbeck R, Dahlweid M, Koch R. Dehydroepiandrosterone decreases mortality rate and improve cellular immune function during polymicrobial sepsis. Critical Care Med 2001;29(2):380–384.

66. Rasmussen KR, Healy MC, Cheng L. Effects of DHEA in immunosuppressed adult mice infected with Cryptosporidium parvum. J Parasitol 1995;8:429–433.

67. Lorie RM, Inge TH, Cook SS. Protection against acute lethal injections with native steroid dehydroepiandrosterone. J Med Virol 1988;26:301–314.

68. Van Vollenhoven RF, Engleman EG, McGuire JL. DHEA in SLE: Results of double blind, placebo controlled trial. Arthritis Rheum 1995;38:(12):1826–1831.

69. Van Vollenhoven RF, Park JL. A double blind, placebo controlled, and clinical trial of DHEA in severe SLE. Lupus 1999;8(3):181–187.

70. Petri M, Lahita R, McGuire J. Results of GL 701(DHEA) multicenter steroid sparing SLE study. Arthritis Rheum 1997;40:S327.

71. Chatterton RT, Green D, Harris S, et al. longitudinal study of adrenal steroids in a cohort of HIV-infected patients with hemophilia. J Lab Clin Med 1996;127(6):545–552.

72. Spencer NFL, Poynter ME, Hennebold JD. Does DHEAS restores immune competence in aged animals through its capacity to function as a neutral modulator of peroxisome activities? Ann NY Acad Sci 1995;774:200–216.

73. Daynes RA, Dudly DJ, Araneo BA. Regulation of murine lymphokine production in vivo. II. DHEA is a neutral enhancer of interleukin 2 synthesis by helper t cells. Eur J Immunol 1990;20:793–802.

74. Ben-Nathan D, Lustig S, Kobiler D. Danengerg HD. DHEA protects mice inoculated with West nile virus and exposure to cold stress. J Med Virol 1992;38:159–166.

75. Okabe T, Haji M, Takayanagi R, et al. Up regulation of high affinity DHEA binding activity by DHEA in activated human T lymphocytes. J Clin Endocrinol Metab 1995;80:2993–2996.

76. Meikle Aw, Dorchuck RW, Araneo BA. The presence of DHEA-specific receptor binding complex in murine T cells. J Steroid Biochem Mol Biol 1992;42:293–304.

77. Kamio T, Shingematsu K, Kawai K. Immunoreactivity and receptor expression of insulin-like growth factor I and insulin in human adrenal tumor. An immunohistochemal study study of 94 cases. Am J Pathol 1991;138:83–91.

78. Sonka J. Dehydroepiandrosterone. Metabolic effects, In: Charvat J, ed. Acta universitais Carolinae Universita Krlova Praha, Prague 1976, pp. 1–171.

79. Nafziger AN, Herrington DM, Bush TL. Dehydroepiandrosterone and dehydroepiandrosterone sulfate: their relation to cardiovascular disease. Epidemiol Res 1991;13:267–293.

80. Barrett–Conor E. Lower endogenous androgen levels and dyslipidmia in men with non-insulin dependent diabetes mellitus. Ann Intern Med 1992;117:807–811.

81. Nestler JE, Usiskin KS, Barlascini CO, et al. Suppression of serum dehydroepiandrosterone sulfate levels buy insulin: an evaluation of possible mechanism. J Clin Endocrinol Metab 1989;69:1040–1046.

82. Nestler JE, Beer NA, Jakubowicz DJ, et al. Effects of a reduction in circulating insulin by metformin on serum dehydroepiandrosterone in non diabetic men. J Clin Endocrinol Metab 1994;78:549–554.

83. Nestler JE, Kahwaash Z. Sex-specific action of insulin to acutely increase the metabolic clearance rate of dehydroepiandrosterone in humans. J Clin Invest 1994;94:1484–1489.

84. Nestler JE, McClanahan MA, Clore JN. Insulin inhibits adrenal 17,20-lyase activity in man. J Clin Endocrinol Metab 1992;74:362–367.

85. Nestler JE. Regulation of human dehydroepiandrosterone metabolism by insulin. Ann Ny Acad Sci 1995;774:73–81.

86. Bates GW, Egerman RS, Umstor ES, et al. Dehydroepiandrosterone attenuates study-induced decline in insulin sensitivity in postmenopausal women. Ann NY Acad Sci 1995;774:291–293.

87. Casson PR, Faquin LC, Stenz FB, et al. Replacement of dehydroepiandrosterone enhances T-lymphocyte insulin binding in postmentopausal women. Fertil Steril 1995;63(5):1027–1031.

88. Gennet G-M, Husebye ES, Mallmin H, Helstrom L. Oral dehydroepandrosterone replacement therapy in women with Addison Disease. Clin Endocrinol 2000;52:775–780.

89. Callies F, Fassnacht M, van Vlijmen JC, et al. Dehydroepiandrosterone replacement in women with adrenal insufficiency: effects on body composition, serum leptin, bone turnover, and exercise capacity. J Clin Endocrinol Metab 2001;86(5):1968–1972.

90. Arlt W, Callies F, Allolio B. DHEA replacement in women with adrenal insufficiency-pharmacokinetics, bioconversion and clinical effects on well being, sexuality and cognition. Endocrine Res 2000;26(4):505–511.

91. Arlt W, Callies F, van Vlijmen JC, et al. Dehydroepiandrosterone replacement in women with adrenal insufficiency. N Engl J Med 1999;341(14): 1013-20.

92. SzathmariM, Szues J, Feher T, et al. Dehydroepiandrosterone sulfate and bone mineral density. Osteoporosis Intl 1994;4:84–88.

93. Nordin BE, Robertson A, Seamark RF, et al. The relationship between calcium absorption, serum dehydroepiandrosterone and vertebral mineral density in postmenopausal women. J Clin Endocrinol Metab 1985;60:650–657.

94. Rozenberg S, Ham H, Bosson D, et al. Age, steroids and bone mineral content. Maturitas 1990;12(2):137–143.

95. Baulieu EE, Thomas G, Legrain S, et al. Dehydroepiandrosterone (DHEA), DHEA sulfate, and aging: contribution of the DHEAge Study to a sociobiomedical issue. Proc Natl Acad of Sci USA 2000;97(8):4279–4284 .

96. Flood JF, Morley JE, Robert E. Memory enhancing effects in male mice of pregnenolone and steroids metabolically derived from it. Proc Natl Acad Sci USA 1992;89:1567–1571.

96a. Flood JF, Morley JE, Roberts E. Pregnenolone sulfate enhances post-training memory process when injected in very low doses into limbic system structures: the amygdala is by far the most sensitive. Proc Natl Acad Sci USA 1995;92(23):10,806–10,810.

97. Li PK, Rhodes ME, Burke ME, Johnson DA. Memory enhancement mediated by the steroid sulfatase inhibitor (p-O-sulfamoyl)-N-tetradecanoyl tyramine. Life Sci 1997;60(3):PL45–51.

98. Baulieu EE. Neurosteroids: a novel function of the brain. Psychoneuroendocrinology 1998;23(8):963–987.

99. Kimonides VG, Khatibi NH, Svendsen CN, et al. Dehydroepiandrosterone (DHEA) and DHEA-sulfate (DHEAS) protect hippocampal neurons against excitatory amino acid-induced neurotoxicity. Proc Natl Acad Sci USA 1998;95:1852–1857.

100. Kimonides VG, Spillantini MG, Sofroniew MV, et al. Dehydroepiandrosterone (DHEA) antagonises the neurotoxic effects of corticosterone and translocation of SAPK3 in hippocampal primary cultures. Neuroscience 1999;89:429–436.

101. Debonnel G, Bergeron R, de Montigny C. Potentiation by dehydroepiandrosterone of the neuronal response to N-methyl-D-aspartate in the CA3 region of the rat dorsal hippocampus: an effect mediated via sigma receptors. J Endocrinol 1996;150:S33–42.

102. Nasman B, Olsson T, Backstrom T, et al. Serum dehydroepiandrosterone sulfate in Alzheimer's disease and in multi-infarct dementia. Biol Psychiatry 1991;30:684–690.

103. Dodt C, Dittman J, Hruby J, et al. Different regulation of adrenocorticotropin and cortisol secretion in young mentally healthy elderly and patients with senile dementia of Alzheimer's type. J Clin Endocrinol Metabol 1991d;72:272–276.

104. Sunderland T, Merril CR, Harrington MG, et al. Reduced plasma dehydroepiandrosterone concentrations in Alzheimer's disease. Lancet 1989;570.
105. Hillen T, Lun A, Reischies FM, et al. DHEA-S plasma levels and incidence of Alzheimer's disease. Biol Psych 2000;47(2):161–163.
106. Berr C, Lafont S, Debuire B, et al. Relationships of dehydroepiandrosterone sulfate in the elderly with functional, psychological, and mental status, and short-term mortality: a French community-based study. Proc Natl Acad Sci USA 1996;93:13,410–13,415.
107. Schneider LS, Hinsey M, Lyness S. Plasma dehydroepiandrosterone sulfate in Alzheimer's Disease. Biol Psych 1992;31:205–208.
108. Rudman D, Shetty KR, Mattson DE. Plasma dehydroepiandrosterone sulfate in nursing home men. J Am Geriatr Soc 1990;38:421–427.
109. Wolkowitz OM, Reus VI, Roberts E, et al. Antidepressant and cognition-enhancing effects of DHEA in major depression. Ann NY Acad Sci 1995;774:337–339.
110. Morales AJ, Nolan JJ, Nelson JC, et al. Effects of replacement dose of dehydroepiandrosterone in men and women of advancing age. J Clin Endocrinol Metab 1994;78:1360–1367.
111. Wolf OT, Neumann O, Hellammer DH, et al. Effects of a two-week physiological dehydroepiandrosterone substitution on cognitive performance and well-being in healthy elderly women and men. J Clin Endocrinol Metab 1997;82(7):2363–2367.
112. Hunt PJ, Gurnell EM, Huppert FA. Improvement in mood and fatigue after dehydroepiandrosterone replacement in Addison's disease in a randomized, double blind trial. J Clin Endocrinol Metab 2000;85(12):4650–4656.
113. Barnhart KT, Freeman E, Grisso JA, et al. The effect of dehydroepiandrosterone supplementation to symptomatic perimenopausal women on serum endocrine profiles, lipid parameters, and health-related quality of life. J Clin Endocrinol Metab 1999;84(11):3896–3902.
114. Piketty C, Jayle D, Leplege A, et al. Double-blind placebo-controlled trial of oral dehydroepiandrosterone in patients with advanced HIV disease. Clin Endocrinol 2001;55(3):325–330.
115. Huppert FA, Van Niekerk JK. Dehydroepiandrosterone supplementation for cognitive function. The Cochrane Database of Systematic Reviews 2001;4:1–17.
116. Seley H. Correlations between the chemical structure and pharmacological actions of the steroids. Endocrinology 1942;30:437–453.
117. Seley H. The pharmacology of steroid hormones and their derivatives. Rev Can Bio 1942;1:573–632.
118. Morfin R, Courchy G. Pregnenolone and dehydroepiandrosterone as a precursors of native 7-hydroxylated metabolites which increases the immune response in mice. J Steroid Biochem Molec Biol 1994;50:91–100.
119. McGavack TH, Chevalley J, Weissberg J. The use of Δ5 pregnenolone in various clinical disorders. J Clin Endocrinol 1951;11:559–577.
120. Brugsh HG, Manning RA. A comprehensive study of pregnenolone, 21 acetoxypregnenolone and ACTH. N. Eng J Med 1951;d244:628–632.
121. Wu FS, Gibbs TT, Farb DH. Pregnenolone sulfate: a positive allosteric modulator at N-methyl-D-aspartate receptor. Mol Pharmacol 1991;40:333–336.
122. Irwin RP, NJ, Rogawski MA, et al. Pregnenolone sulfate augments NMDA receptor mediated increases in intracellular Ca 2+ in cultured rat hippocampal neurons. Neurosci Lett 1992;141:30–34.
123. Ceccon M, Rumbaugh G, Vicini S. Distinct effects of pregnenolone sulfate on NDMA receptor subtypes. Neuropharamcology 2001;40:4:491–500.
124. Shen W, Mennerick S, Covey DF. Pregnenolone sulfate modulates inhibitory synaptic transmission by enhancing GABA receptor desensitization. J Neuroscience 2000;20:10:3571–3579.
125. Akwa Y, Young J, Kabbadj K, et al. Neurosteroid: biosynthesis, metabolism and function of pregnonelone and dehydroepiandrosterone in the brain. J Steroid Biochem Mol Biol 1991;10(1):71–81.
126. Pincus G, Hoagland H. Effects on industrial production of the administration of 5 pregnonelone to factory workers. I Psychosom Med 1945;7:342–346.
127. Pincus G, Hoagland H, Wilson CH, et al. Effects on industrial production of the administration of 5 pregnenolone to factory workers. II. Psychosom Med 1945;7:347–352.
128. Pincus G, Hoagland H. Effects of administered pregnenolone on fatiguing psychomotor performance. J Aviat Med 1944;15:98–115,135.
129. Stiger A, Trachsel L, Guldner J, et al. Neurosteroid pregnenolone induces sleep-EEG changes in man compatible with inverse agonistic GABAA-receptor modulation. Brain Res 1993;615:267–274.

130. Bitran D, RH, Purdy CK, et al. Anxiolytic effect of progesterone is associated with increase in cortical allopregnenolone and GABA A receptor function. Pharmacol. Biochem. Behav 1993;45:423–428.

131. Vallee M, Mayo W, Darnaudery M, et al. Neurosteroids: deficient cognitive performance in aged rats depends on low pregnenolone sulfate levels in hippocampus. Proc Natl Acad Sci USA 1997;94: 14,865–14,870.

132. Flood JF, Robert E. Dehydroepiandrosterone sulfate improves memory in aging mice. Brain Res 1988;448:178–181.

133. Ladurelle N, Eychenne B, Denton D, et al. Prolonged intracerebroventricular infusion of neurosteroids affects cognitive performances in the mouse. Brain Research 2000;858(2):371–379.

134. Cheney DL, Uzunov D, Guidotti A. Pregnenolone sulfate antagonist dizocilpine amnesia: role of allopregnenolone. Neuroreport 1995;6:1697–1700.

135. Weaver CE Jr, Wu FS, Gibbs TT, et al. Pregnenolone sulfate exacerbates NMDA-induced death of hippocampal neurons. Brain Research.1998;803(1-2):129–136.

136. Gursoy E, Cardounel A, Kalimi M. Pregnenolone protects mouse hippocampal (HT-22) cell against glutamate and amyloid beta protein toxicity. Neurochemical Research 2001;26(1):15–21.

137. Sih R, Morley JE, Kaiser FE, et al. Effects of pregnenolone on aging. J Investig Med 1997;45(7):348A.

138. Morley JE, Kaiser FE, Raum WJ, et al. Potentially predictive and manipulable blood serum correlates of aging in the healthy human male: progressive decreases in bioavailable testosterone, dehydro-epiandrosterone sulfate. Proc Natl Acad Sci USA 1997;94(14):7537–7542.

139. Henderson E, Weinberg M, Wright WA. Pregnenolone. Endocr Rev 1950;10:455–474.

140. Tyler ET, Payne S, Kirsch. Pregnenolone in male infertility. West J Surg 1943;56:459–463.

141. Buster JE, Casson PR, Straughan AB, et al. Postmenopausal steroid replacement with micronized dehydroepiandrosterone: preliminary oral bioavailability and dose proportionality studies. Am J Obstet Gynecol 1992;166(4):1163–1168.

142. Vollenhoven RF, Engelman EG, McGuire JL. Dehydroepiandrosterone in systemic lupus erythromaorosus. Results of a double blind, placebo-controlled, randomized clinical trial. Arthritis Rheum 1995;38(12):1826–1831.

143. Araneo B, Dowell T, Woods ML, et al. DHEAS as an effective vaccine adjuvant Iin elderly humans. Proof-of-principal studies. Ann NY Acad Sci 1995;774:232–248.

144. Dyner TS, Lang W, Geaga J, et al. An open-label dose-escalation trial of oral dehydroepiandrosterone tolerance and pharmakinetics in patients with HIV disease. J AIDS 1993;6:459–465.

145. Friss E, Trachse L, Guldner J, et al. DHE administration increases rapid eye movement sleep and EEG power in the sigma frequency range. Am J Physiol 1995;268:E107–113.

146. Buffington CK, Pourmotabbed G, Kitabchi AE. Case report: amelioration of insulin resistance in diabetes with dehydroepiandrosterone. Am J Med Sci 1993;306(5):320–324.

147. Casson PR, Faquin LC, Stenz FB, et al. Replacement of dehydroepiandrosterone enhances T-lymphocyte insulin binding in postmenopausal women. Fertil Steril 1995;63(5):1027–1031.

148. Usiskin KS, Butterworth S, Clore JN, et al. Lack of effect of dehydroepiandrosterone in obese men. Int J Obese;14(5):457–463.

149. Jones JA, Nguyen A, Straub M, et al. Use of DHEA in a patient with advanced prostate cancer: a case report and review. Urology 1997;50(5):784–788.

150. Labrie F, Diamond P, Cusan L, et al. Effect of 12-month dehydroepiandrosterone replacement therapy on bone, vagina, and endometrium in postmenopausal women. J Clin Endo Metab 1997;82(10):3498–3505.

151. Evans TG, Judd ME, Dowel T, et al. The use of oral dehydroepiandrosterone sulfate as an adjuvant in tetanus and influenza vaccination of the elderly. Vaccine 1996;14(16):1531–1537.

152. Diamond P, Cusan L, Gomez JL, et al. Metabolic effects of 12-month percutaneous dehydro-epiandrosterone replacement therapy in postmenopausal women. J Endocrin 1996;150:S43–50.

VI GONADAL: MEN

19

Androgen Replacement Therapy of Male Hypogonadism

A. Wayne Meikle, MD

INTRODUCTION

Male hypogonadism is a relatively common disorder in clinical practice, particularly in aging men, and has significant effects on the fertility, sexual function, and general health of patients (1–8). Disorders of sperm and testosterone (T) production may be caused by primary, secondary, or tertiary hypogonadism. Some are relatively common and others are rare (9–11). In aging men, a tertiary-like deficiency leads to T deficiency, which affects about 20% of men by age 60 yr (5,12–14). In men with clinical manifestations of primary or secondary hypogonadism, deficiency of T can usually be treated effectively. Fertility in some men with primary testicular disease, such as Klinefelter's syndrome, is irreversible, but those with gonadotropin deficiency resulting in infertility can often be treated successfully (as reviewed in Chapter 24) (15–17). Although both T deficiency and infertility can be corrected using gonadotropin or gonadotropin-releasing hormone (GnRH) therapy in men with hypogonadotropic hypogonadism, this form of therapy is usually restricted to the management of infertility. Otherwise, androgen-replacement therapy is used to correct the chronic T deficiency. Thus, knowledge of the pathophysiology of hypogonadism is needed to plan and use appropriate hormonal replacement therapy in men with deficiency of T and sperm production.

This chapter will focus primarily on androgen-replacement therapy for T deficiency. Androgen-replacement therapy with injectable, oral, and (more recently) transdermal

From: *Endocrine Replacement Therapy in Clinical Practice*
Edited by: A. Wayne Meikle © Humana Press Inc., Totowa, NJ

and injectable pellets preparations has been available to physicians for years. However, an orally active preparation with reliable efficacy may contribute to more widespread acceptance and use of T therapy by many men.

OVERVIEW OF PHYSIOLOGY OF THE TESTES

Pulsatile secretion of GnRH by the hypothalamus stimulates the release of gonadotropins (luteinizing [LH] and follicle-stimulating hormone [FSH]) (1,8). LH stimulates Leydig cells to synthesis and secrete T, which has feedback effects on LH secretion. The seminiferous tubule compartment comprising about 85% of the mass of the testes contains Sertoli cells, which surround developing germ cells that produces mature spermatozoa. FSH binds to receptors on Sertoli cells and stimulates them to produce an androgen-binding protein, enabling the testes to concentrate T many-fold above the serum levels. Inhibin made by Sertoli cells has a feedback influence on FSH secretion (17–21).

Testosterone and its potent 5-α reduced metabolite, dihydroT (DHT), have important physiologic influences during embryogenesis, puberty, and adulthood (8). During fetal development, T and DHT result in normal differentiation of male internal and external genitalia (22,23).

During puberty, T and DHT are required for the development and maintenance of male secondary sexual characteristics. DHT results in growth of the prostate and masculinization of the skin (8,24), and the remaining androgen effects are from the actions of T. In adults, T and DHT are required for the maintenance of libido and potency, muscle mass and strength, fat distribution, bone mass, erythropoiesis, prostate growth, male pattern hair growth, and spermatogenesis.

Pathophysiology of Hypogonadism

Hypogonadism is caused by disorders of the testes (primary, as listed in Table 1), pituitary (secondary), or hypothalamus (tertiary) (1,8). T deficiency may occur as the result of Leydig cell dysfunction from primary disease of the testes, inadequate LH secretion from diseases of the pituitary, or impaired GnRH secretion by the hypothalamus. Pinpointing the cause and extent of hypogonadism makes it possible to tailor successful replacement therapy (see Table 2). Men with primary gonadal failure usually have either isolated azoospermia or oligospermia or azoospermia and T deficiency. T therapy is offered to men with androgen deficiency when successful fertility is improbable or not desired.

General Manifestations

CLINICAL PRESENTATION

The clinical presentation of male hypogonadism depends on the stage of sexual development (1,8). Androgen deficiency occurring during fetal development from defects in androgen synthesis, metabolism, or androgen responsiveness results in various manifestations of male pseudohermaphroditism.

Prepubertal. In boys with prepubertal hypogonadism, expression of the androgen deficiency is seldom recognized before the typical age for onset of puberty except in those with associated growth retardation or other anatomic and endocrine abnormalities. Failure of puberty is well characterized by several clinical features, as shown in Table 3.

Table 1
Causes of Hypogonadism

Gonadal defects
    Genetic Defect-Klinefelter's syndrome, myotonic dystrophy, Prader–Willi syndrome
    Polyglandular autoimmune failure syndromes (e.g., Schmidt syndrome)
    Anatomic defects
    Toxins: cytotoxic agents, spironolactone, alcohol
    Radiation
    Orchitis: usually as a result of mumps
Hormone resistance
    Androgen insensitivity
    Luteinizing hormone insensitivity
Hypopituitarism
    Idiopathic
    Tumor
    Other causes
Hyperprolactinemia
    Usually the result of pituitary adenoma
    Idiopathic increased prolactin production
Gonadotropin deficiency
    Hypogonadotropic hypogonadism
    Isolated congenital idiopathic GnRH deficiency
        GnRH deficiency with anosmia: Kallman syndrome
        Acquired GnRH deficiency is very uncommon
    Respond to pulsatile GnRH administration
    Hypothalamic insufficiency
    LH or FSH deficiency
Systemic diseases
    Chronic diseases
    Malnutrition/starvation
    Massive obesity
    AIDS/HIV

Table 2
Laboratory Testing of Hypogonadism

	Hypothalamic	Primary hypogonadism	Seminiferous tubule disease	Leydig cell failure	Pituitary disease	Hypothalamic disease
T		Low	Normal	Low	Low	Low
LH		High	Normal	High	Low	Low
FSH		High	High	Normal	Low	Low
Sperm count		Low	Low	Low	Low	Low
LH and FSH response to GnRH		Normal	Not done	Not done	Low	Normal

Review: Interpreting the results (1) T low, LH and FSH elevated → primary hypogonadism; order karyotype. (2) T low, LH and FSH normal or low → secondary hypogonadism, obtain PRL and computed tomography scan of head to screen for mass lesion; remaining pituitary hormones must be tested for deficiency. (3) T and LH normal, FSH high → abnormal seminiferous tubule compartment; order semen analysis. (4) T, LH and FSH high → androgen resistance syndrome.

Table 3
Clinical Presentation of Peripubertal Hypogonadism

Small testes, phallus, and prostate (prepubertal testes are between 3 and 4 mL in volume and less
    than 3 cm long by 2 cm wide; peripubertal testes are between 4 and 15 mL in volume and 3–
    4 cm long by 2–3 cm wide)
Lack of male-pattern hair growth
Scant pubic and axillary hair, if adrenal androgens are also deficient
Disproportionately long arms and legs (from delayed epiphyseal closure, eunuchoidism; with the
    crown-to-pubis ratio <1 and an arm span more than 6 cm greater than height)
No pubertal growth spurt
No increase in libido or potency
Reduced male musculature
Gynecomastia
Persistently high-pitched voice

Table 4
Clinical Presentation of Postpubertal Hypogonadism

Progressive decrease in muscle mass
Loss of libido
Impotence
Infertility with oligospermia or azoospermia
Hot flashes (with acute onset of hypogonadism)
Osteoporosis
Anemia
Adult testes are usually between 15 and 30 mL and 4.5–5.5 cm long by 2.8–3.3 cm wide
Mild depression
Reduced energy

Postpubertal. Postpubertal loss of testicular function may be manifested by infertility and androgen deficiency. The clinical symptoms and signs may evolve slowly, making
them relatively subtle, particularly in older men in whom they are incorrectly attributed
to aging. The growth of male pattern body hair often slows, but the change of the voice
and the size of the phallus, testes, and prostate may be undetectable. In younger men, a
delay in temporal hair recession and balding may go unnoticed as a manifestation of T
deficiency. Men with postpubertal hypogonadism may have some or all of these clinical
findings, as summarized in Table 4.

GOAL OF ANDROGEN THERAPY

In androgen-replacement therapy, a safe, general principle is to mimic the normal
concentrations of T (350–1050 ng/dL) and its active metabolites (25–29), thereby avoiding unphysiologically high or low serum T concentrations. (Clearly, patients experience
symptoms with androgen deficiency, but whether unphysiologically high concentrations carry health risks is unknown.) When these goals are met, physiological responses
to androgen-replacement therapy allows virilization in prepubertal males and restoration or preservation of virilization in postpubertal men. The therapy should not have

untoward health hazards on the prostate, serum lipids, and cardiovascular, liver and lung function. Ideally, therapy should allow self-administration, be convenient, cause minimal discomfort, and result in reproducible daily pharmacokinetics at a reasonable cost. None of the currently available androgen-replacement therapies achieves the ideal, but their relative merits will be discussed. A review will be made comparing the pharmacokinetics of different androgen preparations widely used for substitution therapy.

OVERVIEW OF PHARMACOLOGY OF ANDROGENS

Historical Aspects

Evidence that the testes produced virilizing substances initially was observed by Berthold in 1849 *(30)*, who transplanted testes from roosters into the abdomen of capons, which made them behave like normal roosters. Butenandt in 1931 *(31)* was the first to obtain T from urine, and David in 1935 *(32)* crystallized it from the urine of bulls. T was then chemically synthesized by Butenandt and Hanisch in 1935 *(33)* and Ruzick and Wettstein in 1935 *(34)*. After its synthesis, T was introduced for treatment of T deficiency. Because oral pure T was ineffective, subcutaneous T pellets were implanted or T's methyl derivative (methylT) was administered orally. In the 1950s, T ester injections gained widespread acceptance *(35)*. Other derivatives were prepared in an attempt to prepare steroids with anabolic properties. In the 1970s T undecanoate, an oral preparation, became available for clinical use in some countries. Because derivatives of T but not fatty acid esters have hepatic toxicity, the emphasis has recently been on delivering pure T by oral, injectable, or transdermal preparations. Although T is metabolized to potent metabolites by steroid 5-α-reductase to form DHT and aromatase to form estradiol, chemical modification of T results in compounds that are poor substrates for these enzymes.

Oral Testosterone Preparations

PURE TESTOSTERONE

Unesterified pure T administered orally is rapidly metabolized by the liver to inactive products and is therefore an ineffective route of administration *(36–39)*.

17A-METHYLT

17α-MethylT was the first orally active, synthesized derivative of T (Table 6). After oral administration, peak blood levels are achieved between 1.5 and 2 h, and its serum half-life is about 150 min, suggesting that several doses daily would be required to maintain a therapeutic level of the steroid *(40)*. Hepatic toxicity, including cholestasis, peliosis, elevation of liver enzymes, and reduction of HDL cholesterol limit its use *(41–44)*.

FLUOXYMESTERONE

This steroid is a 17α-methylT steroid with fluorine in the 9 position and has a longer half-life in serum than the parent steroid, but its risk of hepatoxicity limits its clinical use *(41,45–47)*.

MESTEROLONE

Mesterolone is a derivative of 5 α-dihydrotestosterone with a methyl group in the 1 position. It is not hepatoxic, but it is not metabolized to estrogen, and dosing is difficult to monitor, making it unsatisfactory for replacement therapy *(35,48–53)*.

Table 6
Structure of Testosterone and Its Derivatives

Generic name	R	X	Other modifications
Natural androgens			
Testosterone	H	H	
5α-DihydroT	H	H	4,5-ane
Unmodified 17α esters			
T propionate	$COCH_2CH_3$	H	
T enanthate	$CO(CH_2)_5CH_3$	H	
T cypionate		H	
T undecanoate	$CO(CH_2)_8CH_2=CH_2$	H	
Modified 17α esters			
Methenolone acetate	$COCH_3$	H	1-CH₃; 1,2-ene; 4,5-ane
Nandrolone phenylpropionate		H	19-nor CH₃
Nandrolone decanoate	$CO(CH_2)_6CH_3$	H	19-nor CH₃
17α-Alkylation			
MethylT	H	CH_3	
Fluoxymesterone	H	CH_3	9-F; 11-OH
Methandrostenolone	H	CH_3	1,2-ene
Oxandrolone	H	CH_3	C_2 replaced by O; 4,5-ane
Oxymethelone	H	CH_3	2=CHOH; 4,5-ane
Stanozolol	H	CH_3	4,5-ane; {3,2-c}pyrazole
Danazole	H	$CH\,CH$	{2,3-d}isoxazole
Norethandrolone	H	CH_2CH_3	19-nor CH₃
Ethylestrenole	H	CH_2CH_3	19-nor CH₃; 3-H
Modified androgen			
Mesterolone	H	H	1-CH₃; 4,5-ane

TESTOSTERONE UNDECANOATE

Adding a 17β long aliphatic side-chain ester to T results in good absorption from the gut and substantial uptake by the lymphatics rather than the hepatic portal system. Consequently, free T enters the systemic circulation (63%) without substantial hepatic transformation, and therapeutic T levels are achieved over the first few hours of administration *(29,54–64)*. This preparation is not currently available in the United States, but an improved formulation now being tested in the United States may overcome some of these deficiencies and make it a more satisfactory preparation for androgen replacement therapy.

Sublingual

Sublingual administration of T complexed with hydroxypropyl-β-cyclodextrin results in a rapid rise in serum T, but adequate serum levels of T are sustained for less than 2 h. Its short serum half-life and bitter taste limit its acceptability *(65–68)*.

TESTOSTERONE CYCLODEXTRIN

A sublingual preparation contains natural T surrounded by a carbohydrate ring (2-hydroxypropyl-β cyclodextrin), a facilitator of absorption of T through the oral mucosa *(65–69)*. This preparation may produce physiologic levels of T without untoward toxicity, but reproducible manufacture of the preparation has limited further clinical study.

Intramuscular Preparations

TESTOSTERONE ESTERS OVERVIEW

Esterification of T at the 17 position with a fatty acid prolongs the intramuscular retention and duration of activity of T in proportion to the length of the fatty acid. When administered intramuscularly *(70)*, the androgen ester is slowly absorbed into the circulation where it is then rapidly metabolized to active unesterified T *(71)*. Intrinsic potency, bioavailability, and rate of clearance from the circulation are determinants of the biological actions of androgens.

Testosterone propionate has a short release phase of only 2–3 d and should not be used for long-term replacement therapy *(72)*. Longer-acting preparations include T enanthate (TE), cypionate (TC) and cyclohexane carboxylate, which all have similar steroid release profiles when injected intramuscularly (*see* Fig. 1). A satisfactory regimen is to administer 200 mg of either T enanthate or cypionate once every 2 wk intramuscularly or 100 mg weekly *(72–76)*. T-*trans*-4-*n*-butylcyclohexyl-carboxylate and T undecanoate are even longer-acting preparations. Blood levels following T-*trans*-4-*n*-butylcyclohexyl-carboxylate administration are sustained for about 12 wk after a large injection of 600 mg in a volume of 2.4 mL *(77)*.

NANDROLONE PHENYLPROPIONATE AND DECANOATE

Nandrolone phenylpropionate and decanoate are 17β-hydroxyl esters of 19-norT *(78,79)*, have prolonged action when injected, and are used to treat refractory anemias primarily rather than for androgen-replacement therapy.

MULTIPLE-DOSE PHARMACOKINETICS

As summarized in Fig. 2 and based on simulation and dosing pharmacokinetics, injections of T enanthate (200–250 mg injected every 2 wk) result in a maximal supraphysiological T serum concentrations as high as 51 nmol/L shortly after injection and T serum levels at the lower range of normal T serum concentration (12 nmol/L) before 2 wk *(74,80,81)*.

TESTOSTERONE ESTER COMBINATIONS

Although the intermediate-acting preparations provide high concentrations of T within hours after their administration (*see* Table 5), no advantage has been shown for combining a short- and an intermediate-acting preparation *(74)*.

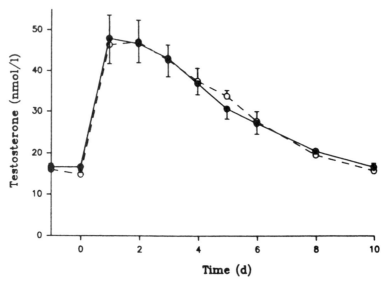

Fig. 1. Comparative pharmacokinetics of 194 mg of T enanthate and 200 mg of T cypionate after intramuscular injection to six normal volunteers. Filled circles: mean ± SEM of T enanthate kinetics; open circles: mean ± SEM of T cypionate kinetics. (From ref. *74*.)

TESTOSTERONE BUCCILATE

Intramuscular injection of 600 mg of T buccilate to hypogonadal men produced serum T concentrations within the normal range for about 8 wk with a terminal elimination half-life of 29.5 d *(77)*. Serum DHT concentrations were within the normal range; estradiol was only slightly increased above normal; SHBG did not change; and gonadotropins were significantly suppressed. No adverse biochemical or prostate responses were reported. It is unknown if this preparation will find use for male contraceptive therapy or replacement for hypogonadism.

TESTOSERONE UNDECANOATE

Intramuscular injections of 500 and 1000 mg of testosterone undecanoate (TU) in hypogonadal men resulted in increased mean serum T levels from less than 10 nmol/L to 47.8 ± 10.1 and 54.2 ± 4.8 nmol/L, respectively, after about 1 wk. Thereafter, serum T levels decreased progressively and reached the lower-normal limit for adult men by d 50–60 and had a terminal elimination half-life of 18.3 ± 2.3 and 23.7 ± 2.7 d, respectively *(82,83)*. Estradiol and DHT followed the pattern of T and remained within normal limits. In these short-term studies, no serious side effects were noted. Intramuscular TU appears to be well suited for long-term substitution therapy in hypogonadism and hormonal male contraception *(82,83)*.

SUBCUTANEOUS TESTOSTERONE IMPLANTS

Fused pellets or silastic capsules of pure T implanted subcutaneously release T in sufficient quantities to maintain physiologic concentrations of T for between 4 and 6 mo *(84,85)*. The bioavailability of T from subdermal pellet implants approaches 100% by 6 mo *(see* Fig. 3) and is proportional to the dose administered. T pellets implanted in 43 hypogonadal men (6 × 100 mg, 3 × 200 mg, 6 × 200 mg; total of 111 implants) reproducibly maintained serum T concentrations within the normal range for 4–6 mo *(see* Fig. 3) *(84,85)*.

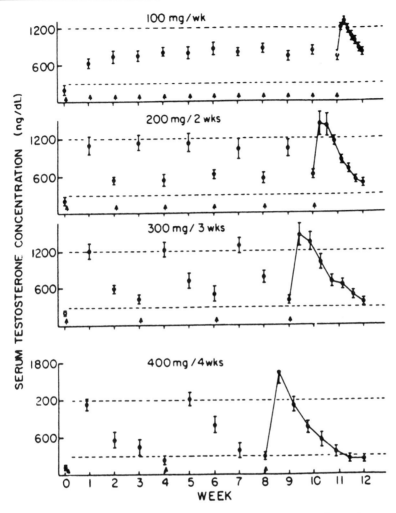

Fig. 2. Serum T concentrations during T replacement therapy in adult primary hypogonadal men. T enanthate was administered by intramuscular injection (arrows) for 12 wk in four dosage regimens: 100 mg weekly; 200 mg every 2 wk; 300 mg every 3 wk; and 4000 mg every 4 wk. Blood was sampled weekly until the last dose and more frequently thereafter. (From ref. *80.*)

Similar results were reported by Jockenhovel et al. *(87)* who implanted 6- to 200-mg fused crystalline T pellets in the subdermal fat tissue of the abdomen in hypogonadal men. An initial peak was observed on the first day of administration; thereafter, a stable plateau lasted for 63 d. On average T values fell below the normal range by 180 d but did not return to baseline for about 300 d. Serum estradiol and DHT were elevated from d 21 to d 105, and SHBG was decreased from d 21 to d 168. Thus, implants of T pellets have potential for both T replacement therapy, as well as reversible male contraception.

Transdermal Testosterone

Transdermal creams containing T have been used in the treatment of microphallus in children *(88)*. The applications probably are effective because of systemic absorption rather than local absorption in the penis. As yet, a widespread clinical trial with these preparations has not been reported *(89)*.

Table 5
Pharmacokinetics and Safety of Androgens

Preparation	Peak	Trough	T monitoring	DHT	Estradiol	Liver dysfunction	HDL cholesterol	Skin irritation
T propionate	1 d	2–3 d	None	Dose depend.	Dose depend.	None	Dose depend.	None
T enanthate	1–2 d	10–14 d	1 wk	Dose depend.	Dose depend.	None	Dose depend.	None
T cypionate	1–2 d	10–14 d	1 wk	Dose depend.	Dose depend.	None	Dose depend.	None
T buccilate	2–4 wk	12–14 wk	4–6 wk	Dose depend.	Dose depend.	None	Dose depend.	None
T pellets	1 mo	6 mo	3–4 mo	Dose depend.	Dose depend.	None	Dose depend.	None
T undeconoate	2–6 h	2–6 h		Increased	Normal	None	Dose depend.	None
T cyclodextrin	1 h	6 h	2–4 h	Normal	Normal	None	Modest	None
MethylT	1.5–2 h	4–5 h	None	Low	Low	Yes	30% dec.	None
Fluoxymesterone				Low	Low	Yes		None
Mesterolone				Low	Low	None		None
T gel	20–24 h	d	24 h	Normal	Normal	None	Modest	Minimal
T scrotal	3–5 h	20–24 h	12 h	Elevated	Normal	None	Modest	Minimal
T nonscrotal	6–8 h	24 h	12 h	Normal	Normal	None	Modest	Yes
DHT topical	4–8 h	20–24 h	DHT 12 h	Elevated	Low	None	Modest	Minimal

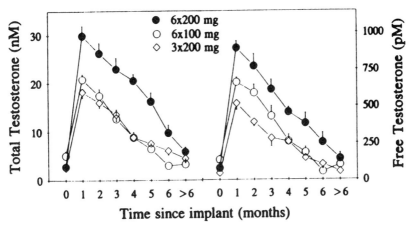

Fig. 3. Plasma total (left) and free (right) T following a single implantation in 43 hypogonadal men. (From ref. *86*).

PERCUTANEOUS DHT IN HYPOGONADAL MEN

A 125-mg dose of hydroalcoholic gel of DHT applied twice daily to the skin can produce sustained concentrations of DHT *(90–92)*. The ratio of DHT/T ratio increased to around 5 (normal ranges between 0.1 and 0.2), and serum T, estradiol, and SHBG concentrations did not increase; no change in gonadotropins was observed *(92)*. Treatment of hypogonadal men reportedly improved virilization and sexual function *(93)*, and a moderate decrease in plasma low-density lipoprotein (LDL) and high-density lipoprotein (HDL) cholesterol levels was observed. DHT therapy did not result in enlargement of the prostate as determined by ultrasound study *(92,94)*.

Transdermal Testosterone

TRANS-SCROTAL TESTOSTERONE

Scrotal skin is at least five times more permeable to T than other skin sites. Testoderm® or Testoderm® With Adhesive will only produce adequate serum T concentrations if applied to scrotal skin. The 60-cm² and 40-cm² Testoderm patches applied to the scrotum of hypogonadal men delivers 4 and 6 mg, respectively, of T daily *(95)*. Peak T concentrations increased progressively during the first 3 wk and then remained stable. Although DHT concentrations remained elevated, the normal range androgen concentrations (T plus DHT) and estradiol were achieved in 80% of hypogonadal men *(28,95–101)*.

NONSCROTAL TESTOSTERONE PATCH THERAPY (ANDRODERM)

Pharmacokinetics. After two 2.5-mg or one 5-mg Androderm system(s) was applied daily to nonscrotal skin (back, abdomen, thighs, and upper arms) at about 10 PM, T was continuously absorbed during the 24-h dosing period. The serum T concentration profile mimicked the normal circadian variation observed in healthy young men (*see* Fig. 4) *(26,102,103)*. In addition, bioavailable T, DHT, and estradiol serum T concentrations (BT) measured during Androderm treatment paralleled the serum T profile (*see* Fig. 4) and remained within the normal reference range.

In clinical studies of Androderm, 93% of patients needed a dose of 5 mg daily to maintain normal concentrations of T; 6%, 7.5 mg daily; and 1%, 2.5 mg daily

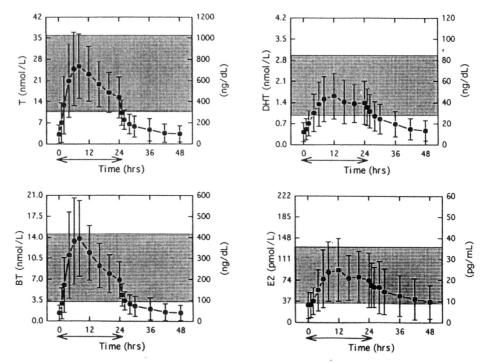

Fig. 4. Serum concentration profiles of T, BT, DHT, and E2 during and after the nighttime application of two TTD systems to the back of 34 hypogonadal men (mean ± SD). The shaded areas represent 95% confidence intervals for morning hormone levels in normal men between the ages of 20–65 yr. The arrow denotes the 24-h duration of TTD system application. (Reproduced with permission from ref. 26.)

(26,102,103). Androderm therapy for 6–12 mo in men with primary hypogonadism had suppressed gonadotropins to normal range in about 50% of men *(26,102–104)*. Androderm therapy had positive effects on fatigue, mood, and sexual function as determined from questionnaires and nocturnal penile tumescence *(26,102–104)*.

Comparison with Intramuscular Testosterone. In a study of 66 patients previously treated with T injections, subjects were randomized to receive either Androderm or intramuscular T enanthate (200 mg every 2 wk) treatment for 6 mo *(102)*. The percent of normal range serum concentrations of T, bioavailable T, DHT, and estradiol was 82, 87, 76, and 81%, respectively, compared with 72, 39, 70, and 35%, respectively, for intramuscular T injections. Sexual function assessment and lipid profiles were comparable between groups.

Management of Skin Irritation. Chronic contact dermatitis resulting mainly from the alcohol component of the patch occurs in about 10% of men following several weeks of use of Androderm. Applying about two drops of 0.1% triamcinolone acetonide cream to the skin under the central drug reservoir has been shown to greatly reduce contact dermatitis and itching without significantly affecting T delivery *(105,106)*. The quantity of glucocorticoid applied and absorbed is insufficient to produce significant alteration of the hypothalamic–pituitary–adrenal axis. Hydrocortisone is less effective, and ointments should not be used because they will diminish T delivery.

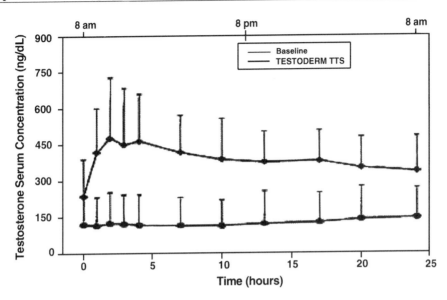

Fig. 5. Serum concentrations of T (mean±SD) during pretreatment baseline or while wearing a Testoderm TTS system on the upper buttocks (*n* = 32). Systems were applied at 0 h (8 AM) and removed 24 h later. (From Physician Desk Reference).

TESTODERM TTS

Testoderm TTS applied each morning to the arm, back, or upper buttocks delivers physiologic amounts of T that exhibits a serum T circadian pattern resembling normal men (*see* Fig. 5). Following skin application, T concentrations peak at 2–4 h, continue to be absorbed during the 24-h dosing period, and return toward baseline within approx 2 h after removal of the system. In clinical trials, 94% of patients on Testoderm TTS treatment had peak (531 ng/dL) and average (366 ng/dL) serum T concentrations within the normal range. Applying two systems also doubles the amount of T delivered. When applied to the skin sites recommended (arm, back, or upper buttocks), the ratio of T to DHT or estradiol was also normal. The most commonly reported adverse events were application site reactions of transient itching (12%) and moderate or severe erythema (3%). All topical reactions decreased with duration of use.

ANDROGEL™

AndroGel™ 5 G, 7.5 G, or 10 G contain packets of 50 mg, 75 mg, or 100 mg of T, respectively. Approximately 10% of the applied T dose is absorbed across skin of average permeability during a 24-h period, resulting in circulating concentrations of T observed in normal men (*107*). Figure 6 summarizes the 24-h pharmacokinetic profiles of T for patients maintained on 5 G or 10 G of AndroGel (to deliver 50 or 100 mg of T, respectively) for 30 d. The average (± SD) daily T concentration produced by AndroGel 10 G on d 30 was 792 (± 294) ng/dL and by AndroGel 5 G, it was 566 (± 262) ng/dL.

AndroGel dries quickly when applied to the skin surface, and the skin serves as a reservoir for the sustained release of T into the systemic circulation (*107*). After the first 10 G dose, increases in serum T are observed within 30 min; and by 4 h of application, most patients have a serum T concentration within the normal range. Absorption of T into

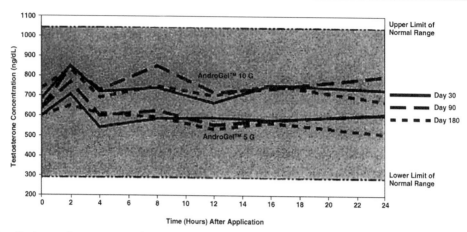

Fig. 6. shows the mean steady-state serum T concentrations in patients applying 5 g or 10 g Androgel once daily. (Data on file. Unimed Pharmaceuticals.)

the blood is sustained for the 24-h dosing interval, resulting in serum T concentrations approximating the steady-state level by the end of the first 24 h and achieving steady state by the second or third day of dosing.

Serum T levels decrease sharply after withdrawal of the patches, but serum T concentrations remain in the normal range for 24–48 h after the last application, and it take 5 d to return to baseline. Eighty-seven percent achieved an average serum T level within the normal range on treatment d 180.

Potential Partner Testosterone Transfer. Studies of the potential for dermal T transfer following AndroGel use between males dosed with AndroGel and their untreated female partners indicated that unprotected female partners had a serum T concentration more than twice the baseline value at some time during the study. When a barrier, such as a shirt, covered the application site(s), no transfer of T from the males to the female partners was observed.

Following AndroGel doses of 5 G/d and 10 G/d, DHT and estradiol concentrations increased in parallel with T concentrations, and the DHT/T ratio and estradiol levels stayed within the normal range. During AndroGel treatment, decreases of serum levels of SHBG were modest (1–11%), and serum levels of LH and FSH in men with hypergonadotropic hypogonadism fell in a dose- and time-dependent manner during treatment with AndroGel. Although skin reactions were reported in 3–5% of patients using AndroGel for up to 6 mo, none was severe enough to require treatment or discontinuation of drug.

TOSTREX

A new T gel (Cellegy Pharmaceuticals, Inc.) has undergone clinical trials in about 200 hypogonadal men. The initial dose applied to the skin daily raises the serum concentrations of T on the first day of application, and reaches steady state by 14 d. A metered-dose canister allows adjusting the dose in 10-mg increments. Following adjustment of the dose based on the testosterone concentrations on d 14, over 90% of men achieved a 24-h concentration average within the normal physiologic range, as was the ratio of estradiol to T and DHT to T. Its safety profile in terms of chemistries, lipid profiles, polycythemia, and prostate-specific antigen were comparable to other transdermal testosterone preparations on the market. Tostrex therapy for 6 mo resulted in improvement of hip and spine bone mineral density (BMD) of about 4%.

Human Chorionic Gonadotropin

Human chorionic gonadotropin (hCG) is a polypeptide hormone produced by the human placenta and is composed of an α-subunit essentially identical to the α-subunits of the human pituitary gonadotropins (LH and FSH) and TSH. A specific α-subunit of hCG binds to the LH receptors on Leydig cells and stimulates endogenous T production from the testes. hCG also has some FSH activity that differs from pure LH.

In prepubertal boys between the ages of 4 and 9 yr with cryptorchidism not caused by anatomical obstruction, hCG treatment is done with the following regimen: 4000 USP units of hCG three times weekly for 3 wk; then 5000 U every 2 d for 4 injections followed by 15 injections of 500 to 1000 U for 6 wk; and then, 500 U three times a week for 4–6 wk.

Human chorionic gonadotropin is an alternative to T therapy in inducing pubertal development in boys and treating androgen deficiency in men with gonadotropin deficiency. In young prepubertal boys (e.g., 13–14 yr of age) presenting with hypogonadotropic hypogonadism and delayed puberty, hCG may be begun at a dosage of 1000–2000 IU intramuscularly. It is then slowly increased during the next 1–2 yr to the adult dosages of 1000–2000 IU intramuscularly, two to three times weekly (*see* Table 7). Some men with gonadotropin deficiency require either higher or lower dosages of hCG. Therapy in prepubertal boys can be monitored by assessing the clinical response to treatment by following the progression of virilization and growth and the serum T concentration, which should be maintained within the normal range for the desired Tanner stage of sexual development *(108)*.

Human chorionic gonadotropin therapy has two major advantages over T replacement therapy. Firstly, it stimulates growth of the testes, which may be important to boys with delayed puberty *(108)*. Secondly, it may stimulate sufficient intratesticular T production to facilitate initiation of spermatogenesis. hCG treatment has several disadvantages. It requires frequent injections, is expensive, elevates estradiol relative to T and may cause gynecomastia. If neutralizing antibodies to hCG are induced, they may reduce the efficacy of hCG or make it completely ineffective *(1,8)*.

POTENTIAL BENEFITS OF ANDROGEN THERAPY

Testosterone Replacement Therapy in Andropause (Aging Men)

(This topic will be covered in detail in Chapter 21.) Most studies have confirmed an age-related decline in T beginning in the fourth decade of life, and about 20% of men by age 60 have serum T concentrations of less than 300–350 ng/dL *(2–5,14,27,28,109–113)*. Because SHBG rises in aging men, bioavailable T (non-SHBG-bound) or free T concentrations may better reflect the deficiency of T than the total T concentration. Thus, free or bioavailable T measurements are recommended when the total T concentration is between 200 and 400 ng/dL.

Testosterone Effects on Body Composition

Studies in older men treated with T replacement have generally confirmed that body fat mass declines and lean body mass increases. Several forms of therapy have been used and

Table 7
Treatment of Male Hypogonadism

Group	Goal of therapy	Plasma T	Preparation	Usual dose
Delayed adolescence	Short-term maintenance, initial	100–300 ng/dL	hCG	500 IU im 1–2 times/wk
			Androderm	2.5 mg patch, 12 h at night
			TE or TC	50–100 mg q 3–4 wk
	Subsequent	300–400 ng/dL	Androderm	2.5 mg/daily
			TE or TC	100 q 2 wk
Adult	Long-term maintenance	400–1000 ng/dL		
Hypogonadotropic			GnRH[a]	5–30 μg sc q 2 h
hypogonadism				
Hypogonadism			hCG	1000–4000 IU im 1–3 times/wk
			Androderm, Testoderm, Androgel	5 mg/d
			Testoderm, Scrotal	4 or 6 mg/d
			TE or TC	200 mg q 2 wk or 100 q 1 wk im
	Subreplacement		Fluoxymesterone	5–10 mg/d po
			Methyltestosterone	5–25 mg daily
			T undecanoate[b]	200 po q 2 wk

[a]Experimental, requires programmed pump.
[b]Not available in the United States.
Abbreviations: hCG, human chorionic gonadotropin; GnRH, gonadotropin-releasing hormone; TE, T enanthate; TC, T cypionate.

include T esters, the scrotal patch, and a gel preparation. In addition, some aspects of muscle strength, fat-free mass, and visceral fat improved. These studies were relatively short and ranged in length between 3 and 18 mo. The studies are too small and of inadequate length to make it possible to compare one treatment modality to another (114–117).

Muscle Performance and Wasting

In addition, the measurement of the triceps and quadriceps increased significantly as did muscle strength measured by one repetition maximum of weight lifting. These results are in agreement with cross-sectional studies in men with the AIDS wasting syndrome (118). Testosterone therapy is used for management of weight loss and wasting associated with AIDS (119–121). Administration of replacement doses of T to healthy hypogonadal and HIV-infected men improves lean body mass, muscle size, and maximal voluntary strength (122). Sih et al. (123) reported improvement of bilateral grip strength in older hypogonadal men treated with T at 3, 6, 9, and 12 mo of therapy.

Mood

In elderly and younger hypogonadal men, T therapy improves spatial cognition, sense of well being, libido, fatigue, self-reported sense of energy ($49 \pm 19\%$ to $66 \pm 24\%$; $p = 0.01$) and sexual function ($24 \pm 20\%$ to $66 \pm 24\%$; $p < 0.001$) within the first 3 mo of initiation of therapy (68,114,115,124–127).

Testosterone therapy (68) significantly decreases anger, irritability, sadness, tiredness, and nervousness while improving energy level, friendliness, and sense of well-being. Sih et al. (123) did find an improvement of memory with of T replacement.

Impotence

Impotence in hypogonadal men may be corrected in about 75% of men if the cause of impotence is androgen deficiency (128). Some men have androgen deficiency and impotence caused by other factors. If several months of T therapy does not correct their impotence, other causes should be sought.

Leptin

Although serum T is negatively associated with leptin in men, the association is confounded with visceral and subcutaneous adipose tissue, fasting insulin, and sex hormones. Thus, T does not appear to be the major determinate of serum leptin in men (129). In aging men, a rise of serum leptin levels occurs, and a strong association between serum leptin and adiposity is maintained (130). Furthermore, T ester therapy significantly reduced leptin concentrations in elderly men (123), normalizes elevated *ob* gene product leptin (OB) levels in hypogonadal men (131) and also decreases leptin concentrations in boys with delayed puberty (132). The studies suggest the hypothalamic–pituitary–gonadal–adipose tissue axis is involved in body weight maintenance and reproductive function (131,133).

Osteoporosis

Androgen Deficiency and Osteoporosis

Effects of Androgens in Normal Men. Androgens affect both by the peak bone mass achieved during development and the subsequent amount of bone lost. The dramatic increase in both cortical and trabecular bone density during puberty in boys (134,135) is attributed to the pubertal rise in T or one of its metabolites. During puberty, an increase in serum alkaline phosphatase heralds a rise in osteoblast activity and subsequent bone density increases. In normal boys, peak trabecular bone density is usually achieved by the age of 18 yr (135), and peak cortical bone density is often reached a few years later. Bone density remains relatively stable in young adult males and then declines slowly after age 35 yr (136); the bone loss is regulated by genetic, endocrine, mechanical, and nutritional factors.

BONE DENSITY IN HYPOGONADAL MEN

Studies in Men with Primary Hypogonadism. Surgical or medical castration in men results in a reduction in BMD and elevated biochemical markers of bone turnover (137,138). These findings suggest that gonadal steroid deficiency is associated with increased bone turnover and loss, leading to osteoporosis (*see* Fig. 7); other secondary causes are glucocorticosteroid therapy, skeletal metastases, multiple myeloma, gastric surgery, and anticonvulsant and neuroleptic treatment (139–142).

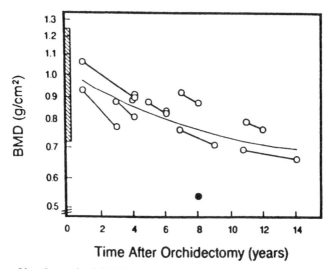

Time After Orchidectomy (years)

Fig. 7. Scattergram of lumbar spinal BMD as a function of time after orchidectomy in 12 men. In eight patients, the measurement was repeated after 1–3 yr. The hatched bar indicates the normal range for 20 men matched for age. The solid circle represents the value for one man who developed a hip fracture. (Reproduced with permission from ref. *137*.)

Although hypogonadism is found in up to 20% of men with vertebral crush fractures or osteoporosis, the clinical features of T deficiency may be subtle.

Aging and Osteoporosis

Osteoporosis is one of the leading causes of morbidity and mortality in the elderly. Bone is lost with advancing age in both men and women, leading to an increased incidence of osteoporotic fractures of the forearm, vertebral body, and femoral neck. Although aging women lose more bone than men, aging men still lose 30% of their trabecular bone and 20% of their cortical bone *(136)*. Thus, despite lower rates of osteoporosis in men than in women, one-fifth of all hip fractures occur in men and hypogonadism is one of the most common underlying causes *(143,144)*. Further study is needed to clarify this association between bone loss and T deficiency, but androgen replacement in aging hypogondal men does improve BMD *(115,123)*.

Men with acquired hypogonadism, idiopathic hypogonadotropic hypogonadism (IHH) and constitutionally delayed puberty have reduced BMD and may be at increased risk for osteoporosis. In boys with delayed puberty or IHH, T may not result in normal bone accretion in adulthood *(145–147)*. Finkelstein et al. *(147)* postulated that inadequate bone accretion rather than accelerated bone loss may account for the diminished adult bone mass of patients with delayed puberty or IHH. Both radial and spinal bone mineral density were significantly lower in men with histories of delayed puberty than in normal controls (see Fig. 8A,B). These results establish that T replacement in young or elderly hypogonadal men improve BMD.

Glucocorticoids, Androgens, and Osteoporosis

Osteoporosis is associated with both hypogonadism and corticosteroid therapy. In addition, glucocorticoid therapy may cause a variety of adverse systemic effects, including adrenal suppression, dermal thinning, and a reduction in total bone calcium. Test-

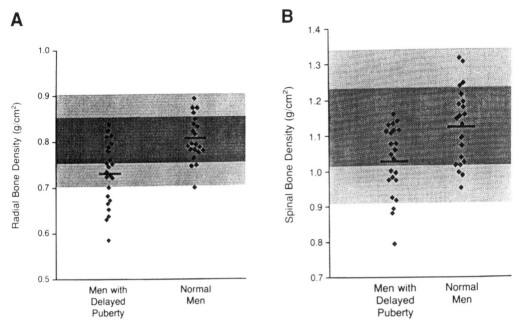

Fig. 8. Radial bone density (**A**) and spinal bone density (**B**) in 23 men with histories of delayed puberty and 21 normal controls. The horizontal lines indicate the group means, and the shaded areas indicate the mean ± 1 SD and ± 2 SD. for the normal men. (Reproduced with permission from ref. *147*.)

osterone levels are reduced about 33% by long-term oral prednisolone treatment, but are minimally affected by therapeutic doses of inhaled corticosteroids *(148–152)*.

HYPOGONADISM, OSTEOPOROSIS, AND TESTOSTERONE THERAPY

Recently, Behre et al. *(153)* reported on the long-term effects of androgen-replacement therapy on BMD in hypogonadal men. During the first year of therapy, BMD increased 26% (see Figs. 9 and 10). In 72 hypogonadal men, long-term therapy maintained BMD in the age-dependent reference range independent of whether the patients had primary or secondary hypogonadism. Adequate T-replacement therapy with injection of T esters, oral or transdermal preparations will improve BMD, markers of bone formation and resorption and also treat osteoporosis in hypogonadal men *(115,116,154,155)*.

MECHANISM OF ACTION OF ANDROGENS ON BONE

The mechanism(s) whereby androgens affect bone density is still unclear. Testosterone can be converted to DHT by human bone in vitro. However, inhibition of DHT formation by administration of an inhibitor of 5α-reductase has no effect on bone mass in humans *(156)* or rats. The aromatization of T into estrogens may be important for many of the effects of T on bone: (1) Estrogen receptors are present in human osteoblasts *(157–164)*; (2) estrogens appear to maintain bone mass in castrated male-to-female transsexuals; (3) men with complete estrogen resistance as a result of a genetic defect in the estrogen receptor or aromatase deficiency have severe osteopenia despite normal T levels and complete virilization *(165)*. These findings provide compelling evidence that

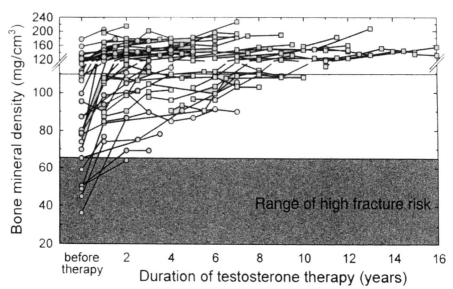

Fig. 9. Increase in BMD during long-term T-substitution therapy up to 16 yr in 72 hypogonadal patients. Circles indicate hypogonadal patients with first QCT measurement before initiation of T-substitution therapy, squares show those patients already receiving T therapy at the first QCT. The dark shaded areas indicates the range of high fracture risk, the unshaded area shows the range without significant fracture risk, and the light shaded area indicates the intermediate range where fractures may occur. (Reproduced with permission from ref. *153*.)

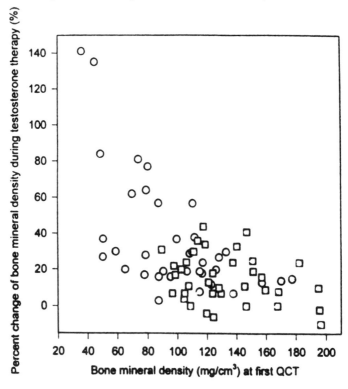

Fig. 10. Correlation between BMD at the first QCT measurement and percent change in BMD during T-substitution therapy. Circles indicate hypogonadal patients with first QCT measurement before initiation of T-substitution therapy; squares show those patients already receiving T therapy at the first QCT. (Reproduced with permission from ref. *153*.)

estrogens are required for a normal peak bone mass in men. However, cortical bone mineral density is higher in men than in women (135); whether this is secondary to the larger muscle mass in men (than in women) is unknown.

THERAPY OF ANDROGEN-DEFICIENCY BONE LOSS

Androgen-replacement therapy has been shown to increase in BMD in hypogonadal men and particularly those with skeletal immaturity (147,166). The studies of Snyder et al. (115) suggest that improvement in BMD is achieved with a eugonadal serum concentration of T (>350 ng/dL) (115), so even in men with modest decreases of serum T concentrations, osteoporosis is observed. Long-term studies are needed to determine if T therapy will prevent osteoporosis without causing undue risks. Although it appears that normalization of serum T concentrations is satisfactory therapy for osteoporosis of hypogonadism, studies comparing various forms of androgen-replacement therapy on management and prevention of osteoporosis should be conducted. For some men, androgens are contraindicated and designer estrogens or bisphosphonates may provide benefits in preventing bone loss after induction of hypogonadism with medical or surgical therapy.

PRECAUTIONS OF ANDROGEN THERAPY IN AGING MEN

Several complications of androgen replacement therapy have been reported. With T preparations, the risk of adverse influences on water retention, polycythemia, hepatotoxicity, sleep apnea, prostate enlargement, and cardiovascular appear small.

Water Retention

Some weight gain is common with androgen-replacement therapy, but the occurrence of peripheral edema, hypertension, and congestive heart failure is uncommon (167).

Polycythemia

Androgens stimulate erythropoiesis, which accounts for higher hematocrits in normal men compared to hypogonadal men. Because older men tend to have lower hematocrits than younger men, the risk of polycythemia is low (167). Although Sih et al. (123) reported that 24% of older men treated with injections of T cypionate (200 mg every 2 wk) had hematocrits above 52%, T-patch therapy appears to have a lower risk for hematocrit elevation than injections of 200 mg of T esters given every 2 wk (168). Men with a history of polycythemia should be monitored closely, and those without a history of polycythemia should have periodic screening of the hematocrit.

Sleep Apnea

Testosterone-replacement therapy has been associated with worsening of sleep apnea, apparently without affecting upper airway dimension (169,170).

Recent studies of T therapy in older men have not reported sleep apnea as a complication. However, men with a history of sleep apnea were generally excluded from participation (166).

Serum Lipids

An elevation of total cholesterol and a suppression of HDL are known risk factors for cardiovascular disease. Many studies have shown a reduction in total cholesterol and

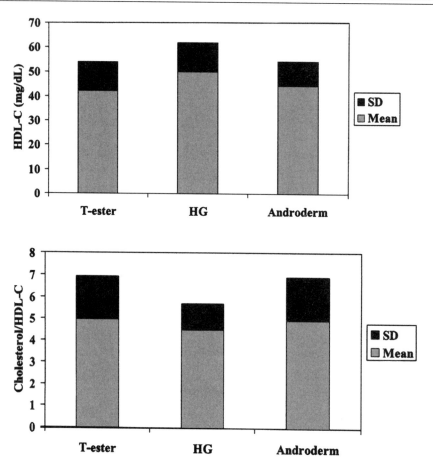

Fig. 11. Lipid changes during Androderm and T enanthate therapy in hypogonadal men. Mean ± SE. (Reproduced with permission from ref. *26*.)

LDL cholesterol in response to androgen replacement therapy without an adverse profile for HDL cholesterol. Higher than usual replacement doses of T have been associated with adverse lipid profiles *(171–174)*.

ANDROGEN EFFECTS ON PLASMA LIPIDS

Compared to an androgen-withdrawal interval of 8 wk, Androderm treatment for 1 yr decreased cholesterol 1.2% and HDL 8%, but increased the ratio of cholesterol to HDL 9% *(102)* (*see* Fig. 11). Other studies with transdermal (patches and gel systems) androgen-replacement therapy have shown comparable results *(114,115,175)*. However, these results were not significantly different from those measured during the intramuscular injection baseline treatment phase. In the study of Dobs et al. *(175)*, during the T replacement phases, serum HDL levels showed a strong negative correlation with BMI and other obesity parameters. Thus, the results of transdermal T replacement on serum lipids were consistent with physiologic effects of T observed in eugonadal men.

In other studies in healthy younger men, Golderberg et al. *(176)* reported that treatment with a GnRH agonist produced elevation of HDL cholesterol, apo AI, and apo B levels, and no change in triglycerides. If androgen replacement is done along with GnRH therapy, the rise in HDL cholesterol can be aborted *(171–174,177)*. GnRH plus 100 mg/ wk of TE produced only a slight decrease in HDL cholesterol without a significant change in HDL2 or 3 and apo AI. Estradiol was shown to be important in preventing the drop in HDL2 in men treated with T *(173)*. The relationship between androgen therapy and changes in plasma lipids is complex because androgens also are associated with changes in body composition and metabolic variables *(178)*. In older men treated with T cypionate or enanthate, no adverse effects of therapy were reported for cholesterol, LDL, HDL, or triglycerides *(179,180)*.

Oral methylT replacement therapy decreases HDL by more than 30%, with striking changes in the HDL2 subfraction and apo AI and AII. LDL cholesterol rises about 30–40% with a decrease of 65–80% in Lp(a) levels (at least in women) *(181,182)*. The more profound influence of anabolic androgens compared with parenteral T preparations appears to be related to the metabolism of T to estradiol and to lack of first-pass liver effects. Thus, oral nonaromatizable androgens have a greater suppression of HDL cholesterol than do aromatizable androgens such as T.

Prostate Disease

Benign Prostate Enlargement

Progressive growth of the prostate occurs in both the transition and peripheral zones of the prostate as men age *(183–186)*. In both normal and hypogonadal aging men, androgen withdrawal results in a significant reduction in prostate volume of both zones *(see* Fig. 12) *(185)*. Meikle et al. *(185)* found a high correlation with the volume of the prostate and age in men receiving T enanthate during androgen withdrawal and during androgen therapy with Androderm. Following 8 wk of androgen withdrawal, Androderm treatment resulted in growth of the prostate to the size observed during T enanthate therapy. Over the next 9 mo, further enlargement was not observed. In a cross-sectional study, Behre et al. *(187)* reported that in untreated hypogonadal men, no significant correlation existed between prostate volume and age. In contrast, T-treated men and normal men showed a positive correlation with prostate volume and age, and no significant age-adjusted differences were observed between the T-treated men and normal controls *(see* Fig. 13) consistent with the studies of Meikle et al. *(185)*. Serum concentrations of PSA were not elevated above those expected in men of comparable age, which is consistent with results reported recently by Sih et al. *(123)*. Jin and associates *(188)* observed that despite adequate long-term androgen-replacement therapy in men with androgen deficiency, they had reduced volumes of the central and peripheral zones as well as the total volume compared to age-matched controls, suggesting that age combined with T is important for prostate growth in mid-life. Because lower urinary tract symptoms are strongly influenced by hereditary factors and prostate volume *(189)*, it is not surprising that androgen-replacement therapy is associated with symptomatic prostate symptoms. Although there are limitations in study design, these observations do not suggest that androgen-replacement therapy will cause growth of the prostate beyond what will occur in men with normal gonadal function.

Prostate Cancer

Prostate cancer is an androgen-responsive cancer, but evidence that T therapy causes prostate cancer is lacking *(190,191)*. An undiagnosed prostate cancer may grow in response to T therapy. A PSA and digital rectal examination is recommended in men age

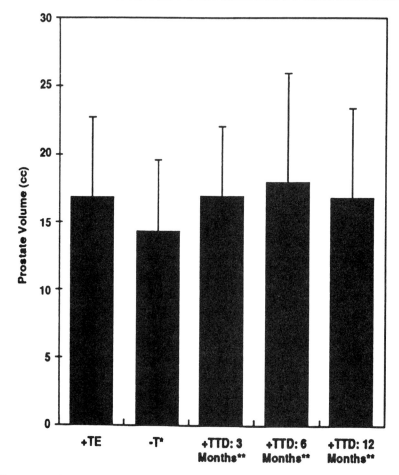

Fig. 12. Prostate volumes measured by TRUS. (T = T; TE = T enanthate; TTD = T transdermal system.) (Reproduced with permission from ref. *185.*)

40 and over before initiation of androgen-replacement therapy for hypogonadism. Further, screening for prostate cancer in men on T therapy should follow the usual guidelines for normal men of comparable age. None of the studies of androgen-replacement of men has shown an increased risk of prostate cancer. However, long-term controlled studies are needed in aging men.

OTHER CONSIDERATIONS OF TREATMENT OF ANDROGEN DEFICIENCY

The main use of androgen-replacement therapy is in the management of men with T deficiency. The cause of the hypogonadism should be established to determine if it might be reversible. If so, therapy should be directed at correction of the underlying cause. For example, hyperprolactinemia from a pituitary tumor can be treated with bromocryptine, which will often correct the T deficiency. Some tumors of the pituitary or hypothalamus may require surgical or irradiation therapy. Thus, in addition to secondary or tertiary hypogonadism, other deficiencies, such as ACTH, growth hormone, and thyroid-stimu-

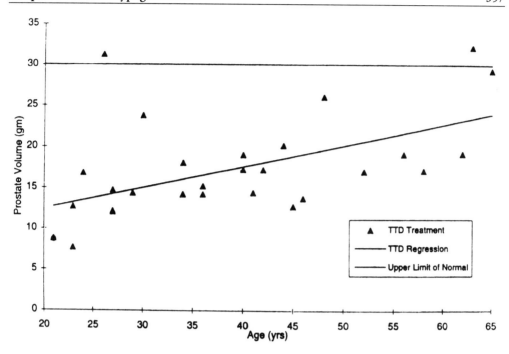

Fig. 13. Linear regression of prostate volume with age. Prostate volume correlated significantly with age during 1 yr of T transdermal system treatment ($r = 0.55$, $p < 0.01$). (IM = IM; TTD = T transdermal system.) (Reproduced with permission from ref. *185*.)

lating hormone (TSH) may exist and require management. Systemic illness and gluco-corticoid therapy will cause hypogonadism, and depending on the clinical situation, androgen-replacement therapy may be considered in such patients. In aging men, andro-gen replacement therapy requires the usual monitoring for diseases incident to age but may offer benefits in bone preservation, lean body mass, mood, and intellectual and sexual function. For men who desire fertility at some time in their life, hormonal therapy directed at enhancing spermatogenesis may be successful. After fertility therapy is deemed a success or a failure, resumption of conventional T therapy is then indicated.

Severe gynecomastia or small testes may contribute to psychological problems or social embarrassment for some hypogonadal boys and men. Gynecomastia usually does not regress and may worsen during hormonal replacement therapy of hypogonadism; plastic surgery (reductive mammoplasty) is a reasonable alternative. Some patients with secondary hypogonadism may have enlargement of the testes in response to gonadotro-pin therapy, but such therapy is not indicated in men with primary hypogonadism, such as those with Klinefelter's syndrome who have extremely small testes. Surgical implan-tation of testicular prostheses is an option for some men and may have psychological benefits.

SUMMARY OF ANDROGEN-REPLACEMENT THERAPY

The hormone replacement goals for management of male hypogonadism depend on both the cause and the stage of sexual development in which gonadal failure occurs (Table 7). Androgen-replacement therapy is indicated to stimulate and sustain normal secondary sexual characteristics, sexual function, and behavior in prepubertal boys and men with either primary or secondary hypogonadism. Several options for replacement therapy are available in various countries, and the availability of those preparations should be taken into consideration by the clinician before therapy is instituted. The goal is to normalize physiology as closely as possible and at the lowest cost. All of these factors influence the decision, which is shared with the physician and patient.

The available T esters for intramuscular injection (T propionate, T enanthate, T cypionate, and T cyclohexane carboxylate) do not achieve physiologic serum T profiles for the treatment of male hypogonadism (*see* Table 7). However, they do achieve therapeutic responses when administered in appropriate doses and intervals. Doses and injection intervals frequently prescribed in the clinic result in initial supraphysiologic androgen levels and subnormal levels prior to the next injection. Injections of 100 mg of T enanthate or cypionate intramuscular at weekly intervals would more closely approximate normal physiology than 200–250 mg every 2–3 wk. However, an injection frequency more often than 2 wk may be unacceptable to many patients. Further, because both the short-acting and intermediate-acting esters show maximal serum concentrations shortly after injection, there is no advantage in combining short-acting T esters (i.e., T propionate) and longer-acting esters (i.e., T enanthate) for T-replacement therapy.

Of the clinically available injectable androgen esters, 19-norT hexoxyphenyipropionate shows the best pharmacokinetic profile. However, as a derivative of the naturally occurring T, 19-norT might not possess its full pharmacodynamic spectrum and, therefore, is not an ideal drug for treatment of male hypogonadism *(78,79)*.

Oral administration of T undecanoate is easy to administer, and a new formulation may reduce the need for multiple daily doses. The most favorable pharmacokinetic profiles of T are observed using either the transdermal patch or gel systems. The scrotal system has the disadvantage of supraphysiologic DHT concentrations and is not easy to use for many patients. Daily administration of Androderm, in the evening results in serum T concentrations in the normal range, mimicking the regular circadian rhythm. The nontranscrotal system has the disadvantage of local skin reactions, which can often be successfully managed with topical glucocorticoid administration. Testoderm, TTS also produces a circadian variation of T delivery and satisfactory replacement therapy. Patch adherence is a problem for many patients, which reduces its therapeutic efficacy. Skin reactions are much less with Testoderm, TTS than with Androderm. Androgel, also produces T levels within the normal range but does not have a distinct diurnal delivery pattern. A newer gel preparation should be available soon. Skin reactions are much less frequent with gels than with patch systems, and because the gels are transparent after application, they are more discreet. Person-to-person transfer is a potential problem with gels, but this problem can be avoided with appropriate precautions. Currently, several satisfactory options for T-replacement therapy are available to clinicians in various countries. Of course, the treatment must be tailored for each patient, and important considerations include ease of use, physiologic replacement, few side effects, and cost. All of these should be discussed with the patient before making the selection. Although T esters, T enanthate, and T cypionate are effective, safe, and the least expensive androgen preparations available (particularly if self-administered), they require administration by injection into a large muscle. Testosterone enanthate and cypionate are considered equally effective and have been popular in the past for treatment of hypogonadal men (*see* Table 7).

Prepubertal

Androgen-replacement therapy in prepubertal hypogonadism is usually started at about 14 yr of age. The earliest sign of puberty in boys is enlargement of the testes. Increases in serum LH and T levels (initially at night) are the hormonal signals that also indicate the onset of puberty *(1,8)*. Growth, virilization, and psychological adjustment are evaluated clinically during androgen-replacement therapy. Severe emotional and psychological distress in affected boys and their families makes earlier institution of androgen replacement therapy a prudent choice. It is often difficult to accurately distinguish between simple delayed puberty and hypogonadism. Therefore, only transient androgen therapy is used until permanent hypogonadism is established, which then dictates continuous treatment to induce puberty and maintain sexual function *(1,8)*. In young boys with delayed puberty and also markedly retarded bone age and short stature, excessive androgen treatment causes rapid virilization and increases in long bone growth and also may lead to premature closure of epiphyses, resulting in compromised adult height *(1,8)*.

In boys with simple delayed puberty, gradual replacement therapy with T is usually begun using a 50 or 100 of T enanthate or cypionate intramuscularly monthly *(1,8)* or 2.5 mg daily of transdermal T. The design of the regimen in boys is to duplicate the changes in T that occur with puberty in normal boys and thus gradual virilization and progression of secondary sexual development. This regimen will stimulate long bone growth and initiate virilization without interfering with the onset of spontaneous puberty. If simple delayed puberty or hypogonadism is diagnosed, the dosage of T ester is increased to 50–100 mg every 2 wk or 2.5 mg of Androderm, nightly for 12 h for approx 6 mo. It is then stopped for 3–6 mo for assessment of the spontaneous onset and progression of puberty. If spontaneous pubertal development and growth do not occur, androgen therapy is reinstituted for another 6 mo with 100 mg of T ester every 2 wk or 2.5 mg of Androderm, daily. This will produce further virilization; full virilization can be achieved over the next few years with full adult replacement doses. Full adult replacement dosages are seldom needed in those with simple delayed puberty.

Adults

In adults with hypogonadism, androgen-replacement therapy is begun by administering a 5 mg delivery dose of a patch or gel system or 200 mg of either T enanthate or cypionate, intramuscularly every 2 wk. Figures 1 and 2 display the fluctuations of serum T concentrations after intramuscular injection of 200 mg of either ester. Injectable T preparations result in T levels at or above the normal range 1–4 d after administration and then gradually fall over the subsequent 2 wk and may be below the normal range before the next injection. Administering 100 mg of T enanthate or cypionate intramuscularly weekly produces a better pattern of T levels, but higher doses at less frequent intervals deviate much more from physiologic normal T range *(74,80)*. Patients, family members, or friends can be taught to give deep intramuscular injections of T esters; otherwise, injections by nursing personnel in the clinic are needed.

The therapeutic efficacy of androgen replacement is assessed by monitoring the patient's clinical and serum T responses *(1,8)*. Variability in response to T therapy in hypogonadal men in libido, potency, sexual activity, feeling of well-being, motivation, energy level, aggressiveness, stamina, and hematocrit is considerable and may occur during the first few weeks to months of androgen-replacement therapy. Body hair, muscle mass and strength, and bone mass increase over months to years. In a sexually immature, eunuchoidal man, androgen replacement also stimulates development of secondary sexual characteristics and long bone growth. Many months to years may be required to achieve the mature adult status.

If injectable forms of T are used, T levels during therapy should be in the mid-normal range 1 wk after an injection and above the lower limit of the normal range preceding the next injection. In some hypogonadal men treated with T esters, disturbing fluctuations in sexual function, energy level, and mood are associated with fluctuations in serum T concentrations between injections. Thus, some patients may complain of reduced energy level and sexual function a few days before their next T injection and have serum T levels below the eugonadal range at that time. Shortening the dosing interval of T ester administration from every 2 wk to every 10 d is recommended in these patients.

With patch and gel systems, a beginning dose of 5 mg of T is recommended for adults; however, a smaller dose may be appropriate for some elderly men. Therapeutic efficacy of patch and gel systems can be monitored by measurement of serum T concentrations about 12 h after application and continued daily for 7–14 d. If levels are not in the eugonadal range, then the dose should be adjusted. Men who have been hypogonadal for prolonged intervals may experience alarming changes in sexual desire and function, which may cause stress in a sexual relationship *(1,8)*. Counseling of patients and their partners before beginning androgen replacement is recommended to help reduce or alleviate these adjustment problems. Beginning with a lower replacement dose may be wise, particularly in an elderly hypogonadal man.

As discussed in detail elsewhere, men with prepubertal hypogonadotropic hypogonadism require the combined treatment with hCG plus human menopausal gonadotropins to initiate sperm production and fertility (refer to Chapter 24). In those with a selective deficiency of GnRH, such as Kallmann's syndrome, pulsatile GnRH therapy has been shown to stimulate T production and spermatogenesis.

ACKNOWLEDGMENTS

This work was supported by grants DK-45760, DK-43344, and RR-00064 from the National Institute of Health USPHS and Department of Internal Medicine and Pathology funds.

REFERENCES

1. Santen RJ. Testis: function and dysfunction. In: Yen SSC, Jaffe RB, Barbieri RL, eds. Reproductive Endocrinology. Saunders, Philadelphia, 1999, pp. 632–668.
2. Korenman SG. Androgen function after age 50 years and treatment of hypogonadism. Curr Ther Endocrinol Metab 1994;5:585–587.
3. Korenman S, Morley J, Mooradian A, et al. Secondary hypogonadism in older men: its relation to impotence. J Clin Endocrinol Metab 1990;71:963–969.
4. Mastrogiacomo I, Feghali G, Foresta C, Ruzza G. Andropause: incidence and pathogenesis. Arch Androl 1982;9:293–296.
5. Vermeulen A, Kaufman JM. Ageing of the hypothalamo-pituitary-testicular axis in men. Horm Res 1995;43:25–28.
6. Ou Y, Hwang T, Yang C, et al. Hormonal screening in impotent patients. J Formos Med Assoc 1991;90:560–564.
7. Wortsman J, Rosner W, Dufau M. Abnormal testicular function in men with primary hypothyroidism. Am J Med 1987;82:207–212.
8. Griffin JE, Wilson JD. Disorders of the testes and male reproductive tract. In: Wilson JD, Foster DW, eds. William's Textbook of Endocrinology. Saunders, Philadelphia, 1998, pp. 819–875.

9. Nielsen J, Wohlert M. Chromosome abnormalities found among 34,910 newborn children: results from a 13-year incidence study in Arhus, Denmark. Hum Genet 1991;87:81–83.

10. Tunte W, Niermann H. Incidence of Klinefelter's syndrome and seasonal variation. Lancet 1968;1:641.

11. Luciani J, Guichaoua M. Chromosome abnormalities in male infertility. Ann Biol Clin (Paris) 1985;43:71–74.

12. Morley JE, Kaiser FE, Perry HM, 3rd, et al. Longitudinal changes in testosterone, luteinizing hormone, and follicle- stimulating hormone in healthy older men. Metabolism 1997;46:410–413.

13. Tenover JL. Testosterone and the aging male. J Androl 1997;18:103–106.

14. Harman SM, Metter EJ, Tobin JD, Pearson J, Blackman MR. Longitudinal effects of aging on serum total and free testosterone levels in healthy men. Baltimore Longitudinal Study of Aging. J Clin Endocrinol Metab 2001;86:724–731.

15. McClure RD. Endocrine investigation and therapy. Urol Clin North Am 1987;14:471-88.

16. Huang CC, Huang HS. Successful treatment of male infertility due to hypogonadotropic hypogonadism—report of three cases. Chang Keng I Hsueh 1994;17:78–84.

17. Nachtigall LB, Boepple PA, Pralong FP, Crowley WF, Jr. Adult-onset idiopathic hypogonadotropic hypogonadism—a treatable form of male infertility. N Engl J Med 1997;336:410–415.

18. Nachtigall LB, Boepple PA, Seminara SB, et al. Inhibin B secretion in males with gonadotropin-releasing hormone (GnRH) deficiency before and during long-term GnRH replacement: relationship to spontaneous puberty, testicular volume, and prior treatment—a clinical research center study. J Clin Endocrinol Metab 1996;81:3520–3525.

19. Seminara SB, Boepple PA, Nachtigall LB, et al. Inhibin B in males with gonadotropin-releasing hormone (GnRH) deficiency: changes in serum concentration after shortterm physiologic GnRH replacement—a clinical research center study. J Clin Endocrinol Metab 1996;81:3692–3696.

20. Anawalt BD, Bebb RA, Matsumoto AM, et al. Serum inhibin B levels reflect Sertoli cell function in normal men and men with testicular dysfunction. J Clin Endocrinol Metab 1996;81:3341–3345.

21. McLachlan RI, Finkel DM, Bremner WJ, Snyder PJ. Serum inhibin concentrations before and during gonadotropin treatment in men with hypogonadotropic hypogonadism: physiological and clinical implications. J Clin Endocrinol Metab 1990;70:1414–1419.

22. MacDonald PC, Wilson JD. Familial incomplete male pseudohermaphroditism, type 2. N Engl J Med 1974;291:944–949.

23. Walsh PC, Harrod MJ, Goldstein JL, MacDonald PC, Wilson JD. Familial incomplete male pseudohermaphroditism, type 2, decreased dihydrotestosterone formation in pseudovaginal perineoscrotal hypospadias. N Engl J Med 1974;291:944–949.

24. Imperato-McGinley J, Peterson RE, Gantier T, et al. Hormonal evaluation of a large kindred with complete androgen insensitivity: evidence of a secondary 5 alpha-reductase deficiency. J Clin Endocrinol Metab 1982;54:931–941.

25. Meikle AW, Mazer NA, Moellmer JF, et al. Enhanced transdermal delivery of testosterone across nonscrotal skin produces physiological concentrations of testosterone and its metabolites in hypogonadal men. J Clin Endocrinol Metab 1992;74:623–628.

26. Meikle AW, Arver S, Dobs AS, Sanders SW, Rajaram L, Mazer NA. Pharmacokinetics and metabolism of a permeation-enhanced testosterone transdermal system in hypogonadal men: influence of application site—a clinical research center study. J Clin Endocrinol Metab 1996;81:1832–1840.

27. Matsumoto AM. Clinical use and abuse of androgens and antiandrogens. In: Becker KL, ed. Prinicples and Practice of Endocrinology and Metabolism. J.B. Lippincott, Philadelphia, 1995, pp. 1110–1122.

28. Matsumoto AM. Hormonal therapy of male hypogonadism. Endocrinol Metab Clin North Am 1994;23:857–875.

29. Cantrill J, Dewis P, Large D, Newman M, Anderson D. Which testosterone replacement therapy? Clin Endocrinol (Oxf) 1984;21:97–107.

30. Berthold A. Transplantation der Hoed. Archiv fur Anatomie, Physiologie und wissenschaftliche Medicin, Berlin 1849:42–46.

31. Butenandt A. Uber die chemische Untersuchung des Sexualhomons. A angew Chem 1931;44:905–908.

32. David k, Dingermanse E, Freud J, Laqure E. Uber krystallinisches mannliches Hormon aus Hoden (Testosteron), wirksamer als aus Harn oder aus Cholesterin bereitetes Androsteron. Hoppe-Seyler's Z physiol Chem 1935;233:281,282.

33. Butenandt A, Hanisch G. Uber Testosteron, Umwandlung des Dehydro-androsterons in Androstendiol und Testosteron;ein Weg zur Darstellung des Testosterons aus Cholesterin. Hoppe-seyler's Z Physiol Chem 1935;237:89–98.

34. Ruzick L, Wettstein A. synthetische Darstellung des Testishormons, Testosteron (androsten 3-on-17ol). Helv chim Acta 1935;18:1264–1275.

35. Nieschlag E, Behre HM. Pharmacology and clinical uses of testosterone. In: Nieschlag E, Behre HM, eds. Testosterone: Action, Seficiency, Substitution. Springer-Verlag, New York, 1990, pp. 92–108.

36. Daggett P, Wheeler M, Nabarro J. Oral testosterone, a reappraisal. Horm Res 1978;9:121–129.

37. Johnsen S, Bennett E, Jensen V. Therapeutic effectiveness of oral testosterone. Lancet 1974;2:1473–1475.

38. Nieschlag E, Hoogen H, Bolk M, Schuster H, Wickings E. Clinical trial with testosterone undecanoate for male fertility control. Contraception 1978;18:607–614.

39. Nieschlag E, Cuppers H, Wickings E. Influence of sex, testicular development and liver function on the bioavailability of oral testosterone. Eur J Clin Invest 1977;7:145–147.

40. Alkalay D, Khemani L, Wagner WE J, Bartlett M. Sublingual and oral administration of methyltestosterone. A comparison of drug bioavailability. J Clin Pharmacol New Drugs 1973;13:142–151.

41. Lie J. Pulmonary peliosis. Arch Pathol Lab Med 1985;109:878,879.

42. Westaby D, Ogle S, Paradinas F, Randell J, Murray-Lyon I. Liver damage from long-term methyltestosterone. Lancet 1977;2:262,263.

43. Paradinas F, Bull T, Westaby D, Murray-Lyon I. Hyperplasia and prolapse of hepatocytes into hepatic veins during longterm methyltestosterone therapy: possible relationships of these changes to the developement of peliosis hepatis and liver tumours. Histopathology 1977;1:225–246.

44. Pezold F. Anabolic hormones in chronic hepatitis. Oral therapy with 1 alpha, 17 alpha-bis(acetylthio)-17 alpha-methyltestosterone. Munch Med Wochenschr 1968;110:2663–2668.

45. Doerr P, Pirke K. Regulation of plasma oestrogens in normal adult males. I. Response of oestradiol, oestrone and testosterone to HCG and fluoxymesterone administration. Acta Endocrinol (Copenh) 1974;75:617–624.

46. Jones TM, Fang VS, Landau rL, Rosenfield RL. The effects of fluoxymesterone administration on testicular function. Clin Endocrinol Metab 1977;43:121–129.

47. Nadell J, Kosek J. Peliosis hepatis. Twelve cases associated with oral androgen therapy. Arch Pathol Lab Med 1977;101:405–410.

48. Kovary P, Lenau H, Niermann H, Zierden E, Wagner H. Testosterone levels and gonadotrophins in Klinefelter's patients treated with injections of mesterolone cipionate. Arch Dermatol Res 1977;258:289–294.

49. Wang C, Chan C, Wong K, Yeung K. Comparison of the effectiveness of placebo, clomiphene citrate, mesterolone, pentoxifylline, and testosterone rebound therapy for the treatment of idiopathic oligospermia. Fertil Steril 1983;40:358–365.

50. Ros A. Our experience with mesterolone therapy. Evaluation of 22 hormonal steroids constituting the gas chromatographic picture in the total neutral urinary fraction. The effectiveness of mesterolone in the therapy of oligoastenospermias. Attual Ostet Ginecol 1969;15:37–53.

51. Gerhards E, Nieuweboer B, Richter E. On the alkyl-substituted steroids. V. Testosterone excretion in man after oral administration of 1alpha-methyl-5alpha-androstane-17beta ol-3-one(mesterolone) and 17-alpha-methyl-androst-4-en-17beta-ol-3-one (17 alpha-methyltestosterone). Arzneimittelforschung 1969;19:765,766.

52. Komatsu Y, Tomoyoshi T, Okada K. Clinical experiences with mesterolone, an orally administered androgen, in male urology. Hinyokika Kiyo 1969;15:663–669.

53. Aakvaag A, Stromme S. The effect of mesterolone administration to normal men on the pituitary-testicular function. Acta Endocrinol (Copenh) 1974;77:380–386.

54. Schurmeyer T, Wickings E, Freischem C, Nieschlag E. Saliva and serum testosterone following oral testosterone undecanoate administration in normal and hypogonadal men. Acta Endocrinol (Copenh) 1983;102:456–462.

55. Tauber U, Schroder K, Dusterberg B, Matthes H. Absolute bioavailability of testosterone after oral administration of testosterone-undecanoate and testosterone. Eur J Drug Metab Pharmacokinet 1986;11:145–149.

56. Luisi M, Franchi F. Double-blind group comparative study of testosterone undecanoate and mesterolone in hypogonadal male patients. J Endocrinol Invest 1980;3:305–308.
57. Maisey N, Bingham J, Marks V, English J, Chakraborty J. Clinical efficacy of testosterone undecanoate in male hypogonadism. Clin Endocrinol (Oxf) 1981;14:625–629.
58. Tax L. Absolute bioavailability of testosterone after oral administration of testosterone-undecanoate and testosterone (letter). Eur J Drug Metab Pharmacokinet 1987;12:225,226.
59. Gooren L. Long-term safety of the oral androgen testosterone undecanoate. Int J Androl 1986;9:21–26.
60. Frey H, Aakvaag A, Saanum D, Falch J. Bioavailability of oral testosterone in males. Eur J Clin Pharmacol 1979;16:345–349.
61. Coert A, Geelen J, de Visser J, van der Vies J. The pharmacology and metabolism of testosterone undecanoate (TU), a new orally active androgen. Acta Endocrinol (Copenh) 1975;79:789–800.
62. Nieschlag E, Mauss J, Coert A, Kicovic P. Plasma androgen levels in men after oral administration of testosterone or testosterone undecanoate. Acta Endocrinol (Copenh) 1975;79:366–374.
63. Skakkebaek N, Bancroft J, Davidson D, Warner P. Androgen replacement with oral testosterone undecanoate in hypogonadal men: a double blind controlled study. Clin Endocrinol (Oxf) 1981;14:49–61.
64. Conway A, Boylan L, Howe C, Ross G, Handelsman D. Randomized clinical trial of testosterone replacement therapy in hypogonadal men. Int J Androl 1988;11:247–264.
65. Salehian B, Wang C, Alexander G, et al. Pharmacokinetics, bioefficacy, and safety of sublingual testosterone cyclodextrin in hypogonadal men: comparison to testosterone enanthate—a clinical research center study. J Clin Endocrinol Metab 1995;80:3567–3575.
66. Stuenkel CA, Dudley RE, Yen SS. Sublingual administration of testosterone-hydroxypropyl-beta-cyclodextrin inclusion complex simulates episodic androgen release in hypogonadal men. J Clin Endocrinol Metab 1991;72:1054–1059.
67. Wang C, Eyre DR, Clark R, et al. Sublingual testosterone replacement improves muscle mass and strength, decreases bone resorption, and increases bone formation markers in hypogonadal men—a clinical research center study. J Clin Endocrinol Metab 1996;81:3654–3662.
68. Wang C, Alexander G, Berman N, et al. Testosterone replacement therapy improves mood in hypogonadal men—a clinical research center study. J Clin Endocrinol Metab 1996;81:3578–3583.
69. Pitha J, Anaissie E, Uekama K. gamma-Cyclodextrin:testosterone complex suitable for sublingual administration. J Pharm Sci 1987;76:788–790.
70. Junkmann K. Long-acting steroids in reproduction. Recent Prog Horm Res. 1957;13:389–419.
71. Fujioka M, Shinohara Y, Baba S, Irie M, Inoue K. Pharmacokinetic properties of testosterone propionate in normal men. J Clin Endocrinol Metab 1986;63:1361–1364.
72. Nieschlag E, Cuppers H, Wiegelmann W, Wickings E. Bioavailability and LH-suppressing effect of different testosterone preparations in normal and hypogonadal men. Horm Res 1976;7:138–145.
73. Nankin H. Hormone kinetics after intramuscular testosterone cypionate. Fertil Steril 1987;47:1004–1009.
74. Behre HM, Oberpenning F, Nieschlag E. Comparative pharmacokinetics of testosterone preparations: application of computer analysis and simulation. In: Nieschlag E, Behre HM, eds. Testosterone: Action, Deficiency, Substitution. Springer-Verlag, New York, 1990, pp. 115–134.
75. Schulte-Beerbuhl M, Nieschlag E. Comparison of testosterone, dihydrotestosterone, luteinizing hormone, and follicle-stimulating hormone in serum after injection of testosterone enanthate of testosterone cypionate. Fertil Steril 1980;33:201–203.
76. Schurmeyer T, Nieschlag E. Comparative pharmacokinetics of testosterone enanthate and testosterone cyclohexanecarboxylate as assessed by serum and salivary testosterone levels in normal men. Int J Androl 1984;7:181–187.
77. Behre HM, Nieschlag E. Testosterone buciclate (20 Aet-1) in hypogonadal men: pharmacokinetics and pharmacodynamics of the new long-acting androgen ester. J Clin Endocrinol Metab 1992;75:1204–1210.
78. Knuth U, Behre H, Belkien L, Bents H, Nieschlag E. Clinical trial of 19-nortestosterone-hexoxyphenylpropionate (Anadur) for male fertility regulation. Fertil Steril 1985;44:814–821.
79. Belkien L, Schurmeyer T, Hano R, Gunnarsson P, Nieschlag E. Pharmacokinetics of 19-nortestosterone esters in normal men. J Steroid Biochem 1985;22:623–629.
80. Snyder PJ, Lawrence DA. Treatment of male hypogonadism with testosterone enanthate. J Clin Endocrinol Metab 1980;51:1335–1339.
81. Demisch K, Nickelsen T. Distribution of testosterone in plasma proteins during replacement therapy with testosterone enanthate in patients suffering from hypogonadism. Andrologia 1983;15:536–541.

82. Nieschlag E, Buchter D, Von Eckardstein S, Abshagen K, Simoni M, Behre HM. Repeated intramus-
    cular injections of testosterone undecanoate for substitution therapy in hypogonadal men. Clin
    Endocrinol (Oxf) 1999;51:757–763.
83. Zhang GY, Gu YQ, Wang XH, Cui YG, Bremner WJ. A pharmacokinetic study of injectable test-
    osterone undecanoate in hypogonadal men. J Androl 1998;19:761–768.
84. Handelsman D, Conway A, Boylan L. Suppression of human spermatogenesis by testosterone im-
    plants. J Clin Endocrinol Metab 1992;75:1326–1332.
85. Handelsman DJ, Conway AJ, Boylan LM. Pharmacokinetics and pharmacodynamics of testosterone
    pellets in man. J Clin Endocrinol Metab 1990;71:216–222.
86. Handelsman DJ. Androgen delivery systems: testosterone pellet implants. In: Bhasin S, HL
    Gabelnick, JM Spieler, RS Swerdloff, C Wang, ed. Pharmacology, Biology and Clinical Applica-
    tions of Androgens. Wiley-Liss, New York, 1996, pp. 459–469.
87. Jockenhovel F, Vogel E, Kreutzer M, Reinhardt W, Lederbogen S, Reinwein D. Pharmacokinetics
    and pharmacodynamics of subcutaneous testosterone implants in hypogonadal men. Clin Endocrinol
    Oxf 1996;45:61–71.
88. Choi S, Kim D, de Lingnieres B. Transdermal dihydrotestosterone therapy and its effects on patients
    with microphallus. J Urol. 1993;150:657–660.
89. Cutter CB. Compounded percutaneous testosterone gel: use and effects in hypogonadal men. J Am
    Board Fam Pract 2001;14:22–32.
90. Chemana D, Morville R, Fiet J, et al. Percutaneous absorption of 5 alpha-dihydrotestosterone in man.
    II. Percutaneous administration of 5 alpha-dihydrotestosterone in hypogonadal men with idiopathic
    haemochromatosis;clinical, metabolic and hormonal effectiveness. Int J Androl 1982;5:595–606.
91. Kuhn J, Laudat M, Roca R, Dugue M, Luton J, Bricaire H. Gynecomastia: effect of prolonged
    treatment with dihydrotestosterone by the percutaneous route. Presse Med 1983;12:21–25.
92. Schaison G, Nahoul K, Couzinet B. Percutaneous dihydrotestosterone (DHT) treatment. In: Nieschlag
    E, Behre HM, eds. Testosterone: Action, Deficiency, Substitution. Springer-Verlag, New York,
    1990, pp. 155–164.
93. Vermeulen A, Deslypere J. Long-term transdermal dihydrotestosterone therapy: effects on pituitary
    gonadal axis and plasma lipoproteins. Maturitas 1985;7:281–287.
94. De Lignieres B. Transdermal dihydrotestosterone treatment of 'andropause'. Ann Med 1993;25:235–241.
95. Place VA, Atkinson L, Prather DA, Trunell N, Yates FE. Transdermal testosterone replacement
    through genital skin. In: Nieschlag E, Behre HM, eds. Testosterone: Action, Deficiency, Substitu-
    tion. Springer-Verlag, New York, 1990, pp. 165–180.
96. Ahmed SR, Boucher AE, Manni A, Santen RJ, Bartholomew M, Demers LM. Transdermal testoster-
    one therapy in the treatment of male hypogonadism. J Clin Endocrinol Metab 1988;66:546–551.
97. Bals-Pratsch M, Knuth UA, Yoon YD, Nieschlag E. Transdermal testosterone substitution therapy
    for male hypogonadism. Lancet 1986;2:943–946.
98. Cunningham GR, Cordero E, Thornby JI. Testosterone replacement with transdermal therapeutic
    systems. Physiological serum testosterone and elevated dihydrotestosterone levels. JAMA
    1989;261:2525–2530.
99. Findlay JC, Place V, Snyder PJ. Treatment of primary hypogonadism in men by the transdermal
    administration of testosterone. J Clin Endocrinol Metab 1989;68:369–373.
100. Carey PO, Howards SS, Vance ML. Transdermal testosterone treatment of hypogonadal men. J Urol
    1988;140:76–89.
101. Findlay JC, Place VA, Snyder PJ. Transdermal delivery of testosterone. J Clin Endocrinol Metab
    1987;64:266–268.
102. Meikle AW, CardosaDeSousa JC, Dacosta N, Bishop DK, Samlowski WE. Direct and indirect
    effects of Murine Interleukin-2, Gamma interferon, and tumor necrosis factor on Testosterone syn-
    thesis in mouse leydig cells. J Androl 1992;13:1–7.
103. Meikle AW, Arver S, Dobs AS, Sanders SW, Mazer NA. Androderm: a permeation enhanced non-
    scrotal testosterone transdermal system for the treatment of male hypogonadism. In: Bhasin S, HL
    Gabelnick, JM Spieler, RS Swerdloff, C Wang, ed. Pharmacology, Biology and Clinical Applica-
    tions of Androgens. Wiley-Liss, New York, 1996.
104. Arver S, Dobs AS, Meikle AW, Allen RP, Sanders SW, Mazer NA. Improvement of sexual function
    in testosterone deficient men treated for 1 year with a permeation enhanced testosterone transdermal
    system. J Urol 1996;155:1604–1608.
105. Meikle AW, Annand D, Hunter C, et al. Pre-treatment with a topical corticosteroid cream improves
    local tolerability and does not significantly alter the pharmacokinetics of the androderm testosterone
    transdermal system in hypogonadal men. Endocrine Soc 1997;79:P01–322.

106. Wilson DE, Kaidbey K, Boike SC, Jorkasky DK. Use of topical corticosteroid cream in the pretreat-ment of skin reactions associated with Androderm testosterone transdermal system. Endocrine Soc 1997;79:P01–323.

107. Wang C, Berman N, Longstreth JA, et al. Pharmacokinetics of transdermal testosterone gel in hypogonadal men: application of gel at one site versus four sites: a General Clinical Research Center Study. J Clin Endocrinol Metab 2000;85:964–969.

108. Finkel D, Phillips J, Snyder P. Stimulation of spermatogenesis by gonadotropins in men with hypogonadotropic hypogonadism. N Engl J Med 1985;313:651–655.

109. Baker HW, Hudson B. Changes in the pituitary-testicular axis with age. Monogr Endocrinol 1983;25:71–83.

110. Carter HB, Pearson JD, Metter EJ, et al. Longitudinal evaluation of serum androgen levels in men with and without prostate cancer. Prostate 1995;27:25–31.

111. Tenover JS, Matsumoto AM, Plymate SR, Bremner WJ. The effects of aging in normal men on bioavailable testosterone and luteinizing hormone secretion: response to clomiphene citrate. J Clin Endocrinol Metab 1987;65:1118–1126.

112. Nankin HR, Calkins JH. Decreased bioavailable testosterone in aging normal and impotent men. J Clin Endocrinol Metab 1986;63:1418–1420.

113. Bremner WJ, Vitiello MV, Prinz PN. Loss of circadianrhythmicity in blood testosterone levels with aging in normal men. J Clin Endocrinol Metab 1983;56:1278–1281.

114. Wang C, Swedloff RS, Iranmanesh A, et al. Transdermal testosterone gel improves sexual function, mood, muscle strength, and body composition parameters in hypogonadal men. Testosterone Gel Study Group. J Clin Endocrinol Metab 2000;85:2839–2853.

115. Snyder PJ, Peachey H, Berlin JA, et al. Effects of testosterone replacement in hypogonadal men. J Clin Endocrinol Metab 2000;85:2670–2677.

116. Katznelson L, Finkelstein JS, Schoenfeld DA, Rosenthal DI, Anderson EJ, Klibanski A. Increase in bone density and lean body mass during testosterone administration in men with acquired hypogo-nadism. J Clin Endocrinol Metab 1996;81:4358–4365.

117. Bhasin S, Storer TW, Berman N, et al. Testosterone replacement increases fat-free mass and muscle size in hypogonadal men. J Clin Endocrinol Metab 1997;82:407–413.

118. Grinspoon S, Corcoran C, Lee K, et al. Loss of lean body and muscle mass correlates with androgen levels in hypogonadal men with acquired immunodeficiency syndrome and wasting. J Clin Endocrinol Metab 1996;81:4051–4058.

119. Klein SA, Klauke S, Dobmeyer JM, et al. Substitution of testosterone in a HIV-1 positive patient with hypogonadism and Wasting-syndrome led to a reduced rate of apoptosis. Eur J Med Res 1997;2:30–32.

120. Rabkin JG, Rabkin R, Wagner GJ. Testosterone treatment of clinical hypogonadism in patients with HIV/AIDS. Int J STD AIDS 1997;8:537–545.

121. Holzman D. Testosterone wasting and AIDS [news]. Mol Med Today 1996;2:93.

122. Bhasin S, Javanbakht M. Can androgen therapy replete lean body mass and improve muscle function in wasting associated with human immunodeficiency virus infection? JPEN J Parenter Enteral Nutr 1999;23:S195–201.

123. Sih R, Morley J, Kaiser F, Perry HM, Patrick P, Ross C. Testosterone replacement in older hypogonadal men: a 12-month randomized controlled trial. J Clin Endocrinol Metab 1997;82:1661–1667.

124. Morales A, Johnston B, Heaton J, Clark A. Oral androgens in the treatment of hypogonadal impotent men. J Urol 1994;152:1115–1118.

125. Burris AS, Banks SM, Carter CS, Davidson JM, Sherins RJ. A long-term, prospective study of the physiologic and behavioral effects of hormone replacement in untreated hypogonadal men. J Androl 1992;13:297–304.

126. O'Carroll R, Shapiro C, Bancroft J. Androgens, behaviour and nocturnal erection in hypogonadal men: the effects of varying the replacement dose. Clin Endocrinol 1985;23:527–538.

127. Hubert W. Psychotropic effects of testosterone. In: Nieschlag E, HM Behre, ed. Testosterone: Action, Deficiency, Substitution. Springer-Verlag, New York, 1990, pp. 51–65.

128. Jain P, Rademaker AW, McVary KT. Testosterone supplementation for erectile dysfunction: results of a meta-analysis. J Urol 2000;164:371–375.

129. Baumgartner RN, Ross RR, Waters DL, et al. Serum leptin in elderly people: associations with sex hormones, insulin, and adipose tissue volumes. Obes Res 1999;7:141–149.

130. Van Den Saffele JK, Goemaere S, De Bacquer D, Kaufman JM. Serum leptin levels in healthy ageing men: are decreased serum testosterone and increased adiposity in elderly men the consequence of leptin deficiency? Clin Endocrinol (Oxf) 1999;51:81–88.

131. Jockenhovel F, Blum WF, Vogel E, et al. Testosterone substitution normalizes elevated serum leptin levels in hypogonadal men. J Clin Endocrinol Metab 1997;82:2510–2513.

132. Adan L, Bussieres L, Trivin C, Souberbielle JC, Brauner R. Effect of short-term testosterone treatment on leptin concentrations in boys with pubertal delay. Horm Res 1999;52:109–112.

133. Soderberg S, Olsson T, Eliasson M, et al. A strong association between biologically active testosterone and leptin in non-obese men and women is lost with increasing (central) adiposity. Int J Obes Relat Metab Disord 2001;25:98–105.

134. Krabbe S, Christiansen C. Longitudinal study of calcium metabolism in male puberty. I. Bone mineral content, and serum levels of alkaline phosphatase, phosphate and calcium. Acta Paediatr Scand 1984;73:745–749.

135. Bonjour J, Theintz G, Buchs B, Slosman D, Rizzoli R. Critical years and stages of puberty for spinal and femoral bone mass accumulation during adolescence. J Clin Endocrinol Metab 1991;73:555–563.

136. Scane AC, Sutcliffe AM, Francis RM. Osteoporosis in men. Baillieres Clin Rheumatol 1993;7:589–601.

137. Stepan JJ, Lachman M, Zverina J, Pacovsky V, Baylink DJ. Castrated men exhibit bone loss: effect of calcitonin treatment on biochemical indices of bone remodeling. J Clin Endocrinol Metab 1989;69:523–527.

138. Goldray D, Weisman Y, Jaccard N, Merdler C, Chen J, Matzkin H. Decreased bone density in elderly men treated with the gonadotropin-releasing hormone agonist decapeptyl (D-Trp6-GnRH). J Clin Endocrinol Metab 1993;76:288–290.

139. Baillie S, Davison C, Johnson F, Francis R. Pathogenesis of vertebral crush fractures in men. Age Ageing 1992;21:139–141.

140. Halbreich U, Palter S. Accelerated osteoporosis in psychiatric patients: possible pathophysiological processes. Schizophr Bull 1996;22:447–454.

141. Halbreich U, Rojansky N, Palter S, et al. Decreased bone mineral density in medicated psychiatric patients. Psychosom Med 1995;57:485–491.

142. Keely E, Reiss J, Drinkwater D, Faiman C. Bone mineral density, sex hormones, and long-term use of neuroleptic agents in mem. Endocr Pract. 1997;3:209–213.

143. Seeman E, Melton LJd, WM OF, Riggs BL. Risk factors for spinal osteoporosis in men. Am J Med 1983;75:977–983.

144. Seeman E. The dilemma of osteoporosis in men. Am J Med 1995;98:76s–88s.

145. Finkelstein JS, Klibanski A, Neer RM, Greenspan SL, Rosenthal DI, Crowley WF, Jr. Osteoporosis in men with idiopathic hypogonadotropic hypogonadism. Ann Intern Med 1987;106:354–361.

146. Finkelstein JS, Klibanski A, Neer RM, et al. Increases in bone density during treatment of men with idiopathic hypogonadotropic hypogonadism. J Clin Endocrinol Metab 1989;69:776–783.

147. Finkelstein JS, Neer RM, Biller BM, Crawford JD, Klibanski A. Osteopenia in men with a history of delayed puberty. N Engl J Med 1992;326:600–604.

148. Kuhn JM, Gay D, Lemercier JP, Pugeat M, Legrand A, Wolf LM. Testicular function during prolonged corticotherapy. Presse Med 1986;15:559–562.

149. Lukert BP. Glucocorticoid-induced osteoporosis. South Med J 1992;85:48–51.

150. Reid IR, Veale AG, France JT. Glucocorticoid osteoporosis. J Asthma 1994;31:7–18.

151. MacAdams MR, White RH, Chipps BE. Reduction of serum testosterone levels during chronic glucocorticoid therapy. Ann Intern Med 1986;104:648–651.

152. Praet JP, Peretz A, Rozenberg S, Famaey JP, Bourdoux P. Risk of osteoporosis in men with chronic bronchitis. Osteoporos Int 1992;2:257–261.

153. Behre HM, Kliesch S, Leifke E, Link TM, Nieschlag E. Long-term effect of testosterone therapy on bone mineral density in hypogonadal men. J Clin Endocrinol Metab. 1997;82:2386–2390.

154. Wang C, Swerdloff RS, Iranmanesh A, et al. Effects of transdermal testosterone gel on bone turnover markers and bone mineral density in hypogonadal men. Clin Endocrinol (Oxf) 2001;54:739–750.

155. Katznelson L, Finkelstein J, Baressi C, Klibanski A. Increase in trabecular bone density and altered body composition in androgen replaced hypogonadal men. Endocrine Soc 1994;75:1524A.

156. Matzkin H, Chen J, Weisman Y, et al. Prolonged treatment with finasteride (a 5 alpha-reductase inhibitor) does not affect bone density and metabolism. Clin Endocrinol (Oxf.) 1992;37:432–436.

157. Pederson L, Kremer M, Foged N, et al. Evidence of a correlation of estrogen receptor level and avian osteoclast estrogen responsiveness. J Bone Miner Res 1997;12:742–752.

158. McDonnell D, Norris J. Analysis of the molecular pharmacology of estrogen receptor agonists and antagonists provides insights into the mechanism of action of estrogen in bone. Osteoporos Int 1997;7:S29–34.

159. Hoyland J, Mee A, Baird P, Braidman I, Mawer E, Freemont A. Demonstration of estrogen receptor mRNA in bone using in situ reverse-transcriptase polymerase chain reaction. Bone 1997;20:87–92.

160. Grese T, Cho S, Finley D, et al. Structure-activity relationships of selective estrogen receptor modulators: modifications to the 2-arylbenzothiophene core of raloxifene. J Med Chem 1997;40:146–167.

161. Fiorelli G, Gori F, Frediani U, et al. Membrane binding sites and non-genomic effects of estrogen in cultured human pre-osteoclastic cells. J Steroid Biochem Mol Biol 1996;59:233–240.

162. Kobayashi S, Inoue S, Hosoi T, Ouchi Y, Shiraki M, Orimo H. Association of bone mineral density with polymorphism of the estrogen receptor gene. J Bone Miner Res 1996;11:306–311.

163. Frolik C, Bryant H, Black E, Magee D, Chandrasekhar S. Time-dependent changes in biochemical bone markers and serum cholesterol in ovariectomized rats: effects of raloxifene HCl, tamoxifen, estrogen, and alendronate. Bone 1996;18:621–627.

164. Mano H, Yuasa T, Kameda T, et al. Mammalian mature osteoclasts as estrogen target cells. Biochem Biophys Res Commun 1996;223:637–642.

165. Smith EP, Boyd J, Frank GR, et al. Estrogen resistance caused by a mutation in the estrogen-receptor gene in a man (see comments) (published erratum appears in N Engl J Med 1995 Jan 12;332:131). N Engl J Med 1994;331:1056–1061.

166. Greenspan SL, Neer RM, Ridgeway EC, Klibanski A. Osteoporosis in men with hyperprolactinemic hypogonadism. Ann Intern Med 1986;104:777–782.

167. Tenover J. Androgen therapy in aging men. In: Bhasin S, Galelnick H, Spieler J, swerdloff R, Wang C, eds. Pharmacology, Biology, and Clinical Applications of Androgens. Wiley-Liss, New York, 1996, pp. 309–318.

168. Arver S, Meikle AW, Dobs AS, Sanders S, Mazer NA. Hypogonadal men treated with the Androderm testosterone transdermal system had fewer abnormal hematocrit elevations than those treated with testosterone enanthate injections. Endocrine Soc. 1997;79:P01–327.

169. Matsumoto AM, Sandblom RE, Schoene RB, et al. Testosterone replacement in hypogonadal men: effects on obstructive sleep apnoea, respiratory drives, and sleep. Clin Endocrinol 1985;22:713–721.

170. Schneider BK, Pickett CK, Zwillich CW, et al. Influence of testosterone on breathing during sleep. J Appl Physiol 1986;61:618–623.

171. Bagatell CJ, Bremner WJ. Androgen and progestagen effects on plasma lipids. Prog Cardiovasc Dis 1995;38:255–271.

172. Bagatell CJ, Heiman JR, Matsumoto AM, Rivier JE, Bremner WJ. Metabolic and behavioral effects of high-dose, exogenous testosterone in healthy men. J Clin Endocrinol Metab 1994;79:561–567.

173. Bagatell CJ, Knopp RH, Rivier JE, Bremner WJ. Physiological levels of estradiol stimulate plasma high density lipoprotein2 cholesterol levels in normal men. J Clin Endocrinol Metab 1994;78:855–861.

174. Bagatell CJ, Knopp RH, Vale WW, Rivier JE, Bremner WJ. Physiologic testosterone levels in normal men suppress high-density lipoprotein cholesterol levels. Ann Intern Med 1992;116:967–973.

175. Dobs AS, Bachorik PS, Arver S, et al. Interrelationships among lipoprotein levels, sex hormones, anthropometric parameters, and age in hypogonadal men treated for 1 year with a permeation-enhanced testosterone transdermal system. J Clin Endocrinol Metab 2001;86:1026–1033.

176. Goldberg RB, Rabin D, Alexander AN, Doelle GC, Getz GS. Suppression of plasma testosterone leads to an increase in serum total and high density lipoprotein cholesterol and apoproteins A-1 and B. J Clin Endocrinol Metab 1985;60:203–207.

177. Byerley L, Lee WN, Swerdloff RS, et al. Effect of modulating serum testosterone levels in the normal male range on protein, carbohydrate, and lipid metabolism in men: implications for testosterone replacement therapy. Endocrine J 1993;1:253–262.

178. Mooradian AD, Morley JE, Korenman SG. Biological actions of androgens. Endocr Rev 1987;8:1–28.

178. Zgliczynski S, Ossowski M, Slowinska-Srzednicka J, et al. Effect of testosterone replacement therapy on lipids and lipoproteins in hypogonadal and elderly men. Atherosclerosis 1996;121:35–43.

180. Rabijewski M, Adamkiewicz M, Zgliczynski S. [The influence of testosterone replacement therapy on well-being, bone mineral density and lipids in elderly men]. Pol Arch Med Wewn 1998;100:212–221.

181. Hromadova M, Hacik T, Malatinsky E, Sklovsky A, Cervenakov I. Some measures of lipid metabolism in young sterile males before and after testosterone treatment. Endocrinol Exp 1989;23:205–211.

182. Friedl K, Hannan CJ J, Jones R, Plymate S. High-density lipoprotein cholesterol is not decreased if an aromatizable androgen is administered. Metabolism 1990;39:69–74.

183. Meikle AW, Stephenson RA, McWhorter WP, Skolnick MH, Middleton RG. Effects of age, sex steroids, and family relationships on volumes of prostate zones in men with and without prostate cancer. Prostate 1995;26:253–259.

184. Meikle AW. Endocrinology of the prostate and of benign prostate prostatic hyperplasia. In: Degroot LJ, ed. Endocrinology, 3rd ed. Saunders, Philadelphia, 1995, pp. 2459–2473.

185. Meikle AW, Arver S, Dobs AS, et al. Prostate size in hypogonadal men treated with a nonscrotal permeation-enhanced testosterone transdermal system. Urology 1997;49:191–196.

186. Meikle AW, Stephenson RA, Lewis CM, Middleton RG. Effects of age and sex hormones on transition and peripheral zone volumes of prostate and benign prostatic hyperplasia in twins. J Clin Endocrinol Metab 1997;82:571–575.

187. Behre HM, Bohmeyer J, Nieschlag E. Prostate volume in testosterone-treated and untreated hypogonadal men in comparison to age-matched normal controls. Clin Endocrinol (Oxf) 1994;40:341–349.

188. Jin B, Conway AJ, Handelsman DJ. Effects of androgen deficiency and replacement on prostate zonal volumes. Clin Endocrinol (Oxf) 2001;54:437–445.

189. Meikle AW, Bansal A, Murray DK, Stephenson RA, Middleton RG. Heritability of the symptoms of benign prostatic hyperplasia and the roles of age and zonal prostate volumes in twins. Urology 1999;53:701–706.

190. McWhorter WP, Hernandez AD, Meikle AW, et al. A screening study of prostate cancer in high risk families. J Urol 1992;148:826–828.

191. Meikle AW, Smith J. Epidemiology of prostate cancer. Urol Clin North Am 1990;17:709–718.

20
Androgen Replacement
Sexual Behavior, Affect, and Cognition

Max Hirshkowitz, PhD,
Claudia A. Orengo, MD, PhD,
and Glenn R. Cunningham, MD

CONTENTS

INTRODUCTION

An awareness of the relationship between erectile function and testicular integrity has existed since antiquity *(1)*. However, some castrated men retain potency and erectile function for many years *(2)*. Most authors attribute this to the complexity of human sexual function, the importance of learned behavior, or both. Clinicians began using testosterone (T) to restore libido and erectile function in the late 1930s when a synthetic form became available. It was not until 1979 that T's ability to restore libido was more rigorously demonstrated. Subsequently, investigators have examined if a "threshold" for androgen's effects on erectile function exists and whether there is a progressive beneficial effect even when levels are in the "normal" range. Another issue concerns the possibility that some components of sexual behavior are androgen dependent, whereas others are not. Even today the literature contains relatively few randomized, placebo-controlled, double-blind studies comparing more than one delivery system. Nonetheless, much progress has been made in the last 25 years. Here, we review the effects of T deficiency on sexual behavior and function and the beneficial effects of T replacement in T-deficient men.

From: *Endocrine Replacement Therapy in Clinical Practice*
Edited by: A. Wayne Meikle © Humana Press Inc., Totowa, NJ

Findings from animal studies link androgen and aggressive behavior in our minds. Male sexuality, even in humans, apparently involves aggressive behavioral features, thereby perpetuating this notion. Decreased aggressiveness reported in sex offenders after castration is considered by many as supporting evidence. However, controlled studies in normal men typically do not confirm the association between T and aggression. A model is evolving that considers such aggressive behavior as an interaction between androgen and an impulse-control deficit. Finally, recent data indicate possible relationships among androgen, mood, and cognition. Testosterone's potential beneficial effects on mood and cognitive function have attracted clinical interest and are explored in a number of studies.

NEUROPHYSIOLOGY

Research from a variety of mammalian species has suggested that the steroid hormones T and 17β-estradiol may play a variety of regulatory roles in the central nervous system (CNS). During brain development, sex steroids appear to have a fine-tuning function in certain regions of the brain, modifying events related to neuronal survival and synapse formation (3,3a). In the adult brain, sex steroids are capable of modulating synaptic transmission or neurosecretion in numerous hypothalamic and extrahypothalamic brain areas by interacting with specific receptors (4). Therefore, it is reasonable to expect that these brain-related events have some functional or behavioral consequences. Figure 1 illustrates CNS areas implicated in sexual behavior and androgen receptor localization.

Androgen receptors (ARs) are found in the pituitary, hypothalamus, and preoptic areas. Using ^{3}H-T, Michael and colleagues (5) identified ARs in the amygdala, lateral septum, and premammillary bodies of nonhuman primates. Studies in intact, adult rats using double-label immunocytochemistry indicate the distribution of AR immunoreactivity is similar in males and females (6). The vast majority of AR$^+$ cells in the ventral tegmental area and substantia nigra (SN) pars compacta were tyrosine hydroxylase immunopositive, approximately half in the SN pars lateralis and one-third in the lateral retrorubral fields. The authors argue that receptor alignments are consistent with "estrogen influence over motor behaviors and androgen involvement in motivational functions." In rams, ARs have been found in many ventromedial somatostatin (+) neurones; however, the neurochemical phenotype of most AR+ cells in the arcuate nucleus remains unknown (7).

An antiandrogen can inhibit male copulatory activity in rat when injected systemically (8). Medial preoptic area (MPOA)-implanted hydroxyflutamide (OHF) prevented restoration of sexual behavior by systemically administered T. The greatest effect occurred at the ventromedial nucleus of hypothalamus (VMN), a partial effect was found at the medial amygdala (AME), and no effect at the lateral septum (SEPT). Upon discontinuation of OHF, sexual activity was restored in most animals. Thus, male sexual behavior is affected by blockade of specific androgen-containing brain sites.

Apomorphine (APO) increases erectile behavior in intact adult rats (9). Castration prevents this response and T replacement (testosterone propionate >60 μg/kg) restores it within 24 h. This effect is thought to be mediated centrally and probably involve dopaminergic receptors (10). Dopamine antagonists that cross the blood-brain barrier antagonize the APO response; whereas dopamine antagonists with only peripheral effects (e.g., domperidone) do not block APO-induced erections (11). Lesions of the

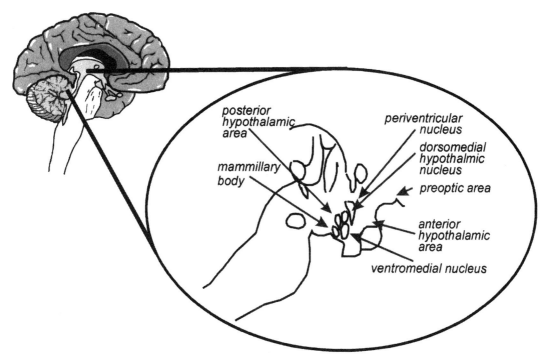

Fig. 1. Brain areas associated with sexual activity. The human brain with an inserted parasagittal section of rhesus monkey brain. Electrical stimulation and lesion sites shown to affect sexual behavior include dorsomedial hypothalamic nucleus, preoptic, anterior hypothalamic, and posterior hypothalamic areas. In nonhuman primates, androgen receptors are found in amygdala, lateral septum, and premammillary bodies.

periventricular nucleus in the hypothalamus prevent APO-induced erections *(12)*, and applying APO to this nucleus increases erectile responses *(13)*.

In general, studies using electrical brain stimulation and brain lesions to localize areas mediating sexual activity in animals correlate well with AR mapping. Stimulation of forebrain, hippocampus, dorsomedial, and lateral hypothalamic nuclei produce penile erections, mating behavior, or both in laboratory animals *(14–18)*. Similar activities are evoked by anterior cingulate gyrus and tegmental stimulation. Lesioning the medial preoptic areas are associated with cessation of male mating activity *(19)*. Implantation of crystalline T in the anterior hypothalamic preoptic areas restored sexual behavior that ceased after rats were castrated; however, implants in other areas had significantly less or no effect *(20)*.

More recent data implicate the hypothalamic paraventricular nucleus (PVN) as possibly the major source of direct descending spinal erection generator excitation *(21,22)*. PVN oxytocinergic neurons send long descending projections to sacral spinal parasympathetic preganglionic neurons that govern erectile activity *(23,24)*. Through this mechanism, the PVN may directly or indirectly increase penile parasympathetic drive. Schmidt *(25)* argues that this oxytocinergic PVN (excitatory) in conjunction with the serotinergic nPGi (inhibitory) system constitute a final common path from brain to spinal cord in the control of the spinal erection generator.

Higher central mechanisms also appear to exert context-related influences on erections *(26,27)*. For example, olfactory cues may involve the olfactory bulbs *(28)*, amygdala

(29), and bed nucleus of the stria terminalis (BNST) *(30)*. Copulatory behaviors likely involve MPOA (27); whereas the hippocampus and cortex may be more involved when erections are elicited from memory or fantasy. Imaging studies were performed using positron-emission tomography (PET) and regional cerebral blood flow (rCBF) in nine healthy men. Visual sexual stimuli were presented and correlated with brain activation. PET revealed activation in the claustrum, paralimbic areas, striatim (caudate nucleus and putamen), and the posterior hypothalamus. By contrast, rCBF showed increases in several temporal areas *(31)*.

PERIPHERAL PHYSIOLOGY

Reflexes

The importance of lower motor neurons and of neurons in the major pelvic ganglion (MPG) in erections is illustrated by midthoracic transection of the spinal cord in castrated rats. Rats were castrated at age 120 d, and 5 d later the spinal cord was completely transected at the midthoracic level; penile erections and penile flips were markedly influenced by T treatment *(32)*. When rats were castrated and the spinal cord was transected at age 30 d, animals that survived had autonomic bladders, but remained healthy *(33)*. Capsules containing T were implanted at 90 d of age. Penile reflexes were observed when rats were 100–110 d of age. Removal of the T capsules caused a reduction in penile erections ($p < 0.05$) and penile flips ($p < 0.01$) and these parameters increased ($p < 0.025$) within 12 h of initiating T treatment. In a second experiment, the investigators demonstrated that these reflexes were T-dose dependent. Subsequently other investigators have demonstrated that enzymes required for synthesis of neurotransmitters in both the sympathetic hypogastric ganglion *(34)* and the parasympathetic major pelvic ganglion (MPG) are regulated by androgen *(35)*. However, some of the erectile response remains in long-term castrate rats *(36)*. Figure 2 provides a schematic representation of neural circuits and ARs involved in rat penile erections.

Autonomic nervous system enervation of the corpora cavernosa is considered the major effector of penile erections. Electrical stimulation of the MPG evokes erection. Preganglionic neurons of the parasympathetic pathway are located in the intermediolateral column of the sacral spinal cord. Their axons are in the pelvic nerves, synapsing with neurons in the MPG. Castration of adult rats reduces intracavernosal pressure, reversible with androgen replacement *(37a)*. Interestingly, pelvic nerves axotomy does not impair the response; however, the response is reduced by concurrent castration and is restored by androgen replacement *(22)*. Furthermore, sectioning pelvic nerves in castrated rats further reduces intracavernosal pressure during MPG stimulation. ARs and nitric oxide synthase (NOS) I (neuronal nitric oxide synthase) colocalize to these neurons *(38)*. Castration reduces NOS I mRNA levels in these neurons and NADPH-diaphorase, which is linked to nitric oxide synthase *(39)*.

Nitric Oxide Synthase

Nonadrenergic, noncholinergic nerves whose neurons are located in the MPG release nitric oxide (NO), vasoactive polypeptide (VIP), and calcitonin gene regulated peptide (CGRP) in the corpora cavernosa. These agents relax smooth muscle cells in arterioles and in the trabeculae of the corpora cavernosa. NO is the most important smooth muscle relaxant but under some circumstances, as demonstrated by the *n*-nitric oxide synthase

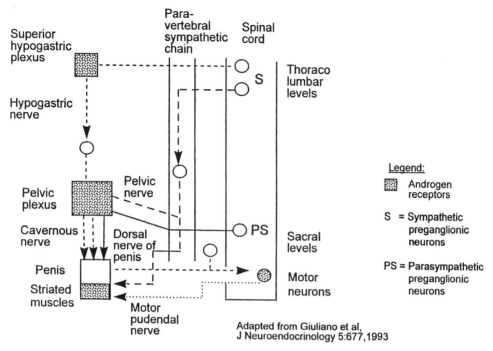

Fig. 2. Neural innervation of rat penile erections. Neurons and skeletal muscle demonstrated to possess androgen receptors are identified. Because little specific binding of androgen is observed in the corpora cavernosa of adults, the penis is not labeled to have androgen receptors; however, androgen receptors are present and responsive during development of the penis. (Adapted from ref. *37a*.)

knockout rat, other mediators may maintain erectile function. Studies in eNOS (–/–) mice indicate that approx 40% of NOS activity in the penis is lost when compared with wild-type mice *(40)*. NO works via a cGMP mechanism to lower intracellular calcium concentrations and cause smooth muscle relaxation.

Nitric oxide synthaste in the corpora cavernosa is partially androgen regulated. Castration reduces intracavernosal pressure and NOS activity. Both are restored by T replacement *(36,41)*. Castration reduces mRNA and nNOS protein in the cavernosa *(42,43)*. Finasteride, a 5α-reductase inhibitor, reduces the effect of T on NOS activity; thus, DHT may be more important than T. Castration also decreases NOS positive nerve fiber density *(44)*. Interestingly, castration-induced NOS activity reduction can be reversed by MPG stimulation when NOS activity is measured during an erection. This indicates that NOS activity can respond acutely to neural stimulation *(45)*. Reduced intracavernosal pressure observed in castrated rats is not limited by the substrate; it can be increased by combining sodium nitroprusside infusion (a NO donor) and MPG stimulation *(42)*. Not all penile NOS activity is androgen dependent given that infusing a NOS inhibitor into corpora cavernosa of castrate rats further reduces intracavernosal pressure. Thus, there may also be androgen and cGMP pathways that are NO independent.

Androgen-stimulated increases in intracavernosal NOS and androgen potentiation of electrical MPG stimulation might be mediated by ARs in neurons of the MPG or by ARs in the corpora cavernosa. However, penile ARs decline during development and are very sparse in the adult rat *(46,47)* and other species *(48)*. ARs in cultured smooth muscle cells from rat corpora cavernosa appear to be downregulated by estrogen (49). AR presence in MPG neurons argues for the androgen's major effect being at this level.

Penile erections depend on both increasing arterial inflow and decreasing venous outflow. Castration reduces arterial inflow and this can be reversed by administration of a nitric oxide donor drug. Castration-related increases in penile outflow indicate that androgen may have additional effects (36,37). Because, venous outflow normally declines when sinusoids of the corpora cavernosa become engorged, the increased outflow may result from changes in tissue compliance of the corpora or the tunica albuginea. Testosterone appears to decrease sensitivity of the erectile tissues to norepinephrine, a constrictor of smooth muscle (42). This increases inflow and sinusoidal blood volume and decreases outflow.

The fifth and sixth lumbar segments of the rat spinal cord contain motor neurons that innervate bulbospongiosus and ischiocavernosus muscles (3). To identify the motor neurons, investigators stained the axons by injecting these muscles with horseradish peroxidase. These neurons are not developed in androgen-resistant rats or in females; however, they concentrate radioactive T or DHT (but not estradiol) in normal males. Bulbospongiousus muscles in rats augment intracavernosal pressure during penile erection (50) and androgen may directly affect bulbospongiousus and ischiocavernosus striated muscle (51).

In summary, rat models provide data concerning androgen-related mechanisms underlying male sexual behavior. Androgen plays a role at many levels, including hypothalamus, spinal cord (L5–L6) motor neurons to the bulbocavernosus muscles, hypogastric sympathetic ganglion, MPG, bulbospongiousus and ischiocavernosus muscles, and, possibly, corpora cavernosa.

ANDROGEN AND MALE SEXUALITY

Most clinical T-deficiency studies examine adult men with congenital or acquired hypogonadism. Other than Klinefelter's syndrome and myotonic dystrophy, most hypogonadal men age 20–50 yr have secondary hypogonadism. However, the majority of hypogonadal men are 50 yr old, or older (52,53). Except in cases of surgical or chemical castration for stage D prostate cancer, T deficiency typically is partial. Some testicular T production usually remains, and this can reduce effects of T deficiency. Recently, a few studies have experimentally induced T deficiency in young, healthy men using gonadotropin-releasing hormone (GnRH) agonists or antagonists. This paradigm provides an unparalleled opportunity for observing acute effects of complete deficiency of testicular androgens.

Methods

SELF-REPORT

This is a simple and direct approach to assessing sexual function. Quantitative indices can be derived from data collected during interviews, rating scales, diaries, and questionnaires. Information from the sexual partner also is useful. Validated questionnaires have appeared in the literature (54–56). Salient inquiries include the frequency and intensity of sexual thoughts, interest, activity, and enjoyment. However, data obtained through self-report suffer from problems common to all self-reported information. The circumstances, potential gains, and hidden agendas must be considered carefully. Some individuals minimize disclosure of their sexuality because of mistrust, embarrassment, or repression, whereas others eagerly report intimate details of their sex life. Thus, differences in personality and personal style can influence self-report and obscure differences by inflating variance. Nonetheless, proper sampling and experimental design can avoid systematic errors in result profiles.

VISUAL SEXUAL STIMULATION

Visual sexual stimulation (VSS) can be used to objectively assess erectile responsiveness. VSS typically involves continuously measuring penile circumference increase while a subject views explicit material depicting nudity and sexual activities performed by adults. Sometimes penile rigidity is measured. Variations on this approach include having subjects engage in *sexual fantasy* or listen to *auditory sexually arousing* material while monitoring erection. Applying these techniques overcome some limitations of self-reported data; however, personality factors and individual differences still may influence results. In some individuals, the laboratory setting and the presence of monitoring equipment on the penis may inhibit sexual response. In repeated-measure designs, order effects are critical. Initial embarrassment or sympathetic nervous system activity (via peripheral vasoconstrictive response) may decline in subsequent trials as a subject becomes more comfortable with procedures. The subject's sexual orientation and activity preference, compared to that depicted in the material presented, should be considered. Aging studies must consider this carefully because attitudes, mores, and practices have changed considerably in the past six decades. Notwithstanding these factors, VSS provides an objective, physiological index of sexual responsiveness.

SLEEP-RELATED ERECTIONS

Sleep-related erections (SREs) sometimes referred to as nocturnal penile tumescence (NPT), index erectile capacity by evaluating the nonvolitional, naturally occurring erections that occur during sleep in all sexually potent, healthy men *(57,58)*. These erections are tightly coupled with rapid-eye-movement (REM) sleep and appear unaffected by behavioral factors. Sexual abstention, viewing sexually explicit material, masturbation, and increased sexual activity all fail to alter SREs *(59)*. Consequently, SRE testing provides objective, quantitative indices of erectile function. Therefore, failure to attain full erections during consolidated REM sleep is taken to indicate erectile pathophysiology. Strain gages placed around the penis are used to record SREs by continuously measuring penile circumference. Concurrently sleep state assessment is preferred to determine coupling between SREs and REM sleep. Because circumference increase can occur without penile rigidity, penile resistance to buckling is a critical parameter for judging erectile quality. SREs are most commonly summarized according to frequency, magnitude, duration, and quality (rigidity).

Developmental Changes in SREs and Testosterone

Karacan and associates *(60)* studied SREs in young boys, young adults, middle-aged men, and the elderly. Their results have subsequently been replicated *(61,62)*. Except for a sharp increase during adolescence, SREs in men age 3–80 yr are fairly consistent. With advancing age, small statistically reliable total tumescence time (duration) decline is found, accounting for approx 15% of variance *(61)*. Frequency and magnitude measures show little or no decline with age in healthy potent seniors. However, there is an increase in latency time and a decrease in maximum circumference in healthy aging men.

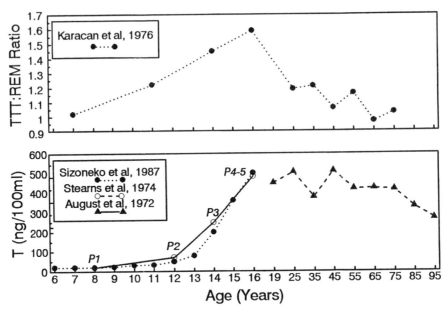

Fig. 3. Age-related changes in total sleep-related tumescence time (TTT) to REM sleep ratio and testosterone (T) levels. Puberty stages (P) 1–5 are shown on the bottom panel. As puberty approaches, the TTT:REM sleep ratio increases to a peak at age 16 yr. The ratio stabilizes slightly higher than 1:1 by age 25 yr. Testosterone rises dramatically during puberty, stabilizing at adult levels by age 16 yr.

At puberty, the ratio of SREs to REM sleep increases dramatically (*see* Fig. 3). This rise in spontaneous erectile activity paralleling increased circulating androgen suggests that T may potentiate erectile activity. In a study investigating SRE association with aging and endocrine function, bioavailable T (but not total T) was found to decline with age (*63*) and SRE frequency and duration correlated with bioavailable T. Overall, age appeared to be the controlling factor; however, SRE duration was related to bioavailable T within the 55- to 64-yr age group but not in younger or older groups. These authors suggest that age alters a central SRE activation threshold to account for the age-related T association with SREs. Finally, another link between SREs and T is the finding that peak levels occur near REM–non-REM sleep transitions.

Testosterone levels are low early during the sleep period and gradually increase toward morning. Sleep-cycle disorganization is marked by T alterations and day sleep is associated with T elevation (*64,65*). In healthy men, three to five REM sleep episodes occur each night. Testosterone peaks were first reported occurring proximal to shifts from non-REM to REM sleep by Evans and colleagues (*65*). This finding was not confirmed by another research group (*66*), who, instead, found that LH rises preceded T peaks (lag time 20–140 min). Similarly, Miyatake and colleagues (*67*) found no sleep stage association with T level; however, mean level rather than peaks were analyzed. Subsequently, the REM–testosterone relationship was quantitatively demonstrated (*68*). Pulsatile peak T levels were concentrated within a 20-min temporal window surrounding transitions from non-REM to REM sleep. Interestingly, the CNS organizational state transition to REM sleep also marks the activation of spontaneous SREs.

If SREs are androgen dependent, prepubescent SRE poses an interesting question. The presence of adrenal androgen during the first 2 yr of life may partially explain SREs in the very young; however, androgen remains low for half a decade or more. The dramatic SRE increase during puberty and then its rapid decline by the end of the next decade to normal adult levels may reflect initial receptor supersensitivity and subsequent downregulation. This model is supported by the finding that spontaneous erectile activation compared to REM sleep declines after puberty, whereas T levels remain high. Another theoretical perspective posits SREs having a very low discrete steplike androgen threshold for occurrence followed by a more continuous correlated association once threshold is met. Finally, SRE may be influenced by both REM sleep and androgen, with one subserving a permissive role and the other a modulating one.

Androgen Deficiency and Replacement in Hypogonadal Men

SELF-REPORT

Davidson and colleagues *(69)* provided the initial scientific evidence for androgen's effects in hypogonadal men. They studied six men between the ages of 32 and 65. Subjects received placebo, 100 mg, or 400 mg of testosterone enanthate (TE) intramuscularly every 4 wk for 5 mo. Treatments were varied at random within and among the subjects; subjects maintained daily logs of sexual activity. Paired *t*-tests comparing placebo and 400 mg TE revealed significant differences for total erections ($p < 0.001$), nocturnal erections ($p < 0.02$), coital frequency ($p < 0.05$), and erections culminating in orgasm ($p < 0.001$). Subsequent reports using different delivery systems confirm these findings (*see* Table 1).

ERECTILE RESPONSE TO VSS, SF, AND AUDITORY STIMULATION

Bancroft and Wu *(70)* studied eight hypogonadal men with T levels <270 ng/dL during VSS. Subjects were studied while hypogonadal and during treatment with TU (160 or 240 mg/d). They reported no visually stimulated (VSS) maximal circumference change or latency to achieving erection difference among normal men, hypogonadal men, or T-treated hypogonadal men. Similar observations were made in a double-blind, crossover study involving six hypogonadal men *(71)*. Subjects were treated with placebo, 200 mg, or 400 mg of TE intramuscularly at monthly intervals. The total duration of erections and the time with maximal circumference were similar in hypogonadal and normal men and were not affected by T treatment. The hypogonadal men had a slower loss of tumescence than the normal controls. A third study evaluated 9 hypogonadal males and 12 eugonadal controls *(72)*. VSS-related penile magnitude and duration did not differ between hypogonadal men and eugonadal controls. Although T replacement failed to alter magnitude or duration, it was associated with increased ($p < 0.01$) penile rigidity. These authors concluded that erectile responses to VSS predominantly involves an androgen-independent system but may be influenced by androgen-sensitive mechanisms.

Subjects also have undergone erection monitoring while fantasizing (SF) about "the most sexually exciting scene." Eight hypogonadal males were studied before and during treatment with TU (160 mg/d) *(70)*. Maximum penile circumference increase was less in the hypogonadal men than in the age-matched normal controls and was not improved by treatment. However, T replacement improved the latency to achieve an erection. Other studies of six *(71)* and nine hypogonadal men *(72)* yielded less consistent results. One investigation found no significant differences in erectile magnitude or duration;

Table 1
Self-Reported Effects of Androgen Deficiency

Investigators	n	Study design	Treatment	Findings
Davidson et al. (69)	6	On and off treatment	Placebo, TE 100 or 400 mg/4 wk	TE 400 mg vs Placebo TE → ↑ total erections ↑ nocturnal erections ↑ coital frequency
Luisi and Franci (141)	26	Double-blind, random	TU (40 mg tid); mesterolone	TU vs baseline or mesterolone TU → ↑ libido ↑ erections ↑ ejaculations
Skakkebaek et al. (142)	12	Double-blind, crossover	Placebo or TU (40 mg qid)	TU vs placebo TU → ↑ sexual thoughts ↑ sexual excitement ↑ sexual acts ↑ ejaculations
Clopper et al. (75)	9	Single blind, crossover	Placebo, hCG 2000 + hMG 75 tiw, or TE (200 mg/2 wk)	Tx vs placebo Tx → ↑ libido ↑ ejaculations TE vs hCG + hMG TE → ↑ ejaculations

however, penile rigidity in hypogonadal men during SF improved ($p < 0.02$) with T replacement *(72)*.

Alexander and colleagues *(73)* evaluated responses to auditory stimuli in 33 hypogonadal men receiving testosterone replacement, 10 eugonadal men receiving testosterone in a contraceptive clinical trial, and 19 untreated eugonadal men prior to and after testosterone treatment. Sexual arousal and sexual enjoyment were increased by testosterone treatment regardless of the pretreatment testosterone levels.

SLEEP-RELATED ERECTIONS

Androgen deficiency and androgen replacement alter SREs (*see* Table 2). Men with severe and previously untreated hypogonadism demonstrate little or no SRE activity *(74)*. All parameters of SRE increased over 1 yr, in which serum T levels were normalized, suggesting SREs in prepubertal males are influenced by even small amounts of T. Nine gonadotropin deficient males (age 16–20 yr) were evaluated in a crossover designed study comparing gonadotropin (2000 U of hCG + 75 IU of hMG tiw) treatment, TE (200 mg for 2 wk), and placebo *(75)*. Similar T levels were achieved with both therapies. Total tumescence time ($p < 0.001$), duration of erections >80% of maximal tumescence ($p < 0.004$), and maximal circumference ($p < 0.001$) improved with both treatments.

Techniques used to monitor SREs and penile rigidity have varied across studies. Researchers employ different study designs and a variety of androgen-replacement regimens; however, all studies indicate androgen-related SREs changes. Androgen deficiency is associated with fewer spontaneous SREs, reduced maximum increase in penile circumference (magnitude), shorter duration of erections, and poorer penile rigidity (quality) during erections. Adequate T replacement in the absence of co-morbid disease increases and sometimes normalizes SREs.

The effects of T on libido in hypogonadal men are best explained by an effect on the CNS. A CNS effect of androgen also could explain the differences in the frequency of SREs and perhaps the duration of SREs observed during androgen replacement. A local effect of T at the level of the spinal cord, pelvic ganglia, and/or corpora cavernosa would help to explain differences in penile circumference and rigidity that have been observed during hypogonadal and androgen replaced states.

Manipulating Testosterone Levels in Eugonadal Men

The effect on sexual behavior of varying serum T levels within the normal or supernormal range interests clinical investigators. At one time, indiscriminant treatment with T was common; however, this practice is much less frequent today. If administering exogenous T produces beneficial effects, one could justify such therapy under specific conditions. It also could help answer the question concerning whether T exerts an effect when levels exceed a threshold or whether there is a continuous effect even when levels are within or exceed the normal range. Bhasin and colleagues *(76)* have convincingly demonstrated anabolic effects of supraphysiological doses of T in young men. Is there a similar effect on sexual behavior?

Buena and co-workers *(77)* administered leuprolide to reduce gonadotropin and T secretion and two doses of T microspheres to restore serum levels of T to low or high normal ranges. Daily logs of sexual activity and SRE studies in a sleep laboratory were conducted before and after 9 wk of treatment. Pretreatment T levels in the two groups were similar (15.5 ± 2.1 and 16.6 ± 2.5 nmol/L). Treatment levels were 10.5 ± 1.7 and

Table 2
Sleep-Related Erections in Androgen Deficient Males

Investigators	n	Study design	Treatment	Findings
Kwan et al. (71)	6	Double-blind, placebo, crossover	Placebo, TE, 200 or 400 mg/1 mo intramuscularly	TE vs placebo TE → ↑ change in penile circumference ↑ SRE duration
O'Carroll et al. (110)	4	Off and on treatment	TU (160 mg/d)	TU vs no treatment TU → ↑ change in penile circumference ↑ SRE duration
Cunningham and Hirshkowitz (73a)	6	On and off treatment	T cypionate (200 mg/2 wk)	TC (1–4 d) vs (7–8 wk): TC (1–4 d) → ↑ number of SREs ↑ max circumference increase ↑ SRE duration ↑ penile rigidity
Burris and Sherins (74)	6	Off and on treatment	TE 200 mg/2 wk intramuscularly or hCG 2000 + hMG 75 tiw	No Tx vs Tx Tx → ↑ number of SREs ↑ max circumference increase ↑ SRE duration ↑ penile rigidity
Arver et al. (143)	20	On TE, off Tx, on transdermal	TE (200 mg/2 wk) or transdermal (7.5 mg/d)	No Tx vs Tx No Tx → ↑ number of SREs ↑ SRE duration ↑ penile rigidity TE vs transdermal no differences
Clopper et al. (75)	9	Single blind, crossover	Placebo, hCG 2000 + hMG 75 tiw or TE (200 mg/2 wk intramuscularly)	Tx vs placebo Tx → ↑ SRE duration ↑ change in penile circumference ↑ max circumference increase TE vs hCG + hMG no differences

| Carini et al. (72) | 8 | Off and on treatment | Multiple treatments | Tx vs no Tx
Tx → ↑ number of maximum SREs ($p < 0.07$)
↑ rigidity ($p < 0.07$) |
| Dobs et al. (144) | 13 | Double-blind, placebo controlled | Placebo, TE, T cyclodextrin 10 mg tablets | TE vs bucal T
Similar max rigidity
Similar max duration
Bucal T vs P
↑ max rigidity
↑ max duration |

26.5 ± 3.4 nmol/L (*p* < 0.05). No differences in sexual behavior were observed when comparing parameters prior to and during treatment or during the two treatments. Similarly, no SRE differences were noted in the number, the magnitude, or duration of nocturnal erections.

The effects of TE (150 mg intramuscularly) vs placebo on SRE in normal men has been examined *(78)*. Subjects were studied in a sleep laboratory 2 d after the injection, a time when T levels would be supernormal or high normal. There were no significant differences in the number, magnitude or duration of sleep related erections. However, penile rigidity and the duration of maximal rigidity were increased by T injections (*p* < 0.0025 and *p* < 0.025, respectively).

To explore possible benefits of T therapy in men with normal serum levels of T but who complained of sexual dysfunction, O'Carroll and Bancroft *(79)* conducted a double-blind, crossover study using placebo or Sustanon, 250 mg intramuscularly per week (T propionate 30 mg; T phenylproprionate 60 mg; T isocaproate 60 mg; T decanoate 100 mg). There was a 4-wk baseline period followed by 6 wk of placebo and 6 wk of T therapy or 6 wk of T therapy and 6 wk of placebo. Patients were divided into two groups: those complaining principally of loss of sexual interest or those complaining primarily of erectile failure. Treatment increased T levels (*p* < 0.01). The frequency of sexual thoughts was increased (*p* < 0.02) by T treatment in the group with low sexual interest; however, there was no increase in sexual activity and in mood. Testosterone therapy provided no benefit to the group of men complaining of erectile dysfunction. In a double-blind, placebo-controlled, crossover study, Schiavi and co-workers *(80)* observed the effects of administering testosterone enanthate 200 mg intramuscularly every 2 wk to eugonadal men with erectile dysfunction. Subjects reported a significant increase in frequency of ejaculations with testosterone treatment. As previously noted, Alexander and colleagues *(73)* noted testosterone treatment increased sexual arousal and sexual enjoyment in eugonadal men.

These studies support the concept that a T threshold exists for sexual behaviors. The threshold seems to be somewhat below the normal serum T level range for young adult men. One cannot justify T treatment of erectile dysfunction when serum T levels are normal. Whether T treatment improves libido within the normal serum T range will require further studies.

Sexuality and 5α-Reductase Deficiency and Inhibition

Associations between T level and sexual function could be mediated directly by T or indirectly by its metabolites (DHT and estradiol). There are at least two 5α-reductase enzymes; therefore, inhibiting both would be necessary to ascertain if DHT is necessary for sexual function. The effects of a 5α-reductase inhibitor or an aromatase inhibitor on CNS would depend on it crossing the blood-brain barrier. Many of these inhibitors are steroids; therefore, they likely cross this barrier in sufficient quantities to influence CNS activity.

Males with an inherited defect in type 2 5α-reductase reportedly develop normal libido and have normal penile erections *(81)*. Penile development in these individuals is delayed but occurs at puberty *(82)*. These men have rudimentary prostates; consequently, pharmaceutical type 1 and type 2 5α-reductase activity inhibitors have been developed in an effort to treat or prevent benign prostatic hyperplasia, male pattern baldness, and, possibly, prostate cancer. Three to four percent of men treated with finasteride *(83)*, a type 2 inhibitor, or with devtasteride (unpublished data), an inhibitor of both the type 1 and type 2 enzymes, report reduced libido or potency. In a double-blind, placebo-controlled trial conducted at our laboratory we gave 20 sexually active men (age 41–64 yr) finasteride 5 mg or placebo for 12 wk (85). A sexual function questionnaire was administered weekly and no loss of libido or erectile dysfunction was found. We also studied these men for four nights in the sleep laboratory—twice during baseline and twice at the end of the treatment period. No consistent SRE frequency, magnitude, duration, or quality differences were observed with finasteride treatment compared to placebo. Thus, it appears that either T or DHT can provide normal men with androgenic stimulation required for normal libido and erectile function. However, the possibility that a longer treatment period could adversely affect sexual function in some men remains. Finasteride is a type 2 inhibitor; therefore, it also is possible that type 1 5α-reductase activity in the brain could be responsible for maintaining libido and erectile function. Studies with devtasteride (unpublished) indicate a comparable incidence of erectile problems, making it likely that some men have a preexisting condition that, in conjunction with 5α-reductase inhibition, causes the problem. As previously noted, animal studies suggest DHT is more potent than T with respect to potentiating neural stimulation of erections.

Sexuality and Aromatase Deficiency and Inhibition

Whereas estrogen is thought to be the major steroid required by the CNS for sexual behavior in the rat, estrogen treatment of men usually reduces libido and potency (86). Few patients with aromatase deficiency or estrogen insensitivity have been evaluated. A recent report describes a male with congenital aromatase deficiency. His psychosexual orientation was male and heterosexual (87). Estrogen treatment increased libido, frequency of sexual intercourse, masturbation, and erotic fantasies. Estrogen treatment also decreased depression and anxiety scores. However, no consistent changes in libido or in sexual function have been noted in men treated with either an aromatase inhibitor (88,89) or with an antiestrogen (90).

Surgical and Chemical Castration

In Men with Normal Sexuality

Surgical or medical (GnRH agonist treatment) castration for stage D prostate cancer reportedly reduces libido. Of 11 men studied, post-treatment libido was absent in 5, poor in 3, and fair in 3 (91). All reported satisfactory erectile function before treatment; however, after 5 or more months, no patient reported spontaneous erections and none had attempted intercourse following treatment. Four subjects had VSS-induced erections with a 10-mm or more circumference increased.

A double-blind study of the GnRH antagonist Nal-Glu randomized 50 men, age 20–40 yr into five groups: Nal-Glu alone, Nal-Glu + TE 50 mg intramuscularly per week, Nal-Glu + TE 100 mg intramuscularly per week, Nal-Glu + TE 100 mg intramuscularly per week + testolactone (an aromatase inhibitor) 250 mg po qid, and placebo (89). After a 4-wk pretreatment phase, there were 6 treatment weeks and 4 recovery weeks. Men receiving Nal-Glu alone experienced less frequent sexual desire ($p < 0.05$), fewer sexual fantasies, less sexual intercourse, fewer spontaneous erections ($p < 0.55$ compared to baseline and $p < 0.05$ compared to post-treatment), and less frequent masturbation ($p < 0.05$). These parameters normalized within 3 wk of treatment cessation. Other groups did not differ from baseline on these parameters. Mean nadir T levels in subjects receiving 50 mg of TE per week were in the borderline low range (8.9 ± 0.6 nmol/L). Because testolactone blocks the conversion of T to estradiol, at least in peripheral tissues, it did not appear that estrogen is required for normal sexual function in the adult male.

The GnRH agonist leuprolide, initially stimulates, and subsequently decreases gonadotropin secretion. Usually T levels are suppressed within 3 wk. In a double-blind, placebo-controlled study involving 10 normal men 21–35 yr of age, Hirshkowitz and colleagues (92) treated 5 men with leuprolide and 5 men with placebo injections. Subjects were studied for two successive nights in a sleep laboratory during a control period, and after 4, 8, and 12 wk of treatment. Second-night data were used for the analysis. REM sleep measures and sleep efficiency were similar in the two groups. Significant ($p < 0.05$) reduction in total tumescence was observed at 8 and 12 wk. There was a trend for the number of SREs to decrease ($p < 0.14$) and a tendency toward reduced maximal penile circumference increase at 8 wk.

In Sex Offenders

Surgical castration of sex offenders was common practice in some European countries after World War II (93). A survey of 39 sex offenders (mean age: 49.3 yr) revealed that although sexual activity declined after castration, 31% still reported ability to engage in sexual intercourse (94). The strongest diminution of sexuality occurred when castration was performed later in life (age: 46–59 yr). Heim compared these data to previously published work and found less cessation of coitus (69%) than previously reported by Cornu (90%) or Langeluddeke (82%).

Antiandrogens that suppress LH and T secretion and/or antagonize T action have been used to treat sex offenders. In one study (95), 19 paraphilic men were administered cyproterone acetate. Significantly decreased sexual fantasies and masturbation were found; however, no decline occurred in self-reported libido, potency, or coitus. A placebo-controlled study of cyproterone acetate (CPA) on hypersexual men found that it reduced sexual drive and arousal (96). Medroxyprogesterone acetate (MPA), a synthetic progestin with gonadotropin-suppressing and antiandrogen properties, and CPA blunted a variety of sexual behaviors in seven pedophiles (97). Both drugs reduced self-reported sexual thoughts, sexual fantasies, number of early morning erections, frequency of masturbation, pleasure derived from masturbation, and level of sexual frustration. MPA also was found to dramatically reduce SREs in three sex offenders (98).

ANDROGEN AND AGGRESSIVE BEHAVIOR

In many species, androgens appear to increase aggressive behavior. Attempts to find analogous androgen-related increases in man have yielded mixed results. In a case report, MPA reduced aggressive sexual behavior and sexual acting out in a male schizophrenic (99). Interestingly, it also suppressed SREs. Sex hormone administration is part of sex change protocols. Fifteen male-to-female transsexuals treated with estrogen and antiandrogens were less prone to aggression and anger (100). By contrast, androgens given to 35 female-to-male transsexuals increased aggression and sexual arousability.

Anabolic steroid abuse is anecdotally implicated in aggressive behavior and violent crime. A prospective double-blind, placebo-controlled study examined whether T would increase aggressive tendencies in normal men (101). After excluding competitive athletes and men with psychiatric disturbances, 600 mg TE or placebo were administered weekly for 6 wk to 43 eugonadal men. Subgroups with and without strength-training exercise regimens also were formed. No treatment-related changes were found on any subscales of the Multi-Dimensional Anger Inventory, the Mood Inventory, or the subjects' significant-others' rating of mood or behavior on the Observer Mood Inventory. By contrast, double-blind, placebo-controlled T injection in 35 hypogonadal adolescents increased aggression scores on the Olweus Multifaceted Aggression Inventory *(102)*. Elevation was found for self-reported physical aggressive behaviors and aggressive impulses; however, verbal aggression did not increase. In school children, T level was found to correlate with aggression during social interactions among boys *(103)*. Testosterone level also correlated with rated aggressiveness of 28 men competing in a judo competition. Ratings of aggressiveness were made from videotapes, and T was sampled before and after the bout *(104)*.

The androgen-disinhibition model can explain these apparently discrepant findings. Some theorists believe that T-related aggressive behavior becomes manifest when impulse-control problems occur. Thus, under normal circumstances, aggression is inhibited; however, when disinhibition occurs, it is unmasked. As such, the data showing no relationship between substantial T supplementation and aggression in normal men does not rule out exacerbation of aggression among individuals prone to violence. The androgen-disinhibition model is supported by studies in squirrel monkeys *(105)*. Dominant males' T level rose to 202.9 during mating season compared to 28 ng/mL in subordinates. Although alcohol (0.1–1.0 g/kg, po) reduced T in a dose-response manner in dominant males, low doses (0.1 and 0.3 g/kg) also increased aggressive behaviors. At time periods other than mating season, alcohol had no effect on aggressive behavior or T.

ANDROGEN AND AFFECT

The relationship between androgen and affect is the subject of several recent reviews *(106–108)*. Data derive mainly from three sources: (1) studies involving T supplementation in eugonadal men, (2) mood assessment during androgen-replacement therapy in hypogonadal men, and (3) cross-sectional and intervention research on men with depression.

Testosterone enanthate administered to healthy eugonadal men appears not to consistently alter mood. No significant change from placebo baseline was found in 31 men (age 21–41 yr), given TE (200 mg, intramuscularly, weekly) for 4 wk *(109)*. Ratings were made on scales for cheerfulness, lethargy, relaxation, tension, energy, unhappiness, irritability, readiness to fight, and easiness to anger. Tricker et al. *(101)* randomized 43 eugonadal men (age 19–40) to receive either TE (600 mg, weekly) or placebo for 10 wk. They found no change in self-reported or observer rated scales of mood, anger or hostility. O'Carroll and Bancroft *(79)* similarly found no change in mood scales when intramuscular testosterone or placebo injection was administer to 20 eugonadal men 19–64 yr of age with sexual dysfunction, in a double-blind crossover trial. Similarly, no change in Profile of Mood States (POMS) or Symptom Checklist 90 revised (SCL-90r) was found when intramuscular testosterone (TE, 200 mg, biweekly) was administered to 12 eugonadal men (age 46–67 yr) with erectile dysfunction in a double-blind, placebo-controlled, crossover trail *(80)*.

Hypogonadal men often exhibit prominent psychiatric symptoms, including dysphoria, fatigue, irritability, and appetite loss. These symptoms generally diminish after testosterone replacement. In an early study, six men (age 32–65 yr) with hypogonadism received two doses of TE (100 and 400 mg/mo) for 5 mo *(69)*. Subjects completed the POMS at weekly intervals throughout most of the study and were seen monthly by a psychologist. No significant androgen-related changes were found in mood. By contrast, TU administered double blind in four successive, 1-mo periods (40, 80, 120, and 160 mg/d in crossover design) reportedly improved mood *(110)*. Eight subjects recorded their mood states daily in diary format and completed visual analog scales rating 10 separate mood states. Significant T-related improvements were found on several scales, including: cheerful–happy, tense–anxious, and relaxed. Burris and colleagues *(74)*, used a self-reported measures and found that hypogonadal men (age 25–40 yr) scored higher on ratings of depression, anger, fatigue, and confusion than did controls. After TE treatment (200 mg every 2 wk), mood scores improved, suggesting testosterone can elevate mood and decrease anger. In a similar study *(111)*, mood was evaluated 58 men (age 22–60 yr) with hypogonadism that were treated with either TE (200 mg every 20 d) or sublingual testosterone cyclodextrin (2.5 mg or 5 mg, three times per day). After 60 d of T-replacement therapy, there reportedly were increases in energy, well/good feelings, and friendliness and decreases in anger, nervousness, and irritability. Similar mood and energy improvements were found in men administered T transdermally using scrotal patches *(112)*.

Androgen-replacement therapy has also been applied to men with low T levels associated with Klinefelter's syndrome. No mood or energy differences were reported for four men given TU (160 mg) or placebo in a double-blind, crossover study *(113)*. By contrast, in a larger trial, 30 men with Klinefelter's syndrome that were given T showed improved mood, less irritability, more energy and drive, less fatigue, more endurance and strength, less need for sleep, better concentration, and better relations with others *(114)*.

Neuroendocrine studies of the hypothalamic–pituitary–gonadal (HPG) axis among men with well-diagnosed major depression have yielded mixed results, largely as a result of the variation in the studies. This variability stems from the different populations studied, different androgen assays used, and differences in the timing of phlebotomy to obtain blood draws. Some studies find lower T levels in depressed compared to nondepressed men *(115–118)*. However, other studies report no difference related to depression *(118a–122)*. Other studies have found a negative correlation between T levels and severity of depression *(115,122,123)*. For example, Vogel and colleagues *(116)* reported that in 27 men with unipolar depression, total and free T were significantly lower (approx 30%) compared to 13 age-matched controls. Rubin and colleagues *(119)* studied the HPG axis in 16 depressed men and 16 healthy age-matched controls. They found a statistically significant negative correlation between age and total T levels in depressed patients, suggesting that in depressed males, the decline in total serum T is correlated with advancing age and depression. Additionally, a significant negative correlation between salivary T levels and severity of depression was found in 11 men (mean age: 52.4 yr) studied *(122)*. Thus, some men with major depression may have significantly lower free and bioavailable T than their age-matched controls. Furthermore, T levels decline as subjects age and appear to decline as a function of the severity of depression.

The Rancho Bernardo Study, a cross-sectional population-based study, examined the association between endogenous sex hormones and depressed mood in community-dwelling older men *(124)*. Eight hundred fifty-six men (age 50–89 yr) completed the Beck Depression Inventory (BDI) and had assays for total and free T, dihydrotestosterone (DHT), and estradiol (E$_2$). Overall, free T decreased with age and the prevalence of depressive symptoms increased with age. However, multiple-linear regression revealed a graded stepwise decrease in free T with increasing levels of depressed mood, independent of age, weight change, and physical activity.

Notwithstanding mixed results in correlational studies, T administration has been used experimentally to treat patients with depression. In the older literature, T reportedly alleviated depressive symptoms (125). The therapeutic effect of a synthetic weak androgen (mesterolone) was compared to the tricyclic antidepressant (amitriptyline) in men with depression (126). Mesterolone relieved depression as effectively as amitriptyline. Additionally, a double-blind, placebo-controlled study reportedly found mood enhancement with the weak androgen dehydroepiandrosterone (127).

A few recent studies have examined T's efficacy in depressed men. Rabkin and colleagues (127,127a,128) conducted two studies of T administration to human immunodeficiency virus (HIV)-positive men. The first study was an open-label, 8-wk, clinical trial of intramuscular T (400 mg, biweekly) that included 34 hypogonadal HIV-positive men who had mood problems. Of the 34 men, 79% were significantly improved by wk 8, compared to baseline. In the second study, 74 HIV-positive men were enrolled in the double-blind, placebo-controlled, 6-wk trial of biweekly testosterone vs placebo, followed by 12-wk open-label treatment (128). Based on Clinical Global Impressions Scale ratings, improved libido was found for 74% of men treated with T compared to 19% of men treated with placebo ($p < 0.001$). Among 26 study completers with Axis I depressive disorders, 58% of those randomized to testosterone vs 14% of placebo-treated patients were judged to have much or very much improved mood. There was no difference in response rate between men with T levels below vs within normal range. In another study, hypogonadal men with AIDS wasting had higher depression scores. In these patients, T administration (300 mg intramuscularly, every 3 wk) significantly improved depression inventory scores (129).

Testosterone openly administered for 8 wk to five men with SSRI-refractory major depression and T levels below 350 ng/dL had rapid, dramatic recoveries (130). All five patients improved; mean Hamilton Rating Scale of Depression (HAM-D) decrease from 19.2 to 7.2 by wk 2 and to 4.0 by wk 8. More recently, a randomized, placebo-controlled, clinical-trail examined the effects of TE (200 mg, intramuscularly) versus placebo in 32 men with DSM-IV-diagnosed Major Depressive Disorder and a low testosterone (107). Hamilton depression scores decreased in both the 13 subjects receiving T and in the 17 subjects receiving placebo and there were no significant group differences. Thus, it is uncertain whether T-related mood improvements in hypogonadal men with depression are placebo, regression, or intermittent effects. Nonetheless, the overall pattern of results suggests a potential utility for T as an antidepressant for augmenting therapy in some men with depression.

In summary, T supplementation may improve mood in patients with depression, hypogonadism, or both. The lack of change in normal eugonadal men may represent a "ceiling effect" inherent in mood assessment tools or a threshold effect for T. Alternatively, T may reduce an inhibitory depressogenic factor and have no effect when such is not present. Additional work focused on T supplementation and depressive disorder type and depth will likely elucidate the apparent interaction.

ANDROGEN AND COGNITION

Well-established sex differences exist for verbal fluency and visuo-spatial tasks. Although nature vs nurture issues remain unresolved, some evidence implicates a role of androgen in certain cognitive abilities. The classic sex-difference literature concerning cognition derives from IQ tests.

Snow and Weinstock *(131)* reviewed the Wechsler Adult Intelligence Scale (WAIS) literature to compare non-brain-injured males and females on specific subtests. Women tend to outperform men by 0.33 of the standard deviation on the Digit Symbol subtest. By contrast, men outperform women, to the same extent or more, on the Arithmetic and Information subtests. Several studies also found male superiority on Block Design and Comprehension subtests. Notwithstanding subtest differences, overall IQ scores do not differ. Hormonal differences between men and women have been suggested as one of many possible underlying biological mechanisms to account for differential cognitive abilities.

Correlational approaches provide some evidence for a relationship among androgen, visuo-spatial abilities, and verbal abilities. In 117 healthy young men, serum T correlated positively with measures of spatial ability and field dependence–independence *(132)*. By contrast, a significant negative correlation was found between T and measures of verbal production. Five spatial and six verbal test scores determined cognitive function. Another study examined the relationship among serum T, estradiol, and adrenocorticotropin (ACTH) levels and spatial, verbal, and musical abilities *(133)*. For the 26 men (mean age: 19 yr) and 25 women (mean age: 18.7 yr), T and estradiol levels were not significantly related to any cognitive or musical tests; however, the T/estradiol ratio was significantly negatively correlated with spatial tests, and ACTH was significantly positively correlated with spatial and musical tests. Correlations were stronger for woman than men. Other cognitive abilities assessed in 59 men also reportedly correlated with bioavailable T; sensitive tests included the Folstein Mini Mental Status examination, animal naming, Rey visual design learning test, and Rey auditory verbal learning test *(134)*.

Although some researchers report simple correlations, others find more complex relationships. For example, cognitive performance was explored in normal men and women grouped according to relatively high or low salivary T concentrations *(135)*. Men with lower salivary T performed better than other groups on spatial–mathematical tasks. Women with higher T scored higher than low-T women on these same measures. Testosterone concentration did not significantly relate to scores on tests that usually favor women. The authors suggest a nonlinear relationship exists between T and spatial ability. In two studies, moderate levels of androgens were associated with better spatial performance *(136,137)*.

Beyond cross-sectional descriptive and correlational investigations, several reports describe cognitive changes associated with T administration. Eight treated hypogonadal men tended to have better picture identification ability than 12 untreated hypogonadal men *(138)*. Superior verbal fluency and verbal memory occurred when patients were hypogonadal compared to when they were treated.

In the study of transsexuals previously mentioned with reference to aggression *(100)* the contribution of sex hormones to cognitive functioning was assessed. Administering androgens to females was associated with increased spatial ability performance and deterioration in verbal fluency. Male-to-female hormone therapy improved verbal fluency, suggesting that sex hormones quickly and directly influence sex-specific cognitive abilities. Moreover, in a placebo-controlled study, WAIS block design subtest scores in elderly men (not selected for hypogonadism) improved after T administration compared to placebo *(139)*. The same researchers *(140)* more recently reported improved working memory in older men administered TE (150 mg, weekly). By contrast, working memory did not improve in older women treated with estrogen (625 mg/d, po). Finally, Cherrier and colleagues *(140)* found improved spatial and verbal memory in older men treated with TE (100 mg/wk) compared to placebo. Subjects were studied for 6 wk and were evaluated with a neuropsychological test battery at baseline, wk 3, and wk 6. Active treatment was associated with improvement compared to baseline and compared to placebo.

These data, when considered together, suggest a CNS role of T facilitating visuospatial abilities and decreasing verbal abilities. Although an oversimplification, the results provide a fascinating clue about central actions of T. It also establishes a basis for exploring T replacement as a means to improve cognitive function, as well as mood, in men with primary or secondary hypogonadism.

SUMMARY

As our knowledge base expands, it is becoming apparent that T influences both central and peripheral nervous system mechanisms. Although a role for T in sexual behavior has long been known, its relationship with aggression, mood, and cognition are being uncovered. Some simple notions require modification based on systematic experimentation (e.g., T's role in aggression). The availability of clinical paradigms, most notably androgen replacement in hypogonadal men, provide an opportunity to observe and measure changes as the hormonal levels are therapeutically normalized. We see not only self-reported increases in the level of sexual desire but also objective improvements in erectile capability indexed using SREs. Emotion and learned behavior have long been known to modulate human sexual response. Correlational and some experimental studies find mood and specific cognitive abilities affected by T. Experimental models involving surgical castration in animals and androgen blockade or androgen suppression in humans open additional avenues to explore how changes in T alter sexual function, mood, and intellect. Finally, AR localization and its relationship with other neurotransmitter systems add important pieces to the complex puzzle of androgenic influence on human sexuality.

REFERENCES

1. Newerla GJ. The history of the discovery and isolation of the male hormone. N Engl J Med 1943;228(2):39–47.
2. Hammond TE. The function of the testes after puberty. Br J Urol 1943;6:128–141.
3. Breedlove SM, Arnold AP. Hormone accumulation in a sexually dimorphic motor nucleus of the rat spinal cord. Science 1980;210:564–566.
3a. Breedlove SM. sexual dimorphism in the vertebrate nervous system. J Neurosci 1992;12:4133–4142.
4. McEwen BS. Our changing ideas about steroid effects on an ever-changing brain. Sem Neurosci 1991;3:497–507.
5. Michael RP, Rees HD, Gonsall RW. Sites in the male primate brain at which testosterone acts as an androgen. Brain Res 1989;502:11–20.
6. Kritzer MF. Selective colocalization of immunoreactivity for intracellular gonadal hormone receptors and tyrosine hydroxylase in the ventral tegmental area, substantia nigra, and retrorubral fields in the rat. J Comp Neurol 1997;379(2):247–260.
7. Herbison AE. Neurochemical identity of neurones expressing oestrogen and androgen receptors in sheep hypothalamus. J Reprod Fertil Supp 1995;49:271–283.
8. McGinnis MY, Williams GW, Lumia AR. Inhibition of male sex behavior by androgen receptor blockade in preoptic area or hypothalamus, but not amygdala or septum. Physiol Behav 1996;60(3):783–789.

9. Heaton JPW, Varrin SJ. Effects of castration and exogenous testosterone supplementation in an animal model of penile erection. J Urol 1994;151:797–800.

10. Yamada K, Furukawa T. The effects of APO on penile erection/stretching yawning are thought to be mediated by the CNS. They probably involve dopaminergic receptors. Psychopharmacology 1980;617:39.

11. Pehek E, Thompson J, Eaton R, et al. Apomorphine and haloperidol, but not domeridone, affect penile reflexes in rats. Pharmacol Biochem Behav 1988;31:201.

12. Argiolas A, Melis MR, Mauri A, et al. Paraventricular nucleus lesion prevents yawning and penile erection induced by apomorphine and oxytocin but not by ACTH in rats. Brain Res 1987;421(1-2):349–352.

13. Melis MR, Argiolas A, Gessa GL. Apomorphine-induced penile erection and yawning: site of action in brain. Brain Res 1987;415(1):98–104.

14. MacLean PD, Denniston RH, Dua S. Further studies on cerebral representation of penile erection: caudal thalamus, midbrain, and pons. J Neurophysiol 1963;26:274–293.

15. Malsbury CW. Facilitation of male rat copulatory behaviour by electrical stimulation of the medial preoptic area. Physiol Behav 1971;7:707–805.

16. Perachio AA, Marr LD, Alexander M. Sexual behavior in male rhesus monkeys elicited by electrical stimulation of preoptic and hypothalamic areas. Brain Res 1979;177:127–144.

17. Robinson BW, Mishkin M. Penile erections evoked by forebrain structures in macaca mulatta. Arch Neurol 1968;19:184–189.

18. Chen K-K, Chan JYH, Chang LS, et al. Elicitation of penile erection following activation of the hippocampal formation in the rat. Neurosci Lett 1992;141:218–222.

19. Slimp JC, Hart BL, Goy RW. Heterosexual, autosexual and social behavior of adult male rhesus monkeys with medial preoptic-anterior hypothalamic lesions. Brain Res 1978;142:105–122.

20. Davidson JM. Hormones and sexual behavior in the male. Hosp Prac 1975;126.

21. Melis MR, Stancampiano R, Argiolas A. Penile erection and yawning induced by paraventricular NMDA injection in male rats are mediated by oxytocin. Pharmacol Biochem Behav 1994;48:203–207.

22. Giuliano F, Rampin O. Central neural regulation of penile erection. Neurosci Biobehav Rev 2000;24:517–533.

23. Luiten PGM, ter Horst GJ, Karst H, et al. The course of paraventricular hypothalamic efferents to autonomic structures in medulla and spinal cord. Brain Res 1985;392:374–378.

24. Tang Y, Rampin O, Calas A, et al. Oxytocinergic and serotonergic innervation of identified lumbosacral nuclei controlling penile erection in the male rat. Neuroscience 1998;82:241–254.

25. Schmidt MH. Sleep-related penile erections. In: Kryger MH, Roth T, Dement WC, eds. Principles and Practice of Sleep Medicine. Saunders, Philadelphia, 2000, pp. 305–318.

26. Sachs BD. Placing erection in context: the reflexogenic-psychogenic dichotomy reconsidered. Neurosci Biobehav Rev 1995;19:211–224.

27. Liu YC, Salamone JD, Sachs BD. Lesions in medial preoptic area and bed nucleus of stria terminalis: Differential effects on copulatory behavior and noncontact erection in male rats. J Neurosci 1997;17:5245–5253.

28. Fernandez-Fewell GD, Meredith M. Facilitation of mating behavior in male hamsters by LHRH and AcLHRH5-10: interaction with the vomeronasal system. Physiol Behav 1995;57:213–221.

29. Kondo Y. Lesions of the medial amygdala produce severe impairment of copulatory behavior in sexually inexperienced male rats. Physiol Behav 1992;51:939–943.

30. Valcourt RJ, Sachs BD. Penile reflexes and copulatory behavior in male rats following lesions in the bed nucleus of the stria terminalis. Brain Res 1979;4:131–133.

31. Redoute J, Stoleru S, Gregoire MC, et al. Brain processing of visual sexual stimuli in human males. Hum Brain Map 2000;11:162–177.

32. Hart BL. Testosterone regulation of sexual reflexes in spinal male rats. Science 1997;155:1283,1284.

33. Hart BL, Wallach SJR, Melese-D'Hospital PY. Differences in responsiveness to testosterone of penile reflexes and copulatory behavior of male rats. Horm Behav 1983;17:274–283.

34. Melvin JE, Hamil RW. Gonadal hormone regulation of neurotransmitter synthesizing enzymes in the developing hypogastric ganglion. Brain Res 1986;383:38.

35. Melvin JE, Hamill RW. The major pelvic ganglion: androgen control of postnatal development. J Neurosci 1987;7(6):1607–1612.

36. Mills TM, Stopper VS, et al. Effects of castration and androgen replacement on the hemodynamics of penile erection in the rat. Biol Reprod 1994;51:234–238.

37. Mills TM, Wiedmeier VT, Stopper VS. Androgen maintenance of erectile function in the rat penis. Biol Reprod 1992;46:342–348.

37a. Giuliano F, Rampin O, Schirart A, et al. Autonomic control of penile erection: modulation by testosterone in the rat. J Neuroendocrinol 1993;5:677–683.

38. Schirar A, Chang C, Rousseau JP. Localization of androgen receptor in nitric oxide synthase and vasoactive intestinal peptide-containing neurons of the major pelvic ganglion innervating the rat penis. J Neuroendocrinol 1997;5:677.

39. Schirar A, Bonnefond C, Meusnier C, et al. Androgens modulate nitric oxide synthase messenger ribonucleic acid expression in neurons of the major pelvic ganglion in the rat. Endocrinology 1997;138(8):3093–3102.

40. Burnett AL, Chang AG, Crone JK, et al. Noncholinergic penile erection in mice lacking the gene for endothelial nitric oxide synthase. J Androl 2002;23:92–97.

41. Lugg JA, Rajfer J, Gonzalez-Cadavid NF. Dihydrotestosterone is the active androgen in the maintenance of nitric oxide-mediated penile erection in the rat. Endocrinology 1995;36(4):1495–1501.

42. Reilly CM, Zamorano P, Stopper VS, et al. Androgenic regulation of NO availability in rat penile erection. J Androl 1997;18(2):110–115.

43. Chamness SL, Ricker DD, Crone JK, et al. the effect of androgen on nitric oxide synthase in male reproductive tract of the rat. Feril Steril 1995;63:1101–1107.

44. Zvara P, Sioufi R, Schipper HM, et al. Nitric oxide mediated erectile activity is a testosterone dependent event: a rat erection model. Int J Impotence Res 1995;7:209–219.

45. Lugg J, Ng C, Rajfer J, et al. Cavernosal nerve stimulation in the rat reverses castration-induced decrease in penile NOS activity. Am J Physiol 1996;271:E354–E361.

46. Rajfer J, Namkung PC, Petra PH. Identification, partial characterization and age-related changes of a cytoplasmic androgen receptor in the rat penis. J Steroid Biochem 1980;13:1489.

47. Takane KK, George FW, Wilson JD. Androgen receptor of rat penis is downregulated by androgen. Am J Physiol 1990;258:E46–E50.

48. Nonomura K, Sakakibara N, Demura T, et al. Androgen binding activity in the spongy tissue of mammalian penis. J Urol 1990;144:152.

49. Lin M-C, Rajfer J, Swerdloff RS, et al. Testosterone down-regulates the levels of androgen receptor mRNA in smooth muscle cells from the rat corpora cavernosa via aromatization to estrogens. J Steroid Biochem Mol Biol 1993;45(5):333–343.

50. Leipheimer RE, Sachs BD. Relative androgen sensitivity of the vascular and striated-muscle systems regulating penile erection in rats. Physiol Behav 1993;54:1085–1090.

51. Max SR, Toop J. Androgens enhance in vivo 2-deoxyglucose uptake by rat striated muscle. Endocrinology 1983;113(1):119–126.

52. Harman SM, Metter EJ, Tobin JD, et al. Longitudinal effects of aging on serum total and free testosterone levels in healthy men. Baltimore Longitudinal Study of Aging. J Clin Endocrinol Metab 2001;86:724–731.

53. Morley JE, Charlton E, Patrick P, et al. Validation of a screening questionnaire for androgen deficiency in aging males. Metabolism 2000;49(9):1239–1242.

54. Reynolds CF, Frank E, Thase ME, et al. Assessment of sexual functioning in depressed, impotent, and healthy men: factor analysis of a brief sexual function questionnaire for men. Psychiatry Res 1988;24:231–250.

55. Derogatis LR, Melisanatos N. The DSFI: a multidimensional measure of sexual functioning. J Sex Marital Therapy 1979;5:244.

56. Geisser ME, Jefferson TW, Spevak M, et al. Reliability and validity of the Florida Sexual History Questionnaire. J Clin Psychology 1991;47(4):519–528.

57. Hirshkowitz M, Moore CA, Karacan I. NPT/Rigidometry. In: Kirby RS, Carson C, Webster GD, eds. Impotence: Diagnosis and Management of Male Erectile Dysfunction. Butterworth-Heinemann, Oxford, 1991, pp. 62–71.

58. Ware JC, Hirshkowitz M. Monitoring penile erections during sleep. In: Kryger MH, Roth T, Dement WC, eds. Principles and Practice of Sleep Medicine. Saunders, Philadelphia, 1994, pp. 967–977.

59. Ware JC, Hirshkowitz M, Thornby J, et al. Sleep-related erections: absence of change following presleep sexual arousal. J Psychosom Res 1997;42:547–553.

60. Karacan I, Williams RL, Thornby JI, et al. Sleep-related penile tumescence as a function of age. Am J Psychiatry 1975;132:932–937.

61. Reynolds CF, Thase ME, Jennings JR, et al. Nocturnal penile tumescence in healthy 20- to 59-year olds: a revisit. Sleep 1989;12:368–73.

62. Ware JC, Hirshkowitz M. Characteristics of penile erections during sleep recorded from normal subjects. J Clin Neurophysiol 1992;9:78–87.
63. Schiavi RC, White D, Mandeli J, et al. Hormones and nocturnal penile tumescence in healthy aging men. Arch Sex Behav 1993;22:207–215.
64. Takahashi Y, Kipnis DM, Daughaday WH. Growth hormone secretion during sleep. J Clin Invest 1968;47:2079.
65. Evans JI, MacLean AW, Ismail AAA, et al. Concentration of plasma testosterone in normal men during sleep. Nature 1971;229:261,262.
66. Judd HL, Parker DC, Rakoff JS, et al. Elucidation of mechanism(s) of the nocturnal rise of testosterone in men. J Clin Endocrinol Metab 1973;38:134.
67. Miyatake A, Morimoto Y, Oishi T, et al. Circadian rhythm of serum testosterone and its relation to sleep: comparison with the variation in serum luteinizing hormone, prolactin, and cortisol in normal men. J Clin Enocrinol 1980;51:1365–1371.
68. Roffwarg HP, Sachar EJ, Halpern F, et al. Plasma testosterone and sleep: relationship to sleep stage variables. Psychosomatic Med 1982;44:73–84.
69. Davidson JM, Camargo CA, Smith ER. Effects of androgen on sexual behavior in hypogonadal men. J Clin Endocrinol and Metab 1979;48:955.
70. Bancroft J, Wu FCW. Changes in erectile responsiveness during androgen replacement therapy. Arch Sex Behav 1983;12(1):59–66.
71. Kwan M, Greenleaf WJ, Mann J, et al. The nature of androgen action on male sexuality: a combined laboratory-self-report study on hypogonadal men. Clin Endocrinol Metab 1983;57(3):557–562.
72. Carani C, Granata J, Bancroft P, et al. The effects of testosterone replacement on nocturnal penile tumescence and rigidity and erectile response to visual erotic stimuli in hypogonadal men. Psychoneuroendocrinol 1995;20(7):743–753.
73. Alexander GM, et al. Androgen-behavior correlations in hypogonadal men and eugonadal men. mood and response to auditory sexual stimuli. Horm Behav 1997;31:110–119.
73a. Cunningham GR, Hirshkowitz M, Korenman SG, et al. Testosterone replacement therapy and sleep-related erections in hypogonadal men. J Clin Endocrinol Metab 1990;70:792–797.
74. Burris AS, Banks SM, Carter CS, et al. A long-term, prospective study of the physiologic and behavioral effects of hormone replacement in untreated hypogonadal men. J Androl 1992;13(4):297–304.
75. Clopper RR, Voorhess ML, MacGillivray MH, et al. Psychosexual behavior in hypopituitary men: a controlled comparison of gonadotropin and testosterone replacement. Psychoneuroendocrinol 1993;18(2):149–161.
76. Bhasin S, Storer TW, Berman N, et al. The effects of suprophysiologic doses of testosterone on muscle size and strength in normal men. N Engl J Med 1996;335:1.
77. Buena F, Swerdloff RS, Steiner BS, et al. Sexual function does not change when serum testosterone levels are pharmacologically varied within the normal male range. Fertil Steril 1993;59:1118–1123.
78. Carani C, Scuteri A, Marrama R, et al. Brief Report - The effects of testosterone administration and visual erotic stimuli on nocturnal penile tumescence in normal men. Hormones Behav 1990;24:435–441.
79. O'Carroll R, Bancroft J. Testosterone therapy for low sexual interest and erectile dysfunction in men: A controlled study. Br J Psychiatry 1984;145:146–151.
80. Schiavi RC, White D, Mandeli J, et al. Effect of testosterone administration on sexual behavior and mood in men with erectile dysfunction. Arch Sex Behav 1997;26(3):231–241.
81. Peterson RE, Imperato-McGinley J, Gautier T, et al. Male pseudohermaphroditism due to steroid 5-alpha-reductase deficiency. Am J Med 1977;62(2):170–191.
82. Imperato-McGinley J, Peterson RE, Gautier T, et al. Androgens and the evolution of male-gender identity among male pseudohermaphrodites with 5α-reductase deficiency. N Engl J Med 1979;300:1233–1237.
83. Bartsch G, Rittmaster RS, Klocker H. Dihydrotestosterone and the concept of 5 alpha-reductase inhibition in human benign prostatic hyperplasia. Eur Urol 2000;37(4):367–380.
84. Gormley GJ, Stoner E, Bruskewitz RC, et al. The effect of finasteride in men with benign prostatic hyperplasia. The Finasteride Study Group. N Engl J Med 1992;327:1185–1191.
85. Cunningham GR, Hirshkowitz M. Inhibition of steroid 5α-reductase with finasteride: sleep-related erections, potency, and libido in healthy men. J Clin Endocrinol Metab 1995;80(6):1934–1940.
86. Bergman B, Damber JE, Littbrand B. Sexual function in prostatic cancer patients treated with radiotherapy, orchiectomy or oestrogens. Br J Urol 1984;56(1):64–69.
87. Carani C, et al. Role of oestrogen in male sexual behaviour: insights from the natural model of aromatase deficiency. Clin Endocrinol 1999;51:517–524.

88. Radlmaier A, Eickenberg HU, Fletcher MS, et al. Estrogen reduction by aromatase inhibition for benign prostatic hyperplasia: results of a double-blind, placebo-controlled, randomized clinical trial using two doses of the aromatase-inhibitor atamestane. Prostate 1996;29:199–208.

89. Bagatell CJ, Heiman JR, Rivier JE, et al. Effects of endogenous testosterone and estradiol on sexual behavior in normal young men. J Clin Endocrinol Metab 1994;7:711–716.

90. Gooren LJ. Human male sexual functions do not require aromatization of testosterone: a study using tamoxifen, testolactone, and dihydrotestosterone. Arch Sex Behav 1985;14(6):539–548.

91. Greenstein A, Plymate SR, Katz PG. Visually stimulated erection in castrated men. J Urol 1995;153:650–652.

92. Hirshkowitz M, Moore, CA, O'Connor S, et al. Androgen and sleep-related erections. J Psychosom Res 1997;42:541–546.

93. Heim N, Hursch CJ. Castration for sex offenders: treatment or punishment? A review and critique of recent European literature. Arch Sex Beh 1979;8(3):281–304.

94. Heim N. Sexual behavior of castrated sex offenders. Arch Sex Behav 1981;10(1):11–19.

95. Bradford JMW, Pawlak A. Double-blind crossover study of cyproterone acetate in the treatment of the paraphilias. Arch Sex Behav 1993;22:383–402.

96. Cooper AJ. A placebo controlled trial of the antiandrogen cyproterone acetate in deviant hypersexuality. Compreh Psychiatr 1981;22:458.

97. Cooper AJ, Sandhu S, Losztyn S, et al. A double-blind placebo controlled trial of medroxyprogesterone acetate and cyproterone acetate with seven pedophiles. Can J Psychiatr 1992;37:687–693.

98. Wincze JP, Bansal S, Malamud M. Effects of medroxyprogesterone on subjective arousal, arousal to erotic stimulation, and nocturnal penile tumescence in male sex offenders. Arch Sex Behav 1986;15:293–305.

99. Cooper AJ, Losztyn S, Russell NC, et al. Medroxyprogesterone acetate, nocturnal penile tumescence, laboratory arousal, and sexual acting out in a male with schizophrenia. Arch Sex Behav 1990;19:361.

100. Van Goozen SH, Cohen-Kettenis PT, Gooren LJ, Frijda NH, Van de Poll, NE. Gender differences in behaviour: activating effects of cross-sex hormones. Psychoneuroendocrinology 1995;20(4):343–363.

101. Tricker R, Casaburi R, Storer TW, et al. The effects of supraphysiological doses of testosterone on angry behavior in healthy eugonadal men—a clinical research center study. J Clin Endocrinol Metab 1996;81(10):3754–3758.

102. Finkelstein JW, Susman EJ, Chinchilli VM, et al. Estrogen or testosterone increases self-reported aggressive behaviors in hypogonadal adolescents. J Clin Endocrinol Metab 1997;82:2433–2438.

103. Sanchez-Martin JR, Fano E, et al. Relating testosterone levels and free play social behavior in male and female preschool children. Psychoneuroendocrinology 2000;25:773–783.

104. Salvadora A, Suay F, Martinez-Sanchis S, et al. Correlating testosterone and fighting in male participants in judo contests. Physiol Behav 1999;68:1–15.

105. Winslow JT, Miczek KA. Androgen dependency of alcohol effects on aggressive behavior: a seasonal rhythm in high-ranking squirrel monkeys. Psycholpharmacology 1988;95:92–98.

106. Sternbach H. Age-associated testosterone decline in men: clinical issues for psychiatry. Am J Psychiatr 1998;155:1310–1318.

107. Seidman SN, Walsh BT. Testosterone and depression in aging men. Am J Geriatr Psychiatr 1999;7(1):18–33.

108. Margolese HC. The male menopause and mood: testosterone decline and depression in the aging male—is there a link? J Geriatr Psychiatr Neurol 2000;13(2):93–101.

109. Anderson RA, Bancroft J, Wu FCW. The effects of exogenous testosterone on sexuality and mood of normal men. J Clin Endocrinol Metab 1992;75:1503–1507.

110. O'Carroll R, Shapiro C, Bancroft J. Androgens, behavior and nocturnal erection in hypogonadal men: The effects of varying the replacement dose. Clin Endocrinol 1985;23:527–538.

111. Wang C, Alexander G, Berman N, et al. Testosterone replacement therapy improves mood in hypogonadal men—a clinical research center study. J Clin Endocrinol Metab 1996;81(10):3578–3583.

112. Cunningham GR, Snyder PJ, Atkinson LE. Testosterone transdermal delivery system. In: Bhasin S, Gabelnick HL, Spieler JM, et al., eds. Pharmacology, Biology, and Clinical Applications of Androgen. Wiley-Liss. New York, 1996, pp. 437–447.

113. Wu FCW, Bancroft J, Davidson DW, et al. The behavioural effects of testosterone undecanoate in adult men with Klinefelter's syndrome: a controlled study. Clin Endocrinol 1982;16:489–497.

114. Nielsen FH, Hunt CD, Mullen LM, et al. Effect of dietary boron on mineral, estrogen, and testosterone metabolism in postmenopausal women. FASEB J 1987;1(5):394–397.

115. Rubin RT, Reinisch JM, Haskett RF. Postnatal gonadal steroid effects on human behavior. Science 1981;211(4488):1318–1324.
116. Vogel W, Klaiber EL, Broverman DM. roles of the gonadal steroid hormones in psychiatric depression in men and women. Prog Neuropsychopharmacology 1978;2:487–503.
117. Ettigi PG, Brown GM. Psychoendocrine correlates in affective disorder. In: Muller EE, Agnoli A, eds. Neuroendocrine Correlates in Neurology and Psychiatry. Elsevier, Amsterdam, 1979, pp. 225–238.
118. Mason JW, Giller EL, Kosten TR. Serum testosterone differences between patients with schizophrenia and those with affective disorder. Biol Psychiatr 1988;23:357–366.
118a. Rubin RT, Poland RE. Pituitary-adrenocortical and pituitary-gonadal function in affective disorder. In: Brown GM, Koslow SH, Reichlin S, eds. Neuroendocrinology and Psychiatric Disorder. Raven Press, New York, 1984, pp. 151–164.
119. Rubin RT, Poland RE, Lesser IM. Neuroendocrine aspects of primary endogenous depression VIII. Pituitary-gonadal axis activity in male patients and matched control subjects. Psychoneuroendocrinology 1989;14(3):217–229.
120. Levitt AJ, Joffe RT. Total and free testosterone in depressed men. Acta Psychiatr Scand 1988;77(3):346–348.et alKjellman BF, Wetterberg L. Hypothalamic-pituitary-gonadal axis in major depressive disorders. Acta Psychiatr Scand 1988;78:138–146.
121. Unden F, Ljungsren JG, Beck-Friis J, et al. Hypothalamic-pituitary-gonadal axis in major depressive disorders. Acta Psychiatr Scand 1988;78:138–146.
122. Davies RH, Harris B, Thomas DR,et al. Salivary testosterone levels and major depressive illness in men. Br J Psychiatry 1992;161:629–632.
123. Yesavage JA, Davidson J, Widrow L, et al. Plasma testosterone levels, depression, sexuality, and age. Biol Psychiatry 1985;20(2):222–225.
124. Barrett-Connor E, Von Muhlen DG, Kritz-Silverstein D. Bioavailable testosterone and depressed mood in older men: the Rancho Bernardo Study. J Clin Endocrinol Metab 1999;84(2):573–577.
124a. Barrett-Connor E, Goodman-Gruen D, Patay B. Endogenous sex hormones and cognitive function in older men. J Clin Endocrinol Metab 1999;84(10):3681–3685.
125. Altschule MD, Tillotson KJ. The use of testosterone in the treatment of depression. N Engl J Med 1948;239:1036–1038.
126. Vogel W, Klaiber EL, Broverman DM. A comparison of the antidepressant effects of a synthetic androgen (mesterolone) and amitriptyline in depressed men. J Clin Psychiatr 1985;46:6–8.
127. Morales AJ, Nolan JJ, Nelson JC, et al. Effects of replacement dose of dehydroepiandrosterone in men and women of advancing age. J Clin Endocrinol Metab 1994;78:1360–1367.
127a. Rabkin JG, Wagner GJ, Rabkin R. Testosterone therapy for human immunodeficiency virus-positive men with and without hypogonadism. J Clin Psychopharmacol 1999;19(1):19–27.
128. Rabkin JG, Wagner GJ, Rabkin R. A double-blind, placebo-controlled trial of testosterone therapy for HIV-positive men with hypogonadal symptoms. Arch Gen Psychiatr 2000;57(2):141–147. Discussion 155,156.
129. Grinspoon S, Corcoran C, Parlman K, et al. Effects of testosterone and progressive resistance training in eugonadal men with AIDS wasting. A randomized, controlled trial. Ann Intern Med 2000;133(5):348–355.
129a. Grinspoon S, Corcoran C, Stanley T, et al. Effects of hypogonadism and testosterone administration on depression indices in HIV-infected men. J Clin Endocrinol Metab 2000;85(1):60–65.
130. Seidman SN, Rabkin JG. Testosterone replacement therapy for hypogonadal men with SSRI-refractory depression. J Affect Disord 1998;48(2-3):157–161.
131. Snow WG, Weinstock J. Sex differences among non-brain damaged adults on the Wechsler Adult Intelligence Scales: a review of the literature. J Clin Exp Neuropsychol 1990;12:873–886.
132. Christiansen K, Knussmann R. Sex hormones and cognitive functioning in men. Neuropsychobiology 1987;18(1):27–36.
133. Hassler M, Gupta D, Wollmann H. Testosterone, estradiol, ACTH and musical, spatial and verbal performance. Int J Neurosci 1992;65(1-4):45–60.
134. Morley JE, Kaiser FE, Perry, HM, et al. Longitudinal changes in testosterone, lutenizing hormone, and follicle-stimulating hormone in healthy older men. Metabolism 1997;46:410–413.
135. Gouchie C, Kimura D. The relationship between testosterone levels and cognitive ability patterns. Psychoneuroendocrinology 1991;16(4):323–334.
136. Shute VJ, Pellegrino JW, Hubert L, et al. The relationship between androgen levels and human spatial abilities. Bull Psychonom Soc 1983;21:465–468.

137. Moffat SD, Hampson E. A curvilinear relationship between testosterone and spatial cognition in humans: possible influence of hand preference. Psychoneuroendocrinology 1996;21:323–337.

138. Rich JB, Brandt J, Lesh K, Dobs AS. The effect of testosterone on cognition in hypogonadal men. 1996 ICE the endocrine society page 734 #OR58-6.

139. Janowsky JS, Oviatt SK, Orwoll ES. Testosterone influences spatial cognition in older men. Behav Neurosci 1994;108(2):325–332.

140. Janowsky JS, Chavez B, Orwoll E. Sex steroids modify working memory. J Cogn Neurosci 2000;12:407–414.

140a. Cherrier MM, Asthana S, Plymate S, et al. Testosterone supplementation improves spatial and verbal memory in healthy older men. Neurology 2001;57:80–88.

141. Luisi M, Franchi F. Double-blind group comparative study of testosterone undecanoate and mesterolone in hypogonadal male patients. J Endocrinol Invest 1980;3:305–308.

142. Skakkebaek NE, Bancroft J, Davidson DW, et al. Androgen replacement with oral testosterone undecanoate in hypogonadal men: a double blind controlled study. Clin Endocrinol 1981;14:49–61.

143. Arver S, Dobs AS, Meikle AW, et al. Improvement of sexual function in testosterone deficient men treated for 1 year with a permeation enhanced testosterone transdermal system. J Urol 1996;155:1604–1608.

144. Dobs AS, et al. Pharmacokinetic characteristics, efficacy and safety of buccal testosterone in hypogonadal males: a pilot study. J Clin Endocrinol Metab 1998;83:33–39.

21

Testosterone and the Older Man

J. Lisa Tenover, MD, PhD

CONTENTS

INTRODUCTION

Why Consider Androgen Therapy in the Older Man?

Although sex hormone replacement therapy (HRT) for postmenopausal women has been a standard practice for many years, the idea that an older man might be sex hormone deficient and might benefit from placement therapy has gained significant medical interest only within the past 10–15 years. The first modern era studies of male HRT were reported about a decade ago (1,2), and there are, as yet, no large multicenter randomized placebo controlled trials of male HRT. In addition, there currently is no agreement on what hormonal or clinical criteria should be used to decide which older men might be considered "androgen deficient" and candidates for HRT. The lack of consensus, however, has not lessened the public and media interest in this topic. Testosterone sales, at least in the United States, continue to increase. At the same time, how to identify [partial]androgen deficiency of the aging male (PADAM), and the utility of androgen supplementation for older men continue to be vigorously investigated. The potential interest in male HRT for PADAM is based on two major factors: There is a decline in serum testosterone levels as men age and there are concomitant changes in androgen target organs that are reminiscent of what is seen in hypogonadal young adult men before they receive testosterone replacement.

From: *Endocrine Replacement Therapy in Clinical Practice*
Edited by: A. Wayne Meikle © Humana Press Inc., Totowa, NJ

TESTOSTERONE LEVELS IN OLDER MEN

As shown by both cross-sectional and longitudinal studies, blood levels of testosterone, but not dihydrotestosterone (DHT), decline with age in most men, even those men who are healthy (3–6). This decline seems to begin about the age of 30 yr (6). Most of these data are from Caucasian men of western European descent, but there is some information that the phenomenon occurs, in some manner, in other ethnic groups (7). The rate of decline of serum testosterone can vary greatly between individuals and also can vary by which component of testosterone is measured. The presence of certain chronic medical conditions, such as diabetes mellitus, cardiovascular disease, sleep apnea, or obesity also can negatively impact testosterone levels (8,9). The chronic use of certain medications such as cimetidine, ketoconazole, glucocorticoids, and narcotics have been reported to lead to a decrease in testosterone. Certainly not all men are destined to become "androgen deficient."

In healthy normal-weight older men who are nonsmokers and on no medications, the mechanism of testosterone decline with age has several components. The largest contributor to the decline is reduced production by the testis, which demonstrates blunted testosterone production even when maximally stimulated with luteinizing hormone (LH). The hypothalamus also plays a role in that there is an increased sensitivity to sex steroid negative feedback with age. The ratio of bioactive to immunoreactive gonadotropins made by the pituitary may also decline somewhat with age, but this is only a minor contributor to the decline in testosterone production. Testosterone metabolism slows with normal male aging, but not enough to offset the decline in production.

Although there is now widespread agreement that testosterone levels decline as men age, defining whether this decline results in an androgen-deficient state in many older men has not been firmly established. One of the impediments to defining androgen deficiency in older men is the lack of a practical, clinically useful biochemical parameter of androgen action. The physiological changes and symptoms that might be attributed to PADAM have complicated pathogenesis and could be affected by a variety of factors, low testosterone being only one of them. In addition, it is as yet unknown which component of serum testosterone is the best marker for assessing androgen availability to the androgen receptor in the various target tissues and at what level the measurement of that marker denotes "deficiency." Serum total testosterone is comprised of three fractions (see Fig.1): free testosterone (testosterone not bound to any blood components), testosterone bound loosely to albumin, and testosterone bound rather tightly to sex hormone-binding globulin (SHBG). The combination of free testosterone and albumin-bound testosterone (the non-SHBG-bound testosterone) is denoted as "bioavailable" testosterone. Epidemiological studies have shown that it is the "bioavailable" portion of testosterone that best correlates with parameters such as bone mineral density and sexual function (10,11), but it is not known if this is the component of testosterone that is bioavailable to every androgen target organ. In addition, not all target-organ effects of testosterone likely are the result of the direct effect of the component itself, but may be the result of one of its metabolites, such as estradiol in bone (12) and DHT in the prostate (13). Unlike the thyroid hormone axis, where altered thyroid-stimulating hormone levels can assist in defining thyroid hormone deficiency, serum gonadotropin levels are not helpful in defining an older man as "androgen deficient." Many older men, even with quite low serum testosterone levels, have serum gonadotropin levels within the normal range.

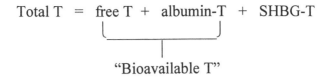

Fig. 1. Components of serum testosterone.

The issue of which component of serum testosterone to use in defining an older man as "androgen deficient" is important for several reasons. One is that the definition will have an ultimate effect on the "prevalence" of PADAM, and the other relates to the cost, availability, and accuracy of the assays used to measure the various components. Because SHBG increases with age, the decline seen in serum non-SBHG-bound testosterone is far greater than that seen with total testosterone. If "androgen deficiency" is defined in older men by a serum total testosterone level below the normal range for young adult men, then about one-quarter of Caucasian men over the age of 65 yr might meet this definition. If non-SHBG-bound testosterone is used, then over 50% of older men may well meet that criterion. The assay for total testosterone is rather straightforward, is widely available, and is the least expensive of the testosterone assays. Analog-free testosterone assays are notoriously inaccurate *(14)*, and "bioavailable" testosterone is difficult to assay, not available except in a few select centers, and the most costly. There is some movement toward using measurements of total testosterone and SHBG, and then calculating "bioavailable" testosterone, but the formulas to use and the value range that defines "testosterone deficiency" have not been definitively determined.

Perhaps there is just not enough information at this time to try to establish one assay measurement that can best define which men are appropriate candidates for HRT. There are no specific androgen target-organ dose-response data for older men and, based on data from young hypogonadal men replaced with testosterone, target organs may vary in their threshold response (e.g., to restore libido may take much lower serum testosterone levels than that needed to restore muscle mass). Given the uncertainties of the testosterone assays vis à vis biological importance of the measured value, along with the insufficient clinical study data to help in defining PADAM, it may be more important at this time to select men for male HRT based on those who have one or more specific androgen target-organ deficiencies and who also have serum testosterone levels that are low enough that meaningful changes in testosterone can be made with physiological replacement therapy.

ANDROGEN TARGET ORGAN CHANGES WITH NORMAL AGING

In young adult males, androgens are known to have many important physiologic actions, including effects on muscle, bone, mood, prostate, bone marrow, cognitive function, and sexual function. Declining lean body mass and strength, loss of stamina, declining bone mineral density, decreased libido and potency, a slight lowering of red blood cell mass, and a decline in a general sense of well-being often are associated with male aging (*see* Table 1).

Both cross-sectional and longitudinal studies have shown that normal male aging is accompanied by an increase in upper and central body fat, a decrease in muscle tissue mass, and a decrease in some aspects of muscle strength *(15,16)*. In healthy older people,

Table 1
Changes in Androgen Target Organs with Normal Aging and with Testosterone (T)
Replacement in Young Hypogonadal Men

Target organ	Changes seen with aging	Changes seen when T given to hypogonadal young
Muscle mass	↓	↑
Muscle strength	↓	↑
Fat mass	↑	↓
Bone mineral density	↓	↑
Libido	↓	↑
Erectile function	↓	↑
Sense of well-being or mood	↔/↓	↑
Cognitive function	↔/↓	↑

Note: ↓, decreased; ↑, increased; ↔, no change.

there is a strong correlation between muscle mass and muscle strength, but the causes of the decline in muscle mass and strength with age are unknown and probably multifactorial. Androgens have long been noted for their anabolic effects, and physiological replacement of testosterone to hypogonadal young men or supraphysiological treatment of eugonadal young adult men can result in increases in lean body mass, muscle size, and strength (17,18).

Osteoporosis is becoming a larger clinical problem as the average life-span of men increases (19). Osteoporosis is a risk factor for hip fracture in the elderly, a major cause of morbidity and mortality. After age 60 yr, hip fracture rates in men increase dramatically, doubling each decade, and by age 80 yr, proximal femur fracture rates in white men approach 1.3% per man-year. In both cross-sectional and longitudinal studies, healthy men have been shown to lose bone mass with age. Typical bone loss rates for vertebral bone in men, aged 30–80 yr, have been 1.2% per year in cross-sectional studies, and just over 2%/ yr in longitudinal studies. Cortical bone is lost less rapidly, with reported rates varying from 0.2 to 1%/yr. Hypogonadism is considered a cause of male osteoporosis, and elderly men who are hypogonadal are at increased risk for minimal trauma hip fracture (20).

Various measures of sexual function seem to change as men age, including a decline in orgasmic frequency, an increase in erectile dysfunction, and a decline in quality and quantity of sexual thoughts and enjoyment (21). Testosterone administration to young hypogonadal men has been shown to increase libido and the frequency of sexual activity (22).

Data to support a relationship between androgen levels and the decline in many aspects of sexual function with age are scarce. Erectile dysfunction (ED) is a common clinical disorder in older men, but only a small percentage of older men with ED have low testosterone levels and the prevalence of low testosterone is not significantly different between older men with and without impotence (23). Testosterone does regulate nitric oxide synthase activity in the smooth muscle of the corpora cavernosa, so it may have some effect on optimal penile rigidity, but the threshold level of testosterone needed for sexual function has not been determined, but may be relatively low. Testosterone administration does not seem to improve ED in men with normal testosterone levels (24).

Androgens improve aspects of mood, such as irritability and depressive affect, when given to young hypogonadal adult men (25). Although supraphysiological doses of androgenic steroids have been associated with aggressive responses, these effects have not been reported with physiologic testosterone replacement. Lower serum bioavailable testosterone levels have been associated with depressed mood in a large cross-sectional study of older men *(26)*.

The relationship between testosterone and cognitive function is not clear because of a lack of data, the many different cognitive processes that can and have been assessed, and the timing of the androgen exposure with regard to age. The effects seem to be domain-specific, with some studies showing a correlation with spatial performance and others reporting improvement in verbal fluency *(27)*. One epidemiological study showed a positive association between total and bioavailable testosterone levels and global cognitive functioning *(28)*.

OVERVIEW OF ANDROGEN-REPLACEMENT TRIALS IN OLDER MEN

When considering testosterone-replacement therapy for older men, it is important to know the various potential benefits, the persons for whom those benefits are most likely to occur, the dose-response profile of the target organ(s) of interest, the potential risks of the therapy, and the relative ratio of risks to benefits. Unfortunately, at this time, these data are limited, and therapeutic decisions by necessity are being made without much of this information. The level of total or bioavailable testosterone used for the entrance criterion into the androgen-replacement studies that have been done have varied significantly. Studies to date also have been in healthy older men, the majority of whom were in the age group of 60 to 75 yr. In addition, these studies have had small study participant numbers, short terms of treatment (most are 12 mo or less), have not always been blinded or placebo controlled, and have utilized various modes of androgen therapy. Nonetheless, by looking at the various study results in terms of target-organ outcomes, it is possible to get an idea as to the relative benefits and risks that might be anticipated, at least in generally healthy men. Definable benefits (and risks) might be present in frail elderly that are not detectable in the healthy younger elderly. Table 2 lists the potential benefits and risks of testosterone replacement therapy in older men.

BENEFICIAL EFFECTS OF TESTOSTERONE THERAPY IN OLDER MEN

BONE

Studies of androgen replacement in older men that have dealt with some aspect of effect on bone have all utilized testosterone as the treatment androgen. These studies have evaluated either biochemical parameters of bone turnover or bone mineral density (BMD). These studies have lasted from 3 to 60 mo, with the shorter studies measuring only turnover parameters. Some, but not all, of the studies enrolled older men who were osteoporotic as baseline. Short-term studies have shown consistent reduction in markers of bone resorption with androgen replacement, but there were inconsistent increases in markers of bone formation *(1,2,29–32)*. There have been at least three peer-reviewed studies *(29,31,32)* and at least five other presented in abstract form that have evaluated the effectiveness of testosterone replacement on BMD. These have generally shown an increase in lumbar spine BMD with therapy, although in at least one study this occurred only in those men with the lowest baseline testosterone. Less than half of the studies that evaluated BMD at other sites showed an increase in BMD at those sites.

Table 2
Potential Benefits and Risks of Testosterone-Replacement Therapy
in Older Men

Benefits
    Maintain or improve bone mineral density and prevent fractures
    Improve body composition
        Increase muscle mass
        Decrease fat mass
    Improve strength and stamina
    Improve or maintain physical function
    Decrease cardiovascular disease risk
    Improve libido
    Improve well-being and mood
    Improve aspects of cognition
Risks
    Develop liver toxicity
    Cause fluid retention
    Develop gynecomastia
    Exacerbate sleep apnea
    Excessively elevate red blood cell mass
    Exacerbate benign or malignant prostate disease
    Increase cardiovascular disease risk

Testosterone is converted to estradiol in vivo, and older men receiving testosterone treatment often show a substantial increase in serum estradiol levels as well. Estradiol or bioavailable estradiol levels have been shown to be better predictors of BMD in older men than testosterone levels in several epidemiological studies. Therefore, it is possible that the effects of testosterone therapy on bone in older men could partly be mediated through its conversion to estradiol. There are, as yet, no data on the effect on fracture rates in older men who are treated with testosterone therapy, and the optimal testosterone dosage to obtain effects on bone is not known.

Body Composition and Strength

There have been a number of published studies in which body composition and muscle strength were evaluated during androgen therapy in older men (1,2,29,32–38). In general, these studies have shown a decline in fat mass and an increase in lean body mass, predominantly muscle mass (see Table 3). The decline in fat mass might be expected to lead to an improvement in insulin sensitivity, as was shown in one study of obese nondiabetic men (33). A recent study, however, reported in abstract form only, did not demonstrate that overtly diabetic men improved their insulin sensitivity with testosterone therapy. When comparing the increase in muscle mass in older men given testosterone-replacement therapy with that seen with physiological replacement in young adult hypogonadal men, the changes are similar in magnitude.

In terms of strength changes with testosterone, the results are inconsistent (see Table 3), and the magnitude of the strength changes in those studies where an effect was shown is not large. More recent studies, as yet unpublished, that have evaluated muscle power rather than isokinetic strength have shown somewhat more robust effects from testoster-

Table 3
Testosterone Replacement Effects on Body Composition
and Strength in Older Men

Months of treatment	No. of men treated	Body fat	Lean mass	Strength[a]
		(trend and mean percent change)		
3	13	↔	↑ (3.2%)	↔ (grip)
3	8	↔	—	↑ (grip)
9	31	↓ (6.4%)	↔	—
1	6	—	—	↑ (LE)
18	29	↓ (14%)	↑ (5%)	—
12	17	↔	—	↑ (grip)
36	54	↓ (14%)	↑ (3.8%)	↔
3	7	—	↔	↔ (LE, grip)
2	9	—	—	↑ (grip)

Note: ↔ = no change; ↑ = increase; ↓ = decrease.
[a]Grip: strength by hand held dynamometry; LE, lower extremity strength, usually by isokinetic testing.

one replacement. For the average older man, the overall clinical relevance of the magnitude of the changes in strength that occur with testosterone therapy alone is uncertain. Only two studies have evaluated the effect of such therapy on some aspect of physical function (36,38) and only one of these showed any effect.

Cardiovascular Disease Risk

In the past, androgens have been categorized as a potential adverse factor with regard to the development of cardiovascular disease (CVD). This has been based primarily on the finding that men are more likely to develop CVD than women of the same age. Over the past decade, however, there has been more evidence to suggest that testosterone may be beneficial in terms of the cardiovascular system (39). Epidemiological studies have reported that men with lower serum testosterone levels have more heart disease. Short-term studies have shown a prolongation of time until ischemia during exercise testing in men with known CVD who are given intravenous testosterone (40), and testosterone infused into coronary arteries seems to have a vasodilatory effect (41). Testosterone has been shown to increase fibrinolysis and lower triglyceride levels. On the other hand, studies of testosterone therapy in young adult men have shown a worsening of the atherogenic lipid profile.

Studies on cardiovascular effects of testosterone therapy in older men have been done by evaluating the response of various CVD risk factors to the treatment, which may not be the most clinically accurate way to assess the true CVD risk and benefits of sex steroids. Nonetheless, until there are large multicenter trials of testosterone replacement in which clinical cardiovascular end points are assessed, these data are all that are available. In terms of changes in cholesterol profiles, the effects of testosterone therapy in older men appear to be generally beneficial. In the studies in which middle-aged or older men were given testosterone, 47% showed a decrease in total cholesterol and low-density lipoprotein (LDL) cholesterol with therapy, whereas the other 53% showed no change in these values. High-density lipoprotein (HDL) cholesterol levels remained unchanged with therapy in most (72%) of the studies, with a small decrease being demonstrated in the other 28% of the trials. Lipoprotein(a) levels decreased with test-osterone therapy in the few studies that have measured this.

Libido and Mood

Studies in older men with low libido have generally reported an improvement in libido and sexual arousal with testosterone therapy *(21,42)*. Several studies have evaluated the effect of testosterone on mood in a blinded placebo-controlled manner and have demonstrated a positive impact *(1,33)*.

Cognitive Function

There have been only a few small clinical trials of testosterone therapy and the effects on cognitive function in older "androgen-deficient" men. One study showed no effects on tested memory *(35)*; another did report a small effect on visual spatial memory *(27)*. Several other studies, as yet presented in only abstract form, have reported improvement in spatial and verbal memory or trail-making ability with testosterone therapy. Inconsistency of findings cannot be interpreted as evidence that there is no effect of testosterone replacement on aspects of cognition in older men. On the other hand, positive effects of testosterone therapy on cognition in older men, even if they do occur, may be rather subtle and, therefore, of questionable clinical and functional relevance.

Risks of Testosterone Therapy in Older Men

In Table 2 are listed the most significant of the potential risks of testosterone therapy in the older man. Liver toxicity is on the list because of the potential of the oral methylated agents to cause hepatomas and liver dysfunction, especially at the doses needed for male replacement therapy. The methylated testosterones are not recommended as a form of testosterone replacement for men, however, and none of the actual studies involving testosterone therapy in older men have used these agents. No problems with liver enzyme abnormalities or other evidence of liver toxicity have been reported with testosterone therapy in older men.

FLUID RETENTION AND GYNECOMASTIA

Fluid retention is possible with androgen replacement, especially within the first few months of therapy. For most men, however, the small amount of fluid retention is not harmful, and no cases of exacerbation of congestive heart failure, development of peripheral edema, or worsening of hypertension have been reported in the trials of replacement therapy in older men. Tender breasts or gynecomastia do occur in a small number of older men on testosterone therapy. Because many older men given testosterone demonstrate a relatively greater percentage increase in serum estradiol levels when compared to serum testosterone levels, this may contribute to the breast changes. Often this adverse effect can be overcome with a downward adjustment in testosterone dose.

SLEEP APNEA

Testosterone appears to play a role in the pathogenesis of obstructive sleep apnea. Testosterone therapy may worsen sleep apnea in some hypogonadal men *(43)* and treatment of sleep apnea may reverse low serum testosterone levels *(9)*. The incidence of testosterone-induced sleep apnea is unknown. A recent study, evaluating 54 older men on testosterone for 3 yr, showed no increase in apneic or hypoapenic episodes during sleep while on therapy *(31)*.

Table 4
Reported Increases in Hemoglobin and/or Hematocrit
Levels with Testosterone Therapy in Older Men

Testosterone patch (scrotal or transdermal)	1–3%
Injectable testosterone enanthate	
50 mg/wk	No change
100 mg/wk	5–12%
200 mg/2 wk	7–17%
300 mg/3 wk	up to 20%

POLYCYTHEMIA

Androgens are known to stimulate red blood stem cells and the production of erythropoietin. Most studies of testosterone replacement in older men have shown a significant increase in red blood cell mass, hemoglobin levels, and hematocrit with therapy. The increases reported are much larger than those usually seen when hypogonadal young adult men are given testosterone replacement. In some cases, it has been necessary with the older men to either terminate therapy or decrease the dose of testosterone given because of the development of frank polycythemia. The exact hematocrit value to warrant discontinuation of testosterone therapy is not known, but hematocrit levels above 54% are associated with increased risk of stroke. Although the coexistence of sleep apnea and elevated body mass index may contribute to the development of polycythemia, this has not been true for many men studied (44). The method of testosterone replacement may affect the magnitude of the change in red blood cell mass, with those methods that provide a more uniform level of testosterone within the physiological range throughout the dosing period demonstrating a smaller increase in red cell mass (see Table 4).

PROSTATE

Androgens are involved in the growth of both benign prostate nodules (BPH) and prostate carcinoma, although whether they play a major role in the initiation of either disease is unclear. Epidemiological studies have not demonstrated consistently that circulating levels of androgens are implicated in the etiology of prostate cancer, although a recent meta-analysis did show a two- to threefold increase in prostate cancer in men with the highest quartile of serum testosterone (45).

Androgen deprivation to castrate levels can cause regression of both of these prostate diseases, but whether increasing testosterone levels from subnormal levels to normal young adult male physiological levels will increase the risk of developing clinically significant disease in men without established prostate cancer or with little to no symptoms of urinary outlet obstruction is a different question. The dose-response range for circulating androgens and the prostate is not known.

There have been at least 32 testosterone-replacement studies in men aged 40–89 yr in which serum levels of prostate-specific antigen (PSA), prostate size, functional urinary parameters such as urine flow rates or urinary bladder residual volumes, or lower urinary tract symptoms have been assessed. Of the 12 testosterone-replacement studies in older men that evaluated parameters of prostate size, prostate function, or lower urinary tract symptoms, none of the studies noted any change in these measures with testosterone therapy. Selection criteria for these studies, however, included exclusion on the basis of significant baseline symptoms of BPH. All 32 of the testosterone trials evaluated PSA; 22 of these studies reported absolutely no change in PSA with testosterone treatment, whereas the other 10 studies reported small, but statistically significant, changes in PSA with therapy. The average change in PSA for the men on testosterone in those 10 studies was 0.61 ng/mL. In 7 of the 10 studies, men were followed for at least 1 yr, and therefore, a PSA velocity can be calculated. The average PSA velocity for those men on testosterone was 0.39 ng/mL/yr, well within the normal range of yearly change due to benign disease (< 0.75 ng/mL/yr). There has been no reported increase in the incidence of prostate cancer in older men on testosterone therapy, but the number of men studied is not large. If PSA production is viewed as a general measure of prostate "activity," the results of the testosterone replacement trials to date suggest that, at least over the period of 3–5 yr, testosterone therapy does not appear to appreciably stimulate most older men's prostates. However, because both prostate cancer and BPH are diseases with long natural histories and the experience thus far with testosterone in older men is limited to just over 1440 man-years of experience, the long-term effects of testosterone therapy on the prostate are still an unknown.

HOW TO DECIDE IF AN OLDER MAN IS A CANDIDATE FOR TESTOSTERONE THERAPY

Given the relative lack of clinical data on testosterone replacement in older men, along with the popularizing of "testosterone" as a potential modality to prevent or reverse the aging process in men, it is likely that men will come to a physician seeking replacement therapy rather than the physician suggesting that "testosterone deficiency" may be a problem. Sometimes men present to the physician with concerns about testosterone deficiency because their wives or significant others have urged them to do so. On the other hand, evaluating for testosterone deficiency should be considered by the physician for those older men who present with certain symptoms or symptom complexes.

Among the symptoms that lead older men to seek evaluation for androgen therapy, or which might suggest to a physician to screen for testosterone deficiency, are decreased libido (with or without erectile dysfunction), lack of energy, decreased "enjoyment in life" or sense of well-being, increased irritability, low dominance (e.g., not liking to direct other people's work), loss of stamina or endurance, persistent sleeplessness, or vasomotor symptoms (see Table 5). Many of these symptoms are vague and could be the results of a number of medical or psychiatric problems. This requires an astute clinician to rule out other possible causes prior to consideration of testosterone-replacement therapy. Other symptoms or findings that may guide a physician to evaluate an older man's androgen status include evidence of other pituitary deficiency, osteopenia, gynecomastia, bilateral small testes, significant obesity, the presence of certain illness such as diabetes mellitus, asthma, or renal insufficiency, and the use of certain medications (see Table 5). There are at least two validated screening questionnaires for testosterone deficiency in older men that have been published (46,47).

In terms of the medical and psychiatric history, it is important to gather information in those areas where androgen replacement may present a potential risk to the patient. A patient history of prostate or breast cancer are the only two absolute contraindications to androgen therapy at this time, but sleep apnea, clinically significant symptoms of BPH, significant cardiovascular disease history, history of elevated hemoglobin levels,

Table 5
Symptoms, Signs, or Conditions That Might Suggest
Evaluation for Testosterone Deficiency in Older Men

Decreased libido (with or without erectile dysfunction)
Lack of energy
Loss of stamina or endurance
Increased irritability
Decreased enjoyment of life or sense of well-being
Low dominance
Persistent sleeplessness
Vasomotor symptoms
Bilateral small testes
Breast enlargement
Significant obesity
Osteoporosis
Other evidence of pituitary hypofunction
Chronic illness
    Diabetes mellitus
    Asthma
    Chronic renal insufficiency
    Liver disease
Chronic use of certain medications
    Ketoconazole
    Glucocorticoids
    Cimetidine
    Opiates

and a family history of prostate cancer should all be considered in the balancing of the possible risks and benefits of therapy.

In addition to a good medical and psychiatric history, a physical examination is an important part of the evaluation of the older man for whom androgen therapy is being considered. This examination is not so much to collaborate findings suggestive of low testosterone but to assess the man for the potential for side effects involved with the therapy. In fact, except for the occasional finding of bilateral small testicles, it is often difficult to ascertain any other clinical findings that reliably predict which older men will have a low serum testosterone level. Particular areas of interest in regard to potential androgen therapy risk include the cardiac/lung exam and the digital rectal examination of the prostate.

With regard to the laboratory evaluation needed in assessing a man for possible androgen therapy, the minimum data obtained should begin with a morning (7–10 AM) serum total testosterone (or alternatively a measured or calculated bioavailable testosterone) level. If the total testosterone level is less than 200 ng/dL (6.9 nmol/L), then the testosterone level need not be repeated (i.e., this level is low enough to warrant treatment). However, if the total testosterone level is between 200 and 400 ng/dL, it should be repeated to ascertain if the value remains in the below normal to low normal range. Alternatively, two measurements of testosterone can be done on the first morning evaluation, but they should be drawn at least 30 min apart. As mentioned previously, there is currently no agreement on the level of total testosterone or bioavailable testosterone that defines an older man as testosterone deficient. The range of suggested values to be used for defining androgen deficiency of the older man vary from <250 ng/dL to <400 ng/dL for total testosterone and from <70 ng/dL to <130 ng/dL for bioavailable testosterone.

Once it is determined that two serum testosterone levels are in the "androgen-deficiency" range, further endocrinological evaluation depends on the history, examination, and the magnitude of the testosterone deficiency. If the serum total testosterone level is <150 ng/dL, then the man should be evaluated for an etiology of the low testosterone other than primary testicular insufficiency. In this case, serum LH and FSH, prolactin, and serum thyroid-stimulating hormone (TSH) should be measured, along with visual field testing and other evaluation for a pituitary tumor. If the total testosterone is over 150 ng/dL, LH and FSH levels usually do not assist in clinical decision making and need not be done. A serum estradiol level could be measured if the man is obese or has significant gynecomastia. Because thyroid disease can affect testicular function and thyroid dysfunction is common in the aging population, measurement of a serum TSH is suggested unless it has been measured within the previous year. In terms of laboratory screening for parameters related to the potential risk of testosterone therapy, it is recommended that hemoglobin/hematocrit and PSA levels be measured.

Further screening that might be considered prior to initiation of therapy would depend on the findings from the history, physical examination, and laboratory studies. Among these additional studies might be sleep studies to evaluate for sleep apnea or a transrectal ultrasound of the prostate (with biopsy) to evaluate an elevated PSA or abnormal digital rectal examination of the prostate.

TESTOSTERONE TREATMENT IN OLDER MEN

The decision to actually place an older man on a trial of testosterone replacement is based on the following:

1. Identifying one or more androgen target-organ symptoms or findings that are present and can be monitored for efficacy of replacement.
2. Having evaluated for minimal short-term risk those areas of potential concern regarding androgen therapy (i.e., ruling out sleep apnea, significant prostate disease, and so forth).
3. Finding that the patient has a serum total or bioavailable testosterone level that is low enough that physiological replacement will make a significant change in serum levels.

Although the androgen dose-response of the various target organs are not known, it has been shown that replacement of endogenous testosterone with equivalent levels of exogenous testosterone has no measurable effect. Therefore, it should be the treatment goal to have some significant increase in testosterone over that at pretreatment. Exactly what that increase should be is yet undetermined, but aiming for about twice pretreatment values seems reasonable. Therefore, if the normal range for serum total testosterone for a young adult male is 350–1100 ng/dL, an older man with two serum testosterone levels below 400 ng/dL could have his serum average testosterone level doubled with replacement therapy and still be well within the normal adult male physiologic range. If his serum testosterone levels were 550 ng/dL, it would be difficult to change serum levels appreciably and still remain in the physiologic range.

Therapeutic Modalities

As with other hormone replacement therapy, choosing the method of testosterone replacement in older men involves consideration of a number of factors. These include the following:

1. Sex steroid serum levels to be obtained
2. Efficacy in management of symptoms for which the therapy is being given
3. Ease and accessibility of the therapy
4. Therapy acceptability
5. Side effects of the particular forms of replacement
6. Cost, both in time and money

Table 6 lists the major delivery forms for androgen therapy currently commercially available in the United States considered generally safe for use in older men. (The oral methylated testosterones are not considered in this category because of their potential for liver toxicity.) Also listed are the recommended initial dose range for older men, the average time to peak serum testosterone value, the recommended time to draw a testosterone level for therapeutic monitoring, and the relative cost of each modality. There are other forms of androgen-replacement therapy that are available outside of the United States, including the following: DHT topical gel; Sustenon, a mixture of testosterone esters for injection; and the oral testosterone undecanoate.

All forms of testosterone listed are probably efficacious if adequate serum testosterone levels are achieved. Selecting the form of therapy largely depends on patient preference with regard to acceptability, dosing regimen, and cost, as well as possible side effects unique to the testosterone delivery form (*see* Table 7).

The two most commonly used injectable esters are the enanthate and the cypionate because they can be given every 1–2 wk. The propionate form needs to be administered about three times per week because of its shorter half-life and, therefore, is generally not recommended for replacement therapy. If the man can learn to give the intramuscular testosterone injections himself (usually given in the thigh) or the injection can be administered by a family member (usually in the buttocks), the cost of this therapy is extremely reasonable. Although most men complain of no or little pain from the testosterone injections, some men do not accept the idea of injections readily. In addition, the serum levels of testosterone obtained are far from physiologic. Especially with the every 2-wk dosing regimens of the enanthate or cypionate esters, serum testosterone levels may be supraphysiologic within the first few days after injection and fall to levels below the normal physiologic range just prior to the next dose. This tends to lead to a larger increase in hemoglobin and estradiol levels than the weekly dosing regimens and is why, if possible, the weekly dosing regimen is the preferred one for older men. Every-3-wk dosing is not recommended for use in most older men. Because testosterone metabolism slows with aging, the recommended initial doses of testosterone for older men are lower than those usually used in younger adults; 75 mg/wk or 150 mg/2 wks of the longer-acting testosterone esters are reasonable starting doses.

The pellet form of testosterone requires a skin incision and a trocar to implant. Local extrusion of the pellets and infection at the site of the pellet are possible problems. Also, because the pellets are active for up to 6 mo, they may give unpredictable serum levels of testosterone, and require pellet removal may be required if dosage adjustment is necessary or adverse events occur. Generally, they are not recommended for use in most older men.

Table 6
Testosterone Delivery Forms Available in the United States for Replacement Therapy
in Older Men—Recommended Dosing, Pharmacokinetics, and Relative Cost

Preparation	Recommended initial regimen	Time to peak (T)	Testosterone monitoring	Relative cost
Injectable esters				
Testosterone enanthate ($100–200$ mg/cm^3; 10 cm^3)	150 mg/2 wk or 75 mg/wk	2–3 d	1 wk	
Generic				$\$^a$
Delatestryl				$\$+^a$
Testosterone cypionate ($100–200$ mg/cm^3; 10 cm^3)	150 mg/2 wk or 75 mg/wk	2–3 d	1 wk	
Generic				$\$^a$
Depo-testosterone				$\$^a$
Virilon				$\$^a$
Testosterone propionate (100 mg/cm^3; 10 cm^3)	15 mg 3X/wk	1 d	d 2	
Generic				$\$+^a$
Testosterone pellets	225 mg/4–6 mo	1 mo	3–4 mo	$\$\$^b$
Patches				
Scrotal				
Testoderm (40 cm^2; 60 cm^2)	40 cm^2; 1 patch/d	3–5 h	12 h	$\$\$+$
Nonscrotal				
Androderm TTS (2.5 mg or 5 mg)	5 mg total/d	6–10 h	12 h	$\$\$\$$
Gel				
Androgel (1%) (2.5 g, 5 g packet)	5 g packet/d	Constant	2–4 wk	$\$\$\$\$$

[a]Relative cost for medication and injection supplies; cost increases if clinic visit needed for each injection.
[b]Relative cost includes cost of implant placement and removal. Requires clinic visit to implant.

The patch forms of testosterone replacement provide physiologic levels of serum testosterone throughout most of the 24-h dosing period and allow for rapid discontinuation of therapy if necessary. The scrotal patch, but not the nonscrotal patch, yields supraphysiologic levels of serum DHT, owing to high 5α-reductase levels in scrotal skin. Whether increased serum DHT levels have deleterious effects in older men has not been proven. It has been suggested that the patches be applied in the evening, so that the serum levels of testosterone more closely mimic testosterone's natural circadian rhythm in blood. However, the clinical importance of mimicking this circadian rhythm has never been demonstrated. The limitations of the various patch forms of delivery include the following:

1. The maximum serum testosterone levels obtainable tend to be in the low normal range and, especially with the scrotal patch, depend heavily on patient compliance with skin preparation (shaving the scrotum) and application instructions. Constancy of adhesion may be variable, even if the patches are applied appropriately.

Table 7
Testosterone Replacement Methods and Some Safety Parameters

Preparation	Estradiol	Hemoglobin	Skin irritation	Other
Injectable esters				
T enanthate or cypionate				
Dose q wk	↑	↑	None	Pain at injection site
Dose q 2 wk	↑↑	↑↑	None	Mood swings
Pellets	↑ or↑↑	↑ or ↑↑	None	Local site infection; extravasation of pellet
Scrotal patch	↔	↔ or ↑	Minimal	Have to shave scrotum; adhesion problems
Nonscrotal patch	↔	↔ or ↑	Minimal to significant	Some adhesion problems
Gel	↑	↔ or ↑	Minimal	Transfer to partner

Note: ↑: Mild increase; ↑↑: moderate to major increase.

2. For cosmetic reasons, some men do not accept the idea of wearing a patch on their scrotum or on their skin.
3. The incidence of skin reactions to the patches is greater in older men than it is in younger men and occurs more frequently with the first-generation nonscrotal patch (Androderm) than with the scrotal patch. Coapplication of 0.1% triamcinolone cream may lessen or negate the skin reaction.
4. There is little flexibility in dosing regimens. Patches should not be cut into smaller units, therefore necessitating only whole-patch dosage adjustments.

The gel form of testosterone is a hydro-alcoholic preparation that provides about 24 h of mid-range physiologic levels of serum testosterone, usually without supraphysiologic levels of DHT. The application of the gel requires a moderate amount of skin area, but the gel is colorless and the exact surface area utilized in application has only a small influence on serum testosterone levels achieved. It is recommended that a man avoid bathing, swimming, or intimate contact during the first several hours after application so as to avoid removal of the testosterone from the skin. After 1–2 h, however, the gel has entered the subcutaneous tissue and transference or loss is no longer a significant issue. Skin reactions to the gel have not proven to be a major problem to date. The gel comes in two different dose packets and application of less than a full packet is possible; this allows for some dosing flexibility. At this time, the major drawback to the gel form of therapy is its cost.

In selecting the method of testosterone replacement to be used, it also may be necessary to consider the potential effect on estradiol or hemoglobin levels. The injectable esters and the subcutaneous pellets tend to result in greater increases in these two measures than do the patch and gel forms of therapy. If the man has a high normal or above normal hemoglobin level at baseline or if he is a heavy smoker or obese, then the preferred method of replacement is other than the injectable esters. Although mood or libido have been reported to fluctuate in parallel with the fluctuations in serum testosterone levels that occur with the injectable esters when used in young adult men, this does not seem to occur very frequently in older men.

Monitoring Treatment and Length of Treatment

Currently, much of the testosterone-replacement therapy in older men is done on a trial basis; that is, the therapy is rendered for a certain period of time, and the efficacy and safety of the therapy is assessed. In general, it is recommended that, in absence of obvious adverse effects, therapy should be continued for at least 6 mo to 1 yr; it often takes that long for the well-known "placebo effect" of sex steroid therapy to dissipate. If after 6–12 mo the treatment is felt to have been beneficial and no significant adverse effects have arisen, then therapy should be continued, but reassessed at least on a yearly basis.

In monitoring for adverse effects, the patient should be seen within the first 3 mo after initiation of therapy. At that point, it would be important to evaluate for weight gain, peripheral edema, gynecomastia or breast tenderness, symptoms of BPH, problems with sleep, and bothersome changes in libido; a digital rectal examination of the prostate also should be done. In addition, it would be important to evaluate the hemoglobin/hematocrit and the PSA levels, as well as the serum testosterone level. If possible, it is best to evaluate serum testosterone levels obtained from the treatment regimen at a time when serum levels should be in the mid-range for that dosing regimen (see Table 6). Unless problems are noted or the testosterone dosing needs readjustment, the next follow-up evaluation should be in another 3–6 mo and then annually. Any persistent increase in PSA by more than 0.75 ng/mL on two consecutive monitoring sessions, a PSA level abnormal for age, or an abnormal prostate on examination should trigger a referral of the patient to a urologist and, in most cases, a prostate biopsy. Any increase in hematocrit to or above 54% warrants temporary discontinuation of therapy or phlebotomy, along with a change in method of testosterone therapy, the dose of testosterone, or both.

CONCLUSION

As with all hormone replacement therapy, the benefits and risks of testosterone therapy for each man need to be continually reassessed. This is especially true for testosterone replacement in the older man, where there is still a need for clinical efficacy and risk data, including long-term evaluations of the effects on the development of bone fractures, cardiovascular disease, BPH, and prostate cancer.

REFERENCES

1. Tenover JS. Effects of testosterone supplementation in the aging male. J Clin Endocrinol Metab 1992;75:1092–1098.
2. Morley JE, Perry HM, Kaiser FE, et al. Effects of testosterone replacement therapy in hypogonadal males: a preliminary study. J Am Geriatr Soc, 1993;41:149–152.
3. Vermeulen A. Clinical Review 24: Androgens in the aging male. J Clin Endocrinol Metab 1991;73:221–224.
4. Gary A, Berlin JA, McKinlay J, et al. An examination of research design effects on the association of testosterone and male ageing: results of a meta-analysis. J Clin Epidemiol 1994;44:671–684.
5. Morley JE, Kaiser FE, Perry HM. Et al. Longitudinal changes in testosterone, luteinizing hormone, and follicle-stimulating hormone in healthy older men. Metabolism 1997;46:410–413.
6. Harman SM, Metter EJ, Tobin JD, et al. Longitudinal effects of aging on serum total and free testosterone in healthy men. J Clin Endocrinol Metab 2001;86:724–731.
7. Perry HM, Miller DK, Patrick P, Morley JE. Testosterone and leptin in older African-American men: relationship to age, strength, function, and season. Metabolism 2000;49:1085–1091.
8. Gray A. Feldman HA, McKinlay JB, Longcope C. Age, disease, and changing sex hormone levels in middle-aged men: results of the Massachusetts male aging study. J Clin Endocrinol Metab 1991;73:1016–1025.

9. Santamaria JD, Prior JC, Fleetham JA. Reversible reproductive dysfunction in men with obstructive sleep apnea. Clin Endocrinol, 1988;28:461–470.

10. van den Beld AW, deJong FH, Grobbee DE, et al. Measures of bio-available serum testosterone and estradiol and their relationship with muscle strength, bone density, and body composition in elderly men. J Clin Endocrinol Metab 2000;85:3276–3282.

11. Nilsson P, Moller L, Solkad K. Adverse effects of psychosocial stress on gonadal function and insulin levels in middle aged males. J Intern Med 1995;237:479–486.

12. Khosla S, Melton LJ, Atkinson EJ, et al. Relationship of serum sex steroid levels and bone turnover markers with bone mineral density in men: a key role for bio-available estrogen. J Clin Endocrinol Metab 1998;83:2266–2275.

13. Geller J, Albert J, Lopez D, et al. Comparison of androgen metabolites in benign prostatic hypertrophy (BPH) and normal prostate. J Clin Endocrinol Metab 1976;43:686–690.

14. Vermeulen A, Verdonck L, Kaufman JM. A critical evaluation of simple methods for the estimation of free testosterone in serum. J Clin Endocrinol Metab 1999;84:3666–3672.

15. Forbes GB, Reina JC. Adult lean body mass declines with age: some longitudinal observations. Metabolism, 1970;19:653–663.

16. Larsson LG, Grimby G, Karlsson J. Muscle strength and speed of movement in relation to age and muscle morphology. J Appl Physiol 1979;46:451–456.

17. Bhasin S, Storer TW, Berman N, et al. Testosterone replacement increases fat-free mass and muscle size in hypogonadal men. J Clin Endocrinol Metab 1997;82:407–413.

18. Bhasin S, Storer TW, Berman N, et al. The effects of supraphysiologic doses of testosterone on muscle size and strength in normal men. N Engl J Med 1996;335:1–7.

19. Orwoll ES, Klein RF. Osteoporosis in men. Endocr Rev 1995;16:87–116.

20. Stanley HL, Schmitt BP, Poses RM, Deiss WP. Does hypogonadism contribute to the occurrence of minimal trauma hip fracture in elderly men? J Am Geriatr Soc 1991;39:766–771.

21. Schiavi RC. Androgens and sexual function in men. In: Oddens BJ, Vermeulen A, eds. Androgens and the Aging Male. New York: Parthenon Press,1996:111–128.

22. Kwan M, Greenleaf WJ, Mann J, et al. The nature of androgen action on male sexuality: a combined laboratory-self-report study on hypogonadal men. J Clin Endocrinol Meab 1983;57:557–562.

23. Korenman SG, Morley JE, Mooradian AD, et al. Secondary hypogonadism in older men: its relation to impotence. J Clin Endocrinol Metab 1990;71:963–969.

24. Carani C, Zini D, Baldini A, et al. Effects of androgen treatment in impotent men with normal and low levels of free testosterone. Arch Sex Behav 1990;19:223–234.

25. Wang C, Alexander G, Berman N, et al. Testosterone replacement therapy improves mood in hypogonadal men—a clinical research center study. J Clin Endocrinol Metab, 1996;81:3578–3583.

26. Barrett-Connor E, Von Muhlen DG, Kritz-Silverstein D. Bioavailable testosterone and depressed mood in older men: the Rancho Bernardo Study. J Clin Endocrinol Metab 1999;84:573–577.

27. Janowsky JS, Oviatt SK, Orwoll ES. Testosterone influences spatial cognition in older men. Behav Neurosci 1994;108:325–332.

28. Barrett-Connor E, Goodman-Gruen D, Patay B. Endogenous sex hormones and cognitive function in older men. J Clin Endocrinol Metab 1999;84:3681–3685.

29. Katznelson L, Finkelstein JS, Schoenfeld DA, et al. Increase in bone density and lean body mass during testosterone administration in men with acquired hypogonadism. J Clin Endocrinol Metab 1996;81: 4358–4365.

30. Jackson JA, Kleerekoper M, Parfitt AM, et al. Bone histomorphometry in hypogonadal and eugonadal men with spinal osteoporosis, J Clin Endocrinol Metab 1987;65:53–58.

31. Snyder PJ, Peachey H, Hannoush P, et al. Effect of testosterone treatment on bone mineral density in men over 65 years of age. J Clin Endocrinol Metab 1999;84:1966–1972.

32. Kenny AM, Prestwood KM, Gruman CA, et al. Effects of transdermal testosterone on bone and muscle in older men with low bioavailable testosterone levels. J Gerontol Med Sci 2001;56A:M266–272.

33. Marin P, Holmang S, Gustafsson C, et al. Androgen treatment of abdominally obese men. Obesity Res 1993;1:245–251.

34. Urban RJ, Bodenburg YH, Gilkison C, et al. Testosterone administration to elderly men increases skeletal muscle strength and protein synthesis. Am J Physiol 1995;269:E820–826.

35. Sih R, Morley JE, Kaiser FE, et al. Testosterone replacement in older hypogonadal men: a 12-month randomized controlled trial. J Clin Endocrinol Metab 1997;82:1661–1667.

36. Snyder PJ, Peachey H, Hannoush P, et al. Effect of testosterone treatment on body composition and muscle strength in men over 65 years of age. J Clin Endocrinol Metab 1999;84:2647–2653.

37. Clague JE, Wu FCW, Horan MA. Difficulties in measuring the effect of testosterone replacement therapy on muscle function in older men. Int J Andrology 1999;22:261–265.
38. Bakhshi V, Elliott M, Gentili A, Godschalk M, Mulligan T. Testosterone improves rehabilitation outcomes in ill older men. J Am Geriatr Soc 2000;48:550–553.
39. Crook D. Androgens and the risk of cardiovascular disease. Aging Male 2000;3:190–195.
40. Webb CM, Adamson DL, deZeigler D, Collins P. Effect of acute testosterone on myocardial ischemia in men with coronary artery disease. Am J Cardiol 1999;83:437–439.
41. Webb CM, McNeill JG, Hayward CS, et al. Effects of testosterone on coronary vasomotor regulation in men with coronary heart disease. Circulation 1999;100:1690–1696.
42. Hajjar RR, Kaiser RE, Morley JE. Outcomes of long-term testosterone replacement in older hypogonadal males: a retrospective analysis. J Clin Endocrinol Metab 1997;82:3793–3796.
43. Matsumoto AM, Sandblom RE, Schoene RB, et al. Testosterone replacement in hypogonadal men: effects on obstructive sleep apnoea, respiratory drives, and sleep. Clin Endocrinol 1985;22:713–721.
44. Drinka PJ, Jochen AL, Cuisinier M, et al. Polycythemia as a complication of testosterone replacement therapy in nursing home men with low testosterone levels. J Am Geriatr Soc 1995;43:899–901.
45. Shaneyfelt T, Husein R, Bubley G, et al. Hormonal predictors of prostate cancer: a meta-analysis. J Clin Oncol 2000;18:847–853.
46. Smith KW, Feldman HA, McKinlay JB. Construction and field validation of a self-administered screener for testosterone deficiency (hypogonadism) in ageing men. Clin Endocrinol (Osf) 2000;53:703–711.
47. Morley JE. Testosterone replacement and the physiologic aspects of aging in men. Mayo Clin Proc 2000;75:583–587.

22 Androgen Administration in Sarcopenia Associated with Chronic Illness

Shalender Bhasin, MD, Atam B. Singh, MD, Keith Beck, MD, and Linda Woodhouse, MS

CONTENTS

INTRODUCTION

The anabolic applications of testosterone in sarcopenia associated with human immunodeficiency virus (HIV)-infection and other chronic illnesses are based on a series of assumptions that are illustrated in Fig. 1. The premise is that these agents increase muscle mass and that androgen-induced changes in muscle mass translate into improvements in skeletal muscle performance, physical function, and other health-related outcomes. Although there is agreement that testosterone supplementation increases muscle mass in a variety of settings (*1–14*), but we do not know whether testosterone improves muscle performance or physical function. The mechanisms by which testosterone increases muscle mass are unknown.

From: *Endocrine Replacement Therapy in Clinical Practice*
Edited by: A. Wayne Meikle © Humana Press Inc., Totowa, NJ

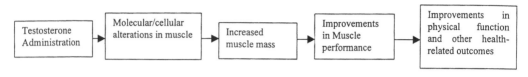

Fig. 1.

There has been a surge of interest in anabolic therapies because of realization that in many chronic illnesses such as that associated with the human immunodeficiency virus, end stage-renal disease, chronic obstructive lung disease, and some types of cancer, we can now achieve disease stability but not cure. In these chronic disorders, muscle wasting occurs frequently and is associated with debility, impaired quality of life, and poor disease outcome *(16–23)*. Therefore, strategies that can reverse muscle wasting and augment muscle function may improve quality of life and reduce utilization of health care resources. Additionally, the human immunodeficiency virus, like many other chronic diseases, produces a heterogeneous, complex, and multisystem syndrome; therefore, anabolic therapy should be viewed as only one component of a multipronged therapeutic strategy.

There is a high frequency of low testosterone levels in chronic illnesses associated with wasting. Low testosterone levels in chronic illnesses are associated with poor disease outcomes and impaired muscle function. Testosterone replacement of healthy, hypogonadal men produces increases in fat-free mass and muscle strength. Emerging data indicate that androgen replacement in chronic illnesses associated with low testosterone levels is also associated with improvements in muscle mass and maximal voluntary strength similar to those observed in healthy, hypogonadal men. The molecular mechanisms of androgen action in the muscle are poorly understood.

HIGH FREQUENCY OF LOW TESTOSTERONE LEVELS IN CHRONIC ILLNESSES

Although the prevalence of androgen deficiency defined solely in terms of low testosterone levels has decreased with the advent of potent antiretroviral therapy, androgen deficiency continues to be a common complication of HIV infection in men. In an earlier survey of 150 HIV-infected men who attended our HIV Clinic in 1997, approximately, a third had serum total and free testosterone levels in the hypogonadal range *(24)*. Other investigators have reported similar prevalence of hypogonadism in HIV-infected men in the pre-HAART era *(19,25–32)*. A more recent survey of HIV-infected drug users found the prevalence of low testosterone levels to be 20% *(33)*. Thus, androgen deficiency continues to be a common occurrence in HIV-infected men.

In our survey, 20% of HIV-infected men with low testosterone levels had elevated luteinizing hormone (LH) and follicle-stimulating hormone (FSH) levels and thus had hypergonadotropic hypogonadism *(24)*. These patients presumably had primary testicular dysfunction. The remaining 80% had either normal or low LH and FSH levels; these men with hypogonadotropic hypogonadism either have a central defect at the hypothalamic or pituitary site or a dual defect involving both the testis and the hypothalamic–pituitary centers. The pathophysiology of hypogonadism in HIV infection is complex and involves defects at multiple levels of the hypothalamic–pituitary testicular axis.

In a recent study, a majority of men with chronic obstructive lung disease had low total and free testosterone levels *(34)*. Similarly, there is a high frequency of hypogonadism in patients with cancer, end-stage renal disease on hemodialysis, and liver disease *(35)*. Previous reports suggest that two-thirds of men with end-stage renal disease have low total and free testosterone concentrations *(36–52)*. In a recent study, of the 39 men with ESRD on hemodialysis who did not have diabetes mellitus, 24 (63%) had serum total and free testosterone levels below the lower limit of normal male range *(53)*. There is a high prevalence of sexual dysfunction and spermatogenic abnormalities in men on hemodialysis *(54)*. Muscle mass is decreased and fat mass increased, and muscle performance and physical function are markedly impaired in men receiving hemodialysis *(55–60)*. Although androgen deficiency might contribute to the complex pathophysiology of sexual dysfunction and sarcopenia in men on hemodialysis, we do not know if any of these physiologic derangements can be reversed by androgen replacement.

The pathophysiology of hypogonadism in chronic illness is multifactorial; defects exist at all levels of the hypothalamic–pituitary–testicular axis *(42,46–50,52,61,62)*. Malnutrition, mediators, and products of the systemic inflammatory response, drugs such as ketoconazole, and metabolic abnormalities produced by the systemic illness all contribute to a decline in testosterone production.

MALNUTRITION AND REPRODUCTIVE FUNCTION

Humans have known since antiquity that energy balance and nutritional status are intimately linked to the reproductive axis in both men and women *(63–67)*. The onset of puberty, the length of the reproductive period, the number of offspring, and the age of menopause have all been linked to body weight and composition, particularly the amount of body fat *(65,66,68)*. Normal reproductive function requires an optimal nutritional intake; both caloric deprivation and consequent weight loss, and excessive food intake and obesity are associated with impairment of reproductive function. In the animal kingdom, during periods of food scarcity, small animals with a short life-span may not even achieve puberty before death *(68)*. In animals with longer life-spans, sexual maturation may be substantially delayed during food deprivation. Undernutrition, caused by famine, eating disorders, and exercise, results in weight loss and changes in body composition and endocrine milieu that can impair reproductive function *(63–71)*. As a general rule, weight loss and body composition changes resulting from undernutrition are associated with reduced gonadotropin (GnRH) secretion; the decrease in FSH and LH levels correlates with the degree of weight loss *(69–71)*. However, both hypogonadotropic and hypergonadotropic hypogonadism have been described in cachexia associated with certain chronic illnesses such as HIV infection *(24)*. Collectively, these observations provide compelling evidence that energy balance is an important determinant of reproductive function in all mammals.

We do not know the precise nature of the biochemical pathways that connect these two-body systems essential for the survival of all species. The prevalent hypothesis is that the metabolic signals that regulate hypothalamic GnRH secretion are mediated through leptin and neuropeptide Y *(68,72–76)*. Leptin, the product of the obesity *(ob)* gene, is a circulating hormone secreted by the fat cells that acts centrally to regulate the activity of central nervous system (CNS) effector systems that maintain energy balance *(75)*. Leptin stimulates LH secretion by activation of the nitric oxide synthase in the gonadotropes *(76)*. Leptin inhibits neuropeptide Y secretion. Neuropeptide Y has a tonic inhibitory effect on both leptin and GnRH secretion. Leptin also stimulates nitric oxide (NO) production in the mediobasal hypothalamus; NO stimulates GnRH secretion by the hypothalamic GnRH secreting neurons *(76)*. Therefore, the net effect of leptin action is stimulation of hypothalamic GnRH secretion *(72–76)*.

Caloric deprivation in experimental animals is associated with reduced leptin levels and a concomitant reduction in circulating LH levels *(72)*. Leptin administration to calorically deprived mice reverses the inhibition of gonadotropin secretion that attends food restriction *(72)*. Similarly, genetically ob/ob mice with leptin deficiency have hypogonadotropic hypogonadism and are infertile; treatment of these mice with leptin restores gonadotropin secretion and fertility *(72)*. Collectively, these observations suggest thatenergy deficit and weight loss are associated with impaired GnRH secretion, in part, because of decreased leptin secretion and a reciprocal increase in neuropetide activity. Although there is agreement that leptin is an important metabolic signal that links energy balance and reproductive axis, it remains unclear whether it is the primary trigger for the activation of the GnRH pulse generator at the onset of puberty. Emerging evidence suggests that leptin is essential but not sufficient for initiation of puberty.

Susser and Stein have described the effects of acute food scarcity on this previously healthy and nutritionally replete population *(72,78)*. Between October 1944 and May 1945, during the German occupation of The Netherlands, the German army restricted food supplies in certain Dutch cities (famine cities), resulting in substantial reduction in average, daily energy intake to less than 1000 kcal *(77,78)*. Some adjacent cities, where food supplies were not curtailed by the Germans, were not affected by the famine (control cities). Fifty percent of women affected by the famine developed amenorrhea. The conception rate dropped to about 53% of that normally expected (based on control cities) and correlated with the decreased caloric ration *(77,78)*. In addition to the decrease in fertility, undernutrition resulted in an increase in perinatal mortality, congenital malformations, schizophrenia, and obesity *(77,78)*. These observations indicate that optimal caloric intake is essential for normal fertility and prenatal growth.

The !Kung San of Botswana were a tribe of hunter–gatherers until about 20 yr ago *(79)*. The body weight of the men and women in the tribe varied substantially throughout the year depending on the availability of food. In the summer months, the food supply was more abundant and the body weight increased; the nadir of body weight was achieved in winter months. The number of births in the tribe peaked about 9 mo after the peak of body weight *(79)*. This is another example of how the availability of food can affect fertility patterns in nature.

These experiments of nature have led to speculation that androgen deficiency might be an adaptive response to malnutrition and illness; therefore, some investigators have questioned whether it is wise to administer anabolic/androgenic therapies to men with chronic illness.

LOW TESTOSTERONE LEVELS CORRELATE WITH POOR DISEASE OUTCOME

Low testosterone levels correlate with adverse disease outcome in HIV-infected men. Serum testosterone levels are lower in HIV-infected men who have lost weight than in those who have not *(31)*. Longitudinal follow-up of HIV-infected homosexual men reveals a progressive decrease in serum testosterone levels *(23)*; this decrease is much greater in HIV-infected men who progress to acquired immune deficiency syndrome (AIDS) than in those who do not. We do not know whether the decrease in testosterone levels is a consequence of weight loss or is a contributory factor that precedes muscle wasting. In a longitudinal study, Dobs et al. *(17)* measured serum testosterone levels in a cohort of HIV-infected men and reported that serum testosterone levels decline early in the course of events that culminate in wasting. Testosterone levels correlate with muscle mass and exercise capacity in HIV-infected men *(18)* leading to speculation that hypogonadism may contribute to muscle wasting and debility. Although, patients with HIV infection may lose both fat and lean tissue, the loss of lean body mass is an important aspect of the weight loss associated with wasting. The magnitude of depletion of nonfat tissues is an important determinant of the time of death in AIDS *(16,21)*. There is a high prevalence of sexual dysfunction in HIV-infected men *(80,81)*. With the increasing life expectancy of HIV-infected men, frailty and sexual dysfunction have emerged as important quality of life issues.

Muscle strength and performance, and physical function are markedly impaired in patients on hemodialysis *(82)*. Exercise tolerance is markedly attenuated *(82–84)*; peak oxygen uptake is typically reduced to roughly half the level predicted for healthy subjects *(82–84)*. Lactic acid threshold is also reduced in both adults and children on maintenance hemodialysis *(82,85)*. Anemia, muscle dysfunction, uremic toxins, cardiovascular dysfunction, and deconditioning collectively produce substantial impairment of exercise tolerance *(82–90)*. Muscle biopsies obtained from patients with end-stage renal disease demonstrate muscle atrophy that predominantly affects the fast twitch, type II fibers *(88,89)*, similar to the changes seen in association with aging. Other abnormalities in the muscle include abnormal morphology, mitochondrial damage, myofilament abnormalities, reduced levels of aerobic enzymes and contractile proteins, and loss of capillaries. Although the etiology of sarcopenia in end-stage renal disease is complex, the decrease in testosterone levels, an important contributor to the loss of muscle mass and dysfunction, is potentially reversible.

DEMONSTRATION THAT TESTOSTERONE HAS ANABOLIC EFFECTS ON THE MUSCLE

Testosterone replacement increases nitrogen retention in castrated males of several animal species *(91)*, eunuchoidal men, boys before puberty, and women *(92)*. Induction of experimental androgen deficiency in healthy men by administration of a GnRH agonist leads to loss of lean body mass, and testosterone replacement reverses the GnRH agonist induced loss of lean body mass *(93)*. Several recent studies *(4,10–12)* have reexamined the effects of testosterone on body composition and muscle mass in hypogonadal men in more detail. We administered 100-mg testosterone enanthate weekly for 10 wk to seven hypogonadal men after a 10- to 12-wk washout *(4)*. Testosterone replacement was associated with a 4.5 ± 0.6-kg ($p = 0.005$) increase in body weight and a 5.0 ± 0.8-kg ($p = 0.004$) increase in fat–free mass, estimated from underwater weight; body fat did not change. Similar increases in fat–free mass were observed using the deuterium water dilution method. Arm and leg muscle cross-sectional areas, assessed by magnetic resonance imaging, increased significantly. Substantial increases in muscle strength were also noted after treatment.

Brodsky et al. *(10)* reported a 15% increase in fat-free mass and an 11% decrease in fat mass in hypogonadal men. The muscle mass increased by 20% and accounted for 65%

of the increase in fat-free mass. The muscle accretion during testosterone treatment was associated with a 56% increase in fractional muscle protein synthesis. Snyder et al. *(14)* have demonstrated that the testosterone-induced gains in lean body mass during test-osterone replacement therapy are maintained for up to 3 yr of replacement therapy.

Intense controversy persisted until recently with respect to the effects of supra-physiologic doses of androgenic steroids on body composition and muscle strength *(3,94,95)*. Many of the previous studies were neither blinded nor placebo-controlled. The doses of androgens used in most studies were relatively low and it is surprising that any effects were seen at all. In some studies, the energy and protein intake was not controlled. The exercise stimulus was not standardized; thus, the effects of andro-gen could not be evaluated independent of the effects of strength training *(34)*. Another confounding factor in some studies was the inclusion of competitive ath-letes whose desire to win might preclude compliance with standardized regimens of diet, exercise, and drug administration *(96,97)*. We conducted a placebo-controlled, double-blind, randomized, clinical trial to separately assess the effects of supraphysiologic doses of testosterone and resistance exercise on fat-free mass, muscle size and strength *(3)*. Healthy men 19–40 yr of age and within 15% of their ideal weight were randomly assigned to one of four groups: placebo but no exercise; testosterone but no exercise; placebo plus exercise; and testosterone plus exercise. The men received 600 mg test-osterone enanthate or placebo weekly for 10 wk. Serum total and free testosterone levels, measured 7 d after each injection, increased fivefold; these were nadir levels and serum testosterone levels at other times must have been higher. Serum LH levels were markedly suppressed in the two testosterone-treated but not placebo-treated men, providing addi-tional evidence of compliance. Men in the exercise groups underwent weight-lifting exercises three times per week; the training stimulus was standardized based on the subjects' initial 1-repetition maximum and supervised. Fat-free mass by underwater weighing, muscle size by magnetic resonance imaging, and muscle strength of the arms and legs in bench press and squat exercises were measured before and after 10 wk of treatment.

The men given testosterone alone had greater gains in muscle size in the arm (mean [± SE] change in triceps area 13.2 ± 3.3 vs $-2.1 \pm 2.9\%$; $p < 0.05$) and leg (change in quadriceps area 6.5 ± 1.3 vs $-1.0 \pm 1.1\%$; $p < 0.05$), than those given placebo injections. Testosterone-treatment was also associated with greater gains in strength in the bench press (increase 10 ± 4 vs $-1 \pm 2\%$; $p < 0.05$) and squat exercise capacity (increase 19 ± 6 vs $3 \pm 1\%$; $p < 0.05$) than placebo injections. Testosterone and exercise, given together, produced greater increase in fat-free mass ($+9.5 \pm 1.0\%$), and muscle size ($+14.7 \pm 3.1\%$ in triceps area and $+14.1 \pm 1.3\%$ in quadriceps area) than either placebo or exercise alone and greater gains in muscle strength ($+24 \pm 3\%$ in bench press strength and $+39 \pm 4\%$ in squat exercise capacity) than either nonexercising group. Serum PSA levels did not change during treatment and no abnormalities were detected in the prostate on digital rectal examination during the 10-wk treatment period. These results demonstrate that supraphysiologic doses of testosterone, especially when combined with strength train-ing, increase fat-free mass, muscle size and strength in normal men.

Griggs et al. *(95)* administered testosterone enanthate at a dose of 3 mg/kg/wk to healthy men, 19–40 yr of age. This was an open-label study that was not placebo con-trolled. Muscle mass, estimated from creatinine excretion, increased by a mean of 20% and ^{40}K mass increased 12% after 12 wk of testosterone treatment. In a separate study

(98), a similar dose of testosterone enanthate given for 12 mo to men with muscular dystrophy was associated with a 4.9-kg increase in lean body mass (approx 10%) at 3 mo; these gains were maintained for 12 mo.

Young et al. *(94)* examined fat-free mass by DXA scan in 13 nonathletic men treated with 200 mg testosterone enanthate weekly for 6 mo during the course of a male contraceptive study. This was an open-label study that included untreated men as controls. Testosterone treatment increased serum testosterone levels by 90% and was associated with a 9.6% increase in fat-free mass and 16.2% decrease in fat mass.

Collectively, these data *(3,94,98)* demonstrate that when dietary intake and exercise stimulus are controlled, supraphysiologic doses of testosterone produce further increases in fat-free mass and strength in eugonadal men. It is likely that strength training may augment androgen effects on the muscle.

EFFECTS OF ANDROGEN REPLACEMENT ON BODY COMPOSITION AND MUSCLE FUNCTION IN HIV-INFECTION AND OTHER CHRONIC ILLNESSES

Several different anabolic interventions have been examined in the treatment of HIV-related wasting including appetite stimulants such as dronabinol *(99)* and megesterol acetate *(100)*; anabolic hormones such as human growth hormone *(101,102)*, insulinlike growth factor-1 *(102)*, and androgens *(1,5,80,103–113)*; and modulators of immune response such as thalidomide. Dronabinol increases appetite but has not been shown to increase lean body mass. Similarly, megesterol acetate treatment produces a modest weight gain but no significant change in lean body mass. This progestational agent decreases serum testosterone levels and may produce symptoms of androgen deficiency.

In the two recently published clinical trials, treatment of HIV-infected men with human growth hormone (hGH) was associated with a 1.5-kg increase in lean body mass *(101,102)*. Although greater gains in weight were recorded after 6 wk of hGH treatment, these gains were not sustained with continued treatment for 12 wk. The reasons for the failure to sustain weight gains during hGH treatment are not clear; it is conceivable that weight gain early in the course of treatment is the result of water retention. Growth hormone administration is associated with a high frequency of side effects including edema, arthralgias, myalgias, and jaw pain. Not surprisingly, the treatment discontinuation rates were high (21–40%) in the two hGH studies. The annual cost of treating HIV-infected men with hGH is substantially greater than that of testosterone-replacement therapy using any of the available androgen formulations.

Several studies on the effects of androgen supplementation in HIV-infected men have been reported *(1,5,80,103–113)*. However, many of these studies were not controlled clinical trials. Most of the studies were of short duration ranging from 12 to 24 wk. Several androgenic steroids have been studied in a limited fashion, including nandrolone decanoate, oxandrolone, oxymetholone, stanozolol, testosterone cypionate, and testosterone enanthate.

Of the five placebo-controlled studies of testosterone replacement in HIV-infected men with weight loss, three *(1,5,103)* demonstrated an increase in fat-free mass and two *(104,110)* did not. The three studies *(1,5,103)* that showed gains in fat-free mass selected patients with low testosterone levels. Coodley et al. *(110)* examined the effects of 200 mg testosterone cypionate given every 2 wk for 3 mo to 40 HIV seropositive patients with weight loss of greater than 5% of usual body weight and CD4 cell counts of $< 2 \times 10^5$/L in a double-blind, placebo-controlled study. Among the 35 patients who completed the first 3 mo of the study, there was no significant difference between the effects of testosterone and placebo treatment on weight gain. However, testosterone supplementation improved overall sense of well-being ($p = 0.03$). The body composition was not assessed.

In a placebo-controlled, double-blind clinical trial, we examined the effects of physiological testosterone replacement by means of the nongenital patch (5). Forty-one HIV-positive men with serum testosterone levels less than 400 ng/dL were randomly assigned to receive either two placebo patches nightly or two testosterone patches, designed to release 5 mg testosterone over a 24-h period. Testosterone replacement was associated with a 1.34-kg increase in lean body mass ($p = 0.02$) as well as a significantly greater reduction in fat mass than that achieved with placebo treatment alone. There were no significant changes in liver enzymes, plasma HIV-RNA copy number, and CD4 and CD8+ T-cell counts. Both placebo and testosterone treatment were associated with significant increase in muscle strength. Because most of the participants in this study had not had prior weight-lifting experience, we hypothesized that the apparent increase in muscle strength in the placebo group reflected the learning effect. Most other studies of testosterone replacement in HIV-infected men have also failed to demonstrate significant increases in muscle strength.

Therefore, in a subsequent study (103), we paid particular attention to having the subjects come back to the Exercise Laboratory on two or more occasions until they were familiar with the equipment and technique and stability of measurement had been achieved. In this study, we determined the effects of testosterone replacement, with or without a program of resistance exercise, on muscle strength and body composition in androgen-deficient, HIV-infected men with weight loss and low testosterone levels. This was a placebo-controlled, double–blind, randomized clinical trial in which HIV-infected men with serum testosterone less than 350 ng/dL, and weight loss of 5% or more in the previous 6 mo were randomly assigned to one of four groups: placebo, no exercise; testosterone, no exercise; placebo plus exercise; or testosterone plus exercise. Placebo or 100 mg testosterone enanthate were given intramuscularly weekly for 16 wk. The exercise program was a three times per week, progressive, supervised strength-training program. Effort-dependent muscle strength in five different exercises was measured by the 1-repetition maximum method. In the placebo-alone group, muscle strength did not change in any of the five exercises (–0.3 to –4.0%). This indicates that this strategy was effective in minimizing the influence of the learning effect. Men treated with testosterone alone, exercise alone, or combined testosterone/exercise, experienced significant increases in maximum voluntary muscle strength in the leg press (+22–30%), leg curls (+18–36%), bench press (+19–33%), and latissimus pulls (+17–33%) exercises. The gains in strength in all the exercises were greater in men receiving testosterone or exercise alone than in those receiving placebo alone. The change in leg press strength was correlated with change in muscle volume ($r = 0.44$, $p = 0.003$) and change in fat-free mass ($r = 0.55$, $p < 0.001$).

We conclude that when the confounding influence of the learning effect can be minimized, as we did in this study, and appropriate androgen-responsive measures of muscle strength are selected, testosterone replacement is associated with demonstrable increase in maximal voluntary strength in HIV-infected men with low testosterone levels.

Strength training also promotes gains in lean body mass and muscle strength (103,114). Supraphysiological doses of androgens augment the anabolic effects of resistance exercise on lean body mass and maximal voluntary strength (111,113).

These data suggest that testosterone can promote weight gain and an increase in lean body mass as well as muscle strength in HIV-infected men with low testosterone levels. We do not know, however, whether physiological androgen replacement can produce meaningful changes in the quality of life, utilization of health care resources, and physical function in HIV-infected men. Emerging data indicate that testosterone does not affect HIV replication, but its effects on virus shedding in the genital tract are not known.

TESTOSTERONE SUPPLEMENTATION IN OTHER CHRONIC ILLNESSES

Patients with autoimmune disorders, particularly those receiving glucocorticoids, often experience muscle wasting and bone loss (115–117). In a placebo-controlled study, Reid et al. (115) administered a replacement dose of testosterone to men receiving glucocorticoids. Testosterone replacement was associated with a greater increase in fat-free mass and bone density than placebo.

Controlled clinical trials of nandrolone decanoate have reported increased hemoglobin levels with androgen treatment in men with end-stage renal disease who are on hemodialysis (118–122). Prior to the advent of erythropoietin, testosterone was commonly used to treat anemia associated with end-stage renal disease. Testosterone increases red cell production by stimulating erythropoieitin, by augmenting erythropoieitin action, and by its direct action on stem cells. Further studies are needed to determine whether testosterone administration can reduce blood transfusion and erythropoieitin requirements in patients with end-stage renal disease on hemodialysis.

In a placebo-controlled study, administration of nandrolone decanoate improved lean body mass in men on hemodialysis. However, there was no significant change in endurance. The strength of lower extremity muscles was not assessed. Physical function was assessed in only a small subset of men and showed modest improvements, using tests that are susceptible to ceiling effect. This important study demonstrated that androgen administration to men on hemodialysis is associated with gains in fat-free mass.

Chronic obstructive lung disease is a chronic debilitating disease for which there are few effective therapies. Muscle wasting and dysfunction are recognized as correctable causes of exercise intolerance in these patients. It has been speculated that low levels of anabolic hormones such as testosterone, growth hormone, and insulinlike growth factor-1 may contribute to muscle atrophy and dysfunction (97). Human growth hormone increases nitrogen retention and lean body muscle in patients with COPD; however, the effects of hGH on respiratory muscle strength and exercise tolerance remain to be established (123,124). Schols et al. (125) examined the effects of a low dose of nandrolone or placebo in 217 men and women with chronic obstructive lung disease; these authors reported modest increases in lean body mass and respiratory muscle strength.

TESTOSTERONE EFFECTS ON FAT METABOLISM

Percent body fat is increased in hypogonadal men (11). Induction of androgen deficiency in healthy men by administration of a GnRH agonist leads to an increase in fat mass (93). Some studies of young, hypogonadal men have reported a decrease in fat mass with testosterone-replacement therapy (10,11); others (4,12) found no change. In contrast, long-term studies of testosterone supplementation of older men are consistent in demonstrating a consistent decrease in fat mass (13). Epidemiologic studies (126,127) have demonstrated that serum testosterone levels are lower in middle-aged men with visceral obesity. Serum testosterone levels correlate inversely with visceral fat area and directly with plasma HDL levels. Testosterone replacement of middle-aged men with visceral obesity improves insulin sensitivity, decreases blood glucose and blood pressure *(128)*. Testosterone is an important determinant of regional fat distribution and metabolism in men *(128)*. Therefore, it has been hypothesized that testosterone supplementation might be beneficial in HIV-infected men with the fat-redistribution syndromes.

TESTOSTERONE DOSE-RESPONSE RELATIONSHIPS

Testosterone increases muscle mass and strength and regulates other physiologic processes, but we do not know whether testosterone effects are dose dependent and whether dose requirements for maintaining various androgen-dependent processes are similar *(7)*. Androgen receptors in most tissues are either saturated or downregulated at physiologic testosterone concentrations *(129–132)*; leading to speculation that there might be two separate dose-response curves: one in the hypogonadal range with maximal response at low normal testosterone concentrations, and a second in supraphysiological range, representing a separate mechanism of action *(7,132)*. However, testosterone dose-response relationships for a range of androgen-dependent functions in humans have not been studied.

To determine the effects of graded doses of testosterone on body composition, muscle size, strength, power, sexual and cognitive functions, PSA, plasma lipids, hemoglobin, and IGF-1 levels, 61 eugonadal men, 18–35 yr of age, were randomized to 1 of 5 groups to receive monthly injections of a long-acting GnRH agonist to suppress endogenous testosterone secretion, and weekly injections of 25, 50, 125, 300, or 600 mg testosterone enanthate for 20 wk. Energy and protein intake were standardized. The administration of GnRH agonist plus graded doses of testosterone resulted in mean nadir testosterone concentrations of 253, 306, 542, 1345, and 2370 ng/dL for the 25-, 50-, 125-, 300-, and 600-mg doses, respectively. Fat-free mass increased dose-dependently in men receiving 125, 300, or 600 mg of testosterone weekly (change +3.4, 5.2, and 7.9 kg, respectively). The changes in fat-free mass were highly dependent on testosterone dose (Tables 1 and 2; $P = 0.0001$) and correlated with log testosterone concentrations ($r = 0.73$, $p = 0.0001$). Changes in leg press strength, leg power, thigh and quadriceps muscle volumes, hemoglobin, and IGF-1 were positively correlated with testosterone concentrations, whereas changes in fat mass and plasma HDL cholesterol were negatively correlated (Tables 1 and 2). Sexual function, visual-spatial cognition and mood, and PSA levels did not change significantly at any dose (Tables 1 and 2). These data demonstrate that changes in circulating testosterone concentrations, induced by GnRH agonist and testosterone administration, are associated with testosterone dose- and concentration-dependent changes in fat-free mass, muscle size, strength and power, fat mass, hemoglobin, HDL cholesterol, and IGF-1 levels, in conformity with a single linear dose-response relationship. However, different androgen-dependent processes have different testosterone dose-response relationships.

MECHANISMS OF TESTOSTERONE'S ANABOLIC EFFECTS ON THE MUSCLE

The prevalent view that testosterone produces muscle hypertrophy by increasing fractional muscle protein synthesis *(9,10)* is supported by a number of studies. However,

Table 1

Placebo-Controlled Studies of Testosterone Supplementation in HIV-Infected Men

Study	Subjects	Treatment regimen	Changes in body composition	Changes in muscle function	Comments
Bhasin et al. (5)	HIV-infected men with serum T <400 ng/dL	Testosterone patch (5 mg daily) vs placebo patch × 10 wk	+1.3 kg gain in FFM after testosterone replacement	Strength gains in placebo- and testosterone-treated men not significantly different	Strength measurements confounded by learning effect
Grinspoon et al. (1)	HIV-infected men with AIDS wasting syndrome and free testosterone levels	300 mg every 3 wk × 6 mo	+2 kg increase in FFM; no change in fat mass	Muscle strength not measured; no change in exercise functional capacity	Testosterone-treated patients reported feeling better, improved quality of life, and appearance
Bhasin et al. (7)	HIV-infected men with >5% weight loss and serum testosterone less than 350 ng/dL	100 mg TE weekly × 16 wk with or without resistance training; placebo-controlled	+2.9 kg gain in testosterone-treated men	Significantly greater gains in muscle strength with testosterone treatment than with placebo	
Grinspoon et al. (18)	HIV-infected men with AIDS wasting syndrome	200 mg TE weekly with or without strength training; placebo-controlled × 12 wk	Greater increments in muscle mass and volume in response to testosterone and resistance exercise training as compared to placebo	Strength gains not significantly greater in testosterone or resistance training groups in comparison to placebo group	
Dobs et al. (17)	HIV-infected men with AIDS and 5–10% weight loss, and baseline testosterone <400 ng/dL or free testosterone <16 pg/mL	Testoderm 6-mg scrotal patch vs placebo patch × 12 wk	Changes in body weight or body cell mass by bioelectrical impedance not significantly different between testosterone and placebo groups	Not measured	Quality of life measure not changed
Coodley et al. (110)	HIV-infected men with >5% weight loss, and CD4 counts <200/cmm	Testosterone cypionate 200 mg every 2 wk × 12 wk vs placebo in a crossover design	No significant differences in change in body weight between testosterone and placebo periods	Not measured	Testosterone treatment associated with improved well-being

Table 2
Controlled Clinical Trials of Other Androgens in HIV-Infected Men

Study	Subjects	Treatment regimen	Changes in body composition	Changes in muscle function	Comments
Sattler et al. (113)	HIV-infected men with CD4+ cell count <400/cmm	Nandrolone 600 mg weekly alone or nandrolone plus resistance training exercise for 12 wk	+3.9 kg gain in FFM after nandrolone treatment alone, and 5.2 kg in combined treatment group	Strength gains greater with combined treatment than with nandrolone alone	No placebo-alone group
Strawford et al. (111)	HIV-infected men with weight loss >5% in the preceding 2 yr	All subjects received resistance exercise training plus TE 100 mg weekly, and randomized to 20 mg oxandrolone or placebo daily	+6.9 kg mean increase in LBM in oxandrolone group; 3.8-kg gain in placebo group	Greater muscle strength gains in oxandrolone group than in placebo group	Significant drop in plasma HDL cholesterol in oxandrolone
Strwaford et al. (112)	HIV-infected men with AIDS wasting syndrome and borderline low testosterone concetrations	Placebo, 65 mg nandrolone weekly, or 200 mg nandrolone weekly	Greater increments in nitrogen retention in both nandrolone groups compared to placebo	LBM increased by 3.1 kg in 10 men in open-label treatment phase	
Batterham and Garsia (XXX)	HIV-infected men with >5% weight loss	Randomized to nutritional supplementation alone, megesterol acetate 400 mg daily or nandrolone 100 mg every 15 d	Greater LBM gain in association with nandrolone than placebo	Muscle strength not measured	Small sample size
Hengge et al. (108)	HIV-infected men with chronic cachexia	Oxymetholone mono-therapy, oxymetholone plus ketotifen, compared to historical controls	8.2-kg weight gain in the oxymetholone group, 6.1-kg gain in combination group, compared with a weight loss of 1.8 kg in historical controls	Body composition and muscle performance not measured	Controls not concurrent; no placebo group

as discussed in this section, recent observations suggest that increase in muscle protein synthesis probably occurs as a secondary event and may not be the sole or the primary mechanism by which testosterone induces muscle hypertrophy *(133)*.

In order to determine whether testosterone-induced increase in muscle size is the result of muscle fiber hypertrophy or hyperplasia, muscle biopsies were obtained from vastus lateralis in 39 men before and after 20 wk of combined treatment with GnRH agonist and weekly injections of 25, 50, 125, 300, or 600 mg testosterone enanthate (TE) *(133)*. Graded doses of testosterone administration were associated with testosterone dose and concentration-dependent increase in muscle fiber cross-sectional area. Changes in cross-sectional areas of both type I and II fibers were dependent on testosterone dose and significantly correlated with total ($r = 0.35$, and 0.44; $p < 0.0001$ for type I and II fibers, respectively) and free ($r = 0.34$ and 0.35; $p < 0.005$) testosterone concentrations during treatment. The men receiving 300 and 600 mg of TE weekly experienced significant increases from baseline in areas of type I (baseline vs 20 wk, 3176 ± 163 vs 4201 ± 163 μm^2, $p < 0.05$ at the 300-mg dose, and 3347 ± 253 vs 4984 ± 374 μm^2, $p = 0.006$ at the 600-mg dose) muscle fibers; the men in the 600-mg group also had significant increments in cross-sectional area of type II (4060 ± 401 vs 5526 ± 544 μm^2, $p = 0.03$) fibers. The relative proportions of type I and type II fibers did not change significantly after treatment in any group. The myonuclear number per fiber increased significantly in men receiving the 300- and 600-mg doses of TE and was significantly correlated with testosterone concentration and muscle fiber cross-sectional area *(133)*. These data demonstrate that increases in muscle volume in healthy eugonadal men treated with graded doses of testosterone are associated with concentration-dependent increases in muscle fiber cross-sectional area and myonulcear number, but not muscle fiber number. We conclude that the testosterone-induced increase in muscle volume is the result of muscle fiber hypertrophy. In our study, the myonuclear number increased in direct relation to the increase in muscle fiber diameter. Therefore, it is possible that muscle fiber hypertrophy and increase in myonuclear number were preceded by testosterone-induced increase in satellite cell number and their fusion with muscle fibers. The mechanisms by which testosterone might increase satellite cell number are not known. An increase in satellite cell number could occur by an increase in satellite cell replication, inhibition of satellite cell apoptosis, and/or increased differentiation of stem cells into the myogenic lineage. We do not know which of these processes is the site of regulation by testosterone. The hypothesis that testosterone promotes muscle fiber hypertrophy by increasing the number of satellite cells should be further tested. Because of the constraints inherent in obtaining multiple biopsy specimens in humans, the effects of testosterone on satellite cell replication and stem cell recruitment would be more conveniently studied in an animal model.

The molecular mechanisms, which mediate androgen-induced muscle hypertrophy, are not well understood. Urban et al. *(9)* have proposed that testosterone stimulates the expression of insulinlike growth factor-1 (IGF-1) and downregulates insulinlike growth factor-binding protein-4 (IGFBP-4) in the muscle. Reciprocal changes in IGF-1 and its binding protein thus provide a potential mechanism for amplifying the anabolic signal.

It is not clear whether the anabolic effects of supraphysiological doses of testosterone are mediated through an androgen receptor mediated mechanism. In vitro binding studies *(134)* suggest that the maximum effects of testosterone should be manifest at about 300 ng/dL; that is, serum testosterone levels that are at the lower end of the normal male range. Therefore, it is possible that the supraphysiological doses of androgen produce muscle hypertrophy through androgen-receptor independent mechanisms, such as through an antiglucocorticoid effect *(135)*. We cannot exclude the possibility that some androgen effects may be mediated through nonclassical binding sites. Testosterone effects on the muscle are modulated by a number of other factors, such as the genetic background, growth hormone secretory status *(136)*, nutrition, exercise, cytokines, thyroid hormones, and glucocorticoids. Testosterone may also affect muscle function by its effects on neuromuscular transmission *(137,138)*.

THE ROLE OF 5-α REDUCTION OF TESTOSTERONE IN THE MUSCLE

Although the enzyme 5-α-reductase is expressed at low concentrations within the muscle *(139)*, we do not know whether conversion of testosterone to dihydrotestosterone is required for mediating the androgen effects on the muscle. Men with benign prostatic hypertrophy who are treated with the 5-α-reductase inhibitor do not experience muscle loss. Similarly, individuals with congenital 5-α-reductase deficiency have normal muscle development at puberty. These data suggest that 5-α reduction of testosterone is not obligatory for mediating its anabolic effects on the muscle. Because testosterone effects on the prostate require its obligatory conversion to DHT, selective androgen receptor modulators that bind the androgen receptor, but are not 5-α reduced would be very attractive; these agents could achieve the desired anabolic effects on the muscle without the undesirable effects on the prostate.

Sattler et al. *(140)* have reported that serum DHT levels are lower and testosterone to dihydrotestosterone levels higher in HIV-infected men than healthy men. These investigators have proposed that a defect in testosterone to dihydrotestosterone conversion may contribute to wasting in a subset of HIV-infected men. If this hypothesis were true, then it would be rational to treat such patients with dihydrotestosterone rather than testosterone. A dihydrotestosterone gel is currently under clinical investigation. However, unlike testosterone, dihydrotestosterone is not aromatized to estradiol. Therefore, there is concern that suppression of endogenous testosterone and estradiol production by exogenous dihydrotestosterone may produce osteoporosis.

CONCLUSION

The loss of muscle mass and function is a common occurrence during the course of many chronic illnesses. These disease states are attended by high prevalence of low testosterone levels. There is agreement that testosterone supplementation of men with chronic illness increases fat-free mass and muscle strength and can promote weight gain. However, further studies are needed to determine whether testosterone supplementation can produce clinically significant benefits such as improved physical function, quality of life, reduced disability, and other health related outcomes. Although short-term administration of testosterone in replacement doses and slightly supraphysiological doses is safe, the long-term risks of testosterone supplementation in men remain largely unknown.

REFERENCES

1. Grinspoon S, Corcoran C, Askari H, et al. Effects of androgen administration in men with the AIDS wasting syndrome: a randomized, double-blind, placebo-controlled trial. Ann Intern Med 1998;129:18–26.

2. Grinspoon. 2000.
3. Bhasin S, Storer TW, Berman N, et al. The effects of supraphysiologic doses of testosterone on muscle size and strength in men. N Engl J Med 1996;335:1–7.
4. Bhasin S, Storer TW, Berman N, et al. A replacement dose of testosterone increases fat-free mass and muscle size in hypogonadal men. J Clin Endocrinol Metab 1997;82:407–413.
5. Bhasin S, Storer TW. Asbel-Sethi N, et al. Effects of testosterone replacement with a non-genital, transdermal system, Androderm, in human immunodeficiency virus-infected men with low testosterone levels. J Clin Endocinol Metab 1998;83:3155–3162.
6. Bhasin S, Woodhouse L, Storer TW. Proof of the effect of testosterone on skeletal muscle. J Endocrinol 2001;170(1):27–38.
7. Bhasin S, Woodhouse L, Casaburi R, et al. Testosterone dose-response relationships in healthy young men. Am J Physiol Endocrinol Metab 2001;281(6):E1172–1181.
8. Tenover JS. Effects of testosterone supplementation in the aging male. J Clin Endocrinol Metab. 1992;75(4):1092–1098.
9. Urban RJ, Bodenburg YH, Gilkison C, et al. Testosterone administration to elderly men increases skeletal muscle strength and protein synthesis. Am J Physiol 1995;269:E820–E826.
10. Brodsky IG, Balagopal P, Nair KS. Effects of testosterone replacement on muscle mass and muscle protein synthesis in hypogonadal men-a Clinical Research Center Study. J Clin Endocrinol Metab 1996;81:3469–3475.
11. Katznelson L, Finkelstein JS, Schoenfeld DA, et al. Increase in bone density and lean body mass during testosterone administration in men with acquired hypogonadism. J. Clin. Endocrinol. Metab. 1996;81:4358–4365.
12. Wang C, Eyre DR, Clark R, et al. Sublingual testosterone replacement improves muscle mass and strength, decreases bone resorption, and increases bone resorption markers in hypogonadal men-a Clinical Research Center Study. J Clin Endocrinol Metab 1996;81:3654–3662.
13. Snyder PJ, Peachey H, Hannoush P, et al. Effect of testosterone treatment on body composition and muscle strength in men over 65. J Clin Endocrinol Metab 1999;84:2647.
14. Snyder PJ, Peachey H, Berlin JA, et al. Effects of testosterone replacement in hypogonadal men. J Clin Endocrinol Metab. 2000;85(8):2670–2677.
15. Wang C, Swerdloff RS, Iranmanesh A, et al. Transdermal testosterone gel improves sexual function, mood, muscle strength, and body composition parameters in hypogonadal men. Testosterone Gel Study Group. J Clin Endocrinol Metab 2000;85(8):2839–2853.
16. Chlebowski RT, et al. Nutritional status, gastrointestinal dysfunction and survival in patients with AIDS. Am J Gastroenterol 1989;84:1288–1293.
17. Dobs AS, Few WL, Blackman MR, et al. Serum hormones in men with human immunodeficiency virus-associated wasting. J Clin Endocrinol Metab 1996;81:4108–4112.
18. Grinspoon S, Corcoran C, Lee K, et al. Loss of lean body and muscle mass correlates with androgen levels in hypogondal men with acquired immunodeficiency syndrome and wasting. J Clin Endocrinol Metab 1996;81:4051–4058.
19. Sellmeyer DE, Grunfeld C. Endocrine and metabolic disturbances in human immunodeficiency virus infection and the acquired immune deficiency syndrome. Endocrine Rev 1996;17:518–532.
20. Hellerstein MK, Kahn J, Mundi H, et al. Current approach to treatment of human immunodeficiency virus associated with weight loss, pathophysiologic considerations and emerging strategies. Sem Oncol 1990;17:17–33.
21. Kotler DP, Tierney AR, Wang J, et al. Magnitude of body cell mass depletion and the timing of death from wasting in AIDS. Am. J. Clin. Nutr. 1989;50:444–447.
22. Linden CP, Allen S, Serufilira A, et al. Predictors of mortality among HIV-infected women in Kigali, Rwanda. Ann. Intern. Med. 1992;116:320–325.
23. Salehian B, Jacobson D, Grafe M, et al. Pituitary-testicular axin during HIV infection: A prospective study. Presented at the 18th annual meeting of the American Society of Andrology. Abstract #9, Tampa, Florida, April 15–19, 1993.
24. Arver SA, Sinha-Hikim I, Beall G, Shen R, Guerrero M, Bhasin S. Serum dihydrotestosterone and testosterone levels in human immunodeficiency virus-infected men with and without weight loss. J Androl 1999;20:611–618.
25. Dobs AS, Dempsey MA, Ladenson PW, et al. Endocrine disorders in men infected with human immunodeficiency virus. Am J.Med 1988;84:611–615.
26. Meremich JA, McDermott MT, Asp AA, et al. Evidence of endocrine involvement early in the course of human immunodeficiency virus infection. J Clin Endocrinol Metab 1990;70:566–571.

27. Villete JM, Bourin P, Dornel C, et al. Circadian variations in plasma levels of hypophyseal, adreno-cortical, and testicular hormones in men infected with human immunodeficiency virus. J Clin Endorinol Metab 1990;70:572–577.
28. Croxon TC, Chapman WE, Miller LK, et al. Changes in the hypothalamic pituitary-gonadal axis in human immunodeficiency virus-infected hypogonadal men. J Clin Endocrinol Metab 1989;68:317–321.
29. Raffi F, Brisseau J-M, Planchon B, et al. Endocrine function in 98 HIV-infected patients: a prospective study. AIDS 1991;5:729–733.
30. DePaepe ME, Vuletin JC, Lee MH, et al. Testicular atrophy in homosexual AIDS patients. Hum Pathol 1989;20:572–578.
31. Coodley GO, Loveless MO, Nelson HD, et al. Endocrine function in HIV wasting syndrome. J Acquir Immune Def Retrovirol 1994;7:46–51.
32. Laudet A, Blum L, Guechot J, et al. Changes in systematic gonadal and adrenal sterods in asymptomatic human immunodeficiency virus-infected men: relationship with CD4 counts. Euro J Endocrin 1995;133:418–424.
33. Rietschel P, Corcoran C, Stanley T, et al.Prevalence of hypogonadism among men with weight loss related to human immunodeficiency virus infection who were receiving highly active antiretroviral therapy. Clin Infect Dis 2000;31(5):1240–1244.
34. Casaburi R, Storer T, Bhasin S. Androgen effects on body composition and muscle performance. In: Bhasin S, Gabelnick H, Spieler JM, et al., eds. Pharmacology, Biology, and Clinical Applications of Androgens: Current Status and Future Prospects. Wiley-Liss, New York, NY, 1996, pp. 283–288.
35. Handelsman DJ, Dong Q. Hypothalamic-pituitary gonadal axis in chronic renal failure. Endocrinol Metab Clin N Am 1993;22:145–161.
36. Handelsman DJ, Spaliviero JA, Turtle JR. Testicular function in experimental uremia. Endocrinology 1985;117:1974–1983.
37. Guevara A, Vidt D, Hallberg MC, et al. Serum gonadotropins and testosterone levels in uremic males undergoing intermittent dialysis. Metabolism 1969;18:1062.
38. Holdsworth J, Atkins RC, Deketser DM. The pituitary-testicular axis in men with chronic renal failure. N Engl J Med 1977;296:1245–1249.
39. Van Kammen E, Thijssen JHH, Schawrtz F. Sex hormones in male patients with chronic renal failure,I. The production of testosterone and of androstenedione. Clin Endocrinol (Oxf). 1987;8:7–15.
40. Lim VS, Fang VS. Gonadal dysfunction in uremic men: a study of hypothalamo-pituitary-testicular axis before and after renal transplantation. Am J Med 1975;58:665–663.
41. Stewart-Bentley M, Gans D, Horton R. Regulation of gonadal function in uremia. Metabolism 1974;23:1065–1075.
42. Sawin CT, Langcope C, Schmidt GW, et al. Blood levels of gonadotropins and gonadal hormones in gynecomastia associated with chronic hemodialysis. J Clin Endocrinol Metab 1973;36:988–994.
43. Gomez F, De LA Cueva R, Wauters J, et al. Endocrine abnormalities in patients undergoing long term hemodialysis. Am J Med. 1985;65:522–529.
44. Zadeh JA, Koutsamainos KG, Roberts AP, et al. The effect of maintenance hemodialysis and renal transplantation on the plasma testosterone levels of male patients in chronic renal failure. Acta Endocrinol. 1975;80:577–582.
45. Lim VS, Auletta F, Kathpalia S. Gonadal dysfunction in chronic renal failure: an endocrinologic review. Dial Transplant 1978;7:896.
46. Tsitsouras PD, Kowatch Ma, Briefel GR, et al. In vivo pretreatment with human chorionic gonadotropin fails to reverse the dysfunction of isolated Leydig cells from chronically uremic rats. Biol Reprod 1985;33:781–785.
47. Wheatley T, Clark PMS, Clark JDA, et al. Pulsatility of luteinizing hormone in men with chronic renal failure: abnormal rather than absent. Br Med J 1987;294:482–483.
48. Veldhius DJ, Wilkowski MJ, Zwart AD, et al. Evidence for attenuation of hypothalamic gonadotropin releasing hormone (GnRH) impulse strength with preservation of GnRH pulse frequency in men with chronic renal failure. J Clin Endocrinol Metab 1993;76:648–654.
49. Wibullaksanakul S, Handelsman DJ. Regulation of hypothalamic gonadotropin-releasing hormone secretion in experimental uremia: In Vitro studies. Neuroendocrinology 1991;54:353–358.
50. Hasegawa K, Matsushita Y, Hirai K, et al. Abnormal response of luteinizing hormone, follicle stimulating hormone and testosterone to luteinizing hormone releasing hormone in chronic renal failure. Acta Endocrnol (Copenh) 1978;87:467–475.

51. Levitan D, Moser S, Goldstein DA, et al. Disturbances in the hypothalamic-pituitary-gonadal axis in male patients with acute renal failure. Am J Nephrol 1984;4:99.

52. Blackman MR, Weintraub BD, Kourides IA, et al. Discordant elevation of the common alpha subunit of the pituitary glycoprotein hormones compared to beta subunits in the serum of uremic patients. J Clin Endocrinol Metab 1981;53:39.

53. Singh AB, Norris K, Modi N, et al. Pharmacokinetics of a transdermal testosterone system in men with end stage renal disease receiving maintenance hemodialysis and healthy hypogonadal men. J Clin Endocrinol Metab 2001;86(6):2437–2445.

54. Lawrence IG, Price DE, Howlet TAt, et al. Correcting Impotence in The Male Dialysis Patients: Experience With Testosterone Replacement and Vacuum Tumescence Therapy. Am J Kidney Dis 1998;31.

55. Woodrow G, Oldroyd B, Turney J, Tomkins L, Brownjohn A, Smith M. 1996 Whole body and regional body composition in patients with chronic renal failure. Nephrol Dial Transplant. 11:1613-8.

56. Pollock C, Allen B, Warden R, et al. Total body nitrogen by neutron activation in maintenance hemodialysis. Am J Kidney Dis. 1990;16:38–45.

57. Coles G. Body composition in chronic renal failure. Q J Med 1972;41:25–47.

58. Hakim R, Levin N. Malnutrition in hemodialysis patients. Am J Kidney Dis 1993;21:125–137.

59. Lazarus J. Nutrition in hemodialysis patients. Am J Kidney Dis 1993;21:99–105.

60. Kopple J. Effect of nutrition on morbidity and mortality in maintenance dialysis patients. Am J Kidney Dis 1994;24:1002–1009.

61. Cowden EA, Ratcliffe JG, Dobbie JW, Kennedy AC. Hyperprolactinemia in renal disease. Clin Endocrinol (Oxf) 1978;9:241.

62. Hagen C, Olgaard C, McNeilly AS, et al. Prolactin and the hypothalamic-pituitary-gonadal axis in male uremic patients on regular dialysis. Acta Endocrinol. 1976;82:29.

63. Van der Spruy ZM. Nutrition and reproduction. Clin Obstet Gynecol 1985;12:579–604.

64. Knuth VA, Hull MGR, Jacobs HS. Amenorrhea and loss of weight. Br J Obstet Gynecol 1977;84:801–807.

65. Frisch RE. Fatness and fertility. Sci Am 1988;258:88–95.

66. Frisch RE. Body weight and reproduction. Science 1989;246:432.

67. Frisch RE, McArthur JW. Menstrual cycles: fatness as a determinant of minimum weight for height necessary for their maintenance or onset. Science 1974;185:949–995.

68. Foster DL, Nagatani S. Physiological perspectives on leptin as a regulator of reproduction: role in timing puberty. Biol Reprod 1999;60:205–215.

69. Penny R, Goldstein IP, Frasier SD. Gonadotropin excretion and body composition. Pediatrics 1978;61:294–300.

70. Rock CL, Curran-Celentano J. Nutritional management of eating disorders. Psychiatr Clin North Am 1996;19:701–713.

71. Bates GW, Bates SR, Whitworth NS. Reproductive failure in women who practice weight control. Fertil Steril 1982;37:373–378.

72. Cunningham MJ, Clifton DK, Steiner RA. Leptin's actions on the reproductive axis: perspectives and mechanisms. Biol Reprod 1999;60:216–222.

73. Aubert ML, Pierroz DD, Gruaz NM, et al. Metabolic control of sexual function and growth: role of neuropetide Y and leptin. Mol Cell Endocrinol 1998;140:107–113.

74. Clarke IJ, Henry BA. Leptin and reproduction. Biol Reprod 1999;4:48–55.

75. Schwartz MW, Baskin DG, Kaiyala KJ, et al. Model for the regulation of energy balance and adiposity by the central nervous system. Am J Clin Nutr 1999;69:584–594.

76. McCann SM, Kimura M, Walczewska A, et al. Hypothalamic control of FSH and LH by FSH-EF, LHRH, cytokines, leptin and nitric oxide. Neuroimmunomodulation 1998;5:193–202.

77. Susser M, Stein Z. Timimg in prenatal nutrition: a reprise of the Dutch Famine Study. Nutr Rev 1994;52:84–92.

78. Stein Z, Susser M. Famine and fertility. In: Mosley WH, ed. Nutrition and Human Reproduction. Plenum Press, New York, 1978, pp. 123–145.

79. Van Der Walt LA, Wilmsen EN, Jenkins T. Unusual sex hormone patterns among desert dwelling hunter gatherers. J Clin Endocrinol metab 1978;46:658–663.

80. Rabkin JG, Rabkin R, Wagner GJ. Testosterone treatment of clinical hypogonadism in patients with HIV/AIDS. Int J STD AIDS 1997;8:537–545.

81. Meyer-Bahlburg FH, et al. HIV positive gay men: sexual dysfunction Proc VI International Conference on AIDS 1989;701.

82. Casaburi R. Rehabilitative exercise training in chronic renal failure. In: Kopple JD, Massry SG, eds. Nutritional Management of Renal Disease. Williams and Wilkins, Baltimore, MD, 1998, pp. 817–841.

83. Barnea N, Drory Y, Iaina A, et al. Exercise tolerance in patients in chronic hemodialysis. Isr J Med Sci 1980;16:17–21.

84. Moore GE, Brinker KR, Tray-Gundersen J, et al. Determinants of VO2 peak in patients with end stage renal disease: on and off dialysis. Med Sci Sports Exerc 1993;25:18–23.

85. Painter PL. Exercise in end-stage renal disease. Exerc Sports Sci Rev 1988;16:305–339.

86. Robertson HT, Haley NR, Gutherie M, et al. Recombinant erythropeoitin improves exercise capacity in anemic hemodialysis patients. Am J Kid Dis 1990;4:325–332.

87. Bradley JR, Anderson JR, Evans DB, Cowley AJ. Impaired nutritive skeletal muscle blood flow in patients with chronic renal failure. Clin Sci (Lond) 1990;79:239–245.

88. Diesel W, Emms M, Knight BK, et al. Morphological features of the myopathy associated with chronic renal failure. Am J Kid Dis 1993;22:677–684.

89. Braubar N. Skeletal myopathy in uremia: abnormal energy metabolism. Kidney Int 1983;24:S81–S86.

90. Garber AJ. Skeletal muscle protein and amino acid metabolism in experimental chroni uremia in the rat. Accelerated alanine and glutamine formation and release. J Clin Invest 1978;61:623–632.

91. Kochakian CD. Comparison of protein anabolic properties of various androgens in the castrated rat. Am J Physiol 1950;60:553–558.

92. Kenyon AT, Knowlton K, Sandiford I, et al. A comparative study of the metabolic effects of testosterone propionate in normal men and women and in eunuchoidism. Endocrinology 1940;26:26–45.

93. Mauras N, Hayes V, Welch S, et al. Testosterone deficiency in young men: marked alterations in whole body protein kinetics, strength and adiposity. J Clin Endocrinol Metab 1998;83:1886.

94. Young NR, Baker HWG, Liu G, et al. Body composition and muscle strength in healthy men receiving testosterone enanthate for contraception. J Clin Endocrinol Metab 1993;77:1028–1032.

95. Griggs RC, Kingston W, Josefowicz RF, et al. Effect of testosterone on muscle mass and muscle protein synthesis. J Appl Physiol 1989;66:498–503.

96. Bardin, CW. The anabolic action of testosterone. N Engl J Med 1996;335:52,53.

97. Casaburi R, Goren S, Bhasin S. Substantial prevalence of low anabolic hormone levels in COPD patients undergoing rehabilitation. Am J Resp Crit Care Med 1996;153:A128.

98. Griggs RC, Pandya S, Florence JM, et al. Randomized controlled trial of testosterone in myotonic dystrophy. Neurology 1989;39:219–222.

99. Beal JE, Oldson R, Laubenstein L, et al. Dronabinol as a treatment for anorexia associated with weight loss in patients with AIDS. J. Pain Symptom Manag 1995;10:89–97.

100. Von Roenn JH, Armstrong D, Kotler DP, et al. Megestrol acetate in patients with AIDS-related cachexia. Ann Intern Med 1994;121:393–399.

101. Schambelan M, Mulligan K, Grunfeld C, et al. Recombinant growth horone in patients with HIV-associated wasting. Ann Intern Med 1996;125:873–882.

102. Waters D, Danska J, Hardy K, et al. Recombinant growth hormone, insulin-like growth factor-1, and combination therapy in AIDS-associated wasting. Ann Intern Med 1996;125:865–872.

103. Bhasin S, Storer TW, Javanbakht M, et al. Effects of testosterone replacement and resistance exercise on muscle strength, and body composition in human immunodeficiency virus-infected men with weight loss and low testosterone levels. JAMA 1999;in press.

104. Dobs A, Cofrancesco J, Nolten WE, et al. The use of a transscrotal testosterone delivery system in the treatment of patients with weight loss related to human immunodeficiency virus infection. Am J Med 1997;107:126–132.

105. Bucher G, Berger DS, Fields-Gardner C, et al. A prospective study on the safety and effect of nandrolone decanoate in HIV positive patients [abstract #Mo.B. 423] Int Conf AIDS 1996;11:26.

106. Gold J, High HA, Li Y, et al. Safety and efficacy of nandrolone decanoate for treatment of wasting in patients with HIV infection. AIDS 1996;10:745–752.

107. Berger JR, Pall L, Hall CD, et al. Oxandrolone in AIDS-wasting myopathy. AIDS 1995;10:1657–1662.

108. Hengge UR, Baumann M, Maleba R, et al. Oxymetholone promotes weight gain in patients with advanced human immunodeficiency virus (HIV-1) infection. Br J Nutr 1996;75:129–138.

109. Engelson ES, Rabkin JG, Rabkin R, et al. Effects of testosterone upon body composition. J AIDS 1996;11:510–511.

110. Coodley GO, Coodley MK. A trial of testosterone therapy for HIV-associated weight loss. AIDS 1997;11:1347–1352.

111. Strawford A, Barbieri T, Neese R, et al. Effects of nandrolone decanoate therapy in borderline hypogonadal men with HIV-associated weight loss. J AAIDS Hum Retrovirol 1999;20:137–146.

112. Strawford A, Barbieri T, Van Loan M, et al. Resistance exercise and supraphysiologic androgen therapy in eugonadal men with HIV-related weight loss. JAMA 1999;281:1282–1290.

113. Sattler FR, Jaque SV, Schroeder ET, et al. Effect of pharmacological doses of nandrolone decanoate and progressive resistance training in immunodeficient patients infected with the human immuno-deficiency virus. J Clin Endocrinol Metab 1999;84:1268–1276.

114. Roubenoff R, McDermott A, Weiss L, et al. Short-term progressive resistance training increases strength and lean body mass in adults infected with human immunodeficiency virus. AIDS 1999;13:231–239.

115. Reid IR, Wattie DJ. Evans MC, et al. Testosterone therapy in glucocorticoid-treated men. Arch. Intern. Med. 1996;156:1173–1177.

116. Reid IR, Ibbertson HK, France JT, et al. Plasma testosterone concentrations in asthmatic men treated with glucocorticoids. Br Med J 1985;291:574–577.

117. McAdams MR, White RH, Chipps BE. Reduction of serum testosrone levels during chronic gluco-corticoid therapy. Ann. Intern. Med. 1986;104:648–651.

118. Berns JS, Rudnick MR, Cohen RM. A controlled trial of recombinant erythropoieitin and nandrolone decanoate in the treatment of anemia in patients on chronic hemodialysis. Clin Nephrol 1992;37:264–267.

119. Buchwal D, Argyres S, Easterling RE, et al. Effect of nandrolone decanoate on the anemia of chronic hemodialysis patients. Nephron 1997;18:232–238.

120. Williams JL, Stein JH, Ferris TF. Nandrolone decanoate therapy for patients receiving hemodialysis. A controlled study. Arch Intern Med 1974;134:289–292.

121. Hendler ED, Goffinet JA, Ross S, et al. Controlled study of androgen therapy in anemia of patients on maintenance hemodialysis. N Engl J Med 1994;291:1046–1051.

122. Neff MS, Goldberg J, Slifkin RF, et al. A comparison of androgens for anemia in patients on hemo-dialysis. N Engl J Med 1981;304:871–875.

123. Pape GS, Friedman M, Underwood LE, et al. The effect of growth hormone on weight gain and pulmonary function in patients with chronic obstructive lung disease. Chest 1991;99:1495–1500.

124. Pichard C, Kyle U, Chevrolet JC. Lack of effects of recombinant growth hormone on muscle function in patients requiring prolonged mechaniscal ventilation: a prospective randomized controlled study. Crit Care Med 1996;24:403–413.

125. Schols AMW, Soeters PB, Mostert R. Physiologic effects of nutritional support and anabolic steroids in patients with chronic obstructive pulmonary disease. Am J Resp Crit Care Med 1995;152:1268–1274.

126. Seidell J, Bjorntorp P, Sjostrom L, et al. Visceral fat accumulation in men is positively associated with insulin, glucose and C-peptide levels, but negatively with testosterone levels. Metabolism 1990;39:897–901.

127. Barrett-Connors E, Khaw K-T. Endogenous sex-hormones and cardiovascular disease in men. A prospective population-based study. Circulation 1998;78:539–545.

128. Marin P, Oden B, Bjorntorp P. Assimilation and mobilization of triglycerides in subcutaneous ab-dominal and femoral adipose tissue in vivo in men: effects of androgens. J Clin Endocrinol Metab 1995;80:239–243.

129. Antonio J, Wilson JD, George FW. Effects of castration and androgen treatment on androgen-receptor levels in rat skeletal muscles. J Appl Physiol 1999;87:2016–2019.

130. Dahlberg E, Snochowski M, Gustafsson JA. Regulation of the androgen and glucocorticoid receptors in rat and mouse skeletal muscle cytosol. Endocrinology 1981;108:1431–1440.

131. Rance NE, Max SR. Modulation of the cytosolic androgen receptor in striated muscle by sex steroids. 1984;115:862–866.

132. Wilson CM, Kimberlin DF, Griffin JE, Wilson JD. Specificity of androgen resistance in Mus caroli kidney. Biochem Genet 1988;26:705–716.

133. Sinha-Hilim I, Artaza J, Woodhouse L, et al. Testosterone-induced increase in muscle size is asso-ciated with muscle fiber hypertrophy. Am J Physiol (Endo Metab). 2002; in press.

134. Saartok T, Dahlberg E, Gustaffsson JA. Relative binding affinity of anabolic-androgenic steroids, comparison of the binding to the androgen receptors in skeletal muscle and in prostate as well as sex hormone binding globulin. Endocrinology 1984;114:2100–2107.

135. Konagaya M, Max SR. A possible role for endogenous glucocorticoid in orchiectomy-induced atro-phy of the rat levator ani muscle: studies with RU38486, a potent glucocorticoid antagonist. J. Steroid Biochem. 1986;25:305–311.

136. Fryburg DA, Weltman A, Jahn LA, et al. Short-term modulation of the androgen milieu alters pulsatile, but not exercise- or growth hormone (GH)-releasing hormone-stimulated GH secretion in

healthy men: impact of gonadal steroid and GH secretory changes on metabolic outcomes. J Clin Endocrinol Metab 1997;82:3710–3719.

137. Leslie M, Forger NG, Breedlove SM. Sexual dimorphism and androgen effects on spinal motoneurons innervating the rat felxor digitorum brevis. Brain Res 1991;561:269–273.

138. Blanco CE, Popper P, Micevych P. Anabolic-androgenic steroid induced alterations in choline acetyltransferase messenger RNA levels of spinal cord motoneurons in the male rat. Neuroscience 1997;78:973–882.

139. Bartsch W, Krieg M, Voigt KD. Quantitation of endogenous testosterone, 5-alpha-dihydrotestosterone and 5-alpha-androstane-3-alpha, 17-beta-diol in subcellular fractions of the prostate, bulbocavernosus/levator ani muscle, skeletal muscle, and heart muscle of the rat. J Steroid Biochem 1980;13:259–267.

140. Sattler FR, Antonipillai I, Allen J, et al. Wasting and sex hormones: evidence for the role of dihydrotestosterone in AIDS patients with weight loss. Abstract Tu.B.2376 presented at the XI International Conference on AIDS. Vancouver, Canada, 1996.

23

Hormonal Male Contraception

Christina Wang, MD and Ronald S. Swerdloff, MD

PREDOMINANCE OF FEMALE-DIRECTED CONTRACEPTIVE METHODS

Currently, available female methods of contraception include the combined estrogen–progesterone oral contraceptive pill, progestin-only pills, 3-monthly depo-medroxyprogesterone acetate (DMPA) injections, levonorgestrel (LNG)-containing implants (Norplant), copper intrauterine devices, vaginal rings, female condoms, tubal ligation, menses inducers (mifepristone [RU486] and misoprostol [prostaglandin E_1]), and emergency contraception using estrogens. Other less effective methods include natural family planning, lactation amenorrhea, and vaginal spermicides. Recent pharmaceutical developments and introductions of new or improved methods include ultra-low-dose estrogen–progestin combination pills, emergency contraception with oral tablets containing LNG or mifepristone alone, combination of estradiol cypionate and DMPA monthly injections, low-dose LNG-releasing intrauterine devices, transdermal skin patches delivering low-dose estrogens plus progestins, single implant systems delivering etonorgestrel, and nesterone (a progestin) vaginal rings. These new methods will provide an even wider choice of contraceptive methods for women. Other female methods under preclinical or early clinical development include the following: immuno-contraception using antisperm antibodies, anti-zona-pellucida antibodies, or anti-hCG vaccine; new injectable progesterone esters; and new vaginal spermicides with antiviral activities that will provide dual protection (against pregnancy and sexually transmitted infections). In contrast, the currently male-controlled methods are limited to coitus interruptus, male condoms, and vasectomy.

From: *Endocrine Replacement Therapy in Clinical Practice*
Edited by: A. Wayne Meikle © Humana Press Inc., Totowa, NJ

CURRENTLY AVAILABLE MALE METHODS

Coitus interruptus requires high motivation and control. Male condoms are used by about 40–50 million men worldwide. They have the added advantage of protection against sexually transmitted diseases. Condoms can be used with spermicides with antiviral properties to increase protection. Although condoms are relatively inexpensive, the user failure rate of condoms is as high as 12% *(1)*, which is related both to lack of compliance as well as breakage. Nonlatex condoms have been developed to increase acceptability; however, condoms are not acceptable to many couples.

Vasectomy is a simple outpatient procedure. The morbidity associated with vasectomy has been dramatically reduced by the "no-scalpel technique" *(2)*. Acceptability of vasectomy as a birth control method has wide geographical variation. About 45 million men have been vasectomized worldwide. A high percentage of these men are from the United States, the United Kingdom, Australia, the Netherlands, China, Korea and Thailand. The contraceptive efficacy of vasectomy is very high, although azoospermia is not reached immediately because of the time required for clearance of the sperm through the ejaculatory system. This usually takes several weeks to months, depending on the frequency of ejaculations. Vasectomy is considered an irreversible method. Re-anastomoses when performed by skilled surgeons lead to reappearance of sperm in the ejaculate in more than 90% of men, but pregnancy in their partners occurs only in about 50% of vasovasostomy. Development of antisperm antibodies is the most likely cause of infertility after re-anastomoses. Newer developments in this field include percutaneous introduction of intravasal devices and percutaneous intravasal injection of cured-in-place silicone to halt sperm transport.

NONHORMONAL METHODS

Gossypol, a chemical agent derived from cottonseed oil, was studied in more than 8000 men in China in the 1970s *(3)*. Gossypol acts directly on the testes, affecting spermatogenesis and leading to spermatogenic arrest and irreversible damage to germ cells. Because of the high incidence of irreversibility and the potential of causing hypokalemia in some men, studies on gossypol have been largely discontinued in China and most other parts of the world *(4)*.

Agents with action in the postmeiotic spermatozoa or in the epididymis may decrease the function and/or number of sperm and cause infertility. Such agents will have a quicker onset of action and will not disturb the subjects' hormonal milieu. Examples of such agents include α-chlorohydrin and the 6 chloro-6-deoxy sugars. Although active in the epididymal spermatozoa leading to infertility, these agents were discarded as potential leads because of unacceptable toxicity. Other agents active in the epididymis or postmeiotic spermatogenesis include the proton pump ATPase inhibitors and imidazoles. There is a research network of investigators who are focusing their efforts on finding a male contraceptive agent that has the target action on the epididymis. No such agent has been tested in clinical studies *(5)*.

In the 1980s, investigators in China noted that a multiglycoside extract of the plant *Tripterygium wilfordii* (used in Chinese traditional medicine for psoriasis, rheumatoid arthritis) caused decrease sperm motility and concentrations in male patients. Studies in rats confirmed that administration of this multiglycoside results in marked reduction in sperm motility, suggesting that tripterygium may have its antifertility effect on the epididymis or postmeiotic sperm *(6,7)*. One of the active principles from *Tripterygium wilfordii*, triptolide has been purified and tested in fertility studies in rats. When the animals were dosed for 70 d with the pure compound triptolide, sperm motility was markedly lowered, with a small decrease in sperm concentration. However, on extending the studies to dosing for two spermatogenic cycles, triptolide caused significant suppressive effects on spermatogenesis in addition to its effect on decreasing motility of epididymal spermatozoa. The infertility of some of the treated animals was not reversible, suggesting permanent damage to the germinal epithelium *(8,9)*. These more recent findings have decreased the potential of triptolide as a reversible male contraceptive.

HORMONAL METHODS

Hormonal methods are based on reversible suppression of gonadotropins, testicular steroid, and sperm production (*see* Fig. 1). Many hormonal methods have been tested in clinical trials and represent the most promising lead in a new method of contraception for men *(10–13)*.

Hormonal Regulation of Spermatogenesis

Spermatogenesis is a highly organized process involving germ cell proliferation, maturation, and death. The spermatogonia undergo multiplication (mitosis) to become spermatocytes. Two meiotic divisions occur yielding haploid spermatids. The spermatids then undergo a complex process of differentiation called spermiogenesis during which the acrosome and flagellum were formed. The developmental processes are arranged in defined cell association or stages of the seminiferous epithelium. These stages follow one another in a regular fashion, giving rise to a wave of germ cell maturation and differentiation. In the human, the average length of the seminiferous epithelium cycle is about 73 d *(14)*. Throughout the process of spermatogenesis, the germ cells are enveloped by the surrounding Sertoli cells. The Sertoli cells and germ cells cross-communicate via hormones, many paracrine factors, and signals, some of which are not clearly defined.

The mature spermatid is then released into the tubular lumen by a process called spermiation. The spermatids pass through the ductus efferentia and rete testes to the epididymis. During the transit through the epididymis, the spermatozoa mature, acquiring both fertilizing capacity and motility, probably through maturational changes in the cell membrane induced by proteins and other substances. The transit of the spermatozoa from the testes through the vas deferens to the ejaculatory ducts takes about 14 d. Secretions from the prostate and seminal fluid contribute about 80% of the seminal fluid volume.

Spermatogenesis in man is regulated by testosterone produced by the Leydig cells in the interstitium and by the gonadotropin, follicle-stimulating hormone (FSH). Both testosterone and FSH act on the germ cells probably indirectly via the Sertoli cells. Testosterone secretion is regulated by luteinizing hormone (LH) produced by the anterior pituitary gland. Both LH and FSH are secreted in a pulsatile fashion under the regulation of the gonadotropin-releasing hormone (GnRH). GnRH secretion by the hypothalamus is, in turn, regulated by a complicated network of neuropeptides and neurotransmitters. In man, it is generally accepted that both FSH and testosterone (LH) are required for initiation of spermatogenesis. Once initial maturation is induced, test-

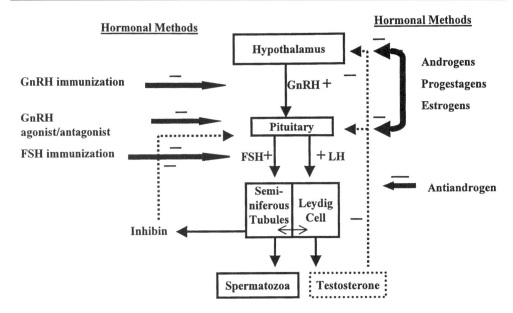

Fig. 1. Hormonal basis of male contraception.

osterone is required for the maintenance of spermatogenesis. Studies in men provided evidence that testosterone alone supports qualitatively normal sperm production, but both FSH and testosterone are required to maintain qualitatively and quantitatively normal spermatogenesis *(15,16)*. Recent studies from FSH-receptor knockout mice and spontaneous FSH-receptor mutations in men cast doubt on the obligatory role of FSH in the regulation of spermatogenesis. In the FSH-receptor-deficient mice/humans, spermatogenesis proceeds normally, albeit in some mice/humans the sperm production is low or compromised *(17,18)*.

Leydig cell dysfunction results in low testosterone production and elevated LH levels because of decreased negative feedback on the hypothalamus–pituitary axis. Similarly, germ cell/Sertoli cell dysfunction results in low inhibin production and elevated FSH secretion because of attenuated negative feedback on the hypothalamic–pituitary system. In addition to the gonadotropins, a large number of growth factors, cytokines and other peptides are secreted by cells within the testis (e.g., Sertoli cells, Leydig cells, peritubular myoid cells, and macrophages) that form a complex cross-communication system between germ cells and their somatic counterparts. The exact role of each of these factors in the regulation of spermatogenesis in vivo is not clear.

Androgens (see Table 1)

Testosterone Enanthate Efficacy Studies

In the 1970s, clinical studies on male hormonal methods of contraception began using testosterone enanthate (TE) as the hormonal prototype. Short-term (4 to 6 mo) studies showed that TE administered at a weekly dose of 200 or 250 mg intramuscularly induced azoospermia in 40–60% of normal men. Oligozoospermia (defined as sperm concentration of less than 5×10^6/mL) was achieved in 90–95% of men *(19–23)*. If the interval between 200 mg intramuscular TE injections was increased to 14 d, then only 45–65%

Table 1
Androgens Alone for Male Contraception

Injectables
 Testosterone enanthate (TE)
 19-Nortestosterone
 Testosterone undecanoate (TU injection)[a]
 Testosterone buciclate (TB)
 Testosterone microspheres
Implants
 Testosterone pellets
 7α-Methyl-19 nortestosterone (MENT)
Oral
 Testosterone undecanoate[b]
 Selective androgen-receptor modulators
Transdermal
 Testosterone patches (nonscrotal)
 Testosterone gel

Note: Agents in italics are not available in the market.
[a]Available in China only.
[b]Not available in the United States.

of the men would reach oligozoospermia. In some studies, suppression of spermatogenesis was initially induced by weekly injections of TE and followed by spacing the frequency of TE injections to 2–4 wk. These regimens were unsuccessful because sperm production increased to above oligozoospermic levels when the interval between injections was increased to more than 10 d *(23)*. In all of these studies, upon discontinuation of treatment, gonadotropins and sperm counts returned to normal.

In 1985, based on the findings of these early studies, the World Health Organization (WHO) started a multicenter study to determine whether testosterone-induced azoospermia would provide effective contraception. TE was chosen as the prototype hormonal method because of its known efficacy, safety, and reversibility in humans. The study included 271 couples in 10 centers in seven countries. During the suppression phase of up to 6 mo, 200 mg of TE was administered weekly by intramuscular injections until azoospermia was demonstrated in three consecutive semen analyses. The couple then entered the 12-mo efficacy phase during which the TE regimen was continued and no other methods of contraception was used. The study showed that at the end of 6 months of TE administration, 64% of the men had persistent azoospermia. When these couples with azoospermic male partners entered the efficacy phase, there was only one pregnancy during 1846 mo of coital exposure. This represented an efficacy rate (Pearl rate) of 0.8 (95% confidence interval: 0.02–4.5) per 100 person-years, which is equivalent or better than existing methods of reversible female or male available contraceptive methods *(24)*. A difference existed in the efficacy rate in centers with predominantly Asian compared to white subjects in that 91% of men in the three Asian centers achieved azoospermia compared to the 50–60% azoospermia in centers whose subjects were predominantly whites *(24)*. The ethnic differences in the suppression of spermatogenesis by androgens were also noted in the androgen plus progestagen combinations. It had been suggested that Asian men may have lower spermatogenic potential *(25)*, and increased germ cell apoptosis *(26)*, as well as an increased sensitivity of the suppression of pulsatile LH secretion in response to exogenous testosterone administration *(27)*.

A second study was designed to determine whether men rendered severely oligozoospermic (defined as sperm concentration less than 3×10^6/mL) by 200 mg weekly intramuscular TE administration would also be infertile. The answer to this question was considered very important because, to date, none of the potential hormonal methods of male contraception tested in adequate numbers of men could completely suppress spermatogenesis (azoospermia) in all men. When the sperm concentration was suppressed to less than 3×10^6/mL in three consecutive semen samples, then the couple would enter an efficacy phase of 12 mo. The testosterone-induced severe oligozoospermia contraceptive efficacy study included 399 couples from 15 centers in nine countries (sponsored by WHO and by Contraceptive Research and Development Program in the United States). Of the subjects, 98% achieved severe oligozoospermia or azoospermia after 6 mo of TE injections and entered the efficacy phase. There were four pregnancies in 49.5 person-years of exposure in men who had a sperm concentration between 0.1 and 3×10^6/mL and none in the 230.4 person-years of observation in men who had persistent azoospermia. The combined contraceptive efficacy rate was 1.4 (95% confidence interval: 0.4–3.7) per 100 person-years. The occurrence of pregnancies was proportional to the sperm concentration in the ejaculate. Once azoospermia or severe oligozoospermia was attained, rebound of sperm concentration to above 3×10^6/mL was very uncommon *(28)*. These two studies *(24,28)* demonstrated for the first time that if a hormonal method of male contraception can render most of the men azoospermic and the remainder severely oligozoospermic, such a method would provide efficacious contraception in the couple. In these studies, as in the previous ones, all couples attained complete recovery of spermatogenesis after withdrawal of TE.

Administration of TE as a weekly injection is clearly not a practical or acceptable method of contraceptive delivery. Moreover, the pharmacokinetic profile of TE with high initial serum testosterone levels followed by troughs is not the ideal for male fertility regulation. It is perceived that steady levels of testosterone might be associated with less side effects, such as acne, oiliness of skin and weight gain.

OTHER ANDROGENS

Other androgen delivery systems are currently being tested or developed that may be more acceptable as a male contraceptive agent. Testosterone implants when inserted into normal volunteers led to suppression of spermatogenesis with similar efficacy as TE weekly injections provided that the serum testosterone levels are maintained in the high normal range with six 200-mg pellets *(29)*. Testosterone biodegradable microspheres when administered to hypogonadal men provided steady serum levels for up to 70 d *(30)*. These microspheres are technically more difficult to produce without batch-to-batch variations and leeching of testosterone from the microspheres. Testosterone buciclate is a product developed jointly by WHO and the National Institutes of Health. Studies in normal men showed that a single 600-mg injection provided testosterone levels within the physiological range for 16–20 wk *(31)*. When a 1200-mg single injection of testosterone buciclate was administered to eight healthy men, azoospermia was achieved in only three men *(32)*. Testosterone buciclate is still undergoing tests to determine the toxicology of the side chain.

With the recent development of transdermal testosterone delivery systems, testosterone patches have been also tested in hormonal contraceptive studies either alone or in combination with progestins. The use of the transdermal patch has not been found to provide sufficient suppression of spermatogenesis either alone or in combination with progestins *(33,34)*. The newly available testosterone gel can maintain serum testosterone levels in the high normal range and has the potential of being exploited in male contraceptive development *(35)*.

TESTOSTERONE UNDECANOATE INJECTIONS

Testosterone undecanoate (TU) as an oral pill was available for many years in Europe, Asia, and Australia as androgen replacement in hypogonadal men. Studies in China showed that when TU was formulated in oil, a single 500- or 1000-mg intramuscular injection resulted in normal serum testosterone levels in hypogonadal men for about 4–6 wk *(36)*. Subsequently studies in Europe showed in repeated dosing studies that after 1000 mg TU, serum testosterone levels in hypogonadal men can be maintained for 8–12 wk *(37,38)*. Investigators in China reported that administration of TU 500 mg and 1000 mg intramuscularly once every 4 wk, led to azoospermia in 11/12 volunteers in the 500-mg group and all volunteers in the 1000-mg group, respectively (39). Serum trough testosterone concentrations remained in the normal range but were significantly higher than baseline in the group receiving TU 1000 mg intramuscularly monthly. The efficacy of TU was confirmed in white men who were administered TU 1000 mg once every 6 wk, and 8 out of the 14 became azoospermic and another 4 severely oligozoospermic *(40)*. After these preliminary studies, an unpublished study with 300 men showed that azoospermia was achieved in almost all men when TU was administered at monthly intervals (Gu, personal communication). These studies lead to the use of TU in combination with other agents in recent clinical trials and prepare the way for a large phase III contraceptive development study to be conducted in China.

POTENTIAL ADVERSE EFFECTS OF ANDROGENS

The common side effects of androgen administration in normal men included weight gain, acne, gynecomastia, decreases in serum high-density lipoprotein (HDL) cholesterol levels and increases in hematocrit *(41)*. Most of the effects are mild and apparently well tolerated by the subjects participating in the clinical studies. The long-term effects of maintaining relatively high serum testosterone levels in normal men are not known. Testosterone administration leads to a decrease in HDL cholesterol levels in some studies without any effect on low-density lipoprotein (LDL) cholesterol levels in white men *(42,43)*. Lower HDL cholesterol levels are associated with increased risk of coronary heart disease. Epidemiological studies, however, showed that lower testosterone levels in men are related to increased risk factors for cardiovascular disease *(44,45)*. There are clearly many factors that may also be involved, such as other lipoproteins, coagulation factors, fibrinolytic pathways, endothelial cell response, and vascular reactivity. The other major concern with use of androgens is the induction of prostate dysfunction. There is no clear evidence that androgens will induce benign prostatic hyperplasia (BPH) or carcinoma of the prostate (CaP) *(46,47)*. Although androgens are required in childhood and adulthood for BPH to develop, there is no evidence that administration of androgens to normal or hypogonadal men will result in BPH. When androgens are given to hypogonadal men, the prostate size and prostate-specific antigen (PSA) levels increased to those of normal men. Prostate size and serum level PSA, however, remained within the normal range *(48,49)*. The development of CaP and the progression from focal to metastatic disease is very complex. Factors that are involved include gene mutations, oncogenes, tumor suppression genes, growth factors, the number of trinucleotide repeats of the androgen receptor, and androgens *(46,50,51)*. There is no clear evidence to demonstrate that exogenous androgens will lead to the development of CaP or progression of histological to clinical disease. These concerns of long-term androgen therapy can only be addressed when male hormonal contraceptive agents become available by long-term follow-up and epidemiological studies.

DESIGNER ANDROGENS

Because of these concerns, an androgen which cannot be 5α reduced but can be aromatized might attenuate the effects on the prostate. One such potential androgen is 7α-methyl-19 nortestosterone (MENT). This androgen is about 10 times as potent as testosterone on gonadotropin suppression but only 4 times as active on stimulation of prostate size in castrated rats and monkeys *(52,53)*. MENT is being formulated as a subcutaneous implant and has been shown to be able to maintain sexual function and mood in hypogonadal men *(54)* and to suppress gonadotropins in healthy young men *(55)*. With the recent advances in the understanding and discovery of coactivators and corepressors regulating the transcription of the androgen receptor, several of selective androgen agonists and antagonists are being developed by industry. These agents may be steroidal or nonsteroidal compounds and may process tissue selectivity similar to the selective estrogen receptor modulators. It is foreseeable that an androgen agonist can be developed that has marked gonadotropin suppressive activity with less potent effects on the prostate and lipoproteins.

Androgen and Progestin Combinations (see *Table 2*)

INJECTABLE PROGESTINS

Progestins suppress the hypothalamic–pituitary axis when administered to normal men. Because of the concomitant suppression of endogenous testosterone production, progestins are always used together with androgens to prevent the manifestation of hypogonadism. Many androgen–progestin combinations were used in single or multicenter, small, clinical trials supported by the WHO or the Population Council *(21,56)*. The most promising progesterone was DMPA in combination with TE or 19-nortestosterone. The combination of injections of DMPA and 19-nortestosterone at 3-weekly intervals led to suppression of spermatogenesis to azoospermia in about 60% of normal white men *(57)* but led to azoospermia in 97% of Indonesian men *(58)*. There were relatively few side effects; libido and erectile functions were retained. The main side effects included weight gain, gynecomastia and lowering of HDL cholesterol levels. DMPA (300 mg) intramuscularly has also been studied in combination with testosterone pellets. The study demonstrated that a single DMPA injection enhanced the suppression of sperm concentration to azoospermia induced by four 200-mg testosterone pellets, a dose that is suboptimal for spermatogenic suppression in white men *(59)*.

More recently, norethisterone (norethindrone in the United States) enanthate (NET-EN) 200 mg intramuscularly was shown to suppress serum gonadotropins and testosterone levels in normal men *(60)*. In combination with TU 1000 mg every 6 wk, NET-EN 200 mg achieved suppression of sperm concentration to azoospermia in 13 out of 14

Table 2
Androgens and Progestin Combinations

Oral
Levonorgestrel + TE or TU injections, T patches, T pellets
Desogestrel + TE, T pellets
Implants
Levonorgestrel (Norplant II) + TE, T patch, T pellets
Etonorgestrel (Implanon) + T pellets
Injectables
Depo-medroxyprogesterone acetate + TE, 19 norT, T pellets
Norethisterone enanthate + TU injections

Androgens and Progestins with Antiandrogenic Activity
Cyproterone acetate + TE, TU tablets and injections

Note: T, testosterone.

volunteers compared to 7 out of 14 in the TU-alone group *(61)*. The combination also caused weight gain and decreased serum HDL-cholesterol levels but has more favorable injection intervals and efficacy. This combination is being studied in other centers to confirm the preliminary results and to seek longer injection intervals and lower doses of both the androgen and the progestin.

ORAL PROGESTINS

The use of androgens plus oral progestins was also demonstrated to have significant advantage over the use of the same dose of androgen alone. The combination of 500 μg daily of oral LNG with 100-mg weekly intramuscular injections of TE, was significantly more effective and had a more rapid suppression of sperm concentration to less than 3×10^6/mL than TE alone *(62)*. It is apparent that combinations of androgens and progestins may allow lowering the doses of both androgens and progestins to achieve equivalent goals. The combination of LNG plus TE suppressed HDL cholesterol by 24% and total cholesterol by 6%. Lowering the dose of LNG reduces the changes in lipoproteins and weight gain without compromising the efficacy of suppression of sperm output *(63)*. These and other investigators also studied desogestrel together with TE injections and found similar effects on spermatogenesis suppression and effects on lipids *(64,65)*. Desogestrel administered orally with testosterone implants were also very efficacious *(66)*. It should be noted that when oral LNG (250 μg) was used with the transdermal testosterone patch delivering 5 mg testosterone per day, the combination was not effective in suppressing spermatogenesis *(33)*. Moreover, when oral LNG was given in combination with 1000 mg TU, the oral LNG had minimal enhancement of gonadotropins and spermatogenesis suppression compared to TU alone *(40)*. These data suggest that the dose or the route of testosterone is important in determining whether androgens have an additive effect on progestins. These studies underscore the importance of the androgen component in androgen–progestin combinations in achieving the optimal spermatogenic suppression.

PROGESTIN IMPLANTS

Long acting progestin implants (Norplant) may attain the same effect but have the added advantage of maintaining steady serum progestin levels and obliterating the first-pass effect of oral progestins on liver lipoprotein metabolism. We have studied Norplant II (four capsules, each releasing approx 40 µg LNG per day) in combination with testosterone patches and showed enhancement of spermatogenic suppression by Norplant but not to optimally low sperm concentration for contraceptive efficacy. The combination of Norplant II with 100 mg TE weekly injections was very effective resulting in azoospermia in most subjects and severe oligozoospermia in all subjects *(34)*. Our study also confirms the important role of androgens for suppression of spermatogenesis in these hormonal combinations. Similar studies using Norplant II and etonorgestrel with testosterone implants are in progress in our center and other centers. These studies aim to develop a long-acting subcutaneous implantable contraceptive for men.

PROGESTINS WITH ANTIANDROGENIC ACTIVITY IN COMBINATION WITH ANDROGENS (*SEE* TABLE 2)

Early studies of cyproterone acetate (CPA; an antiandrogen with progestational activity), showed that when CPA was given alone to normal men, suppression of spermatogenesis was incomplete and a marked decrease in sexual function was associated with the administration of this antiandrogen *(67)*. Subsequent studies in India suggested that the combination of CPA and TE resulted in the alleviation of symptoms of androgen insufficiency and marked suppression of sperm concentration *(68)*. These studies were confirmed in a recent study using a combination of CPA (50 or 100 mg/d) plus TE, which induced azoospermia or near-azoospermia in all subjects. This combination had the advantage of no demonstratable effects on lipid profile and the possibility of lesser effects on the prostate gland *(69)*. However when CPA was combined with oral undecanoate, the suppression of spermatogenesis was reduced, and azoospermia was observed in two out of eight men (70). High-dose CPA, because of its antiandrogenic activity, decreases hematocrit and may have other possible deleterious effects on maintenance of muscle and bone mass. A lower dose of CPA (20 mg/d) had an efficacy similar to a higher dose in suppressing spermatogenesis *(71)*.

Androgens and Estrogens

Androgens in combination with estradiol have been tested in rats and monkeys and induced suppression of spermatogenesis *(72)*. The advantage of using estrogens would be to neutralize the effects of androgens on lipids. Estrogens have been shown to have synergestic effects with testosterone on prostate growth in dogs. Whether estrogens would have synergistic effects with androgens on growth of prostate is not known. A clinical study of androgen plus estrogen implants showed that addition of low-dose estradiol did not significantly enhance the suppressive effects of testosterone. Higher doses of estradiol may produce adverse effects of androgen deficiency or estrogen excess, and the effects of estradiol on sperm suppression had a low therapeutic window *(73)*.

GnRH Analogs and Testosterone (see *Table 3*)

Gonadotropin-releasing hormone agonists cause an initial and transient stimulation of gonadotropin secretion followed by progressive pituitary desensitization to GnRH with consequent suppression of FSH and LH secretion. The use of GnRH agonists (D-

Table 3
Other Nonsteroidal Hormonal Methods
of Contraception (Gonadotropin Suppressors
With or Without Androgens)

GnRH Agonists (D-Trp[6], Buserelin, Nafarelin)
Low dose
High dose
Continuous infusion
GnRH antagonist (Nal-Glu, Cetrorelix)
GnRH immunization
FSH immunization
FSH receptor antagonist
FSH antagonists
Inhibin

Trp[6], Buserelin, Nafarelin) together with testosterone had been studied in 12 clinical studies involving over 106 white normal men. The results of these studies were summarized recently *(10)*. When GnRH agonist was administered with varying doses of TE, spermatogenesis was suppressed to azoospermia in only 20% of subjects; another 30% had sperm concentrations reduced to less than 5×10^6/mL. To determine the role of treatment paradigms, GnRH agonists were administered by daily subcutaneous injections or continuous infusions. The latter was not more successful in suppressing spermatogenesis *(74–76)*. Several possible mechanisms could explain the failure of GnRH agonists to completely inhibit spermatogenesis. First, the highest agonist dose used in human clinical trials was 500 μg/d, (such a dose might not be optimal). Second, serum FSH levels were less suppressed than LH. Moreover, escape of serum FSH sometimes occurred during GnRH agonist treatment. Third, there was controversy over whether androgens when administered with GnRH agonists enhanced or attenuated the spermatogenic suppression induced by GnRH agonists. There was evidence both in primates and humans to demonstrate that exogenous androgens at high doses might interfere with the spermatogenic suppression of GnRH agonists *(77,78)*. On the other hand, synergism between GnRH agonists and testosterone had also been reported to occur in rats and humans *(79,80)*. A two-center study to examine whether higher doses (1–3 mg/d) of GnRH agonist (D-Trp[6]) together with low-dose TE will increase the efficacy of the suppression of spermatogenesis showed insufficient suppression of spermatogenesis to the level of acceptable contraceptive efficacy even with such high doses of GnRH agonists (unpublished data). The advantages of GnRH agonists include the lack of side effects of this group of agents and relative lower costs of synthesis compared with the antagonists.

In contrast to GnRH agonists, the GnRH antagonists interfere with the action of the endogenous hormone by competitive binding at the pituitary receptor sites. Through this action, pituitary FSH and LH secretion is rapidly and completely suppressed, resulting in a reduction of endogenous testosterone production and inhibition of spermatogenesis. These agents were also different from the agonists in that they were expensive to synthesize and frequently gave rise to local reactions at the injection sites, presumably related to the release of histamine from the mast cells. Three human trials studied the potential of the Nal-Glu GnRH antagonists in combination with various doses of TE as male contraceptives *(81–83)*. Azoospermia was achieved in 60–88% of men administered GnRH antagonists. The time to azoospermia appeared to occur earlier than with androgens alone. Upon withdrawal of the GnRH antagonist and TE, complete recovery of spermatogenesis occurred. The Nal-Glu GnRH antagonists induced pain, redness and weal formation at the injection sites. A new GnRH antagonist, Cetrorelix, has been studied in short-term clinical studies *(84,85)*. This GnRH antagonist apparently has little or no local side effects. A recently completed study showed that if azoospermia or severe oligozoospermia was induced by the GnRH antagonist plus TE, the suppression of spermatogenesis could be maintained by the physiological dose of TE (100 mg/wk) alone *(86)*. The results of this study are important because this suggests that once suppression of gonadotropins occurred, continued suppression might require less amounts of hormonally based gonadotropin suppressive agents. A more recent study with fewer men and using a loading followed by a reduced dose of another GnRH antagonist (Cetrorelix) showed failure of maintenance of suppression of gonadotropins and sperm production by a low dose of 19-nor testosterone alone *(87)*. The reason for the failure of maintenance of suppression is not clear but may be related to the use of 19-nor testosterone, which is not aromatizable. Future of studies with GnRH antagonists may be dependent on the development of orally or long-acting, possibly nonpeptide GnRH antagonists by molecular drug modeling which might be safer, more acceptable, and more economical than the peptide analogs.

Gonadotropin-releasing hormone vaccines are also under development and have been tested only in men with prostate cancer. No studies in healthy men had been reported.

Selective FSH Inhibition

Selective FSH inhibition as a male contraceptive is attractive because only spermatogenesis would be suppressed sparing the LH–testosterone axis. This approach has been explored in FSH immunization studies in nonhuman primates. The results were disappointing either because azoospermia was not attained or the suppression of spermatogenesis was not persistent *(88,89)*. Inhibin, which selectively inhibits FSH, has not been examined in humans for sperm suppression. Other investigators are making and studying FSH-receptor antagonists. However, based on the study of men with inactivating mutations of the human FSH receptor, selective inhibition of FSH or FSH action probably would not result in marked or consistent suppression of spermatogenesis. These men with FSH-receptor mutations have varying phenotypes from infertility to proven fertility *(18)*.

FUTURE DEVELOPMENTS IN HORMONAL METHODS OF MALE CONTRACEPTION

In the past decade, significant advances in male contraception development have occurred. It has been shown that if suppression of spermatogenesis to azoospermia (or severe oligozoospermia) is achieved by exogenous administration of hormones, contraceptive efficacy can be attained with rates comparable to female reversible methods. Furthermore, the addition of a gonadotropin-suppressive agent to androgen will enhance the degree and rate of suppression of spermatogenesis by androgen alone, suggesting that lower and close to physiological doses of androgens may be used when administered in a combination regimen. New synthetic steroids with long-acting potential and more selective actions will become available for clinical investigation in the near future.

In the next decade, there will be many new preparations and delivery systems for androgens. Selective orally active androgen receptor modulators will be synthesized that may have strong gonadotropin-suppressive activity, the ability to maintain sexual function and bone and muscle mass but will have little or no effect on serum lipid profile and the prostate gland. Orally active or long-acting nonpeptide GnRH antagonists, with potent receptor-blocking activity but without side effects, may become available. Various mechanisms to shorten the lag time (10–14 wk) between the start of hormone administration and the suppression of spermatogenesis need to be investigated. The combination of an agent acting directly on the epididymis or on spermiogenesis or more mature germ cells (spermatids) might be used concomitantly with a hormonal method initially to accelerate the development of azoospermia. Studies need to be designed to assess which potential method or modes of administration of contraceptive agents might be acceptable to men from different cultural, ethnic, and geographical backgrounds.

ACKNOWLEDGMENTS

This work was supported by the GCRC grant M01 RR00425, NIH training grant DK07571, and the Contraceptive Research and Development Program. We thank Sally Avancena, MA for her assistance in the preparation of the manuscript.

REFERENCES

1. Trussel J, Kost K. Contraceptive failure in the United States: a critical review of literature. Studies Fam Plan 1987;18:237–283.
2. Liu X, Li S. Vasal sterilization in China. Contraception 1993;48:255–265.
3. National Coordinating Group on Male Antifertility Agents. Gossypol: a new antifertility agent for males. Chinese Med J 1978;4:417–428.
4. Meng GD, Zhu JC, Chen ZW, et al. Recovery to normal sperm production following cessation of gossypol treatment: A two center study in China. Int J Androl 1988;11:1–11.
5. Cooper TG. Epididymal approaches to male contraception. In: Robaire B, Chemes H, Morales CR, eds. Andrology in the 21st Century. Medimond, Montreal, 2001, pp. 499–509.
6. Qian SZ. Tripterygium Wilfordii: a Chinese herb effective in male fertility regulation. Contraception 1987;36:247–263.
7. Qian SZ, Xu Y, Zhang JW. Recent progress in research on tripterygium: a male antifertility plant. Contraception 1995;51:121–129.
8. Lue YH, Sinha-Hikim AP, et al. Triptolide: a potential male contraceptive. J Androl 1998;19:479–486.
9. Huynh PN, Sinha Hikim AP, Wang C, et al. Long-term effects of triptolide on spermatogenesis, epididymal sperm function and fertility in male rats. J Androl 2000;21:689–699.
10. Cummings DE, Bremner WJ. Prospects for new hormonal male contraceptives. Endocrinol and Metabol Clin N Am 1994:22:893–922.
11. Wang C, Swerdloff RS, Waites GMH. Male contraception: 1993 and beyond. In: Van Look PFA, Perez-Palacio, eds. Contraceptive Research and Development 1984 to 1994, Oxford University Press, Delhi, 1994, pp. 121–134.
12. Wang C, Swerdloff RSS. Male contraception in the 21st century. In: C Wang, ed, Male Reproductive Function. Kluwer Academic Publishers, Norwell, MA, 1999, pp. 303–319.
13. Nieschlag E, Behre, HM. Testosterone and male contraception. In: Nieschlag E, Behre HM, eds. Testosterone Action, Deficiency and Substitution. Springer-Verlag, Berlin, 1998, pp. 513–528.
14. Clermont Y. The cycle of seminiferous epithelium in man. Am J Anat 1963;112:35–51.
15. Matsumoto AM, Paulsen CA, Bremner WJ. Stimulation of sperm production by human luteinizing hormone in gonadotropin-suppressed normal men. J Clin Endocrinol Metab 1984;59:882–885.
16. Matsumoto AM, Karpas AE, Bremner WJ. Chronic human chorionic gonadotropin administration in normal men: evidence that follicle stimulating hormone is necessary for maintenance of quantitatively normal spermatogenesis in man. J Clin Endocrinol Metab 1986;62:1184–1192.

17. Kumar TR, Wang Y, Lu N, Matzuk MM. Follicle stimulating hormone is required for ovarian follicle maturation but not male fertility. Nat Genet 1997;15:201–204.
18. Tapanainen JA, Ailtomaki K, Min J, et al. Men homozygous for an inactivating mutation of the follicle-stimulating hormone (FSH) receptor gene present variable suppression of spermatogenesis and fertility. Nat Genet 1997;15:205,206.
19. Cunningham GR, Silverman VE, Kohler DO. Clinical evaluation of testosterone enanthate for induction and maintenance of reversible azoospermia in man. In: Patanelli DJ, ed. Hormonal Control of Male Fertility. US DHEW, Bethesda, MD, 1978, pp. 71–92.
20. Mauss J, Borsch G, Bormacher K, et al. Seminal fluid analyses, serum FSH, LH and testosterone in seven males before, during and after 250 mg testosterone enanthate weekly over 21 weeks. In: Patanelli DJ, ed. Hormonal Control of Male Fertility. US DHEW, Bethesda, MD, 1978, pp. 93–122.
21. Paulsen CA, Bremner WJ, Leonard JM. Male Contraception: Clinical Trials. In: Mishell DR Jr, ed. Raven Press, New York, 1982, pp. 157–170.
22. Swerdloff RS, Palacios A, McClure RD, et al. Clinical evaluation of testosterone enanthate in the reversible suppression of spermatogenesis in the human male: efficacy, mechanism of action, and adverse effects. In: Patanelli DJ, ed. Hormonal Control of Male Fertility. US DHEW, Bethesda, MD, 1978, pp. 41–70.
23. Patanelli DJ, ed. Hormonal Control of Male Fertility. US DHEW, Bethesda, MD, 1978.
24. World Health Organization Task Force on Methods for the Regulation of Male Fertility. Contraceptive efficacy of testosterone-induced azoospermia in normal men. Lancet 1990;336:955–959.
25. Johnson L, Barnard JJ, Rodriguez L, et al. Ethnic difference in testicular structure and spermatogenic potential may predispose testes of Asian men to a heightened sensitivity to steroidal contraceptives. J Androl 1998;19:348–357.
26. Sinha-Hikim A, Wang C, Lue YH, et al. Spontaneous germ cell apoptosis in human: evidence for ethnic differences in the susceptability of germ cells to programmed cell death. J Clin Endocrinol Metab 1998;83:152–156.
27. Wang C, Berman NG, Veldhuis JD, Der T, McDonald V, Steiner B, Swerdloff RS. Graded testosterone infusions distinguish gonadotropin negative feedback responsiveness in Asian and White men—a Clinical Research Center Study. J Clin Endocrinol Metab 1998;83:870–876.
28. World Health Organization Task Force on Methods for the Regulation of Male Fertility. Contraceptive efficacy of testosterone-induced azoospermia and oligozoospermia in normal men. Fertil Steril 1996;65:821–829.
29. Handelsman DJ, Conway AJ, Boylan LM. Suppression of human spermatogenesis by testosterone implants in man. J Clin Endocrinol Metab 1992;75:1326–1332.
30. Bhasin S, Swerdloff RS, Steiner B, et al. A biodegradable testosterone microcapsule formulation provides uniform eugonadal levels of testosterone for 10 to 11 weeks in hypogonadal men. J Clin Endocrinol Metab 1992;74:75–83.
31. Behre HM, Nieschlag E. Testosterone buciclate (20 Act-1) in hypogonadal men: pharmacokinetics and pharmacodynamics of the new long-acting androgen ester. J Clin Endocrinol Metab 1992;75:12.
32. Behre HM, Baus S, Kliesch S, et al. Potential of testosterone buciclate for male contraception: endocrine differences betwen responders and non-responders. J Clin Endocrinol Metab 1995;80:2394–2403.
33. Buchter D, von Eckardstein S, von Eckardstein A, et al. Clinical trial of transdermal testosterone and oral levonorgestrel for male contraception. J Clin Endocrinol Metab 1999;84:1244–1249.
34. Gaw Gonzalo IT, Swerdloff RS, Nelson A, et al. Levonorgestrel implants (Norplant II) for male contraception clinical trials combination with transdermal and injectable testosterone. J Clin Endocrinol Metab 2002;87:3562–3572.
35. Swerdloff RS , Wang C, Cunningham G, et al., and the Testosterone Gel Study Group. Long term pharmacokinetics of transdermal testosterone gel in hypogonadal men. J Clin Endocrinol Metab 2000;85:4500–4510.
36. Zhang GY, Gu YO, Wang XH, et al. Pharmacokinetic study of injectable testosterone undecanoate in hypogonadal men. J Androl 1998;19:761–768
37. Behre HM, Abshagen K, Oettel M, et al. Intramuscular injection of testosterone undecanoate for the treatment of male hypogonadism: phase I studies. Euro J Endocrinol 1999;140:414–419.
38. Nieschlag E, Buchter D, von Eckardstein S, et al. Repeated intramuscular injections of testosterone undecanoate for substitution therapy of hypogonadal men. Clin Endocrinol 1999;51:757–763.
39. Zhang G-Y, Gu Y-Q, Wang X-H, et al. A clinical trial of injectable testosterone undecanoate as a potential male contraceptive in normal Chinese men. J Clin Endocrinol Metab 1999;84:3642–3647.

40. Kamischke A, Ploger D, Venherm S, et al. Intramuscular testosterone undecanoate with or without oral levonorgestrel: a randomized placebo-controlled feasibility study for male contraception. Clin Endocrinol 2000;53:43–52.
41. Wu FCW, Farley TMM, Peregoudov A, et al., World Health Organization Task Force on Methods for the Regulation of Male Fertility. Effects of testosterone enanthate in normal men: experience from a multicenter contraceptive efficacy study. Fertil Steril 1996;65:626–636.
42. Freidl KE, Jones RE, Hannan CJ, et al. The administration of pharmacological doses of testosterone or 19-nortestosterone to normal men is not associated with increased insulin secretion or impaired glucose tolerance. J Clin Endocrinol Metab 1989; 68:971.
43. Bagatell CJ, Herman JR, Matsumoto AM, et al. Metabolic and behavioral effects of high-dose, exogenous testosterone in healthy men. J Clin Endocrinol Metab 1994;79:561–567.
44. Barrett-Connor E. Lower endogenous androgen levels and dyslipidemia in men with non-insulin dependent diabetes mellitus. Ann Int Med 1992;117:807–811.
45. Simon D, Charles M-A, Nahoul K, et al. Association between plasma total testosterone and cardiovascular risk factors in healthy adult men: the Telecom Study. J Clin Endocrinol Metab 1997;82:682–685.
46. Meikle AW, Smith JA. Epidemiology of prostate cancer. Urol Clin N Am 1990;17:709–718.
47. McConnell JD (1991). Epidemiology, etiology, pathophysiology, and diagnosis of benign prostatic hyperplasia. In: Walsh K, Retik AB, Vaughan ED, Wein AJ, eds. Campbell's Urology, 7th ed. Saunders, Philadelphia, 1991, pp. 1429–1452.
48. Behre HM, Bohmeyer J, Nieschlag E. Prostate volume in testosterone-treated and untreated hypogonadal men in comparison to age-matched normal controls. Clin Endo 1994;40:341–349.
49. Meikle AW, Arver S, Dobs AS, et al. Prostate size in hypogonadal men treated with a nonscrotal permeation-enhanced testosterone transdermal system. Urology 1997;49:191–196.
50. McConnell JD. Physiologic basis of endocrine therapy for prostatic cancer. Urol Clin N Am 1991;19:1–13.
51. Pienta KJ. Etiology, epidemiology and prevention of carcinoma of the prostate. In: Walsh PC, Retik AB, Vaughan ED, Wein AJ, ed. Campbell's Urology, 7th ed. Saunders, Philadelphia, 1997, pp. 2489–2496.
52. Kumar N, Didolkar AK, Monder C, et al. The biological activity of 7 α-methyl-19-nortestosterone is not amplified in male reproductive tract as is that of testosterone. Endocrinology 1992;130:3677–3683.
53. Cummings DE, Kumar N, Bandin CW, et al. Prostate-sparing effects in primates of the potent androgen 7α-methyl-19nortestosterone: a potential alternative to testosterone for androgen replacement and male contraception. J Clin Endocrinol Metab 1998;83:4212–4219.
54. Anderson RA, Martin CW, Kung AWC, et al. 7α-Methyl-19-Nortestosterone maintains sexual behavior and mood in hypogonadal men. J Clin Endocrinol Metab 1999;84:3556–3562.
55. Noe G, Suvisaari J, Martin C, et al. Gonadotrophin and testosterone suppression by 7α-methyl-19-nortestosterone acetate administered by subdermal implant to healthy men. Hum Reprod 1999;14:2200–2206.
56. Schearer SB, Alvarez-Sanchez F, Anselmo J, et al. Hormonal contraception for men. Int J Androl 1978;2:680–712.
57. Knuth UA, Nieschlag E. Endocrine approaches to male fertility control. Clin Endocrinol Metab 1987;1:113–131.
58. World Health Organization Task Force on Methods for the Regulation of Male Fertility. Comparison of two androgens plus depo-medroxyprogesterone acetate for suppression to azoospermia in Indonesian men. Fertil Steril 1993;60:1062–1068.
59. Handelsman DJ, Conway AJ, Howe CJ, et al. Establishing the minimum effective dose and additive effects of depot progestin in suppression of human spermatogenesis by a testosterone depot. J Clin Endocrinol Metab 1996;81:4113–4121.
60. Kamischke A, Diebacker J, Nieschlag E. Potential of norethisterone enanthate for male contraception: pharmacokinetics and suppression of pituitary and gonadal function. Clin Endocrinol 2000;53:351–358.
61. Kamischke A, Venherm S, Ploger D, et al. Intramuscular testosterone undecanoate and norethisterone enanthate in a clinical trial for male contraception. J Clin Endocrinol Metab 2000;86:303–309.
62. Bebb RA, Anawalt BD, Christiansen RB, et al. Combined administration of levonorgestrel and testosterone induces more rapid and effective suppression of spermatogenesis than testosterone alone: a promising male contraceptive approach. J Clin Endocrinol Metab 1996;81:757–762.
63. Anawalt BD, Bebb RA, Bremner WJ, et al. A lower dosage levonorgestrel and testosterone combinaiton effectively suppresses spermatogenesis and circulating gonadotropin levels with fewer metabolic effects than higher dosage combinations. J Androl 1999;20:407–414.
64. Wu FCW, Balasubramanian R, Mulders TMT, et al. Oral progestogen combined with testosterone as a potential male contraceptive: additive effects between desogestrel and testosterone enanthate in

suppression of spermatogenesis, pituitary-testicular axis, and lipid metabolism. J Clin Endocrinol Metab 1999;84:112–122.

65. Anawalt BD, Herbst KL, Matsumoto AM, et al. Desogestrel plus testosterone effectively suppresses spermatogenesis but also causes modest weight gain and high-density lipoprotein suppression. Fertil Steril 2000;74:707–714.

66. Martin CW, Riley SC, Everington D, et al. Dose-finding study of oral desogestrel with testosterone pellets for suppression of the pituitary-testicular axis in normal men. Human Reprod 2000; 15:1515–1524.

67. Wang C, Yeung KC. Use of low-dosage cyprosterone acetate as a male contraceptive. Contraception 1980;21:245–272.

68. Roy S. Experience in the development of hormonal contraceptive for the male. In: Asch RD, ed. Recent Advances in Human Reproduction.Fondazione per gli Studi Sulla Riproduzione Umana, Rome, 1985, pp. 95–104.

69. Meriggiola MC, Bremner WJ, Paulsen CA, et al. A combined regimen of cyproterone acetate and testosterone enanthate as a potentially highly effective male contraceptive. J Clin Endocrinol Metab 1996;81:3018–3023.

70. Meriggiola MC, Bremner WJ, Costantino A, et al. An oral regimen of cyproterone acetate and testosterone undecanoate for spermatogenic suppression in men. Fertil Steril 1997;68:844–850.

71. Merrigiola MC, Bremner WJ, Costantino A, et al. Low dose cyproterceone acetate and testosterone enmanthate for contraception in men. Hum Reprod 1998;13:1225–1229.

72. Ewing L. Effects of testosterone and estradiol, silastic implants, on spermatogenesis in rats and monkeys. In: Patanelli DJ, ed. Hormonal Control of Male Fertility. US DHEW, Bethesda, MD, 1978, pp. 173–194.

73. Handelsman DJ, Wishart S, Conway AJ. Oestradiol enhances testosterone-induced suppression of human spermatogenesis. Hum Reprod 2000;15:672–679.

74. Bhasin S, Heber D, Steiner BS, et al. Hormonal effects of gonadotropin-releasing hormone (GnRH) agonist and androgen. J Clin Endocrinol Metab 1985;60:998–1003.

75. Bhasin S, Steiner B, Swerdloff R. Does constant infusion of gonadotropin-releasing hormone agonist lead to greater suppression of gonadal function in man than its intermittent administration? Fertil Steril 1985;44:96–101.

76. Pavlou SN, Interlandi JW, Wakefield G, et al. Heterogeneity of sperm density profiles following 16-week therapy with continuous infusion of high-dose LHRH analog plus testosterone. J Androl 1986;7:228–233.

77. Bouchard P, Garcia E. Influence of testosterone substitution on sperm suppression by LHRH agonists. Horm Res 1987;28:175–180.

78. Behre HM, Nashan D, Hubert W, et al. Depot gonadotropin-releasing hormone agonist blunts the androgen-induced suppression of spermatogenesis in a clinical trial of male contraception. J Clin Endocrinol Metab 1992;74:84–90.

79. Heber D, Swerdloff RS. Male contraception: synergism of gonadotropin-releasing hormone analog and testosterone in suppressing gonadotropin. Science 1980;209:936–938.

80. Bhasin S, Heber D, Steiner B, et al. Hormonal effects of GnRH agonist in the human male: II. Testosterone enhances gonadotrophin suppression induced by GnRH agonist. Clin Endocrinol 1984;20:119–128.

81. Pavlou SN, Wakefield GB, Island DP, et al. Suppression of pituitary-gonadal function by a potent new luteinizing hormone-releasing hormone antagonist in normal men. J Clin Endocrinol Metab 1987;64:931–936.

82. Tom L, Bhasin S, Salameh W, et al. Induction of azoospermia in normal men with combined Nal-Glu gonadotropin-releasing hormone antagonist and testosterone enanthate. J Clin Endocrinol Metab 1992;75:476–483.

83. Bagatell CJ, Matsumoto AM, Christensen RB, et al. Comparison of a gonadotropin releasing-hormone antagonist plus testosterone (T) versus T alone as potential male contraceptive regimens. J Clin Endocrinol Metab 1993;77:427–432.

84. Behre HM, Klein B, Steinmeyer E, et al. Effective suppression of luteinizing hormone and testosterone by single doses of the new gonadotropin-releasing hormone antagonist cetrorelix (SB-75) in normal men. J Clin Endocrinol Metab 1992;75:393–398.

85. Behre HM, Kliesch S, Puhse G, et al. High loading and low maintenance doses of a gonadotropin-releasing antagonist effectively suppress serum luteinizing hormone, follicle-stimulating hormone, and testosterone in normal men. J Clin Endocrinol Metab 1997;82:1403–1408.

86. Swerdloff RS, Bagatell CJ, Wang C, et al. Suppression of spermatogenesis in man induced by Nal-Glu gonadotropin releasing hormone antagonist and testosterone enanthate is maintained by testosterone enanthate alone. J Clin Endocrinol Metab 1998;83:749–2757.
87. Behre HM, Kliesch S, Lemcke B, et al. Suppression of spermatogenesis to azoospermia by combined administration of GnRH antagonist and 19-nortestosterone cannot be maintained by this non-aromatizable androgen alone. Hum Reprod 2001;16:2570–2577.
88. Murty GSRC, Rani CSS, Moudgal NR, et al. Effect of passive immunization with specific antiserum to FSH on the spermatogenic process and fertility of male bonnet monkeys (macaca radiata). J Reprod Fertil 1979;26:147–154.
89. Nieschlag E. Reasons for abandoning immunization against FSH as an approach to fertility regulation. In Zatuchini GI, Goldsmith A, Spieler JM, Sciana JJ, eds. Male Contraception: Advances and Future Prospects. Harper & Row, Philadelphia, 1985, pp. 395–399.

24

Hormonal Therapy of the Infertile Man

Peter Y. Liu, MBBS, FRACP
and David J. Handelsman, MBBS, FRACP, PhD

CONTENTS

BACKGROUND
SPECIFIC HORMONAL THERAPY
EMPIRICAL HORMONAL THERAPY
CONCLUSION
REFERENCES

BACKGROUND

About 10% of couples seek infertility assessment when pregnancy does not occur within a year *(1)*. Among these infertile couples, male factors are primarily responsible for 20–25% and contribute to another 30% of cases; no male or female factor can be identified in approx 15% *(2,3)*. Despite over half of all infertile couples having a male factor contributing to their infertility, most have oligo/asthenozoospermia without a specific diagnosis ("idiopathic") so that neither cure nor even logical treatment is possible. Indeed, for male infertility, specific treatment, defined as rational medical treatment aim at rectifying a verifiable and sufficient cause, is effectively limited to hormonal treatment of gonadotropin deficiency.

Where no specific treatment is possible, management options are to (1) accept the natural history of conception *(1,4)*, (2) circumvent male infertility by reproductive technology *(5–7)*, or (3) empirical therapies based on plausible drug or physical treatments *(8,9)*. Natural history studies suggest that unassisted conceptions are unlikely after 3 yr of infertility *(1,4)*. Although the best available evidence suggests no greater prevalence of infertility than previously *(10)*, the progressive shortening of effective reproductive years by the demographic convergence between the increasingly late age at first pregnancy attempt and the age at decline of natural female fertility is dictating an increasing consumer demand for infertility services, including the need for effective treatments for infertile men.

Circumvention of male infertility, once limited to adoption and donor insemination (which did not offer genetic paternity) now focuses on technological fertilization using in vitro fertilization (IVF), with or without intracytoplasmic sperm injection (ICSI), which provide paternity despite bypassing a diagnosis. Nevertheless, IVF/ICSI is expen-

From: *Endocrine Replacement Therapy in Clinical Practice*
Edited by: A. Wayne Meikle © Humana Press Inc., Totowa, NJ

sive, invasive and risks multiple gestation *(11)*, ovarian hyperstimulation *(12)*, congenital abnormalities in the progeny after ICSI *(13–16)*, and testicular damage after testicular sperm extraction *(17)*. Nevertheless, the consistent success rates of IVF/ICSI raises the question of whether future empirical therapies should be judged against the standard of reproductive technologies rather than the natural history of untreated fertility.

This review will focus on studies with pregnancy outcomes, rather than semen variables which are an imprecise surrogate marker of fertility *(18–20)*. Nonhormonal treatments such as kinins, or treatment of varicocele and cryptorchidism are outside the scope of this review.

SPECIFIC HORMONAL THERAPY

Gonadotropin Deficiency

Gonadotropin deficiency is an infrequent (<1%) cause of male infertility *(21)*. It may be congenital, leading to delay or failure of puberty, or be acquired after completion of reproductive maturation, an important distinction for therapeutic prognosis. The underlying causes are functional disorders of hypothalamic gonadotropin-releasing hormone (GnRH) secretion (hypogonadotropic hypogonadism associated without or with anosmia [Kallmann's syndrome]), pituitary tumors and their treatment, hemochromatosis, autoimmune hypophysitis, and genetic defects in GnRH, luteinizing hormone (LH) or follicle-stimulating hormone (FSH) synthesis, secretion, receptors or action *(22–25)*. Treatment aiming to rectify the underlying disorder is only possible with depletion of iron overload *(26)*, dopamine agonist treatment for hyperprolactinemia, and surgery and/or radiotherapy for pituitary tumors; however, none of these is very effective at restoring gonadotropin secretion and normalizing reproductive function. After chronological age of puberty, virilization is usually readily affected by testosterone as for any other cause of androgen deficiency. Androgens alone, however, do not stimulate spermatogenesis, for which gonadotropin-replacement therapy is necessary when fertility is required *(27)*. Gonadotropin-replacement therapy can, in theory, be provided by administration of pulsatile GnRH (where pituitary gonadotroph reserve is intact, usually only in hypothalamic causes *[26]*) or by administration of exogenous gonadotropins, namely hCG (as a naturally occurring, long-acting LH analog) with or without FSH.

Pulsatile GnRH Therapy

Although GnRH was characterized in 1971, effective treatment with GnRH only became feasible a decade later after Knobil *(28)* identified the pivotal role of pulsatility in GnRH action. In men with hypothalamic GnRH deficiency and an intact pituitary, pulsatile GnRH therapy is effective for induction of virilization, spermatogenesis, and fertility *(23,29)*. Typically, GnRH (2.5–20 µg) is administered every 60–120 min via an indwelling iv or sc cannula. Although the iv route of administration has better pharmacokinetics than the sc route *(30)*, whether the superior clinical efficacy of the iv route justifies the more intensive monitoring required for this delivery modality is not clear.

Pregnancy outcomes from pulsatile GnRH therapy for male gonadotropin deficiency are reported in four studies *(31–34)*. Three of these studies, treating altogether 29 men, compared the efficacy of pulsatile GnRH against gonadotropin therapy *(32–34)*; however, none were randomized. One study reported that pulsatile GnRH therapy resulted in faster onset of spermatogenesis compared with gonadotropin therapy *(33)*, but no study has shown any difference in pregnancy outcome.

Complications of pulsatile GnRH therapy are few, apart from infrequent adverse effects related to the delivery system (pump mechanical failure, fever, sepsis, bruising) or the development of anti-GnRH antibodies causing treatment failure *(35–37)*.

In summary, the more intensive monitoring and compliance required for pulsatile GnRH therapy renders it impractical outside large clinical research centers, compared with gonadotropin therapy.

Gonadotropin Therapy

Human gonadotropins have been used effectively for specific treatment of gonadotropin deficiency since the early 1960s *(38)* using regimens including human chorionic gonadotropin (hCG) purified from urine of pregnant women together with FSH purified from human pituitaries *(39)*, urine of menopausal women *(34)*, or recombinant FSH *(40)*. Pituitary extracts that risk transmitting Creutzfeld–Jakob disease were discontinued in 1985 *(41,42)* and urinary preparations are increasingly supplanted by recombinant human FSH. Present evidence suggests that recombinant and urinary FSH are comparable in efficacy *(43)*.

Typically, hCG therapy is initiated alone, at a dose of 1500–2000 IU administered twice weekly by self-administered subcutaneous or supervised intramuscular injections. Adequacy of hCG dosage is evaluated after the first month by whether trough plasma testosterone (measured immediately before the next injection) is in the eugonadal range. If plasma testosterone response is inadequate, the same dose may be increased to three, or rarely four, times weekly. Treatment with hCG alone can continue up to 6 mo. Among those with the best prognosis, hCG alone may be sufficient to induce spermatogenesis without need for FSH (44). If no sperm appear by 4–6 mo, FSH is added initially at 50–75 IU three times weekly, aimed at reconciling in frequency with hCG dosage. FSH may be mixed and administered in the same syringe as hCG. If testis growth and sperm output is inadequate, FSH dosage can be increased to 100–150 IU three times weekly and, rarely, to 150 IU daily.

Among studies reporting pregnancy outcomes *(31,33,34,39,43–54)* only four involve more than 20 men *(34,43,45,46)* with two being multicenter *(45,46)*.

From the limited data available, conception appears to occur after an average of 20 mo of treatment at a sperm density as low as 5 *M*/mL (range 3–8) *(34,39,43,44,47,52)*. The timing of pregnancy seems to parallel attainment of a sperm density of 5 *M*/mL, occurring approx 8 mo afterward *(43)*.

The most consistent positive predictors of response to gonadotropin therapy are higher initial testis volume and postpubertal onset of gonadotropin deficiency (neither of which is modifiable) and prior gonadotropin therapy *(43)*. The observation that prior gonadotropin therapy is the most important modifiable factor of response to gonadotropin therapy suggests that a review of standard treatment for induction of virilization in adolescents with delayed puberty may be warranted. The long-standing policy to initiate puberty with androgens, justified by simplicity and lower cost as well as unavailability of sufficient gonadotropins, may no longer be optimal, particularly because the advent of recombinant gonadotropins means that supply is no longer limiting and self-administered therapy is now feasible *(55,56)*. Initial gonadotropin therapy may be advantageous in timely initiation of spermatogenesis and testis growth, which can lead either to cryostorage of sperm for later use or accelerated induction of spermatogenesis when fertility is desired.

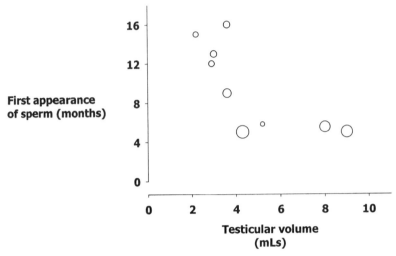

Fig. 1. Bubble plot of central estimates (mean or median) of time to appearance of sperm (months) versus initial testicular volume (mL). Each point represents a single published study of at least seven men. The area of each point is proportional to the square root of the sample size of that study.

In order to evaluate the relationship between testis volume and time to appearance of sperm, a review of literature published since 1966 was undertaken. Thirteen independent studies that had a sample size of seven or more men, provided baseline testis volume and an estimate of time to appearance of sperm were located *(31,33,34,43,45–47,49,50,57–60)*. One study *(58)* was excluded because it was incorporated into a later report *(34)*. A plot (Fig. 1) shows that 5–6 mo of treatment is required to induce spermatogenesis in men with pretreatment testis volumes of 4–9 mL *(34,43,46,50,59)*. A longer duration (9–13 mo) is required in men with smaller (2–4 mL) initial testicular volumes *(31,45,47,60)*. Three studies that represented outlying, longer mean durations of 20 *(33)*, 19 *(57)*, and 27 *(49)* mo. This may be largely the result of design features of the latter two studies, which utilized very sparse semen sampling and lower gonadotropin doses *(49,57)*.

Side effects from gonadotropin therapy in gonadotropin-deficient men are rare. In a few men, particularly with coexisting testicular disorders, hCG at maximal doses may be unable to achieve adequate androgenization. In these cases, gonadotropin induction of spermatogenesis is unlikely to succeed and alternative management of infertility and virilization need to be considered. Rarely, men may develop significant antibodies to hCG or FSH, which may cause treatment failure.

In summary, treatment of gonadotropin-deficient men with gonadotropin therapy is usually successful but relatively slow. Sperm can be expected to appear within 6 mo with a pretreatment testis volume of 4 mL or larger, but over 9 mo for smaller initial testis volume. In addition to pretreatment testis volume, postpubertal onset of gonadotropin deficiency and prior gonadotropin therapy are strong predictors of a speedier outcome. Given the relatively slow time to conception unaided, sperm are increasingly often used in conjunction with reproductive technologies to accelerate achievement of pregnancy.

Growth Hormone Deficiency and Treatment

Although growth hormone (GH) is involved in somatic growth and reproductive maturation *(61)*, claims that GH deficiency adversely affects male fertility and that this can be rectified by GH replacement therapy, remain unproven. Reproductive dysfunction in men with adult GH deficiency is likely due to the associated gonadotropin deficiency and there is no persuasive evidence that the concomitant GH deficiency has any significance for reproductive function. Isolated GH deficiency is not usually associated with infertility. The available clinical studies evaluating GH effects on reproductive function of GH-deficient men (62–67) are small and poorly controlled and constitute unconvincing evidence for significant GH effects. A controlled, non-human primate study (68) fails to support the claim that GH augments gonadotropin action on the testis (62). The remote possibility that pharmacological GH therapy might improve fertility of infertile men without GH deficiency has not been tested.

Glucocorticoids for Sperm Antibodies

High titers of antisperm antibodies in seminal plasma reduces pregnancy rates (69), presumably as a result of inhibition of sperm–egg interaction. Logically treatment can be directed at lowering sperm antibody levels or bypassing the need for natural fertilization by ICSI (70). Immunosuppressive treatment with prednisone has been utilized in men with sperm autoimmunity to reduce antisperm antibodies and improve the pregnancy rate. Six randomized controlled studies have examined the effect of prednisone on pregnancy outcome (71–76). Two examined the effect of prednisone combined with artificial reproductive technologies (71,73). Although dose and duration of therapy as well as selection criteria of sperm antibodies have varied, the two studies where treatment was continued for over 3 mo both reported increased pregnancies for prednisone compared with placebo treatment (72,75). A critical meta-analysis employing criteria for study quality reported no significant improvement with prednisone (77). Aggregating all available data provided an odds ratio of 1.88 (0.94–3.86) in (no-significant) favor of treatment.

In summary, there is a nonsignificant trend toward an improved pregnancy rate with prednisone treatment. This may require prolonged (>3 mo) treatment, a regimen that entails the risk of a rare but devastating complication—aseptic necrosis of the femoral head. Given the proven efficacy of IVF/ICSI, prednisone treatment for sperm autoimmunity can only be justified when IVF/ICSI is not possible and with careful warning and appropriate medical supervision.

EMPIRICAL HORMONAL THERAPY

Among *empirical* treatments for male infertility, no drug, device, or surgical methods have established efficacy in properly controlled clinical trials compared with the natural history of marital fertility (8,9) or reproductive technologies (5–7). Nevertheless, the pivotal importance of hormonal regulation of spermatogenesis has naturally led to plausible hypotheses that various hormonal regimens may be effective empirical treatments for unexplained male infertility. The available properly controlled trials, ideally involving randomization, placebo controls, and pregnancy outcomes, of such empirical hypotheses are reviewed in this section.

GnRH and GnRH Analog Treatment

One randomized study examined the effects of two doses of a GnRH analog (buserelin) or placebo administered twice weekly for 12 wk but failed to show any effect on sperm concentration or gonadotropins *(78)*. No well-controlled studies of pulsatile GnRH therapy in idiopathic male infertility have been reported.

Gonadotropin Treatment

Gonadotropin therapy for gonadotropin deficiency usually involves hCG with or without FSH. Administration of FSH alone to infertile men who were not gonadotropin deficient has been reported in two randomized controlled studies. One used purified urinary human menopausal gonadotropin *(79)* and the other used recombinant human FSH *(80)*. Neither showed any increase in pregnancy rates, although one claimed improved pregnancy rate in a posthoc analysis of a subpopulation *(79)*. Another nonrandomized comparative study reported no significant improvement in pregnancy rates with purified FSH *(81)*.

Only one published study has examined the effects of stimulation with both gonadotropins in a randomized, controlled trial *(82)*, although many uncontrolled studies have been reported *(83)*. In the Knuth study, hCG and hMG or placebo were administered in 3-mo blocks, but there was no significant effect on pregnancy or sperm parameters.

All three randomized studies used a similar FSH dose (150 IU, three times weekly) for at least 3 mo with pregnancy monitoring for at least another 3 mo, a duration and dosage that should suffice to evaluate potential therapeutic effects over a full spermatogenic cycle. Based on the consistent design features, a quantitative pooling of this limited data shows no significant effect (odds ratio = 1.46 [95% confidence interval {CI}: 0.77–2.76]) of gonadotropin therapy on pregnancy rates in 234 couples. Given the high cost and unproven efficacy, FSH therapy cannot be recommended in infertile men without gonadotropin deficiency. Claims of more subtle effects of FSH (e.g., on sperm function) lack substantiation by well-controlled studies.

Androgen Treatment

Testicular Leydig cells, under stimulation by LH secreted from pituitary gonadotropes, are the source of intratesticular, and virtually all circulating, testosterone in men. Intratesticular testosterone is critical for spermatogenesis with ambient levels approx 100 times higher than blood testosterone concentrations, well above the critical threshold required to support spermatogenesis. Reducing intratesticular testosterone, either by direct Leydig cell damage or indirectly via inhibition of LH secretion, is likely to have little effect until the androgen support threshold for spermatogenesis is reached, after which sperm output would likely diminish. Hence, the rationale for the use of exogenous androgens in treatment of male infertility is poor. High doses are likely to inhibit pituitary LH secretion and lower intratesticular testosterone, whereas lower doses are unlikely to add significantly to intratesticular testosterone. Hence, spermatogenesis is only likely to be unaffected or reduced by exogenous androgen therapy. Furthermore, because most of the androgen supply to the epididymis arrives from intratubular sources, it is also unlikely that exogenous androgens would have any significant positive effect on epididymal function. The rationale for "rebound" therapy (that withdrawal of high dose testosterone leads to a rebound increase in gonadotropin secretion) is implausible given the lack of efficacy of direct gonadotropin therapy.

The effects of androgen therapy for male infertility to improve pregnancy outcomes has been examined in 10 randomized controlled studies *(84–93)*, of which 5 used mesterolone *(84,85,88,90,91)*, 4 used oral testosterone undecanoate *(86,87,89,92)*, and

1 used both mesterolone and testosterone enanthate *(93)*. One study examined the use of androgens prior to IVF *(86)* and only one used a sufficiently high androgen dose to examine the "rebound" hypothesis *(93)*. No individual trial reported an improved pregnancy rate, and quantitative pooling of data from all 10 studies including over 1000 men provided a nonsignificant odds ratio of 1.07 [95% CI: 0.75–1.53] which was consistent for mesterolone alone (odds ratio = 1.09 [0.73–1.62]) and testosterone undecanoate (odds ratio = 1.00 [0.46–2.17]). Similar findings were reported in previous quantitative reviews *(77,94)*.

Given the lack of rationale and ineffectiveness from large studies, androgen therapy for male infertility is wasteful and should not be used clinically. Further studies would require a substantially novel and improved rationale, perhaps based on postreceptor pathways of androgen action.

Estrogen Blockade

Aromatization of testosterone to estradiol is involved in the negative feedback regulation of pituitary gonadotropin secretion. Hence, estrogen-receptor blockade or aromatase inhibition cause a reflex rise in pituitary gonadotropin and testicular testosterone secretion. Both tamoxifen and clomiphene, the first two antiestrogenic drugs, have been used to stimulate endogenous gonadotropin and testosterone secretion for empirical treatment of male infertility via increases in sperm output and/or function.

Ten randomized controlled studies treating more than 700 men for 3–9 mo have been performed *(93,95–103)*. No single study reported a beneficial therapeutic effect on pregnancy rates and a pooled quantitative analysis of this data *(104)*, including an analysis of dosage effects, showed no beneficial effect (odds ratio 1.54 [0.99–2.40]). Although a doubling of pregnancy rates could be excluded, a smaller increase in pregnancy rate or a modest improvement in sperm density and motility could not be excluded. Separate analyses of tamoxifen (four studies *[97,99,100,102]*, odds ratio 1.78 [0.87–3.66]) and clomiphene (six studies *[93,95,96,98,101,103]*, odds ratio 1.48 [0.84–2.61]) were similar suggesting the lower intrinsic estrogenic activity of tamoxifen has little significance in this context.

One randomized, placebo-controlled, crossover study of an aromatase inhibitor (testolactone) in men with idiopathic male infertility reported no change in semen variables or pregnancy rates *(105)*. A recent study reported that infertile men have a disproportionately high estradiol-to-testosterone ratio (consistent with excessive aromatase activity) compared with age-matched fertile men *(106)*. A placebo-controlled randomized clinical trial of aromatase inhibitor treatment for infertile men with such evidence of excess aromatase activity would be of interest.

In summary, estrogen blockade by antiestrogens or aromatase inhibition do not appear to be effective treatment for male infertility, although a small effect of antiestrogen drugs, perhaps among men with higher aromatase activity, cannot be fully excluded. At present, the treatments appear safe; however, accumulated evidence highlighting the importance of estrogens in spermatogenesis *(107)* and general health *(108)* suggesting that more complete estrogen blockade could be potentially detrimental if maintained for prolonged periods in healthy, young, but infertile men.

Dopamine Agonist Treatment

Bromocriptine was the first dopaminergic agonist effective in reducing prolactin secretion in all forms of hyperprolactinaemia. When used as primary treatment of prolactinoma, it partially rectifies the associated gonadotropin deficiency *(109)* but frequently fails to normalize pituitary–testicular function. The physiological basis for use of bromocriptine in idiopathic male infertility is, however, dubious and is mostly explained by the modest increases in circulating prolactin concentrations seen in some infertile men with normal pituitary function.

Three randomized placebo-controlled studies examining pregnancy rates have been reported *(110–112)*. No individual study reported a significant treatment effect on pregnancy rates, and a quantitative analysis pooling all data showed no therapeutic effect on pregnancy rates or semen variables *(113)*, suggesting this dopamine agonist offers little promise as an empirical hormonal treatment of male infertility. Newer dopamine agonists such as pergolide and cabergoline have not been studied in this context.

Hormonal Testicular Cytoprotection

Chemotherapy and/or irradiation for cancer and some nonmalignant conditions causes severe testicular damage. These effects vary in outcome from being effectively irreversible to slow and variable recovery over several years to decades. This type of testicular damage is distinctive because the toxin, timing, and dose are known. The elective timing together with the slow and inconsistent recovery raise the issues of developing cytoprotective regimens.

The first hormonal approach to cytoprotection of spermatogenesis was based on the hypothesis that gonadotropin withdrawal, to render the testis "quiescent" comparable to the prepubertal period, would protect against cytotoxic damage *(114)*. Unfortunately, human infancy is not a quiescent period for the testis *(115)*, the clinical impression of prepubertal protection against cytotoxic damage is illusory *(116)*, and the seminal study proposing that GnRH analog treatment protected the mouse testis against cyclophosphamide damage *(117)* proved not reproducible *(118)*, the latter finding being not surprising given the known resistance of mice to the GnRH analog employed *(119)*.

The available clinical studies of the hormonal downregulation/cytoprotection hypothesis using GnRH superactive analogs as adjuvant therapy have not been encouraging. The available studies have design limitations and limited follow-up *(120–123)*. Only one was randomized *(120)* and another lacked any control *(123)*. A major limitation of the superactive GnRH analogs in this setting is their initial flare of gonadotropin secretion lasting the first 2–3 wk. This undermines any opportunity to test the underlying hypothesis, which requires gonadotropin withdrawal, whereas increased gonadotropin secretion is produced at the most critical time. Pure GnRH antagonists, which lack any initial gonadotropin surge, are essential to test the gonadotropin withdrawal/cytoprotection hypothesis in humans definitively, but this class of GnRH analog has not been tested so far.

Gonadal steroids could be used to cause gonadotropin withdrawal through negative feedback. Although these agents are widely available and affordable, their onset of action is slow and the delay in providing life-saving chemotherapy may not be an acceptable trade-off. One recent randomized controlled pilot study reported that androgen administration commencing well before, and continuing during, elective cyclophosphamide therapy for nephrotic syndrome could speed recovery of spermatogenesis *(124)*. This interesting study needs to be interpreted cautiously and replicated before it can be considered to vindicate an androgen-based cytoprotective regimen. This study's limitations in size and the low-intensity cytotoxicity require further evaluation in the setting of more aggressive combination chemotherapy and irradiation used in modern cancer treatment.

Ultimately, long-term studies comparing hormonal cytoprotection regimens for effi-cacy, safety, and cost-effectiveness compared with standard sperm cryopreservation *(125)* in conjunction with reproductive technologies are needed. In the future, autolo-gous germ cell transplantation to repopulate a cytotoxic-damaged testis may preserve genetic paternity potential in such men *(126)*.

CONCLUSION

Similarities in the gamete biology, notably the pivotal importance and commonality of hypothalamo–pituitary regulation of the ovary and testis functions, have led to the tacit assumption that male and female infertility might have similar vulnerabilities to pathology and susceptibilities to hormonal treatments. However, overwhelming evi-dence refutes this naïve assumption. For example, whereas female reproduction is most susceptible to hypothalamic dysfunction (leading to readily treatable anovulation) because of psychological stress and catabolic states, male reproduction is robust with regard to functional hypothalamic defects but is more vulnerable to genetic and environmental (cytotoxic) damage to spermatogenesis, although most causes remain unidentified.

Currently, male infertility remains so poorly understood that nearly all infertile men, mostly characterized descriptively as having "idiopathic oligo/asthenozoospermia," obtain neither a meaningful diagnosis nor specific treatment. This differs from female infertility where nearly all cases have an identifiable cause leading to effective treatment options. Among infertile women, not only is hormonal dysfunction (notably anovulation) a leading and treatable cause of infertility, but the ovulatory mechanisms are readily susceptible to hormonal overdriving (hyperstimulation) to produce up to 20-fold increases in output of fertilizable gametes. In contrast, the hormonal regulation of spermatogenesis, sperm matu-ration, and function are more complex and tightly governed so that hormonal deficiency is rare and hormonal overdrive is not feasible. Hence, hormonal therapy has a major role in the treatment of female infertility both as a specific treatment for functional hormonal deficiency as well as for empirical (hyperstimulation) treatment, whereas for male infer-tility, hormonal treatment has a minor but important role as an effective and specific treatment for gonadotropin deficiency, but no proven role in empirical treatment.

In the future, novel treatments based on a detailed physiological understanding of hormonal action, notably postreceptor mechanisms, may open a new dimension in bio-chemically based, cellular-targeted, hormonal therapy of male infertility. Protein or gene-based therapies directed at well-characterized underlying causes or mechanisms of male infertility could render obsolete the present continuing need for empirical mecha-nistic bypass treatments such as ICSI/IVF for idiopathic male infertility. Such develop-ments await more profound knowledge of the hormonal mechanisms in supporting spermatogenesis of the functional pathophysiology of defects in sperm production and function. In the meantime, technical improvements in artificial reproductive technolo-gies, including enhancing accessibility and conception rates of ICSI/IVF, lessening genetic and procedural risks, and extending the technologies to men lacking haploid spermatogenic cells, are likely to be easier to achieve in the short term.

REFERENCES

1. Snick HK, Snick TS, Evers JL, Collins JA. The spontaneous pregnancy prognosis in untreated subfertile couples: the Walcheren primary care study. Hum Reprod 1997;12:1582–1588.

2. Comhaire FH, de Krester DM, Farley TM, Rowe PJ. Towards more objectivity in diagnosis and management of male fertility. Int J Androl 1987:1–53.

3. Nieschlag E. Classification of andrological disorders. In: Nieschlag E, Behre HM, eds. Andrology: Male Reproductive Health and Dysfunction, vol. 1. Springer, Berlin, 2000.

4. Collins JA, Burrows EA, Wilan AR. The prognosis for live birth among untreated infertile couples. Fertil Steril 1995;64:22–28.

5. Centers for Disease Control and Prevention, American Society for Reproductive Medicine, RE-SOLVE: The National Infertility Association. 1998 Assisted Reproductive Technology Success Rates: National summary and fertility clinic reports. Vol. 1: http://www.cdc.gov/nccdphp/drh/art98/PDF/art1998.pdf, 2000, p. 444.

6. Hurst T, Lancaster P. Assisted conception Australi and New Zealand 1999 and 2000. Sydney: Australian Institute of Health and Welfare National Perinatal Statistics Unit, 2001.

7. Nygren KG, Andersen AN. Assisted reproductive technology in Europe, 1997. Results generated from European registers by ESHRE. European IVF-Monitoring Programme (EIM), for the European Society of Human Reproduction and Embryology (ESHRE). Hum Reprod 2001;16:384–391.

8. O'Donovan PA, Vandekerckhove P, Lilford RJ, Hughes E. Treatment of male infertility: is it effective? Review and meta-analyses of published randomized controlled trials. Hum Reprod 1993;8:1209–1222.

9. Vandekerckhove P, O'Donovan PA, Lilford RJ, Harada TW. Infertility treatment: from cookery to science. The epidemiology of randomised controlled trials. British J Ob Gyn 1993;100:1005–1036.

10. Akre O, Cnattingius S, Bergstrom R, Kvist U, Trichopoulos D, Ekbom A. Human fertility does not decline: evidence from Sweden. Fertil Steril 1999;71:1066–1069.

11. Anonymous. Multiple gestation pregnancy. The ESHRE Capri Workshop Group. Hum Reprod 2000;15:1856–1864.

12. Abramov Y, Elchalal U, Schenker JG. Severe OHSS: An 'epidemic' of severe OHSS: a price we have to pay? Hum Reprod 1999;14:2181–183.

13. Kurinczuk JJ, Bower C. Birth defects in infants conceived by intracytoplasmic sperm injection: an alternative interpretation. Br Med J 1997;315:1260–1265.

14. Bowen JR, Gibson FL, Leslie GI, Saunders DM. Medical and developmental outcome at 1 year for children conceived by intracytoplasmic sperm injection. Lancet 1998;351:1529–1534.

15. Page DC, Silber S, Brown LG. Men with infertility caused by AZFc deletion can produce sons by intracytoplasmic sperm injection, but are likely to transmit the deletion and infertility. Hum Reprod 1999;14:1722–1726.

16. Foresta C, Moro E, Ferlin A. Y Chromosome Microdeletions and Alterations of Spermatogenesis. Endocr Rev 2001;22:226–239.

17. Schlegel PN, Su LM. Physiological consequences of testicular sperm extraction. Hum Reprod 1997;12:1688–1692.

18. Guzick DS, Overstreet JW, Factor-Litvak P, et al. Sperm morphology, motility, and concentration in fertile and infertile men. N Engl J Med 2001;345:1388–1393.

19. Polansky FF, Lamb EJ. Do the results of semen analysis predict future fertility? A survival analysis study. Fertil Steril 1988;49:1059–1065.

20. Glazener CM, Kelly NJ, Weir MJ, David JS, Cornes JS, Hull MG. The diagnosis of male infertility—prospective time-specific study of conception rates related to seminal analysis and post-coital sperm-mucus penetration and survival in otherwise unexplained infertility. Hum Reprod 1987;2:665–671.

21. Baker HWG. Male infertility. In: DeGroot LJ, Jameson JL, eds. Endocrinology, Vol. 3. Saunders, Philadelphia, 2001, 2308–2328.

22. Nachtigall LB, Boepple PA, Pralong FP, Crowley WF. Adult-onset idiopathic hypogonadotropic hypogonadism—a treatable form of male infertility. N Engl J Med 1997;336:410–415.

23. Seminara SB, Hayes FJ, Crowley WF, Jr. Gonadotropin-releasing hormone deficiency in the human (idiopathic hypogonadotropic hypogonadism and Kallmann's syndrome): pathophysiological and genetic considerations. Endocr Rev 1998;19:521–539.

24. de Roux N, Young J, Brailly-Tabard S, Misrahi M, Milgrom E, Schaison G. The same molecular defects of the gonadotropin-releasing hormone receptor determine a variable degree of hypogonadism in affected kindred. J Clin Endocrinol Metab 1999;84:567–572.

25. Layman LC. Genetics of human hypogonadotropic hypogonadism. Am J Med Genet 1999;89:240–248.

26. Wang C, Tso SC, Todd D. Hypogonadotropic hypogonadism in severe beta-thalassemia: effect of chelation and pulsatile gonadotropin-releasing hormone therapy. J Clin Endocrinol Metab 1989;68:511–516.

27. Schaison G, Young J, Pholsena M, Nahoul K, Couzinet B. Failure of combined follicle-stimulating hormone—testosterone administration to initiate and/or maintain spermatogenesis in men with hypogonadotropic hypogonadism. J Clin Endocrinol Metab 1993;77:1545–1549.

28. Belchetz PE, Plant TM, Nakai Y, Keogh EJ, Knobil E. Hypophysial responses to continuous and intermittent delivery of hypopthalamic gonadotropin-releasing hormone. Science 1978;202:631–633.

29. Crowley WF, Jr., Filicori M, Spratt DI, Santoro NF. The physiology of gonadotropin-releasing hormone (GnRH) secretion in men and women. Recent Prog Horm Res 1985;41:473–531.

30. Handelsman DJ, Jansen RPS, Boylan LM, Spaliviero JA, Turtle JR. Pharmacokinetics of gonadotropin-releasing hormone: comparison of subcutaneous and intravenous routes. J Clin Endocrinol Metab 1984;59:739–46.

31. Liu L, Banks SM, Banres KM, Sherins RJ. Two year comparison of testicular responses to pulsatile gonadotropin-releasing hormone and exogenous gonadotropins from the inception of therapy in men with isolated hypogonadotropic hypogonadism. J Clin Endocrinol Metab 1988;67:1140–1145.

32. Delemarre-Van de Waal HA. Induction of testicular growth and spermatogenesis by pulsatile, intravenous administration of gonadotrophin-releasing hormone in patients with hypogonadotrophic hypogonadism. Clin Endocrinol 1993;38:473–480.

33. Schopohl J, Mehltretter G, von Zumbusch R, Eversmann T, von Werder K. Comparison of gonadotropin-releasing hormone and gonadotropin therapy in male patients with idiopathic hypothalamic hypogonadism. Fertil Steril 1991;56:1143–1150.

34. Buchter D, Behre HM, Kliesch S, Nieschlag E. Pulsatile GnRH or human chorionic gonadotropin/human menopausal gonadotropin as effective treatment for men with hypogonadotropic hypogonadism: a review of 42 cases. Eur J Endocrinol 1998;139:298–303.

35. Blumenfeld Z, Frisch L, Conn PM. Gonadotropin-releasing hormone (GnRH) antibodies formation in hypogonadotropic azoospermic men treated with pulsatile GnRH—diagnosis and possible alternative treatment. Fertil Steril 1988;50:622–629.

36. Meakin JL, Keogh EJ, Martin CE. Human anti-luteinizing hormone-releasing hormone antibodies in patients treated with synthetic luteinizing hormone-releasing hormone. Fertil Steril 1985;43:811–813.

37. Lindner J, McNeil LW, Marney S, et al. Characterization of human anti-luteinizing hormone-releasing hormone (LRH) antibodies in the serum of a patient with isolated gonadotropin deficiency treated with synthetic LRH. J Clin Endocrinol Metab 1981;52:267–270.

38. Gemzell C, Kjessler B. Treatment of infertility arter partial hypophysectomy with human gonadotrophins. Lancet 1964;1:644.

39. Burger HG, Baker HWG. Therapeutic considerations and results of gonadotropin treatment in male hypogonadotropic hypogonadism. Ann NY Acad Sci 1984;438:447–453.

40. Liu PY, Turner L, Rushford D, et al. Efficacy and safety of recombinant human follicle stimulating hormone (Gonal-F) with urinary human chorionic gonadotrophin for induction of spermatogenesis and fertility in gonadotrophin-deficient men. Hum Reprod 1999;14:1540–1545.

41. Cochius JI, Burns RJ, Blumbergs PC, Mack K, Alderman CP. Creutzfeldt-Jakob disease in a recipient of human pituitary-derived gonadotrophin. Aust NZ J Med 1990;20:592,593.

42. Healy DL, Evans J. Creutzfeldt-Jakob disease after pituitary gonadotrophins. Br Med J 1993;307:517,518.

43. Liu PY, Gebski VJ, Turner L, Conway AJ, Wishart SM, Handelsman DJ. Predicting pregnancy and spermatogenesis by survival analysis during gonadotrophin treatment of gonadotrophin deficient infertile men. Hum Reprod 2002:17:625–633.

44. Vicari E, Mongioi A, Calogero AE, et al. Therapy with human chorionic gonadotrophin alone induces spermatogenesis in men with isolated hypogonadotrophic hypogonadism—long-term follow-up. Int J Androl 1992;15:320–329.

45. Anonymous. Efficacy and safety of highly purified urinary follicle-stimulating hormone with human chorionic gonadotropin for treating men with isolated hypogonadotropic hypogonadism. European Metrodin HP Study Group. Fertil Steril 1998;70:256–262.

46. Burgues S, Calderon MD. Subcutaneous self-administration of highly purified follicle stimulating hormone and human chorionic gonadotrophin for the treatment of male hypogonadotrophic hypogonadism. Spanish Collaborative Group on Male Hypogonadotropic Hypogonadism. Hum Reprod 1997;12:980–986.

47. Kung AW, Zhong YY, Lam KS, Wang C. Induction of spermatogenesis with gonadotrophins in Chinese men with hypogonadotrophic hypogonadism. Int J Androl 1994;17:241–247.

48. Kirk JMW, Savage MO, Grant DB, Bouloux PMG, Besser GM. Gonadal function and response to human chorionic and menopausal gonadotrophin therapy in male patients with idiopathic hypogonadotrophic hypogonadism. Clin Endocrinol 1994;41:57–63.

49. Okada Y, Kondo T, Okamoto S, Ogawa M. Induction of ovulation and spermatogenesis by hMG/hCG in hypogonadotropic GH-deficient patients. Endocrinologia Japonica 1992;39:31–43.

50. Saal W, Happ J, Cordes U, Baum RP, Schmidt M. Subcutaneous gonadotropin therapy in male patients with hypogonadotropic hypogonadism. Fertil Steril 1991;56:319–324.

51. Mastrogiacomo I, Motta RG, Botteon S, Bonanni G, Schiesaro M. Achievement of spermatogenesis and genital tract maturation in hypogonadotropic hypogonadic subjects during long term treatment with gonadotropins or LHRH. Andrologia 1991;23:285–289.

52. Burris AS, Rodbard HW, Winters SJ, Sherins RJ. Gonadotropin therapy in men with isolated hypogonadotropic hypogonadism: the response to human chorionic gonadotropin is predicted by initial testicular size. J Clin Endocrinol Metab 1988;66:1144–1151.

53. Okuyama A, Nakamura M, Namiki M, et al. Testicular responsiveness to long-term administration of hCG and hMG in patients with hypogonadotrophic hypogonadism. Hormone Res 1986;23:21–30.

54. Finkel DM, Phillips JL, Snyder PJ. Stimulation of spermatogenesis by gonadotropins in men with hypogonadotropic hypogonadism. N Engl J Med 1985;313:651–655.

55. Barrio R, de Luis D, Alonso M, Lamas A, Moreno JC. Induction of puberty with human chorionic gonadotropin and follicle-stimulating hormone in adolescent males with hypogonadotropic hypogonadism. Fertil Steril 1999;71:244–248.

56. Bouvattier C, Tauber M, Jouret B, Chaussain JL, Rochiccioli P. Gonadotropin treatment of hypogonadotropic hypogonadal adolescents. J Ped Endocrinol Metab 1999;12 :339–344.

57. Tachiki H, Ito N, Maruta H, Kumamoto Y, Tsukamoto T. Testicular findings, endocrine features and therapeutic responses of men with acquired hypogonadotropic hypogonadism. Int J Urol 1998;5:80–85.

58. Kliesch S, Behre HM, Nieschlag E. High efficacy of gonadotrophin or pulsatile gonadotrophin-releasing hormone treatment in hypogonadotrophic hypogonadal men. Eur J Endocrinol 1994;131:347–354.

59. Jones TH, Darne JF. Self-administered subcutaneous human menopausal gonadotrophin for stimulation of testicular growth and the initiation of spermatogenesis in hypogonadotropic hypogonadism. Clin Endocrinol 1993;38:203–208.

60. Ley SB, Leonard JM. Male hypogonadotropic hypogonadism: factors influencing response to human chorionic gonadotropin and human menopausal gonadotropin, including prior exogenous androgens. J Clin Endocrinol Metab 1985;61:746–752.

61. Hull KL, Harvey S. Growth hormone: a reproductive endocrine-paracrine regulator? Rev Reprod 2000;5:175–182.

62. Carani C, Granata AR, De Rosa M, et al. The effect of chronic treatment with GH on gonadal function in men with isolated GH deficiency. Eur J Endocrinol 1999;140:224–230.

63. Zalel Y, Draysen E, Goldschmit R, Zadik Z, Shoham Z. A prospective pilot study of co-treatment with growth hormone and gonadotropins for improving spermatogenesis in normogonadotropic patients with severe oligoteratoasthenospermia. Gyn Endocrinol 1996;10:23–28.

64. Zalel Y, Manor M, Zadik Z, Shoham Z. Successful induction of spermatogenesis in a patient with hypogonadotropic hypogonadism following co-treatment with growth hormone. Gyn Endocrinol 1996;10:29–31.

65. Lee KO, Ng SC, Lee PS, et al. Effect of growth hormone therapy in men with severe idiopathic oligozoospermia. Eur J Endocrinol 1995;132:159–162.

66. Radicioni A, Paris E, Dondero F, Bonifacio V, Isidori A. Recombinant-growth hormone (rec-hGH) therapy in infertile men with idiopathic oligozoospermia. Acta Europaea Fertilitatis 1994;25:311–317.

67. Shoham Z, Conway GS, Ostergaard H, Lahlou N, Bouchard P, Jacobs HS. Cotreatment with growth hormone for induction of spermatogenesis in patients with hypogonadotropic hypogonadism. Fertil Steril 1992;57:1044–1051.

68. Crawford BA, Handelsman DJ. Recombinant growth hormone and insulin-like growth factor I do not alter gonadotrophin stimulation of the baboon testis in vivo. Eur J Endocrinol 1994;131:405–412.

69. Abshagen K, Behre HM, Cooper TG, Nieschlag E. Influence of sperm surface antibodies on spontaneous pregnancy rates. Fertil Steril 1998;70:355,356.

70. Clarke GN, Bourne H, Baker HW. Intracytoplasmic sperm injection for treating infertility associated with sperm autoimmunity. Fertil Steril 1997;68:112–117.

71. Grigoriou O, Konidaris S, Antonaki V, Papadias C, Antoniou G, Gargaropoulos A. Corticosteroid treatment does not improve the results of intrauterine insemination in male subfertility caused by antisperm antibodies. Eur J Ob Gyn Reprod Biol 1996;65:227–230.

72. Omu AE, al-Qattan F, Abdul Hamada B. Effect of low dose continuous corticosteroid therapy in men with antisperm antibodies on spermatozoal quality and conception rate. Eur J Ob Gyn Reprod Biol 1996;69:129–134.

73. Lahteenmaki A, Rasanen M, Hovatta O. Low-dose prednisolone does not improve the outcome of in-vitro fertilization in male immunological infertility. Hum Reprod 1995;10:3124–3129.

74. Bals-Pratsch M, Doren M, Karbowski B, Schneider HP, Nieschlag E. Cyclic corticosteroid immunosuppression is unsuccessful in the treatment of sperm antibody-related male infertility: a controlled study. Hum Reprod 1992;7:99–104.

75. Hendry WF, Hughes L, Scammell G, Pryor JP, Hargreave TB. Comparison of prednisolone and placebo in subfertile men with antibodies to spermatozoa. Lancet 1990;335:85–88.

76. Haas GG, Jr., Manganiello P. A double-blind, placebo-controlled study of the use of methylprednisolone in infertile men with sperm-associated immunoglobulins. Fertil Steril 1987;47:295–301.

77. Kamischke A, Nieschlag E. Analysis of medical treatment of male infertility. Hum Reprod 1999;14:1–23.

78. Badenoch DF, Waxman J, Boorman L, et al. Administration of a gonadotropin releasing hormone analogue in oligozoospermic infertile males. Acta Endocrinologica 1988;117:265–267.

79. Matorras R, Perez C, Corcostegui B, et al. Treatment of the male with follicle-stimulating hormone in intrauterine insemination with husband's spermatozoa: a randomized study. Hum Reprod 1997;12:24–28.

80. Kamischke A, Behre HM, Bergmann M, Simoni M, Schafer T, Nieschlag E. Recombinant human follicle stimulating hormone for treatment of male idiopathic infertility: a randomized, double-blind, placebo-controlled, clinical trial. Hum Reprod 1998;13:596–603.

81. Ashkenazi J, Bar-Hava I, Farhi J, et al. The role of purified follicle stimulating hormone therapy in the male partner before intracytoplasmic sperm injection. Fertil Steril 1999;72:670–673.

82. Knuth UA, Honigl W, Bals-Pratsch M, Schleicher G, Nieschlag E. Treatment of severe oligospermia with human chorionic gonadotropin/human menopausal gonadotropin: a placebo-controlled, double blind trial. J Clin Endocrinol Metab 1987;65:1081–1087.

83. Schill WB, Haidl G. Medical treatment of male infertility. In: Insler V, Lunenfeld B, eds. Infertility: Male and Female. Churchill Livingstone, New York, 1993, pp. 575–622.

84. Aafjes JH, van der Vijver JC, Brugman FW, Schenck PE. Double-blind cross over treatment with mesterolone and placebo of subfertile oligozoospermic men value of testicular biopsy. Andrologia 1983;15:531–535.

85. Anonymous. Mesterolone and idiopathic male infertility: a double-blind study. World Health Organization Task Force on the Diagnosis and Treatment of Infertility. Int J Androl 1989;12:254–264.

86. Comhaire F, Schoonjans F, Abdelmassih R, et al. Does treatment with testosterone undecanoate improve the in-vitro fertilizing capacity of spermatozoa in patients with idiopathic testicular failure? (results of a double blind study). Hum Reprod 1995;10:2600–2602.

87. Comhaire F. Treatment of idiopathic testicular failure with high-dose testosterone undecanoate: a double-blind pilot study. Fertil Steril 1990;54:689–693.

88. Gerris J, Comhaire F, Hellemans P, Peeters K, Schoonjans F. Placebo-controlled trial of high-dose Mesterolone treatment of idiopathic male infertility. Fertil Steril 1991;55:603–607.

89. Gregoriou O, Papadias C, Gargaropoulos A, Konidaris S, Kontogeorgi Z, Kalampokas E. Treatment of idiopathic infertility with testosterone undecanoate. A double blind study. Clin Exp Ob Gyn 1993;20:9–12.

90. Hargreave TB, Kyle KF, Baxby K, et al. Randomised trial of mesterolone versus vitamin C for male infertility. Scottish Infertility Group. Br J Urol 1984;56:740–744.

91. Mauss J. [Results of treatment of male fertility disorders with mesterolone or a placebo]. Arzneimittel-Forschung 1974;24:1338–1341.

92. Pusch HH. Oral treatment of oligozoospermia with testosterone-undecanoate: results of a double-blind-placebo-controlled trial. Andrologia 1989;21:76–82.

93. Wang C, Chan CW, Wong KK, Yeung KK. Comparison of the effectiveness of placebo, clomiphene citrate, mesterolone, pentoxifylline, and testosterone rebound therapy for the treatment of idiopathic oligospermia. Fertil Steril 1983;40:358–365.

94. Vandekerckhove P, Lilford R, Vail A, Hughes E. Androgens versus placebo or no treatment for idiopathic oligo/asthenospermia (Cochrane Review). Cochrane Database of Systematic Reviews, vol. 3. Update Software, Oxford, 2001.

95. Ronnberg L. The effect of clomiphene citrate on different sperm parameters and serum hormone levels in preselected infertile men: a controlled double-blind cross-over study. Int J Androl 1980;3:479–486.

96. Abel BJ, Carswell G, Elton R, et al. Randomised trial of clomiphene citrate treatment and vitamin C for male infertility. Br J Urol 1982;54:780–784.

97. Torok L. Treatment of oligozoospermia with tamoxifen (open and controlled studies). Andrologia 1985;17:497–501.
98. Micic S, Dotlic R. Evaluation of sperm parameters in clinical trial with clomiphene citrate of oligospermic men. J Urol 1985;133:221,222.
99. Hargreave T, Sweeting V, Elton R. Randomised trial of tamoxifen versus vitamin C for male infertility. In: Ratman S, Teoh E, Anandaukmar, eds. Advances in Fertility and Sterility Series: Infertility, Male and Female. vol. 4, Partenon Publishing Group, 1986, pp. 51–57.
100. AinMelk Y, Belisle S, Carmel M, Jean-Pierre T. Tamoxifen citrate therapy in male infertility. Fertil Steril 1987;48:113–117.
101. Sokol RZ, Steiner BS, Bustillo M, Petersen G, Swerdloff RS. A controlled comparison of the efficacy of clomiphene citrate in male infertility. Fertil Steril 1988;49:865–870.
102. Krause W, Holland-Moritz H, Schramm P. Treatment of idiopathic oligozoospermia with tamoxifen—a randomized controlled study. Int J Androl 1992;15:14–18.
103. Anonymous. A double-blind trial of clomiphene citrate for the treatment of idiopathic male infertility. World Health Organization. Int J Androl 1992;15:299–307.
104. Vandekerckhove P, Lilford R, Vail A, Hughes E. Clomiphene or tamoxifen for idiopathic oligo/asthenospermia (Cochrane Review). Cochrane Database of Systematic Reviews, vol. 3. Update Software, Oxford, 2001: p. 3.
105. Clark RV, Sherins RJ. Treatment of men with idiopathic oligozoospermic infertility using the aromatase inhibitor, testolactone. Results of a double-blinded, randomized, placebo-controlled trial with crossover. J Androl 1989;10:240–247.
106. Pavlovich CP, King P, Goldstein M, Schlegel PN. Evidence of a treatable endocrinopathy in infertile men. J Urol 2001;165:837–841.
107. O'Donnell L, Robertson KM, Jones ME, Simpson ER. Estrogen and spermatogenesis. Endocr Rev 2001;22:289–318.
108. Grumbach MM. Estrogen, bone, growth and sex: a sea change in conventional wisdom. J Ped Endocrinol Metab 2000;13:1439–1455.
109. Carter JN, Tyson JE, Tolis G, Van Vliet S, Faiman C, Friesen HG. Prolactin-screening tumors and hypogonadism in 22 men. N Engl J Med 1978;299:847–852.
110. Lunglmayr G, Maier U, Spona J. Therapie der idiopathischen Oligozoospermie mit Bromokriptin Resultate einer prospektiv kontrollierten Studie. Andrologia 1983;15:548–553.
111. AinMelk Y, Belisle S, Kandalaft N, McClure D, Tetreault L, Elhilali M. Bromocriptine therapy in oligozoospermic infertile men. Arch Androl 1982;8:135–141.
112. Hovatta O, Koskimies AI, Ranta T, Stenman UH, Seppala M. Bromocriptine treatment of oligospermia: a double blind study. Clin Endocrinol 1979;11:377–382.
113. Vandekerckhove P, Lilford R, Vail A, Hughes E. Bromocriptine for idiopathic oligo/asthenospermia (Cochrane Review). Cochrane Database of Systematic Reviews, vol. 3. Update Software, Oxford, 2001, pp. 3.
114. Morris ID. Protection against cytotoxic-induced testis damage - experimental approaches. Eur Urol 1993;23:143–147.
115. Chemes HE. Infancy is not a quiescent period of testicular development. Int J Androl 2001;24:2–7.
116. Shalet SM, Beardwell CG, Jacobs HS, Pearson D. Testicular function following irradiation of the human prepubertal testis. Clin Endocrinol 1978;9:483–490.
117. Glode LM, Robinson J, Gould SF. Protection from cyclophosphamide-induced testicular damage with an analogue of gonadotrophin-releasing hormone. Lancet 1981;1:1132–1134.
118. da Cunha MF, Meistrich ML, Nader S. Absence of protection by a GnRH analogue against cyclophosphamide induced testicular cytotoxicity in the mouse. Cancer Res 1987;47:1093–1097.
119. Bex FJ, Corbin A, France E. Resistance of the mouse to the antifertility effects of LHRH agonists. Life Sci 1982;30:1263–1269.
120. Waxman JH, Ahmed R, Smith D, et al. Failure to preserve fertility in patients with Hodgkin's disease. Cancer Chemo Pharmacol 1987;19:159–162.
121. Kreusser ED, Hetzel WD, Hautmann R, Pfeiffer EF. Reproductive toxicity with and without LHRHa administration during adjuvant chemotherapy in patients with germ cell tumors. Hormone Metab Res 1990;22:494–498.
122. Brennemann W, Brensing KA, Leipner N, Boldt I, Klingmuller D. Attempted protection of spermatogenesis from irradiation in patients with seminoma by D-Tryptophan-6 luteinizing hormone releasing hormone. Clin Invest 1994;72:838–842.

123. Johnson DH, Linde R, Hainsworth JD, et al. Effect of a luteinizing hormone releasing hormone agonist given during combination chemotherapy on post-therapy fertility in male patients with lymphoma: preliminary observations. Blood 1985;65:832–836.

124. Masala A, Faedda R, Alagna A, et al. Use of testosterone to prevent cyclophosphamide-induced azoospermia. Ann Int Med 1997;126:292–295.

125. Kelleher S, Wishart SM, Liu PY, et al. Long-term outcomes of elective human sperm cryostorage. Hum Reprod 2001;16:2632–2639.

126. Schlatt S, von Schonfeldt V, Schepers AG. Male germ cell transplantation: an experimental approach with a clinical perspective. Br Med Bull 2000;56:824–836.

VII GONADAL: WOMEN

25

Primary and Secondary
Hypogonadism in Women

Daren A. Watts, MD, Howard T. Sharp, MD,
and C. Matthew Peterson, MD

CONTENTS

INTRODUCTION

Hormone replacement in hypogonadal women is a highly effective preventive health care measure. Estrogen replacement results in a nearly 50% reduction in the risks of vertebral and hip fractures and alleviates menopausal symptoms. Hypogonadal symptomatology such as hot flushes, irritability, anxiety, mood disturbances, loss of libido, and genitourinary atrophy are reduced and often alleviated by estrogen replacement. Numerous estrogen formulations and delivery systems are now available. Progestogens are utilized in women with a uterus to reduce the risk of endometrial hyperplasia and endometrial cancer. The role of androgens and phytoestrogens in hormone replacement therapy (HRT) are noted. Dehydroepiandrosterone (DHEA) supplementation is reviewed. Risks and complications of HRT are outlined, including the potential risk of breast cancer, cardiovascular effects, and nuisance side effects. The expanding role of selective estrogen-receptor modulators (SERMs) is highlighted.

HYPOGONADISM

Hypogonadism is characterized by low or undetectable circulating levels of gonadal steroids. In women, this specifically refers to lower than normal levels of estrogens, progesterone, and androgens, the principal steroidal products of the ovary. Hypogo-

From: *Endocrine Replacement Therapy in Clinical Practice*
Edited by: A. Wayne Meikle © Humana Press Inc., Totowa, NJ

nadism may be the result of a variety of different etiologic factors. In primary hypogonadism, patients never or only briefly express normal ovarian steroid synthesis. The classical presentation is gonadal dysgenesis associated with the 45, XO chromosomal abnormality, Turner's syndrome. Secondary hypogonadism may be caused by several different factors, including the aging process (natural menopause), surgical castration (surgical menopause), radiation or chemotherapy (iatrogenic ovarian failure), or autoimmune or genetic factors resulting in the earlier-than-expected cessation of ovarian function (premature menopause). The pathophysiology and differential diagnosis of these conditions have been extensively reviewed in other texts. This chapter will primarily focus on the treatment of these conditions, which may be discussed almost irrespective of the particular diagnosis, because all of these disorders share a common treatment goal: the elimination or attenuation of the complications incurred as a result of sex steroid hormone deficiency.

RATIONALE FOR TREATMENT

Prior to discussing specific hormone replacement regimens, it is important to clearly understand the goals of treatment. In general, these goals may be divided into two categories, immediate and long range. Immediate treatment goals address the present symptomatology of the hypogonadal patient, whereas long-range treatment goals are concerned the prevention of long-term sequellae associated with hypogonadism.

Patients with primary hypogonadism are usually referred by primary care physicians for the purpose of initiating normal pubertal development, secondary sexual characteristics, and the establishment of menstrual bleeding. Patients with secondary hypogonadism, regardless of etiology, will often present with a constellation of symptoms attributed to the loss of sex steroid production. The most widely recognized of these symptoms is the hot flush, commonly referred to as "hot flash." Seventy percent of women will experience hot flushes within 3 mo of natural or surgical menopause *(1)*. Approximately 55% of women will continue to experience these symptoms for the following 5 yr. Thirty-five percent of women will continue to have symptoms after 5 yr, although they are generally less frequent and intense. Other common complaints include irritability, anxiety, insomnia, mood disturbances, and loss of libido. Physical complaints may include vaginal dryness and irritation (as a result of vaginal atrophy) and urinary incontinence.

Hypogonadism is also associated with an elevated risk of osteoporosis and osteoporotic fractures. Currently, just over one-third of postmenopausal women in the United States use HRT in order to reduce the risk of osteoporosis *(2)*. Changes in bone metabolism that lead to osteoporosis are closely related to the decline in ovarian function. Estrogen replacement has been shown to reduce bone turnover and increase bone mineral density. Specifically, HRT with estrogen reduces the risk of vertebral fractures (40%) and hip fractures (>50%) *(3–7)*.

Until 1998, women were advised that HRT might also reduce their risk of cardiovascular disease. Although estrogen-replacement therapy has been associated with the reduction in the risk of cardiovascular disease in observational studies, recent randomized clinical trials have challenged the rationale for prescribing this therapy for the prevention of cardiovascular disease *(8–11)*. It now appears that some of the benefits seen in large observational studies may be the result of differences between women who choose to take hormones after menopause and those who do not, including different educational levels, medical care access, lifestyle, and compliance *(12,13)*. Definitive evidence regarding the risks and benefits of HRT and cardiovascular events are becoming available through the ongoing, large-scale, randomized clinical trials—such as the Women's Health Initiative in the United States (due 2005) and the Women's International Study of Long Duration Estrogens after Menopause (due 2012)—being conducted in 14 countries *(11)*.

Alzheimer's disease has an age-specific incidence that is 1.5–3 times higher in women than men *(14)*. Observational studies have demonstrated nearly a 50% reduction in the incidence of Alzheimer's disease in estrogen users compared to nonusers *(15–19)*. However, a recent observational study has failed to support this finding *(20)*. Furthermore, a recent randomized clinical trial also failed to demonstrate any benefit of estrogen therapy as a treatment for mild to moderate Alzheimer's disease *(21)*. The Women's Health Initiative is presently evaluating the role of estrogen in the prevention of memory loss and cognitive dysfunction. Theoretical explanations for an improvement in cognitive function that could be attributed to estrogen replacement include the following: enhancement of growth proteins associated with axonal elongation, nerve processes and synapse formation *(22)*; increases in choline acetyl transferase, which is critical to acetylcholine production *(23)*; and, antioxidant and anti-inflammatory properties *(24)*.

With the goals of prevention of osteoporotic fractures and the elimination of hypogonadal symptomatology in mind, the remainder of this chapter will review the numerous hormone replacement strategies available. Despite the documented health benefits, only one-third of patients eligible for HRT currently utilize treatment. One study documented that of women prescribed HRT, 20–30% never fill the prescription, 10% only report intermittent use, and 20% discontinue treatment within 9 mo *(25)*. These statistics serve to emphasize the importance of tailoring the treatment and side-effect profiles to the individual.

RISK ASSESSMENT

An individual assessment of risks for each woman considering HRT will include a discussion of each of the following areas of concern.

Cardiovascular Disease

More than 40 observational studies conducted during the past three decades have suggested that women who take estrogen have a 35–50% lower risk of coronary heart disease than those who do not take estrogen *(26)*. The biological plausibility of such an association has been ascribed to an estrogen-induced reduction in low-density lipoprotein (LDL) and Lp(a) lipoprotein, an increase in high-density lipoproteins (HDL), improved endothelial vascular function, and the elimination of the normal postmenopausal increases in fibrinogen and plasminogen-activator/inhibitor type 1. However, randomized trials of estrogen use in women with preexisting cardiac disease have not confirmed the cardiovascular benefits that were previously reported in observational studies *(8–13)*. The Heart and Estrogen/Progesterone Replacement Study designed to evaluate the effect of HRT on the risk of clinical cardiovascular events, found the overall rates of death from coronary causes and nonfatal myocardial infarction among the 2763 women with documented coronary artery disease were similar to those in the hormone-therapy and placebo groups *(8)*. Of most concern was the fact that there was a 50% increase in the risk of coronary events during the first year of the study among women in the hormone-therapy group. This higher first-year risk was eventually offset by a reduced risk, which could be explained by an acceleration of cardiovascular events leaving a lower-risk group for continued follow-up. These adverse events could potentially be explained by some biological activities associated with estrogen, which include an increase in triglyceride levels, activation of coagulation profiles as a result of increases in Factor VII production, prothrombin fragments 1 and 2, and fibrinopeptide A-10, and increasing levels of C-reactive protein—a marker of inflammation associated with an increased risk of cardiac events. In the placebo-controlled Estrogen Replacement and Atherosclerosis Trial, there was no difference in the angiographically determined progression of coronary atherosclerosis in controls versus those who received estrogen alone or estrogen in combination with progestin *(9)*. The Papworth Hormone-Replacement Therapy Atherosclerosis Study, evaluated transdermal estradiol alone versus transdermal estradiol combined with norethindrone. In that study, no cardiovascular benefits of HRT were seen and there was a slight increase in the risk of cardiovascular events during the first 2 yr of the trial *(10)*. It is possible that subgroups of women, such as those with an elevated baseline serum Lp(a) lipoprotein level, might benefit from HRT *(27)*, whereas those with hypertension and/or a prothrombin mutation might be at a higher risk of cardiovascular events *(28)*. The Women's Health Initiative and other studies have suggested a slight increase in the number of myocardial infarctions, strokes and thromboembolic events during the first 1 or 2 yr of use, which has now been confirmed *(11)*.

Therefore, considering the data obtained from randomized clinical trials, HRT does not reduce the risk of cardiovascular events in women with established coronary heart disease and should not be prescribed for the express purpose of preventing coronary artery disease or cardiovascular events in healthy women. Additionally, women with known coronary artery disease who have been on estrogen for more than 1 or 2 yr and are doing well do not necessarily need to discontinue their estrogen.

Endometrial Cancer

Numerous observational studies have demonstrated that long-term use of unopposed estrogen increases the risk of endometrial cancer by 8- to 10-fold *(29)*. This results in an increase of nearly 50 cases per 10,000 in women who use unopposed estrogen for at least 10 yr. During the Postmenopausal Estrogen/Progestin Interventions Trial, atypical endometrial hyperplasia, a premalignant lesion, developed in 24% of the women who were assigned to receive unopposed estrogen for 3 yr. This is compared with a 1% incidence in the women who were assigned to receive placebo *(30)*. The addition of a sufficient progestin dose (which opposes the effects of estrogen on the endometrium) eliminates this risk and is a critical component of HRT in women with an intact uterus.

Venous Thromboembolism

Postmenopausal use of estrogen increases the risk of deep venous thrombosis by a factor of 2–3.5 *(31)*. Because idiopathic venous thromboembolism is extremely uncommon in women over 50 yr of age, the absolute risk associated with the use of postmenopausal estrogen is quite small and is estimated to increase the incidence by 20 cases per 100,000 woman-years.

Breast Cancer

A recent meta-analysis of more than 51 case-controlled and cohort studies that included more than 52,705 women with breast cancer from around the world found no appreciable increase in the risk of breast cancer associated with short-term use of postmenopausal estrogen-replacement therapy (less than 5 yr) *(32)*. In contrast, however, the risk of breast cancer was increased by 35% in women who used postmenopausal estrogen therapy for 5 yr or more. It is further noted that combination therapy using estrogen and progestin may increase the risk of breast cancer more than estrogen therapy alone *(33)*.

Gall Bladder Disease

Observational studies suggest that the risk of gallstones and/or cholescytectomy is increased by a factor of 2–3 in postmenopausal women taking estrogen. In the Heart and Estrogen/Progestin Replacement Study, it was noted that the risk of gallbladder disease was 38% higher among women who were randomly assigned to receive estrogen–progestin therapy than those assigned to receive placebo *(8)*.

Ovarian Cancer

Some observational studies suggest an increased risk of ovarian cancer in postmenopausal women using estrogen *(34,35)*. In contrast, a recent meta-analysis of 15 case-controlled studies found no association of estrogen therapy with ovarian cancer and no evidence of an effect with increasing duration of use *(36)*. One of the major concerns of observational studies is that it is essentially impossible to control for the possibility that hormone users and never-users possess different risks for ovarian cancer because they are not identical populations *(37)*. Studies are ongoing to help clarify any potential risks and to determine the role, if any, of progestin in mitigating any potential risks of ovarian cancer with HRT.

Guidelines

The two validated indications for HRT in secondary hypogonadism are menopausal symptoms and the prevention or treatment of osteoporosis. Short-term use of estrogen, for the relief of menopausal symptoms associated with secondary hypogonadism, seems to be appropriate for women without contraindications (unexplained vaginal bleeding, active liver disease, history of venous thromboembolism, or a history of endometrial cancer, except stage 1 disease without deep invasion, or breast cancer). Relative contraindications include hypertriglyceridemia and active gallbladder disease. In these cases transdermal estrogen may be an appropriate option. The provider should review the risks and benefits of HRT with the patient and emphasize our lack of certainty regarding potential risks (cardiovascular events, strokes, venous thromboembolic phenomenon, and breast cancer). Randomized clinical trials provide no evidence that HRT prevents coronary artery disease or cardiovascular events. In fact, there is a possibility of accelerated short-term risk, particularly in women with coronary artery disease, hypertension, adverse lipid parameters, and prothrombin mutations. Despite these concerns, HRT may still be appropriate in women at increased risk for coronary artery disease if the noncoronary benefits of treatment exceed the risks (treatment of osteoporosis and/or a reduction in menopausal symptoms).

It appears that short-term use (less than 5 yr) of HRT is appropriate for relieving the symptoms of menopause in women without contraindications to their use. Hormone replacement therapy should be considered as a secondary option for women with coronary heart disease because of their higher than baseline risk of cardiovascular events. In women with contraindications or for those who do not wish to take HRT, alternative options may include selective serotonin reuptake inhibitors (SERMs), tibolone, clonidine, soy, and the use of intravaginal estsrogen creams or rings for genitourinary symptoms. Long-term use (5 yr or more) potentially could be reasonable in a small proportion of postmenopausal women with documented osteoporosis or osteopenia or for those who are at significantly increased risk for osteoporosis (personal or family history of nontraumatic fracture, current smokers, or those with a body mass index of less than 22). Poor candidates for long-term use would include those who do not have an increased risk for osteoporosis, those with cardiovascular disease, those with one or more first-degree relatives with breast cancer, a history of breast biopsy demonstrating atypia, or the presence of genetic susceptibility (BRCA-1 or BRCA-2).

Primary hypogonadism requires HRT for the establishment of secondary sexual characteristics and to avoid severe, early-onset osteoporosis and its sequella. Long-term studies in these women, now underway, will help to resolve some of the questions remaining regarding long-term HRT risks.

HORMONE REPLACEMENT STRATEGIES

Estrogens

Primary and secondary hypogonoadotrophic individuals utilize estrogens for the initiation and maintenance of secondary sexual characteristics, to promote bone and genitourinary health, and, to avoid vasomotor symptoms and their related mental and emotional sequella. Numerous preparations are now available for hypoestrogenic states (*see* Table 1). Potency of these preparations is based on molecular-binding constants, as well as activities in various bioassays, the ability to suppress gonadotropins, and/or induce hepatic synthesis (*see* Table 2). The choice between various medications is dependent on the individual patient's particular medical situation, side-effect profiles, and her particular needs and concerns *(25)*.

Classical Estrogen Receptor Concepts: Estrogen Receptor Alpha

Estrogen activity is dependent on binding with the estrogens receptor. This binding facilitates interaction of the DNA-binding region of the receptor with cellular DNA and ultimately results in the protein product of estrogen-responsive genes. The estrogen receptor is a member of the steroid receptor superfamily that contains the vitamin D, retinoic acid, and thyroid hormone receptors. These receptors conserve both the ligand and DNA-binding areas. The ligand or hormone-binding area is approx 250 amino acids and is hydrophobic. The transactivating function-1 (TAF-1) site is both cell- and promotor-specific and has constitutive activity for the receptor. The TAF-2 site in the steroid-binding domain is inducible by the ligand. The DNA-binding region can fold into two dissimilar zinc fingers to interact with the estrogen-responsive gene. The longer the estrogen remains bound to the complex, the more potent the hormone. Proteins transcribed (estrogen-responsive genes) are cell-specific (i.e., hepatocytes increase protein synthesis and cervical cells produce cervical mucous) (*see* Fig. 1) *(38)*.

Table 1
Approximate Serum Estrone and Estradiol Levels After Various Doses and Formulations of Common Estrogens

Brand name	Estrogen	Daily dose[a] (mg)	Average estrone[b] (pg/mL)	Average estradiol[b] (pg/mL)
Oral				
Cenestin®[c]	Synthetic conjugated estrogens	0.625 0.9	40-60	n/a
Estinyl®[d]	Ethinyl estradiol	0.02 0.05 0.5	n/a	n/a
Estrace®[e]	Micronized estradiol	1 2	150 250	40 60
Estradiol®, USP[f]		0.5 1.0 2.0	n/a n/a n/a	n/a
Estratab®[g]	Esterfied estrogens	0.3 0.625 1.25 2.5	n/a	n/a
Estratest®[h]	Esterified estrogens plus 2.5 mg methyltestosterone	1.25	n/a	n/a
Estratest® H.S.[i]	Esterified estrogens plus 1.25 mg methyltestosterone	0.625	n/a	n/a
Estropipate®[j]	Estropipate	0.75 1.5		
Menest®[k]	Esterified estrogens	0.3 0.625 1.25 2.5	n/a	n/a
Ogen®[l]	Piperazine estrone sulfate (estropipate)	0.75 1.5 3.0	125	30

(*continued*)

Table 1 (*continued*)

Brand name	Estrogen	Daily dose[a] (mg)	Average estrone[b] (pg/mL)	Average estradiol[b] (pg/mL)
Ortho-Est®[m]	Estropipate	0.75 1.5	200	40
Premarin®[n]	Conjugated equine estrogen	0.3 0.625 0.9 1.25 2.5	75 150 200	20 40 60
Tace®[o]	Chlorotrianisene	12	n/a	n/a
Oral combination therapy				
Femhrt®[p]	Norethindrone acetate/ethinyl/estradiol	1 mg/5 μg	n/a	20
Orthro-Prefest®[q]	17β-estradiol/Norgestimate	1 mg d 1–3 then 1 mg/0.09 mg d 4–6 of therapy, then repeat	n/a	50
Premphase®[r]	Conjugated estrogens/medroxyprogesterone acetate	0.625 mg d 1–14 0.625/5 mg d 15–28		
Prempro®[s]	Conjugated estrogens/medroxyprogesterone acetate	0.625/2.5 mg 0.625/5 mg		
Transdermal systems		Daily/total patch dose (size)		20
Alora®[t]	Estradiol—biweekly patch	0.025/2.0 mg (6.25 cm²) 0.05/1.5 mg (18 cm²) 0.075/2.3 mg (27cm²) 0.1/3.0 mg (36 cm²)	n/a	n/a

Climara®[u]	Estradiol—biweekly patch		
	0.05/3.8 mg (12.5 cm^2)	20–40	40
	0.075/5.7 mg (18.75 cm^2)		
	0.1/7.6 mg (25 cm^2)	40–60	80
Esclim®[v]	Estradiol—biweekly patch		
	0.025/5 mg (11 cm^2)	39	48
	0.0375/7.5 mg (16.5 cm^2)		
	0.05/10 mg (22 cm^2)	49	102
	0.075/15 mg (33 cm^2)		
	0.1/20 mg (44 cm^2)	64	165
Estraderm®[w]	Estradiol—biweekly patch		
	0.025/2 mg (5 cm^2)	12	30
	0.05/4 mg (10 cm^2)	25	73
	0.1/9 mg (200 cm^2)		
FemPatch®[x]	Estradiol—weekly		
Vivelle®[y]	Estradiol—biweekly patch		
	0.025/10.3 mg (11 cm^2)	25	30
	0.0375/3.3 mg (11 cm^2)	12	
	0.05/4.3 mg (14 cm^2)	25	50
	0.075/6.6 mg (22 cm^2)	35	75
	0.1/8.6 mg (2 cm^2)	50	90

(continued)

Table 1(*continued*)

Brand name	Estrogen	Daily dose[a] (mg)	Average estrone[b] (pg/mL)	Average estradiol[b] (pg/mL)
Vivelle-Dot[®z]	Estradiol—biweekly	0.0375/0.59mg (3.75 cm^2)		30
		0.05/0.78 mg (5.0 cm^2)		60
		0.075/1.17 mg (7.5 cm^2)		80
		0.1/1.56 mg (10 cm^2)		90
Combination patch				
Combipatch[®aa]	Estradiol/ Norethindrone acetate	0.05/0.14 mg (9 cm^2)	49	45
		0.05/0.25 mg (16 cm^2)	58	50
Vaginal creams				
Dienstrol[®bb]	Dienstrol	0.1	n/a	n/a
Estrace[®cc]	Micronized estradiol	0.1	n/a	n/a
Ogen[®dd]	Piperazine estrone sulfate	1.5	n/a	n/a
Premarin[®ee]	Conjugated equine estrogen	1.25	120	35
Vaginal ring system				
Estring[®ff]	Estradiol	2–9 d	60	50
Estradiol pellets	Estradiol pellet (not available in the United States)	25	n/a	n/a

[a]Physicians should consult detail information supplied by the manufacturer before use.
[b]Average steady-state serum concentrations.
[c]Cenestin, Duramed Pharmaceuticals, Inc. Cincinnati, OH.
[d]Estinyl, Schering Corportation, Phoenix, AZ

[e]Estrace Bristol-Myers Squibb, Princeton, NJ.

[f]Estradiol Tablets, USP, Watson, Corona, CA.

[g]Estratab Tablets, Solvay, Marietta, GA.

[h]Estratest Tablets, Solvay, Marietta, GA.

[i]Estratest H.S. Tablets, Solvay, Marietta, GA.

[j]Estropipate Tablets, USP, Watson, Corona, CA.

[k]Menest Tablets, SmithKline Beecham Pharmaceuticals.

[l]Ogen Tablets, Pharmacia-Upjohn, Kalamazoo, MI.

[m]Ortho~Est Tablets, Ortho-McNeil Pharmaceuticals, Raritan, NJ.

[n]Premarin Tablets, Wyeth-Ayerst, Philadelphia, PA.

[o]Tace, Hoechst & Marion Roussel, Kansas City, MO.

[p]Femhrt, Duramed Pharmaceuticals, Inc., Cincinnati, OH.

[q]Ortho-Prefest, Ortho-McNeil Pharmaceuticals, Inc., Raritan, NJ.

[r]Premphase, Wyeth-Ayerst, Philadelphia, PA.

[s]Prempro, Wyeth-Ayerst, Philadelphia, PA.

[t]Alora, Thera Tech, Inc., Salt Lake City, UT.

[u]Climara Transdermal System, Berlex, Wayne, NJ.

[v]Esclim, Fournier Research, Farifield, NJ.

[w]Estraderm Transdermal System, CibaGeneva, Summit, NJ.

[x]FemPatch, Parke-Davis, Morris Plains, NJ.

[y]Vivelle Transdermal System, CibaGeneva, Summit, NJ.

[z]Vivelle-Dot, CibaGeneva, Summit, NJ.

[aa]Combipatch, Rhone-Poulenc Rorer Pharmaceuticals, Inc., Collegeville, PA.

[bb]Dienstrol, Alora, Proctor & Gamble Pharmaceuticals, Cincinnati, OH.

[cc]Estrace Vaginal Cream, Bristol-Myers Squibb, Princeton, NJ.

[dd]Ogen Vaginal Cream, Pharmacia-Upjohn, Kalamazoo, MI.

[ee]Premarin Vaginal Cream, Wyeth-Ayerst, Philadelphia, PA.

[ff]Estring Vaginal Ring, Pharmacia-Upjohn, Kalamazoo, MI.

481

Table 2
Relative Potency of Various Oral Estrogens

Estrogen	Serum FSH	Serum CBG-BC	Serum SHBG	Serum angiotensinogen
Estropipate	1.1	1.0	1.0	1.0
Micronized estradiol	1.3	1.9	1.0	0.7
Conjugated estrogens	1.4	2.5	3.2	3.5
DES	3.8	70	28	13
Ethinyl estradiols	80–200 (est.)	1000 (est.)	614	232

Source: Adapted with permission from ref. *39.*

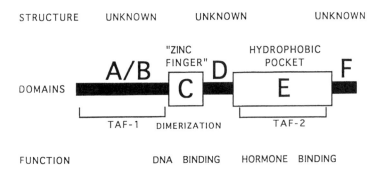

Fig. 1. Structural and functional organization of the estrogen receptor. The different domains perform different functions. The DNA-binding domain (C) and the hormone binding domain (E) are the best characterized, but other important areas must be considered: TAF-1 is both cell- and promoter-specific and can produce constitutive activity for the receptor; the TAF-2 site, in the steroid-binding domain, is inducible by the ligand. There is also a region of a few amino acids that is believed to be essential to dimerize the liganded receptor when it is located at the hormoneresponse element. (Reprinted with permission from ref. *38.*)

CONJUGATED EQUINE ESTROGENS

The most widely utilized estrogens in HRT are conjugated equine estrogens (CEEs). This formulation is a combination of more than 10 different estrogenic compounds found in pregnant mare's urine. By US Pharmacopeia standards, the estrogenic content of CEEs are as follows: sodium estrone sulfate, 52.5–61.5%; sodium equilin sulfate, 22.5–30.5%; 17α-dihydroequilin sulfate, 13.5–19.5%; sodium 17α-estradiol sulfate, 2.5%; and sodium 17β-dihydroequilin sulfate, 0.5–4%. The major components are depicted in Fig. 2. The complexity of the receptor–ligand complexes of the various components and their metabolic derivatives renders a complete understanding of the pharamcokinetics problematic *(39).*

Once absorbed and metabolized through the liver, the estrogens circulate primarily as sulfated conjugates. These conjugated (sulfated) forms are bound primarily to albumin, which significantly prolongs their half-life and establishes a reservoir of estrogens. Only the hepatocyte has a membrane that is permeable to sulfated estrogens. A major portion of the activity of CEEs is attributed to the hepatic regeneration of estradiol from this conjugated estrogen reservoir. The remainder of the biologic activity of CEEs is assigned to the equine estrogens equilin and equilenin. These equine estrogens are chemically

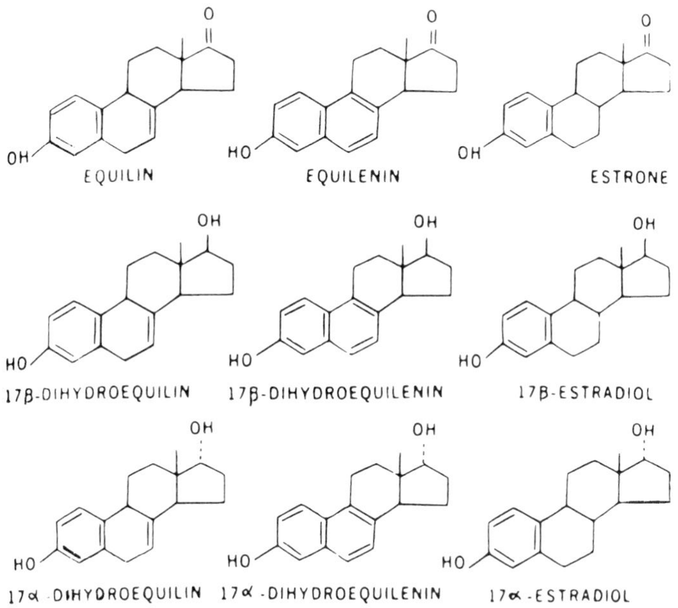

Fig. 2. The estrogenic compounds found in the urine of pregnant mares (conjugated equine estrogens). (Reprinted with permission from ref. *40*.)

referred to as ring B unsaturated estrogens because of the additional one or two double bonds in the B ring (*see* Fig. 2).

ESTERIFIED ESTROGENS

The major difference between esterified estrogens and CEEs is the percentage of estrone sulfate and equilin sulfate. Esterified estrogens have 75–85% estrone sulfate and 6–15% of sodium equilin sulfate (52.5–61.5% and 22.5–30.5% for CEE, respectively). Less than 10% are minor estrogen compounds (ring B unsaturated equine estrogens) compared to CEEs, which contain up to 25% minor estrogens. Esterified estrogens are water soluble and are easily absorbed. The pharmacokinetics and hepatic metabolism resulting in the regeneration of estradiol from the conjugated (sulfated) estrone reservoir are very similar to CEEs.

ESTROPIPATE

Conjugated (sulfated) estrone is soluble and attains stability when combined with a molecule of piperazine. Estropipate is the compound piperazine estrone sulfate (*see* Fig. 3). Piperazine is pharmacologically inert and is utilized only for its ability to stabilize the compound. Piperazine and estrone sulfate are combined in a 1:1 ratio. A dose of 0.75 mg of estropipate is equivalent to 0.625 mg of CEEs. Oral absorption is good and the drug is metabolized in the liver. Estropipate administration results in high serum concentrations of estrone sulfate, just as with CEEs. Likewise, the effects of estropipate are considered to be the result of hepatic regeneration of estradiol from the estrone sulfate reservoir.

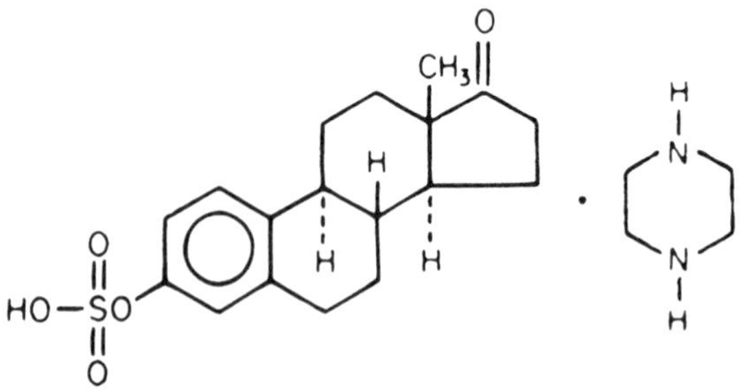

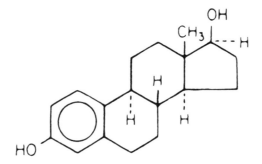

Fig. 3. Estropipate. Equilin is known to be significantly more potent with regard to hepatic protein synthesis relative to estrone sulfate *(41)*. The pronounced hepatic protein synthesis activity of CEEs, particularly equilin, theoretically may be beneficial when considering improved lipid parameters and detrimental when considering renin substrate (angiotensinogen) *(42)*, and clotting factors *(43,44)*. With regard to the risk of deep venous thrombosis (DVT) while on HRT, studies suggest a potentially increased risk in estrogen users, which was restriced solely to the first year of use. This finding may indicate an underlying risk factor that was not controlled for such as Leiden Factor V or prothrombin mutation *(45)*. Generic CEE preparations were removed from the United States market in 1991 owing to the possibility of bioinequivolence and significant differences in chemical composition *(46,47)*.

Fig. 4. Estradiol.

Estradiol

Natural estradiol is the common denominator of biologic activity of most of the administered estrogens *(see* Fig. 4). It is poorly absorbed in its natural form and is metabolized rapidly in a first pass effect through the liver. For this reason, micronization (micronized estradiol) or acetylation (ethinyl estradiol) is required for effective oral preparations. Micronization avoids poor absorption by delivering the drug in particles <20 μ*M* in diameter, which allows the whole intestinal mucosa to absorb the compound *(48)*. Ethinyl estradiol is synthesized by the acetylation of estradiol with an ethinyl group at position C-17 *(see* Fig. 5).

After absorption of any of the micronized estradiol compounds, the majority of the steroid is metabolized within the intestinal mucosa and liver to estrone sulfate (65%) and estrone (15%) *(49,50)*. As in the case of CEEs, esterified estrogens, and estropipate, the circulating reservoir of estrone sulfate and estrone created after the metabolism of absorbed micronized estradiol serves as the pool for the regeneration of estradiol *(51)*. Estrogenic induction of hepatic protein synthesis with the synthetic micronized estradiol

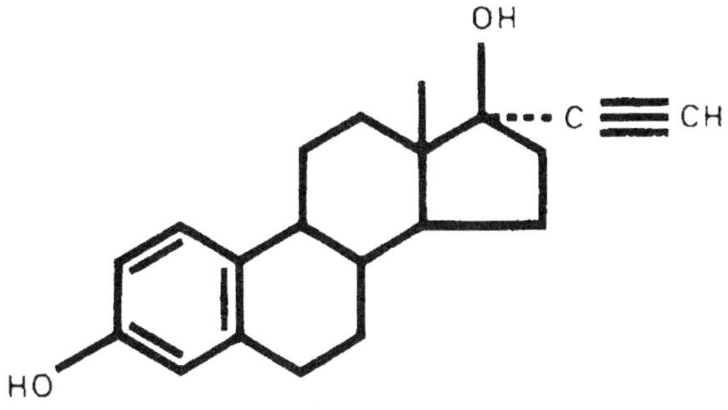

Fig. 5. Ethinyl estradol.

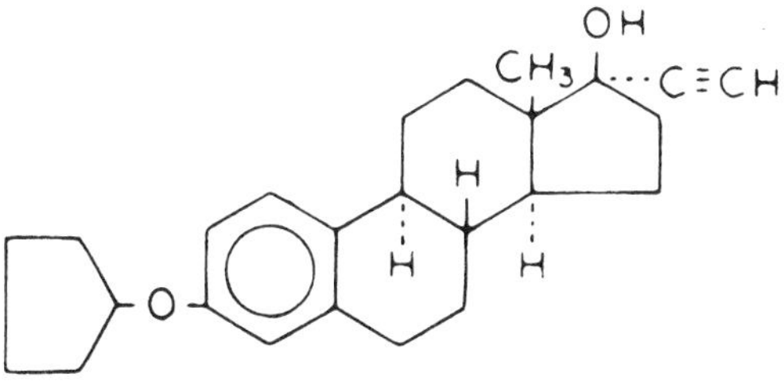

Fig. 6. Quinestrol.

preparations is significantly less than that found with CEEs, which may be of particular benefit when considering some relative contraindication (e.g., clotting factors in an immobilized patient, patient with personal or family history of elevated triglycerides) *(25)*.

Ethinyl estradiol is much more potent than the native steroid estradiol because it is a relatively poor substrate for the activity of 17β-estradiol dehydrogenase, which normally converts estradiol to estrone *(52)* (*see* Table 2). Because it is spared from the rapid D ring metabolism, its potency is prolonged and this effect is present regardless of oral or parenteral administration. Despite the protective C-17 acetylene group, significant metabolism by the gut and liver do occur, resulting in a peripheral conversion bioavailability of somewhere between 38 and 59% *(53,54)*.

Ethinyl estradiol metabolized in the liver is converted to ethinyl estradiol-3-sulfate. This sulfated pool does not serve as a reservoir for the creation of estradiol as estrone sulfate does for CEEs, esterified estrogens, or estropipate. Ethinyl estradiol is also a potent simulator of hepatic protein synthesis as are CEEs.

QUINESTROL

Quinestrol, the 3-cyclopentyl ether derivative of estradiol, is a prodrug with no inherent estrogenic activity of its own (*see* Fig. 6). After nearly complete absorption, intestinal and hepatic metabolism results in the formation of ethinyl estradiol and cyclopentanol. The metabolism and availability of ethinyl estradiol is as described previously.

The alkyl ether group provides resistance to hepatic metabolism and also enhances the prodrug's lipophilicity resulting in adipose storage. This adipose storage provides a half-life of over 120 h. Thus, the alkyl ether group provides a sustained reservoir of available prodrug and allows for 7 d dosing intervals. Because of these properties, quinestrol is two

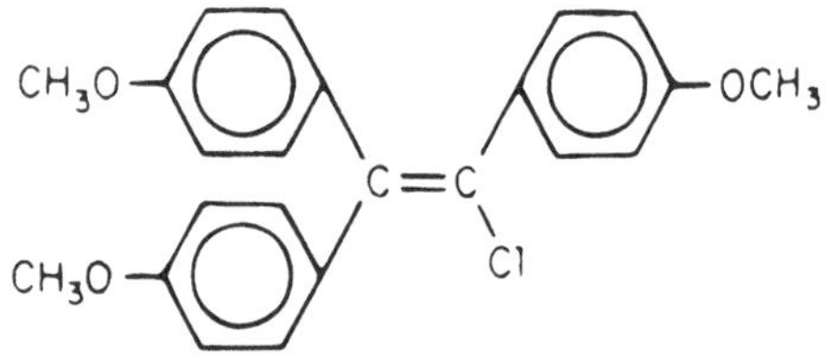

Fig. 7. Chlorotrianisene.

to three times more potent than ethinyl estradiol *(52,55)*. Quinestrol is not presently marketed.

CHLOROTRIANISENE

Chlorotrianisene is a derivative of diethylstilbestrol with only one-eighth the potency of DES (*see* Fig. 7). This drug also has extensive lipophilicity and is metabolized into other estrogenic substances after ingestion. Its potency hence is reduced if given parenterally.

Methods of Estrogen Delivery

Various preparations and their methods of administration are outlined in Table 1. Oral administration is the most common regimen prescribed. Poor absorption of insoluble estrogens requires modification through conjugation (CEEs, esterified estrogens, estropipate) or micronization (micronized estradiol). Additionally, synthetic molecules allow oral administration (ethinyl estradiol, quinestrol, chlorotrianisene). Increased potency and prolonged half-lives make the synthetic forms less commonly utilized for hormone replacement. Oral micronized estradiol administration results in rapid conversion to estrone and estrone-3-glucuronide. Phenytoin can increase this metabolic step and reduce the desired estrogen effects. This does not occur when administered transdermally or vaginally. Transdermally administered estradiol may theoretically reduce some of the beneficial hepatic effects on lipids. Additionally, it may be the preferred method in those with a personal or family history of elevated triglycerides or who are immobilized and at risk for thromboembolic events. Transdermal delivery is particularly convenient and preferred in the postoperative state. Skin sensitivity in transdermal administration occurs in a portion of patients and may preclude their use. Injectable estrogen administration results in higher rates of endometrial hyperplasia and addictive behavior secondary to widely fluctuating estrogen levels and other factors and is not routinely recommended *(56)*.

Vaginal preparations effectively administer estradiol and avoid hepatic effects (increased sex-hormone-binding globulin [SHBG], renin substrate [angiotensinogen], and hepatic coagulation factors). Concerns over the removal of estrogen containing implants has kept this delivery system from the market in the United States.

The Breast in the Treatment of Primary Hypogonadism

Particular attention to a near-physiologic addition of estrogen is required for some duration (often up to 2 yr) in order to maximize breast development in the woman with primary hypogonadism. If progestogens are added immediately with the onset of replacement therapy, breast development is abnormal and often minimal. Our approach has been to initiate low-dose estrogen (0.3 mg CEEs or equivalent) while monitoring breast development. Once adequate development is attained, a progestogen is added. The period of isolated low-dose estrogen required can be as long 1–2 yr. It is rare to induce uterine bleeding with low-dose estrogen alone , but should it occur, endometrial sampling and progestogen administration is indicated.

The Future: Estrogen Receptors Alpha and Beta and Selective Estrogen Receptor Modulators

Interactions of the estrogen receptor–ligand complexes with the DNA estrogen response element results in estrogen-responsive gene transcription. In 1995, a second estrogen receptor (estrogen receptor-β) was discovered and cloned (57,58). Although the two receptors appear similar physically, their distribution and subsequent gene transcriptions are very different depending on the site and substance, or ligand, binding to the receptor. Specific conformations of each of the receptor–ligand complexes are postulated to influence unique subsets of estrogen-responsive genes resulting in differential modulation and, hence, tissue-selective outcomes. The selective estrogen receptor modulators (SERMs) have been formulated to capitalize on these differential effects. Raloxifene (Evista) is approved for osteoporosis prevention. It has no apparent effect on the uterus or breast. Investigational SERMs include droloxifene, idoxifene, LY353381 HCl, CP336156, and tiboline (Livial). This generation and subsequent generations of SERMs may assist in maintaining the beneficial effects of estrogen while avoiding its adverse effects. Estrogen receptor–ligand complexes of both estrogen receptor-α and -β will also allow further selection of effects. The isolation and enhancement of these selective activities will hopefully provide an improved safety profile for HRT and will be a major area of research and development in the future.

Progestogens

Unopposed estrogen therapy increases the risk of endometrial cancer five- to 10-fold. The addition of a progestogen to estrogen replacement negates and may actually reduce this risk (59,60). Other potential concerns with long-term estrogen and estrogen–progestogen use include a potential increase in the risk of breast cancer (61–65), reduced cardiovascular benefits after long-term estrogen–progestogen replacement in low-risk women (66), and side effects that reduce compliance (breast tenderness, PMS-like symptoms, edema, bloating, irritability and depression, and lethargy) (25). Despite these concerns regarding estrogen and estrogen–progestogen regimens, present data provide little evidence of an adverse effect of the combined estrogen–progestin regimen as compared with estrogens alone on mortality (67).

Thus, in postmenopausal women with and without uteri and no contraindications, presently available data indicate that the use of an estrogen–progestogen or estrogen-alone regimen, respectively, of less than 5 yr duration is beneficial for bone and genitourinary health and to avoid vasomotor symptoms and their related mental and emotional sequella. After more than 5 yr use, SERMs may play an increasingly important role in maintaining the beneficial effects on the bone system without creating adverse outcomes on the breast or uterus. For women with primary hypogonadism, the initiation of secondary sexual characteristics and subsequent health benefits of long-term HRT appear to outweigh potential long-term risks. Studies are underway to determine the actual risks associated with the long-term use of estrogen–progestogen regimens in these women.

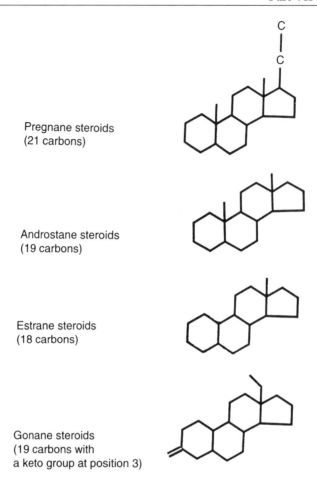

Pregnane steroids
(21 carbons)

Androstane steroids
(19 carbons)

Estrane steroids
(18 carbons)

Gonane steroids
(19 carbons with
a keto group at position 3)

Fig. 8. Pregnane steroids have 21 carbons and include progesterone, glucocorticoids, mieralcorticoids, and synthetic progestogens. Androstane steroids have 19 carbons and include testosterone and related steroids. Estrane steroids have an 18-carbon backbone and include estradiol and many of the 19-nortestosterone derivatives used as pregestogens that have an ethinyl group at position 17 (20 carbons) and the absence of a methyl group between the A and B rings. 17-Ethinyl-19 nortestosterone (norethindrone) is the estrane steroid that serves as the compound to which many estrane progestogens are metabolized. They are the second most commonly utilized progestogens in HRT. The more biologically active gonane steroids possess the structure of the estrane steroids and, additionally, have an ethyl group at position 13 and a keto group at position 3. The newer gonane progestogens may have reduced adverse effects (acne, hirsutism, weight gain, altered lipid, and glucose metabolism).

SYNTHETIC PROGESTOGENS

Synthetic progestogens are classified into three groups: pregnanes, estranes, and gonanes *(68)* (*see* Fig. 8). Their unique characteristics are discussed.

Pregnanes. Pregnanes are derived from I 7-hydroxy-progesterone. The pregnane progestogens are synthesized from natural precursor steroids (*see* Fig. 9). The most widely used progestogen in HRT is the pregnane medroxyprogesterone acetate. It is also used as a long-term injectable contraceptive (depo-medroxyprogesterone acetate given 150 mg intramuscularly every 3 mo) and for the treatment of endometrial hyperplasia (30 mg/d). Hydroxyprogesterone caproate (250 mg intramuscularly weekly through

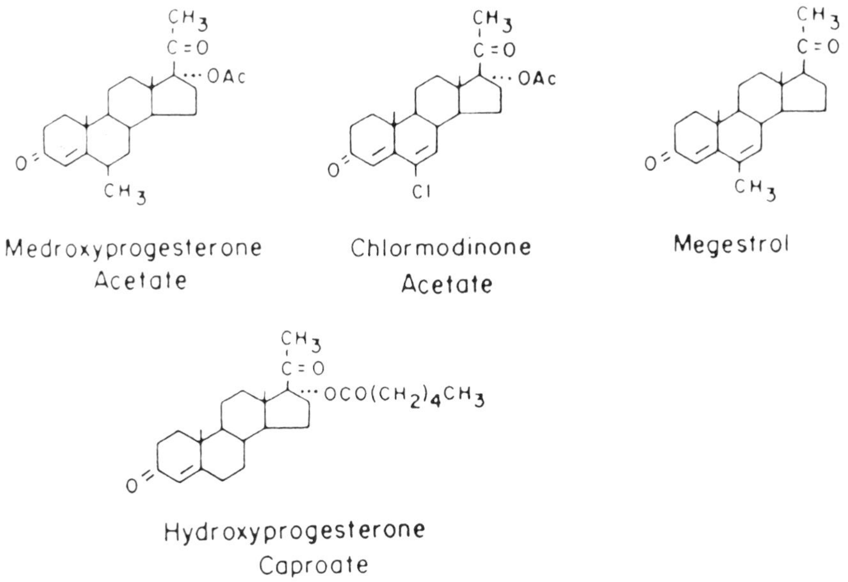

Medroxyprogesterone
Acetate

Chlormodinone
Acetate

Megestrol

Hydroxyprogesterone
Caproate

Fig. 9. The pregnane pregestogens: medroxy-progesterone acetate, chlormodinone acetate megestrol, and hydroxy-progesterone caproate.

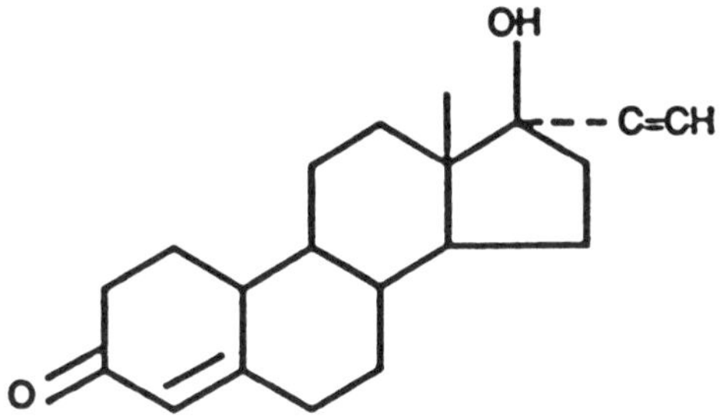

Fig. 10. The estrane progestogen norethindrone.

12 wk) is occasionally used to maintain progesterone levels in women who undergo removal of the corpus luteum during pregnancy. Megestrel is often used in cases of endometrial carcinoma.

Estranes. Estrane and gonane progestogens are derived from 19-nortestosterone, the progestogenic parent compound used in oral contraceptives in the United States. Estranes are characterized by the presence of an ethinyl group at position 17 and by the absence of a methyl group between the A and B rings (*see* Fig. 10). The estrane progestogens that are related structurally to norethindrone (norethynodrel, lynestrenol, norethindrone acetate, ethynodiol diacetate) are converted to this parent compound. Norethindrone is the second most commonly used progestogen in the United States for HRT.

Gonanes. The gonanes share the structural modifications found in the estranes and also possess an ethinyl group at position 13 and a keto group at position 3 (*see* Fig. 11). Norgestrel was synthesized in 1963 and is a racemic mixture of dextro and levorotatory forms. The levorotatory form, levonorgestrel, provides the biologic activity. Third-generation gonanes (desogestrel, gestedene, and norgestimate) have been developed to

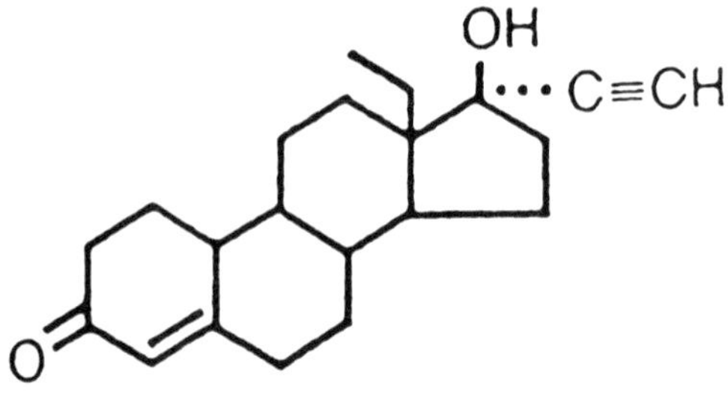

Fig. 11. The gonane progestogen levonorgestrel.

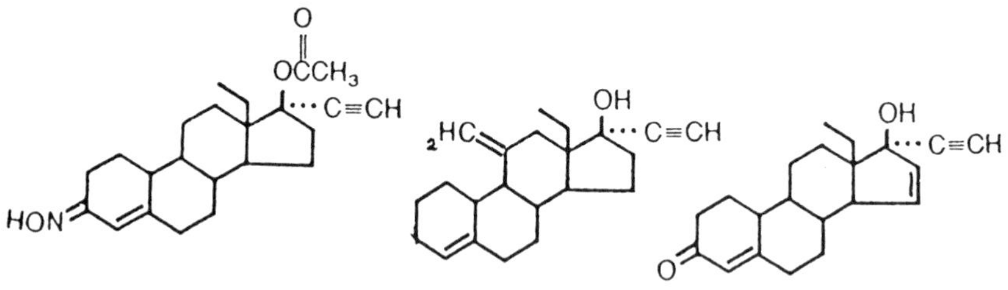

Fig. 12. Other gonane progestogens: norgestimate, desogestrel, and gestodene.

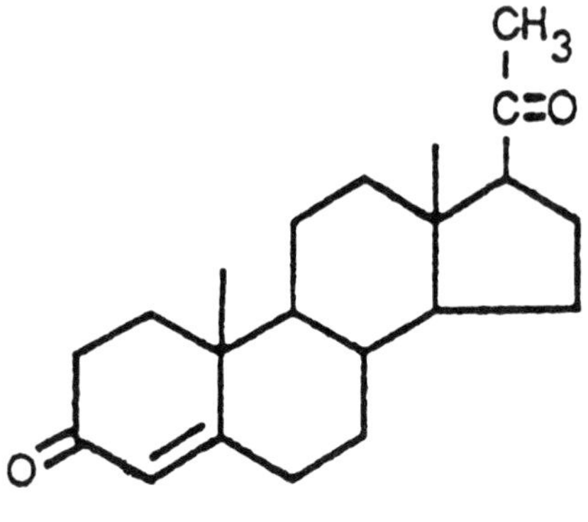

Fig. 13. Progesterone.

reduce unwanted side effects of progestogens, such as acne, altered glucose and lipid metabolism, weight gain, and hirsutism (*see* Fig. 12). They may be utilized in estrogen–progestogen regimens of the future.

PROGESTERONE

Progesterone preparations are synthesized from stigmasterol or diosgenin (derived from soy beans or Mexican yams, respectively) and occasionally from animal ovaries (*see* Fig. 13). Progesterone was first synthesized for commercial uses in 1934. Its use is hampered by poor oral absorption and rapid first-pass liver metabolism. It has been used orally (micronized and unaltered), intramuscularly, rectally, and vaginally (micronized or carried in cocoa butter or polyethylene glycol vehicle in estrogen–progestogen regimens). Micronization of the progesterone in combination with lipophilic vehicles enhances oral absorption and has become increasingly popular. Orally administered micronized progesterone at 100 mg twice to three times per day for 12 d each month in estrogen–progestogen regimens reveals rates of endometrial hyperplasia similar to that for medroxyprogesterone acetate (69,70). In continuous combined regimens, doses of 100 mg of oral micronized progesterone have been shown to cause an inactive endometrium and amenorrhea (71).

Vaginal delivery of micronized progesterone has been shown to enhance progesterone delivery to the uterus compared to the standard intramuscular regimen and results in a synchronous secretory endometrial histologic pattern in agonadal women preparing for embryo donation (72). The recommended dosage of vaginal micronized progesterone for estrogen–progestogen replacement in this setting is 800 mg/d (prior to embryo transfer in in vitro fertilization).

Only recently have studies been conducted utilizing a progesterone gel formulation. This preparation places progesterone in a 2% polycarbophil base that produces a controlled and sustained release of medication when given intravaginally. This approach takes advantage of the first uterine pass effect so that the desired endometrial impact can be obtained with lower systemic progesterone levels that could reduce progesterone–related side effects. Preliminary data have shown that in women on estrogen replacement for hypogonadism, a dose of 45–90 mg given every other day for up to 12 d induces complete secretory transition of the endometrium. Long-term studies are underway to confirm the efficacy of this approach (73).

Strong arguments for the use of natural progesterone, rather than synthetic, as the progestogen in estrogen–progestin replacement are being made and include the absence of adverse lipid alterations (70,74) and the absence of unwanted androgenic or estrogenic properties and their side effects (75).

Progestogen Regimens

When progestogens use is indicated (intact uterus) in hormone replacement for women, the therapy is individualized to meet each woman's particular needs and desires. The most commonly used administration regimen is cyclic sequential, which has the lowest incidence of adverse effects, excluding vaginal bleeding. Cyclic sequential therapy results in withdrawal bleeding in 97% of women. After 65 yr of age, 60% continue to have bleeding on cyclic sequential delivery schedule. Continuous sequential regimens have similar rates of bleeding (see Table 3).

For sequentially delivered regimens, endometrial sampling and transmission electron microscopy of ultrastructural elements have documented that the minimum progestin dose required to produce complete endometrial regression and a zero incidence of hyperplasia is 10 mg of medroxyprogesterone acetate (MPA) given daily for 12 d (76). A 2% incidence of hyperplasia has been reported with the use of 10 mg MPA for 10 d and a 4% incidence was noted for patient's receiving MPA for 7 d. With respect to protection against endometrial hyperplasia, based on recent clinical trials, it has been proposed that a dose of 5 mg of MPA prescribed for 14 d may be equivalent to a 10-mg dose taken over the same interval (76). Clearly, one needs to consider both the dose, duration, and formulation (i.e., endometrial activity) of the progestogen. Given the lack of a clearly preferred drug formulation and regimen, most practitioners will utilize progestogens in the dose range listed in Table 4, for 12–14 d per cycle, often modified according to the patient's tolerance of progestin-related side-effects. If less than customary doses are used, endometrial surveillance by endometrial biopsy is recommended.

Women routinely object to the prospect of vaginal bleeding, even if scheduled. This may be one of the reasons for the poor compliance rates seen with HRT. This has

Table 3
Common Progesterone Administration Regimens

Oral-administration regimens	Estrogens	Progestogens
Cyclic sequential	1st–25th d of mo	12th–25th d of mo
Continuous sequential	Daily	1st–14th d of mo
Continuous combined	Daily	Daily
Cyclic combined	1st–25th d of mo	1st–25th d of mo
Continuous estrogen/interrupted progestin	Daily	3 d on, 3 d off

prompted the development of continuous combined and cyclic combined regimens aimed at inducing amenorrhea. Continuous combined regimens, such as CEE (0.625 mg/d) or micronized estradiol (1 mg/d) given with medroxyprogesterone acetate or norethindrone acetate (2.5 mg/d for both), produce spotting and bleeding in the first 3–6 mo but by 6 mo 60–65% are amenorrheic. Breakthrough bleeding may occur and, if persistent, a sequential (cyclic or continuous) will be required (*see* Table 3). Patient acceptance of this regimen is high *(77–79)*.

Since its introduction over a decade ago, continuous combined HRT has been studied in numerous clinical trials with over 10 yr of follow-up. These studies reveal dropout rates averaging only 20% and nearly uniform resolution of vasomotor symptoms. Approximately three-quarters of the women receiving treatment for more than 6 mo report no uterine bleeding. Irregular uterine bleeding during the initial months of treatment is common and may reduce patient compliance and acceptance. Endometrial atrophy is most commonly noted on endometrial biopsy. However, two symptomatic patients (return of uterine bleeding after the establishment of amenorrhea) with a history of atypical endometrial hyperplasia developed endometrial carcinoma *(80)*.

A meta-analysis of patients on combined continuous conjugated equine estrogen and medroxyprogesterone acetate demonstrated a significant decrease in the circulating levels of total and LDL cholesterol and a significant increase in circulating HDL cholesterol posttreatment. Although such changes may be cardioprotective, no studies document decreased cardiovascular morbidity or mortality on this regimen. Bone density appears to be spared or increased *(70)*.

Because of concerns regarding potential unknown risks of the continuous combined regimens, some clinicians have recommended a cyclic combined regimen. This regimen results in minimal controlled spotting for 1–3 mo followed by amenorrhea in three-quarters of patients *(81,82)*. A continuous estrogen/interrupted progestin regimen has also been developed (3 d on, 3 d off of progestin), which is theorized to reduce the metabolic effects of progestogens and also caused amenorrhea in more than 75% of study participants *(83)*. To further reduce the patient exposure to progestogens, the quarterly administration of progestogens has been investigated in limited studies. Endometrial protection was shown to be adequate, although further study is required.

Continuous combined, cyclic combined, and continuous estrogen with interrupted progestogen regimens have not demonstrated unequivocal differences in terms of the incidence of PMS-like side effects, reduction in vasomotor symptoms, improvement of lipid profile, maintenance of bone density, or patient compliance compared to cyclic sequential or continuous sequential regimens.

Progestogens presently available or soon to be released are included in Tables 4 and 5.

Table 4
Commonly Available Progestogen

Brand name	Progestogen	mg Available	Minimal effective dosage[a]
Oral			
Amen[®][b]	Medroxyprogestrone acetate	10	10 mg daily
Aygestin[®][c]	Norethindrone acetate	5	2.5 mg daily
Cycrin[®][d]	Medroxyprogestroone acetate	2.5, 5, 10	10 mg daily
Megace[®][e]	Megstrol acetate	20, 40	40 mg daily
MicroNor[®][f]	Norethindrone	0.35	1.05 mg daily
Nor-QD[®][g]	Norethindrone	0.35	1.05 mg daily
Ovrette[®][h]	Norgestrel	0.075	0.150 mg daily
Prometrium[®][i]	Micronized progestrone	100, 200	200 mg daily
Provera[®][j], generic	Medroxyprogestrone acetate	2.5, 5, 10	10 mg daily
Vaginal			
Progesterone[®][k]	Micronized progesterone	50, 100	800 mg in divided doses
Progesterone	Progesterone vaginal suppositories	25, 50	25 mg tid
Injectable			
Depo-Provera[®][l]	Medroxyprogestrone acetate	100	
Hydroxyprogesterone caproate	Hydroxyprogesterone caproate	125	
Progesterone	Progesterone	100	

[a]All progestogens listed have not been Food and Drug Administration-approved for use in HRT regimens and are not recommended for use. Physicians should consult detail information supplied by the manufacturer before use.

[b]Amen, Carnick Labs, Inc., Cedar Knolls, NJ.

[c]Aygestin, ESI-Lederle,Philadelphia, PA.

[d]Cycrin, ESI-Lederle,Philadelphia, PA.

[e]Megace Bristol-Myers, Syracuse, NY.

[f]MicroNor, Ortho Pharmaceutical, Raritan, NJ.

[g]Nor-QD, G. D. Searle, Chicago, IL.

[h]Ovrette, Wyeth-Ayerst Laboratories, Philadelphia, PA.

[i]Prometrium, Solvay Pharmaceuticals, Inc., Marietta, GA.

[j]Provera, Pharmacia-Upjohn Co., Kalamazoo, MI.

[k]Crinone, Serono Laboratories, Inc., Randolph, MA.

[l]Depo-Provera, Pharmacia-UpJohn Co., Kalamazoo, MI.

Delivery Systems for Progestogens

Similar to estrogens, the oral route of progestin administration is the most common. Micronization has vastly improved the erratic absorption pattern seen with oral progesterone administration. The potential to reduce adverse side effects through the use of natural micronized progesterone is gaining greater appeal and vaginal delivery formulations have recently been released which, despite fluctuating serum levels, provide sustained and reliable endometrial effects. Depo-medroxyprogesterone acetate is infrequently given with continuous estrogen administration as a combined continuous regimen. Injectable biopolymer delivery techniques and patch systems are under development.

Table 5
Additional Estrogen and Progestogens in Development

Product	Manufacturer
Estradiol/norethindrone acetate patches for hormone replacement	RWJohnson Pharmaceuticals, Raritan, NJ
Estradiol/progestin transdermal patches	
17β-Estradiol transdermal patches	TheraTech, Salt Lake City, UT
Norethindrone acetate and ethinyl estradiol (Fem HRT)	Novo Nordic, Princeton, NJ
Conjugated estrogen and trirnegesterone	Warner-Lambert, Morris Plain, NJ
Cyclophasic hormone replacement	Wyeth-Ayerst, Philadelphia, PA
ERT/HRT transdermal patches	RW Johnson Pharmaceuticals, Raritan, NJ
Estradiol	Wyeth-Ayerst, Philadelphia, PA
β-Estradiol transdermal patches	G. D. Searle, Skokie, IL
Estradiol/norethindrone acetate	RW Johnson Pharmaceuticals, Raritan, NJ
Estradiol/norethindrone acetate transdermal patches	G. D. Searle, Skokie, IL
Estradiol/progestin transdermal patches	Cygnue, Redwood City, CA
Estradiol/testosterone transdermal patches	TheraTech, Salt Lake City, UT
Testosterone transderrnal patches	TheraTech, Salt Lake City, UT
17β-estradiol and norethindrone transdermal patches	Novo Nordic, Princeton, NJ
Estropipate and medroxyprogesterone acetate	Pharmacia-Upjohn

HRT: Contraindications and Adverse Effects

There are several contraindications for the use of HRT. These include coronary heart disease, active thrombophlebitis or thromboembolic disorders, known or suspected estrogen-dependent neoplasia, and known or suspected cancer of the breast. Patients with a past history of these disorders have a relative contraindication to treatment and deserve a careful assessment of risk versus benefits prior to the institution of treatment. Other contraindications include undiagnosed abnormal genital bleeding, pregnancy, and hypersensitivity to the drugs in question. Caution must be used in treating patients with impaired liver function owing to a concern for poor estrogen metabolism. Additionally, patients with hypertriglyceridemia (e.g., familial defects of lipoprotein metabolism) need to be carefully evaluated because they may be at risk for pancreatitis as a result of an estrogen associated rise in serum triglyceride levels. Other patients who warrant special consideration include those with a history of preexisting uterine fibroids, which may enlarge with estrogen therapy, and patients with hypercalcemia and renal insufficiency in which the prolonged use of estrogens can alter the metabolism of calcium and phosphorus.

There are numerous side effects that may be associated with the use of HRT in menopausal women, many of which are thought to be linked to the overall poor long-term compliance rates with this treatment (often reported as less than 25%). Women may experience bloating, breast tenderness, weight gain, headaches, nausea, irritability and premenstruallike symptoms. Additionally, most women can expect uterine bleeding unless a combined continuous regimen is utilized.

Complications associated with the use of HRT are commonly attributed to the effects of estrogen on the liver. These complications include an increase, albeit small, in the incidence of venous thromboembolism, an increase in serum triglyceride levels (of possible significance to cardiac disease risk), and an increase in gallbladder disease. The effect of estrogen replacement on carbohydrate economy is unclear, but, in general, HRT is not contraindicated in diabetics. HRT is not associated with detrimental effects in patients with a history of cancer of the cervix, ovary, or vulva. If a progestogen is used, there is no increased risk in endometrial cancer expected, although the use of HRT in patients with a history of endometrial cancer is somewhat controversial.

One of the most publicly debated issues surrounding adverse events related to HRT is whether or not treatment is linked to an increase in the risk of breast cancer. The fear of breast cancer remains one of the primary reasons women do not use HRT. The availability of SERMs that do not stimulate breast tissue (or that may even be protective against breast cancer) but provide some of the benefits of estrogen in other target organs such as the bone will be an important treatment option or maintenance regimen for patients who avoid HRT because of a concern regarding breast cancer, as well as those with a history or family history of breast cancer.

The Women's Health Initiative confirms an increased relative and absolute risk of heart attack, stroke, breast cancer, and venous thromboembolic phenomenon when using a combination of conjugated equine estrogens (0.625 mg/d) combined with medroxy-progesterone acetate (2.5 mg/d) (11). These recent finding confirm that, at present, the only two validated indications for HRT in secondary hypogonadism are menopausal symptoms and the prevention or treatment of osteoporosis. Short-term use may be indicated after the provider reviews the risks and benefits of HRT with the patient and emphasizes our lack of certainty regarding potential risks (cardiovascular event, stroke, venous thromboembolic phenomenon, and breast cancer). Randomized clinical trials provide no evidence that HRT prevents coronary artery disease or cardiovascular events. In fact, there is a possibility of accelerated short-term risk, particularly in women with coronary artery disease, hypertension, adverse lipid parameters, and prothrombin mutations. Despite these concerns, HRT may still be appropriate in women at increased risk for coronary artery disease if the noncoronary benefits of treatment exceed the risks (treatment of osteoporosis and/or a reduction in menopausal symptoms).

In women with contraindications or for those who do not wish to take HRT, alternative options may include SERMs, selective serotonin reuptake inhibitors, tibolone, clonidine, soy, and the use of intravaginal estsrogen creams or rings for genitourinary symptoms. Long-term use (more than 5 yr) potentially could be reasonable in a small proportion of postmenopausal women with documented osteoporosis or osteopenia or for those who are at significantly increased risk for osteoporosis (personal or family history of nontraumatic fracture, current smokers, or those with a body mass index of less than 22). Poor candidates for long-term use would include those who do not have an increased risk for osteoporosis, those with cardiovascular disease, those with one or more first-degree relatives with breast cancer, a history of breast biopsy demonstrating atypia, or the presence of genetic susceptibility (BRCA-1 or BRCA-2).

Androgens

The beneficial effects from the replacement of estrogen and progesterone because of nonfunctional or absent ovarian follicles has prompted a re-evaluation of ovarian androgen effects. In the United States, 130,000–195,000 women per year have their ovaries removed in conjunction with a hysterectomy.

Within the first day after total abdominal hysterectomy and bilateral salpingo-oophorectomy (TAH/BSO), plasma levels of estradiol and testosterone decrease significantly. Although estrogen levels in the premenopausal female fall from peak levels of 150–400 pg/mL to less than 20 pg/mL, testosterone levels fall in proportion to the production fraction of the premenopausal ovary, approx 25%. In postmenopausal women, however, the fall in testosterone production may be more than the 25% total production fraction usually attributed to the premenopausal ovary *(84)*. Vermilion et al. also demonstrated the ovary to be a major contributor to the production of postmenopausal androgen levels *(85)*.

Because the number of women seeking HRT after oophorectomy, the rationale for the use of androgens in women should be understood. Studies of sexual behavior in bilaterally oophorectomized females reveals that estrogen-replacement therapy alleviates atrophic vaginitis and dyspareunia, but does not affect motivational aspects, such as sexual desires and fantasies *(86)*.

EFFECTS OF ANDROGENS IN SURGICALLY CASTRATED ANIMALS

Animal studies have supported a role for androgens in surgically castrated primates. Testosterone propionate given to castrated rhesus monkeys increased the activity of sexually related behaviors *(87)*. Pharmacologic *(88)*, but not physiologic, doses *(89)* of testosterone administered to ovariectomized female monkeys increased their sexual invitational behavior and increased lever pressing, which allowed access to a male partner *(90)*. Human studies suggest a potential benefit for sexual motivation in women, but results of such therapy in castrated females vary in the premenopausal versus postmenopausal state *(91)*.

ANDROGENS FOR WOMEN

Premenopausal Oophorectomized Women. Studies suggest that the addition of androgens to standard estrogen-replacement therapy in the premenopausal woman may play a beneficial role for women who experience serious difficulty in stabilizing on standard estrogen-replacement therapy and/or for those who have specific complaints regarding libido. Psychosomatic complaints are rarely improved with treatment *(92–94)*.

Postmenopausal Oophorectomized and Naturally Menopausal Women. With regard to postmenopausal oophorectomized and naturally menopausal women, the published work to date suggests that the addition of androgens to estrogen-replacement regimen does not significantly enhance sexual activity or reduce depression over standard estrogen replacement alone *(95–98)*.

NEW INDICATIONS FOR ANDROGENS: OSTEOPOROSIS

Androgenic steroids are known to play a role in the maintenance of bone mass in men and women *(99,100)*. The beneficial effects of androgens, specifically dihydrotestosterone, on bone cell differentiation appears to be mediated by transforming growth factor-cx, and the induction of bone cell proliferation is the result of an enhanced response of osteoblastic cells to growth factors (fibroblast growth factor and insulin-like growth factor II) *(101)*.

For many years, nandrolone decanoate has been shown to increase the vertebral bone mineral density (BMD) in postmenopausal women with osteoporosis *(102)*. Raisz et al.

compared the effects of estrogen given alone to those of estrogen plus androgen therapy on biochemical markers of bone formation and resorption in postmenopausal women. Urinary excretion of the markers of bone resorption decreased equally in both groups. The estrogen-only group had a reduction in serum markers of bone formation; however, in women treated with the combination of estrogen and testosterone, the markers of bone formation increased *(103)*.

It does appear, however, that testosterone's effects on BMD are highly dependent on the actions of estrogen in skeletal maturation and mineralization. Examples of this interaction include the finding of severe osteoporosis in a male with normal testosterone levels but a defective estrogen receptor and an increase in BMD in postmenopausal women using combination estrogen and testosterone *(104–107)*.

It would appear that androgen replacement may potentially play a role in the treatment of women with or at high risk for osteoporosis in the future. Studies are in progress to characterize appropriate candidates and identify the potential risks (i.e., cardiovascular).

INDICATIONS/CONTRAINDICATIONS/ADVERSE EFFECTS OF METHYL TESTOSTERONE

The only Food and Drug Administration-approved combination for androgen-containing HRT in the United States is Estratest (Solvay, Marietta, GA). Estratest is a combination of esterified estrogens (1.25 mg) and methyl testosterone (2.5 mg), whereas EstratestHS (half-strength) is esterified estrogens (0.625 mg) and methyl testosterone (1.25 mg).

Androgens are responsible for the normal growth and development of male secondary sexual characteristics, including growth and development of the prostate, seminal vesicles, penis, scrotum, male hair patterns (beard, chest, axillary), laryngeal enlargement, vocal cord thickening, and alterations in musculature and body fat distribution. They cause retention of nitrogen, sodium, potassium, and phosphorus and decrease urinary excretion of calcium. Protein anabolism is increased and erythropoiesis is stimulated. Testosterone, which is metabolized by the gut, is 44% cleared by the liver on the first pass. Methyl testosterone is less extensively metabolized by the liver.

PRECAUTIONS

Patients should be observed for signs of virilization (voice deepening, hirsutism, acne, clitoromegaly). Prolonged use may result in fluid and sodium retention, and hypercalcemia may occur. Because of the known hepatotoxicity of 17α-alkylated androgens, liver function tests should be obtained periodically. Hemoglobin and hematocrit also should be evaluated on a periodic basis to check for polycythemia. Additionally, androgens may decrease the oral anticoagulant requirements of patients receiving such drugs, reduce insulin requirements, and lower blood glucose levels. There are rare reports of hepatocellular carcinoma in women receiving long-term high-dose therapy. Androgens decrease thyroid-binding globulin, causing lower T_4 and higher T_3RU.

Although the addition of androgens to postmenopausal estrogen-replacement is apparently not accompanied by a significant bone-sparing effect *(108)*, further research in this area may indicate positive effects. Parental androgen administration has been associated with hirsutism, hot flushes, decreased libido, mood changes, depression, and clitoromegaly. In some patients, testosterone levels have remained elevated with the occurrence of virilizing symptoms of 12–20 mo after an intramuscular injection *(109)*. (This parenteral [intramuscular] product is not available in the United States.)

Finally, potential adverse effects on cholesterol, high-density lipoprotein, high-density lipoprotein 2, high-density lipoprotein 3, and apolipoprotein A_2 have been noted in women receiving esterified estrogens plus methyl testosterone compared to estrogen alone *(110)*.

Although these concerns are valid, retrospective and prospective studies involving the use of androgen alone and in combination with estrogens demonstrate that concerns about the adverse effects of androgen use associated with supraphysiologic, self-escalated doses in men do not apply to the much lower doses combined with estrogens for hormone replacement in postmenopausal women *(111)*.

Recent clinical studies indicate that approx 5% will have a serious adverse event while taking an estrogen/androgen combination. The most commonly reported adverse events were those known to be associated with estrogen therapy (weight gain, headache, nausea, and vasodilatation) and androgen treatment (alopecia, acne, and hirsutism) *(112)*.

Summary of Androgen Use

In conclusion, androgens may be of some use in premenopausally castrated females with difficulty adjusting to estrogen replacement alone or for those with specific complaints regarding decreased libido. The studies cited, and clinical experience suggests that early sexual experiences impact greatly on sexuality in later life and particular attention should be addressed to such historic factors. Interventions should address apparent causal factors. The benefit of treatment in postmenopausal females is controversial at present. Further studies to evaluate the effects on bone mineral density in this group of women may define other appropriate roles for androgens in hormone-replacement regimens.

Androgen Delivery Systems

Injectable androgen administration has not been approved in the United States; thus, the oral route is utilized. New transdermal delivery systems are being actively developed. The chemical structure of methyl testosterone is shown in Fig. 14.

Phytoestrogens

Despite the major health benefits derived from HRT, compliance is relatively poor. Factors associated with patient noncompliance include concerns over an increased risk of breast cancer (RR 1.2–1.4) *(25)*, progestogen use with an intact uterus resulting in vaginal bleeding, PMS-like symptoms, and mood swings *(25)*.

Recent work suggests that soybean phytoestrogens may provide some of the health benefits attributed to estrogens without adverse events. Phytoestrogens are found in the legumes, particularly soy. The phytoestrogens found in soy are genistein, daidzein, and glycitein. Soybean phytoestrogens appear to be estrogen agonists for bone in experimental situations but act significantly less effectively than estrogen (CEEs) *(113)*.

In cynomolgus monkeys, soy phytoestroogens, however, failed to maintain bone density *(114)*. However, advantageous effects have been noted in cynomolgus monkeys in serum lipids (decreased plasma cholesterol and LDL, with increased HDL, and Apo A_1) and coronary artery atherogenesis *(115–118)*. Epidemiologic data would suggest that soy intake may reduce the risk of breast cancer *(119)*, potentially through a reduction in circulating ovarian steroids and adrenal androgens *(120)*. Phytoestrogens do not appear to stimulate the endometrium or genitourinary tissues *(121)*.

The selective activities of the phytoestrogens may potentially be explained by selective estrogen-receptor modulatory activities and different gene transcriptional activities

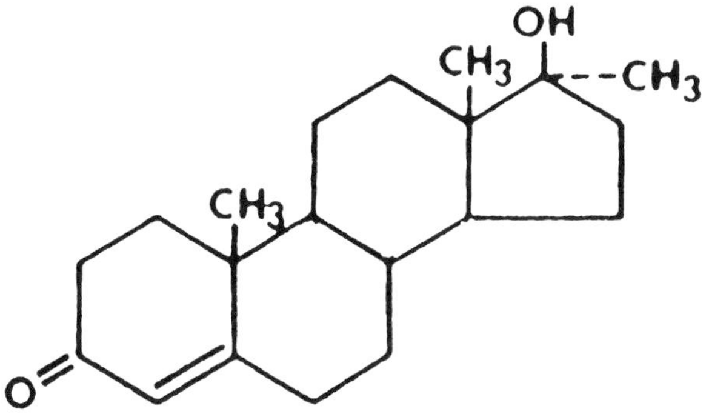

Fig. 14. Methyl testosterone.

of estrogen receptors-α and -β–ligand complexes. It does appear that phytoestrogens do not increase the risks of breast and endometrial cancers and may play a supportive role in sustaining healthy bone and cardiovascular systems in women. Further research will more clearly define the potential role of the phytoestrogens in health maintenance.

DHEA

Dehydroepiandrosterone sulfate (DHEAS) is the most abundant steroid in the body. It is primarily produced by the adrenal gland, with small amounts produced by the ovary. DHEA levels vary with age. Levels are low until adrenarche and then peak at 20–30 yr; thereafter, levels progressively decrease with age *(122)*.

By the seventh decade, DHEA levels are 10% of peak values. The decline in DHEAS with age results in a reduction in the formation of androgens and estrogens in peripheral target tissues.

Clinically, declining DHEA, and DHEAS levels have been associated with reduced protein synthesis, decreased body mass, and increased body fat *(123)*, cardiovascular disease in men *(124)*, various cancers *(125)*, and attenuation of the immune system *(126,127)*.

Clinical studies with appropriate controls are underway, and clear recommendations should be forthcoming. Documented side effects with use include hirsutism, decreased breast size, acne, hair loss, deepening voice, gastrointestinal discomfort, and reversible hepatitis *(128)*. Prudence suggests awaiting the results of the prospective clinical trials. For those who have self-initiated the medication, the dose should certainly be less than or equal to 50 mg. Additionally, lipids, liver function tests, and testosterone levels should be monitored periodically. There is no evidence that DHEA could be used in place of estrogen replacement.

CONCLUSIONS

Regardless of the etiology of hypogonadism, treatment goals are similar. Immediate goals address the present symptomatology of the patient. This may include the treatment of osteoporosis, hot flushes, and urogenital atrophy in patients with secondary hypogonadism or the lack of secondary sexual characteristics, as in primary hypogonadal women. Treatment of primary hypogonadism attempts to mimic normal physiology (low-dose isolated estrogen therapy) to allow normal breast maturation. Long-range treatment goals are concerned with the reduction of osteoporosis that is associated with prolonged hypogonadism. For women with a uterus, treatment utilizes an estrogen compound to directly address symptomatology and long-range concerns and a progestogen to protect against the increased risk of endometrial hyperplasia and cancer observed in women receiving unopposed estrogen therapy. In some situations, patients may benefit from an expansion of HRT to include the use of androgens and or phytoestrogens. DHEA is not considered an alternative to HRT. All women should be educated regarding adequate calcium (1000 mg/d) and vitamin D (400–800 IU/d) intake. Those choosing not to take HRT should increase their calcium to 1500 mg/d.

Based on data currently available, there is no clear justification to recommend the use of one hormonal formulation, delivery system, or treatment regimen over another. Rather, there are relative benefits that may be achieved with the various options available that are dependent on the particular characteristics of the individual patient. Medication choices will likely be even more complex in the future as the availability and activities of SERMs expands.

Many of the hormonal preparations being developed rely on transdermal delivery systems (*see* Table 5). This expansion in technology and information will result in improved health and well-being for hypogonadal women.

REFERENCES

1. Hagstad A, Janson PO. The epidemiology of climacteric symptoms. ACTA Obstet Gynecol Scand 1986;134:59–65.
2. Keating NL, Cleary PD, Rossi AS, et al. Use of hormone replacement therapy by postmenopausal women in the United States. Ann Intern Med 1999;130:545–553.
3. Seeman E. Osteoporosis: trials and tribulations. Am J Med 1997;18;103:74S–87S.
4. Eiken F, Kolthoff N, Nielsen SF. Effect of 10 years' hormone replacement therapy on bone mineral content in postmenopausal women. Bone 1996;5 (Suppl):191S–193S.
5. Daly E, Roche M, Barlow D, Gray A, McPherson K, Vessey M. HRT: An analysis of benefits, risks and costs. Br Med Bull 1992;48:368–400.
6. Van derLoos M, Paccaud F, GutzwillerF, Chrzanowski R. Impact of hormonal prevention on fractures of the proximal femur in postmenopausal women: a simulation study. Soz Praventivmed 1988;33:162–166.
7. Speroff L, Lobo RA. Postmenopausal hormone therapy and the cardiovascular system. Heart Dis Stroke 1994;3:173–176.
8. Hulley S, Grady D, Bush T, et al. Randomized trial of estrogen plus progestin for secondary prevention of coronary heart disease in postmenopausal women. JAMA 1998;280:605–613.
9. Herrington DM, Reboussin VN, Brosnihan KB, et al. Effects of estrogen replacement therapy on the progression of coronary-artery atherosclerosis. N Engl J Med. 2000;343:522–529.
10. Clarke S, Kelleher J, Lloyd-Jones H, et al. Transdermal hormone replacement therapy for secondary prevention of coronary artery disease in postmenopausal women. Eur Heart J 2000;21(Suppl):212.
11. Writing Group for the Women's Health Initiative Investigators. Risks and benefits of estrogen plus progestin in healthy opstmenopausal women. Principal results from the Women's Heath initiative Randomized Controlled Trial. JAMA 2002;288:321–333; L'Enfant C. Preliminary trends in women's health in the Women's Health Initiative. National Heart, Lung, and Blood Institute Communications Office, Bethesda, MD, 2000.
12. Mansen JE. Postmenopausal hormone therapy and atherosclerotic disease. Am Heart J 1994; 128:1337–1343.
13. Barrett-Connor E, Grady D. Hormone replacement therapy, heart disease, and other considerations. Annu Rev Public Health 1998;19:55–72.
14. Jorm AF, Korten AE, Henderson AS. The prevalence of dementia: a quantitative integration of the literature. Acta Psychiatr Scand 1987;76:465–479.
15. Paganini-Hill A, Henderson VW. Estrogen deficiency and risk of Alzheimer's disease in women. Am J Epidemiol 1994;140:256–261.

16. Paganini-Hill A, Henderson VW. Estrogen replacement therapy and risk of Alzheimer's disease. Arch Intern Med 1996;156:2213–2217.
17. Brenner De, Kukull WA, Stergachis A, et al. Postmenopausal estrogen replacement therapy and the risk of Alzheimer's disease: a population-based case-control study. Am J Epidemiol 1994;140:262–267.
18. Mortel KF, Meyers JS. Lack of postmenopausal estrogen replacement therapy and the risk of dementia. J Neuropsychiat Clin Neurosci 1996;7:334–337.
19. Kawas C, Resnick 5, Morrison A, et al. A prospective study of estrogen replacement therapy and the risk of development of Alzheimer' s disease: the Baltimore Longitudinal Study of Aging. Neurology 1997;48:1517–1521.
20. Grodstein F, Chen J, Pollend A, et al. Postmenopausal hormone therapy and cognitive function in healthy older women. J Am Geriatri Soc 2000;48:746–752
21. Mulnard RA, Cotman CW, Kawas C, et al. Estrogen replacement therapy for treatment of mild to moderate Alzheimer's disease: a randomized controlled trial: Alzheimer's Disease Cooperative Study. JAMA 2000;283:1007–1015.
22. Gould E, Wooley CS, Frankfurt M, McEwen BS. Gonadal steroids regulate dendritic spine density in hippocampal pyramidal cells in adulthood. J Neurosci 1990;l0:1286–1291.
23. Luine VN. Estradiol increases choline acetyltransferase activity in specific basal forebrain nuclei and projection areas of female rats. Exp Neurol 1985;89:484–490.
24. Behl C, Davis JB, Lesley R, Schubert D. Hydrogen peroxide mediates amyloid beta protein toxicity. Cell 1994;77:817–827.
25. Ravnikar VA. Compliance with hormone therapy. Am J Obstet Gynecol 1987;156:1332–l334.
26. Grodstein F, Manson JE, Colditz GA, Willett WC, Speizer FE, Stampfer MJ. A prospective, observational study of post menopausal hormone therapy and primary prevention of cardiovascular disease. Ann Intern Med 2000;133:933–941.
27. Chae CU, Manson JE. Postmenopausal hormone replacement therapy. In: Hennekens CH, ed. Clinical Trials in Cardiovascular Disease: A Companion to Braunwald's Heart Disease. Saunders, Philadelphia, 1999, pp. 399–414.
28. Pstay BM, Smith NL, LeMaitre RN, et al. Hormone replacement therapy prothrombotic mutations and the risk of incident non-fatal myocardial infarctions in postmenopausal women. JAMA 2001;285:906–913.
29. Grady D, Gebretsadik T, Kerlikowske K, Ernster V, Petitti D. Hormone replacement therapy and endometrial cancer risk: a meta-analysis. Obstet Gynecol 1995;85:304–313.
30. The Writing Group for the PEPI Trial. Effects of estrogen or estrogen/progestin regimens on heart disease risk factors in postmenopausal women: the Postmenopausal Estrogen/Progestin Intervention (PEPI) Trial. JAMA 1995;273:199–208 (with Erratum, JAMA 1995;274:1676).
31. Grady D, Wenger NK, Herrington D, et al. Postmenopausal hormone therapy increases risk for venous thromboembolic disease: the heart and estrogen/progestin replacement study (HEPRS). Ann Intern Med 2000;132:689–696.
32. The Collaborative Group on Hormonal Factors in Breast Cancer. Breast cancer and hormone replacement therapy: collaborative reanalysis of data from fifty-one epidemiologic studies of 52,705 women with breast cancer and 108,411 women without breast cancer. Lancet 1997;350:1047–1059.
33. Schairer C, Lubin J, Troisi R, Sturgeon S, Brinton L, Hoover R. Menopausal estrogen and estrogen-progestin replacement therapy in breast cancer risk. JAMA 2000;283:485–491.
34. Rodriguez C, Patel AV, Calle E, et al. Estrogen replacement therapy in ovarian cancer mortality in a larger prospective study of US women. JAMA 2001;285:1460–1465.
35. Garg PP, Kerlikoeske K, Subak L, et al. Hormone replacement therapy in the risk of epithelial ovarian carcinoma: a meta-analysis. Obstet Gynecol 1998;92:472–479.
36. Coughlin SS, Giutozzi A, Smith SJ, et al. A meta-analysis of estrogen replacement therapy and risk of epithelial ovarian cancer. J Clin Epidemiol 2000;53:367–375.
37. Negri E, Tzonou A, Beral V, et al. Hormone therapy for menopause and ovarian cancer in a collaborative reanalysis of European studies. Int J Cancer 1999;80:848–851.
38. Jordan CV. Estrogen receptor antagonists. In: Adashi EY, Rock JA, Rosenwaks, eds. Reproductive Endocrinology, Surgery, and Technology. Lippencott-Raven, Philadelphia, PA, 1996, p. 535.
39. Mashchak CA, Lobo RA, Dozono-Takano R, et at. Comparison of pharmacodynamic properties of various estrogen formulations. Am J Obstet Gynecol 1982;144:511–518.
40. Eighth Supplement to U.S.P. XXII. Easton, PA. Mack;l990;3256–3258.
41. Lobo RL, Nguyen HN, Eggena P, Brenner PF. Biologic effects of equilin sulfate in postmenopausal women. Fertil Steril 1988;49:234–238.

42. Brosnihan KB, Weddle D, Anthony MS, Heise C, Li F, Ferrario CM. Effects of chronic hormone replacement on the renin-angiotensin system in cynomolgus monkeys. J Hypertens 1997;15:719–726.

43. Aylward M, Maddock J, Rees PL. Natural estrogen replacement therapy and blood clotting. Br Med J 1976;1:220–222.

44. Varma TR. Effect of estrogen replacement on blood coagulation factors in postmenopausal women. Int J Gynaecol Obstet 1983;21:291–296.

45. Perez-Gutthan. Hormone replacement therapy and risk of venous thromboembolism: a population-based case controlled study. BMJ 1997;314:796–800.

46. Wash Drug Lett. 1991:6.

47. Bhavnani BR. Pharmacokinetics and pharmacodynamics of conjugated equine, estrogens: chemistry and metabolism. Proc Soc Exp Biol Med 1998;217:6–16.

48. Yen SCC, Martin FL, Burnier AM, et at. Circulating estradiol, estrone, and gonadotropin levels following the administration of orally active 17 beta estradiol in post-menopausal women. J Clin Endocrinol Metab 1975;40:518–521.

49. Ryan KJ. Engel LL. Endocrinology 1953;52:287.

50. LoboRA, Cassidenti DL. Pharmacokinetics of oral 17 beta estradiol . J Reprod Med 1992;37:77–84.

51. Kuhl H. Pharmacokinetics of oestrogens and progestogens. Maturitas 1990;12:171–197.

52. McEvoy GK, et al., eds. American Hospital Formulary Service. American Society of Hospital Pharmacists, Bethesda, MD, 1991.

53. Orme M, Back DJ, Ward S, Green S. The pharmacokinetics of ethinyl estradiol in the presence and absence of gestodene and desogestrel. Contraception 1991;43:305–316.

54. Mandel FP, Geoia Fl, Lu KH, Biologic effects of various doses of ethinyl estradiol in postmenopausal women. Obstet Gynecol J 982;59:673–679.

55. Hammond CB, Maxon WS. Estrogen replacement therapy. Clin Obstet Gynecol 1986;29:407–430.

56. Bewley S, BewleyTH. Drug dependence with estrogen replacement therapy. Lancet 1992;339:290,291.

57. Kuiper GGJM, Enmark E, Pelto-Huikko M, Nilsson S, Gustafsson J-A.Cloning of a novel receptor expressed in rat prostate and ovary. Proc Natl Acad Sci USA 1996;93:5925–5930.

58. Mosselman S, Polman J, Dijkema R.ER beta: identification and characterization of a novel human estrogen receptor. FEBS Lett 1996;392:49–53.

59. Gambrel RD Jr. Use of progestogen therapy. Am J Obstet Gynecol 1987;156:1304–1313.

60. Persson I. Cancer risk in women receiving estrogen-progestin replacement therapy. Maturitas 1996;23:S37–S45.

61. Persson I, Thurfjell E, Bergstrom R, Holmberg L. Hormone replacement therapy and the risk of breast cancer. Nested case-control study in a cohort of Swedish women attending mammography screening. Int J Cancer 1997;72:758–761.

62. von Schoultz B. HRT and breast cancer risk, what to advise? Eur J Obstet Gynecol Reprod Biol 1997;71:205–208.

63. Persson I, et al. Cancer incidence and mortality in women receiving estrogen and estrogen-progestin replacement therapy: long-term follow-up of a Swedish cohort. Int J Cancer 1996;67:327–332.

64. Caldas GA, Hankinson SE, Hunter DJ, Willett WC, Manson JE, Stampfer MJ, Hennekens C, Rosner B, Speizer FE. The use of estrogens and progestins and the risk of breast cancer in postmenopausal women. N Engl J Med 1995;332:1589–1593.

65. Colditz GA, Egan KM, Stampfer MJ. Hormone replacement therapy and risk of breast cancer: results from epidemiologic trials. Am J Obstet Gynecol 1993;168:1473–1480.

66. Grodstein F, Stampfer MJ, Caldas GA, et al. Postmenopausal hormone therapy and mortality. N Engl J Med 1997;336:1769–1775.

67. Scarier C, Adami HO, Hoover R, Persson I. Cause-specific mortality in women receiving hormone therapy. Epidemiology 1997:1:59–65.

68. Peterson CM. Progestogens, progesterone antagonists, progesterone and androgens: Synthesis, classification, and uses. Clin Obstet Gynecol 1995;38:813–820.

69. Moyer DL, de Lignieres B, Driguez P, Fez JP. Prevention of endometrial hyperplasia by progesterone during long term estradiol replacement: influence of bleeding pattern and secretory changes. Fertil Steril 1993;59:992–997.

70. The Writing Group for the PEPI Trial. Effects of estrogen and estrogen/progestin regimens on heart disease risk factors in postmenopausal women: the postmenopausal estrogen/progestin interventions (PEPI). JAMA 1995;273:199–208.

71. Gillet JY, Andre G, Fauger B, Erny R, Buvat-Herbaut MA, et al. Induction of amenorrhea during hormone replacement therapy: optimal micronized progesterone dose. A multicenter study. Maturitas 1994;19:103–116.

72. Miles RA, Paulson RJ, Lobo RA, Press MF, Dahmoush L, Sauer MV. Pharmacokinetics and endometrial tissue levels of progesterone after administration by intramuscular and vaginal routes: a comparative study. Fertil Steril 1994;62:485–490.

73. Casanas-Roux F, Nisolle M, Marbaix E, Smets M, Bassil 5, Donnez J. Morphometric, immunohistological and three-dimensional evaluation of the endometrium of menopausal women treated by oestrogen and Crinone, a new slow-release vaginal progesterone. Hum Reprod 1996;11:357–363.

74. Jensen J, Riis BJ, Strin V, Nilas L, Christiansen C. Long term effects of percutaneous estrogens and oral progesterone on serum lipoproteins in postmenopausal women. Am J Obstet Gynecol 1987;156:66–71.

75. Shangold MM, Tomai TP, Cook JD, Jacobs SL, Zinaman MJ, Chin SY, Simon JA. Factors associated with withdrawal bleeding after administration of oral micronized progesterone in women with secondary amenorrhea. Fertil Steril 1991;56: 1029–1033.

76. Whitehead MI, HillardTC, CrookD. The role and use of progestogens. Obstet Gynecol 1990;75:559–576.

77. Woodruff JD, Pickar JH for The Menopause Study Group. Incidence of endometrial hyperplasia in postmenopausal women taking conjugated estrogens with medroxyprogesterone acetate or conjugated estrogens alone. Am J Obstet Gynecol 1994;170:1213.

78. Ulrich LG, Barlow DH, Sturdee DW, Wells M, Campbell Mi, Nielsen B, Bragg AJ, Vessey MP. Quality of life and patient preference for sequential versus continuous combined HRT: the UK Kliofem multicenter study experience. UK Continuous Combined HRT Study Investigators. Int J Gynaecol Obstet 1997;59:S11–S17.

79. Piegsa K, Calder A, Davis JA, McKay-Hart D, Wells M, Bryden F. Endometrial status in postmenopausal women on long-term continuous combined hormone replacement therapy (Kliofem). A comparative study of endometrial biopsy, outpatient hysteroscopy and transvaginal ultrasound. Eur J Obstet Gynecol Reprod Biol 1997;72:175–180.

80. Leather AT, Savvas IA, Studd JWW. Endometrial histology and bleeding patterns after eight years of continuous combined estrogen and progestogen therapy in postmenopausal women. Obstet Gynecol 1991;78:1008–1010.

81. Darj F, Nilsson S, Axelsson O, et al. Clinical and endometrial effects of estradiol and progesterone in postmenopausal women. Maturitas 1991;13:109–115.

82. Gambrell RD Jr. Progestogens in estrogen-replacement therapy. Clin Obstet Gynecol 1995;38:890–901.

83. Casper RF, Chapdelaine A. Estrogen and interrupted progestin: a new concept for menopausal replacement therapy. Am J Obstet Gynecol 1993;168:1188–1196.

84. Judd HL, Judd GE, Lucas WF, Yen S.S. Endocrine function of the postmenopausal ovary: concentration of androgens and estrogens in ovarian and peripheral vein blood. J Clin Endo Metab 1974;39:1020–1024.

85. Vermilion A. The hormonal activity of the postmenopausal ovary. J Clin Endo Metab 1976;42:247–252.

86. Furuhjelm M, Karlgren F, Carstrom K. The effect of estrogen therapy on somatic and psychical symptoms in postmenopausal women. Acta Obstet Gynecol Scand 1984;63:655–661.

87. Wallem K, Goy RW. Effects of estradiol benzoate, estrone, and proprionates of testosterone or dihydrotestosterone on sexual and related behaviors of ovariectomized rhesus monkeys. Horm Behav 1977;9:228–248.

88. Michael RP, Zumpe D. Effects of androgen administration on sexual invitations by female rhesus monkeys. Anim Behav 1977;25:936–944.

89. Michael RP, Richter MC, Cain IA, et al. Artificial menstrual cycles, behavior and the role of androgens in female rhesus monkeys. Nature 1978;175:439–440.

90. Michael RP, Zumpe D, Keverne EB, et al. Neuroendocrine factors in the control of primate behavior. Rec Frog Horm Res. 1972;28:665–706.

91. Sherwin BB, Gelfand MM, Brender W. Androgen enhances sexual motivation in females: a prospective, crossover study of sex steroid administration in the surgical menopause. Psychosom Med 1985;47:339–351.

92. Sherwin BB, Gelfand MM. The role of androgen in the maintenance of sexual functioning in oophorectomized women. Psychosom Med 1987;49:397–409.

93. Sherwin BB, Gelfand MM. Differential symptoms response to parenteral estrogen and/or androgen administration in the surgical menopause. Am J Obstet Gynecol 1985, 151:153–160.

94. Young R, Wilta B, Dabbs I, et al. Comparison of estrogen plus androgen and estrogen on libido and sexual satisfaction in recently oophorectomized women. North American Menopause Society Meeting, September 17–20, 1992.

95. Dow MTG, Hart DM. Hormonal treatments of sexual unresponsiveness in postmenopausal women. Br J Obstet Gynaecol 1983;90:361–366.

96. Sherwin BB, Gelfand MM. Sex steroids and affect in "the surgical menopause: a double blind, crossover study. Psychoneuroendocrinology 1985;10:325–335.

97. Myers LS, Dixon J, Morrissette M, Carmichael M, Davidson JM. Effects of estrogen, androgen, and progestin on sexual psychophysiology and behavior in postmenopausal women. J Clin Endo Metab 1990;70:1124–1131.

98. Notelovitz M, Watts N, Timmons MC, et al. Effects of estrogen plus low dose androgen versus estrogen alone on menopausal symptoms in oophorectomized-hysterectomized women. North American Menopausal Society Meeting, September 17–20, 1992.

99. Colvard DS, Erickson, EF, Meeting FE et al, Identification of androgen receptors in normal human osteoblast-like cells. Proc Natl Acad Sci USA 1989;86:854–857.

100. Kasperk CH, Wergedeal JE, et al. Androgens directly stimulate proliferation of bone cells in vitro. Endocrinology 1989;124:1576,1577.

101. Kasperk C, Fitzsimmons R, Strong D, et al. Studies of the mechanism by which androgens enhance mitogenesis and differentiation in bone cells. J Clin Endocrinol Metab 1990;71:1322–329.

102. Need AG, Horowitz M, Bridges A, Morris H, Nordic BE. Effects of nandrolonedecanoate and antiresorptive therapy on vertebral density in osteoporotic, postmenopausal women. Arch Am Med 1989;149:57–60.

103. Raisz LG, Wiita B, Artis A, et al. Comparison of the effects of estrogen alone and estrogen plus androgen on biochemical markers of bone formation and resorption in postmenopausal women. J Clin Endocrinol Metab 1995;81:37–43.

104. Smith EP, Boyd I, Frank GR, et al. Estrogen resistance caused by a mutation in the oestrogen-receptor gene in a man. N Engl J Med 1994;331:1056–1061.

105. Savvas M, Studd JWW, Fogelman I, et al. Skeletal effects of oral oestrogen compared with subcutaneous oestrogen and testosterone in postmenopausal women. Br Med J 1988;297:331–333.

106. Savvas M, Studd JWW, Norman S, et al. Increase in bone mass after one year of percutaneous oestradiol and testosterone implants in post-menopausal women who have previously received long-term oral oestrogens. Br J Obstet Gynaecol 1992;757–760.

107. Davis SR. McCloud F, Strauss BJG, Burger HG. Testosterone enhances estradiol effects on postmenopausal bone density and sexuality. Maturitas 1995;21:227–236.

108. Garnet T, Studd, J, Watson N, Savvas M. The effects of plasma estradiol levels on increases in vertebral and femoral bone density following therapy with estradiol and estradiol with testosterone implants. Obstet Gynecol 1992;79:968–972.

109. Urman B, Pride SM, Ho Yeun BH. Elevated serum testosterone, hirsutism, and virilism associated with combined androgen-estrogen hormone replacement therapy. Obstet Gynecol 1991;77:595–598.

110. Hickok LR, Toomey C, Speroff L. A comparison of esterified estrogens with and without methyltestosterone: effects on endometrial histology and serum lipoproteins in postmenopausal women. Obstet Gynecol 1993;82:924–927.

111. Gelfand MM, Wiita B. Int J Fertil Menopausal Stud 1996;41:412–422.

112. Phillips F, Bauman C. Safety surveillance of esterified estrogens-methyltestosterone (Estratest and Estratest HS) replacement therapy in the United States. Clin Ther 1997;19:1070–1084.

113. Arjmandi BH, Alkel L, Hollis BW, Amin D, Stacewicz-Sapuntzakis M, Guo P, Kukreja SC. Dietary soybean protein prevents bone loss in an ovariectomized rat model of osteoporosis. J Nutr 21 1996;126: 161–167.

114. Jayo MI, Anthony MS, Register TC, Rankin SE, Vest T, Clarkson TB. Dietary soy isoflavones and bone loss: a study in ovariectomized monkey. J Bone Miner Res 1996;11:8228.

115. Anthony MS, Clarkson TB, Hughes CL, Morgan TM, Burke CL. Soybean isoflavones improve cardiovascular risk factors without affecting reproductive system of peripubertal rhesus monkeys. J Nutr 1996;126:43–50.

116. Anthony MS, Burke GL, Hughes CL, Clarkson TB. Does soy supplementation improve coronary heart disease risk? Circulation 1995;91:925–929.

117. Anthony MS, Clarkson TB, Hughes CL. Plant and mammalian estrogen effects on plasma lipids of female monkeys. Circulation 1994;90:1235–1239.

118. Williams 1K, Honore EK, Washburn SA, Clarkson TB. Effects of hormone replacement therapy on reactivity of atherosclerotic coronary arteries in cynomolgus monkeys. J Am Coll Cardiol 1994;24:1757–1761.

119. Messina MI, Persky V, Setchell KDR, Barnes S. Soy intake and cancer risk: a review of the in vitro and in vivo data. Nutr Cancer I 994;21:113–131.

120. Lu U, Anderson KE, Grady JJ, Nagamani M. Effects of soya consumption for one month on steroid hormones in premenopausal women: implications for breast cancer risk reduction. Cancer Epidemiol Biomarkers Prey 1996;5:63–70.

121. Knight DC, Eden IA. A review of the clinical effects of phytoestrogens. Obstet Gynecol 1996;87:897–904.

122. Orentreich N, Brind I, Rizer R, Vogelmen J. Age changes and sex differences in serum dehydro-epiandrosterone sulfate concentration throughout adulthood. J Clin Endocrinol Metab 1 984;59:551–555.

123. Nestler JE, Barlascini CO, Clore JN, Blackard WG. Dehydroepiandrosterone reduces serum low density lipoprotein levels and body fat but does not alter insulin sensitivity in normal men. J Clin Endocrinol Metab 1988;66:57–61

124. Barrett-Conner F, Khaw KT. Absence of an inverse relation of dehydroepiandrosterone sulfate with cardiovascular mortality in postmenopausal women. N Engl J Med 1987;317:711–715.

125. Casson PR, Buster IE. DHEA administration to humans: panacea or palaver? Sem Repro Endo 1995;13:247–256.

126. Casson PR, Anderson RN, Herod HG. Oral dehydroepiandrosterone in physiologic doses modulates immune function in postmenopausal women. Am J Obstet Gynecol 1993;169:1536–1539.

127. Khorramo, Vu L, Yen SS. Activation of immune function by dehydroepiandrosterone (DHEA) in age-advanced men. J Gerontol 1997;52:M1–7.

128. Buster IF, Casson PR, Stroaughn AB, et al. Postmenopausal steroid replacement with micronized dehydroepiandrosterone: preliminary oral bioavailability and dose proportionnality studies. Am J Obstet Gynecol 1992;166:1163–1168.

26 Androgen Replacement in Women

Susan R. Davis, MBBS, FRACP, PhD
and Henry G. Burger, MD, FRACP

INTRODUCTION

There is increasing awareness of the significant and varied actions of endogenous androgens in women and acknowledgment that women may experience symptoms secondary to androgen deficiency. There is also substantial evidence that prudent testosterone replacement is effective in relieving both the physical and psychological symptoms of androgen insufficiency and is indicated for clinically affected women. Testosterone replacement for women is now available in a variety of formulations. It appears to be safe, with the caveat that doses should be restricted to the "therapeutic window" for androgen replacement in women in which the beneficial effects on well-being and quality of life can be achieved without incurring undesirable virilizing side effects.

The predominant complaint of women experiencing androgen deficiency is loss of sexual desire. Because of the complex hormonal–psychological etiology of this symptom, clinicians prescribing a hormone replacement therapy (HRT) regimen that includes an androgen component must be sensitive to the sexual and emotional needs of the affected woman and her partner, and care for the totality of the woman, not just her hormonal status. Many women who have the clinical symptoms of androgen insufficiency and low testosterone levels will respond to a replacement regimen and require no further intervention. However, a significant proportion of affected women have additional psychosocial issues that must be addressed, especially those who have undergone

From: *Endocrine Replacement Therapy in Clinical Practice*
Edited by: A. Wayne Meikle © Humana Press Inc., Totowa, NJ

a premature menopause, or a menopause secondary to surgery or cancer therapy, and body image issues, symptoms of posttraumatic stress, depression and other partnership problems may complicate their response to hormonal therapy. Identification of such factors and appropriate professional referral will clearly optimize the overall health of such women and their response to any therapeutic intervention.

ANDROGEN PHYSIOLOGY IN THE PREMENOPAUSAL YEARS

Androgens are produced by both the ovaries and the adrenals, which both synthesize androstenedione (A) and dehydroepiandrosterone (DHEA). The ovaries are a primary site of testosterone production; however, whether there is direct secretion of testosterone from the adrenals is controversial. The adrenals also produce DHEA sulfate (DHEAS). Conversion of the preandrogens to testosterone peripherally accounts for at least 5% of circulating testosterone, with A being the main preandrogen precursor (1). Androgens are produced by the ovary under the control of luteinizing hormone (LH). The preovulatory phase of the menstrual cycle is associated with a rise in intrafollicular and circulating androgen levels, such that peripheral A and testosterone increase 15–20% at mid-cycle, followed by a secondary rise in A in the late luteal phase (2). The mean daily production rate of testosterone in young healthy women is 0.43 ± 0.14 mg/d when measured in the follicular phase, with a diurnal variation, the highest rate of production occurring between 4 AM, and midday (3).

Only 1–2% of total circulating testosterone is free or biologically active; the rest is bound by sex-hormone-binding globulin (SHBG) and albumin. SHBG levels do not vary across the menstrual cycle; hence, there is a mid-cycle increase in free-testosterone in ovulating women (4). SHBG binds, in decreasing order of affinity, dehydrotestosterone (DHT) > testosterone > androstenediol > estradiol > estrone. In addition, SHBG weakly binds DHEA, but not DHEAS (5).

Changes in SHBG levels in women can have dramatic effects on free circulating sex steroid levels. SHBG levels are suppressed by increases in circulating testosterone, glucocorticosteroids, growth hormone, and insulin (as in obesity), and increased by thyroxine and estrogens.

CHANGES IN ANDROGENS
WITH MENOPAUSAL TRANSITION AND AGE

In contrast to estrogens, androgen levels do not fall precipitously at the menopause (6,7), but decline with increasing age, such that total circulating testosterone levels in women in their forties are approx 50% of those of women in their 20s (8). Furthermore, as SHBG also declines with age, the ratio of testosterone to SHBG, also known as the free-androgen index (FAI), does not change. However the absolute amount of circulating free testosterone in older women is less (8,9). The changes in testosterone and SHBG appear to be partly the result of the decline in the adrenal production of DHEA and DHEAS with increasing age (10,11), and as one would expect, the DHEA to testosterone and DHEAS to testosterone ratios are age invariant (8).

Reproductive aging also contributes to the gradual waning of testosterone observed in the premenopausal years. The mid-cycle rise in free testosterone and A seen in younger women is absent in older reproductive women in their mid-40s who continue to have regular menstrual cycles with a measurable LH surge (4). In postmenopausal women.

total testosterone levels are positively correlated with LH, which most probably reflects ongoing stimulation of ovarian interstitial cells by LH in the postmenopausal ovary *(12)*. This is of clinical significance because the administration of exogenous estrogen, either as HRT or the oral contraceptive pill, may not only precipitate relative testosterone deficiency by increasing SHBG and hence lowering the absolute amount of free testosterone *(13–15)*, but also by suppressing the LH stimulus to the ovary for interstitial cell testosterone production *(15–17)*.

Indeed, clinical studies have demonstrated that following the introduction of a standard dose of 0.625 mg of conjugated equine estrogen daily, the mean testosterone-to-SHBG ratio and measured free testosterone each fall by approx 30% *(13,14)*. Similarly, administration of the oral contraceptive pill suppresses circulating total testosterone, with normalization of levels during the pill-free menstrual phase *(15)*. The latter is less likely to be clinically manifest in younger reproductive women, but in the background of declining testosterone production with age, the oral contraceptive pill may be associated with the reporting of diminished libido in women in their later reproductive years.

In evaluating women for androgen deficiency, it is therefore important to measure either SHBG in addition to total testosterone to calculate the FAI or free testosterone directly. Because measured and estimated bioavailable testosterone are strongly correlated *(18)*, calculation of the FAI is adequate for clinical practice. The key point is that detection of a total testosterone level within the normal reproductive female range in any woman taking exogenous thyroid replacement or estrogen in any form does not exclude a physiological deficiency of bioavailable testosterone.

EVIDENCE FOR THE ROLE OF ANDROGENS IN FEMALE HEALTH AND WELL-BEING

Androgens and Female Sexuality

Satisfactory sexual function is an essential component of health and well-being, with "satisfactory" being an evaluation made by the individual in the context of her or his personal expectations and desires. Sexuality and libido are undoubtedly determined by many factors that all interact. These include a person's physiological state, his or her physical and social environment, personal knowledge, past experiences, current expectations and, of major influence, his or her cultural milieu. Thus, the complexity of human sexuality extends far beyond the biology of procreation.

There is a prevailing misconception that women's sexuality declines with increasing age and that older women who continue to engage in intercourse do so to please their partner. The majority of women who undergo a natural menopause maintain their capacity for sexual desire, erotic pleasure, and orgasm, although there is a general age-related decline in sexual frequency in women. However, there is a strong association between menopause and lessening sexual and coital frequency, which is independent of age *(19)*. Compared with premenopausal women, women after menopause report fewer sexual thoughts or fantasies, have less vaginal lubrication during sex, and are less satisfied with their partners as lovers, with a low testosterone level being most closely correlated with reduced coital frequency *(20)*. Clearly, the effects of age on the health and sexual interest of men and availability of a sexual partner contributes to the observed decreases in women. Research addressing the effects of women anticipating an adverse influence of their menopause on their sexuality has shown that the correlation between anticipated changes in sexuality and what is actually experienced is weak *(21)*. The greatest predictor of women having satisfying sexual relationships or experiences after menopause is the quality of the sexual aspects of their lives before menopause, with those most content with their premenopausal sexuality less likely to report problems. Despite this general trend, it is not uncommon for a woman to express frustration that she has had a very satisfying sexual relationship, but since menopause her sexuality has declined dramatically, with no other identifiable factors.

Androgens appear to play a key role in female sexuality in that diminished androgen levels in the postmenopausal years appear to contribute to the decline in sexual interest expressed by many women. Bachmann and Leiblum studied sexuality in sexagenarian women and observed that of the hormones studied, serum free testosterone was positively correlated with increased sexual desire *(22)*. Estrogen replacement will improve vasomotor symptoms, vaginal dryness, and general well-being, but has little effect on libido *(23,24)*. Oral estrogen replacement therapy improves sexual satisfaction in women with atrophic vaginitis causing their dyspareunia, but women without coital discomfort appear to benefit little or not at all *(25,26)*.

Several studies have shown improvements in a number of parameters of sexuality in postmenopausal women treated with exogenous testosterone over and above the effects achieved with estrogen alone. Both estradiol and testosterone are present in the human female brain. The highest concentrations of estradiol have been reported in the hypothalamus and the preoptic area, and that of testosterone, in the substantia nigra, hypothalamus, and the preoptic area *(27)*. The concentration of testosterone is several-fold higher than estradiol in each of these regions, with the highest ratio of testosterone to estradiol occurring in the hypothalamus and preoptic area, which corresponds with the high aromatase activity found in these regions *(28)*. This provokes the question of whether androgens act directly on the brain or only after conversion to estrogen by aromatization to estrogen within the central nervous system. Support for specific direct androgen actions within the brain comes from studies of the effects of cross-sex hormone therapy in transsexuals *(29)*, whereas the administration of androgens to female-to-male transsexuals leads to an increase in sexual motivation and arousability, the combination of anti-androgens and high-dose estrogen given to male-to-female transsexuals has the opposite effect. Androgen treatment of female-to-male transsexuals also results in improved visuospatial ability, a deterioration in verbal fluency, and increased anger readiness, whereas the reverse, including an increased tendency to indirect angry behavior, is seen in the male-to-female subjects *(30)*.

Exogenous androgen replacement in the form of testosterone, as an injection, subcutaneous implant, or transdermal patch enhances sexual motivation *(25,26,31–35)*. Improvements in intensity of sexual drive, arousal, frequency of sexual fantasies, satisfaction, pleasure, and relevancy have all been documented. Transdermal testosterone therapy is also associated with improved mood and well-being measured using the psychological index of well-being *(35)*.

In contrast to the consistently observed increases in sexual motivation, improvements in coital frequency and orgasm vary considerably between studies. Certainly, the failure for androgen therapy to improve coital frequency has been attributed to the relevant studies involving women with very long-term relationships, such that sexual patterns are very established with a reluctance toward change. Frequency of sexual activity as a measure of efficacy of androgen therapy in women can be misleading, as traditionally it is more a measure of a male partner's sexual appetite rather than the woman's. The only study in which the addition of testosterone did not show any benefit over estrogen alone was of women being treated for generalized menopausal symptoms rather than low libido *(36)*.

Testosterone replacement will only be of benefit to women who have a significant hormonal component to their sexual dysfunction. Discerning this can be quite straight-forward in many instances (e.g., post ovariectomy), but extremely complex in some women.

When considering whether a woman may be a candidate for androgen replacement, it is essential to take a reasonably detailed, although not overly intrusive sexual history. The main feature to establish is whether there are other significant aspects of the woman's life or relationship contributing to her apparent sexual difficulties.

Androgens and Bone Function

Androgenic steroids have an important physiologic role in the development and maintenance of bone mass in women and men. Human osteoblastic cells possess andro-gen receptors and androgens have been shown to directly stimulate bone cell prolifera-tion and differentiation *(37,38)*. Clinical research has demonstrated positive relationships between bone density and androgens in young, premenopausal and perimenopausal women. Premenopausal bone loss is significantly associated with circulating testoster-one levels, but not with estradiol *(39,40)*. Women who experience bone loss confined to the hip in their premenopausal years, which is not an uncommon finding, have lower total and free testosterone concentrations (by 14 and 22%, respectively) than those who do not have significant bone loss *(40)*. Consistent with these findings, hyperandrogenic women have higher bone mineral density (BMD), after correction for body mass index (BMI), than their normal female counterparts *(41)*. In the premenopausal years, BMD is also strongly positively correlated with body weight *(39)*. Obesity suppresses SHBG with a resultant increase in free testosterone *(42)*. This may partially explain the relationship among obesity, free testosterone, and increased BMD, with the greater endogenous levels of biologically active free testosterone directly enhancing bone mass.

Studies of both oral and parenteral estrogen and estrogen-plus-testosterone therapy in postmenopausal women have shown beneficial effects of androgens on BMD *(43,44)*. An oral esterified estrogen–methyltestosterone combination lead to increased spinal bone mineral density over a 2-yr period, in contrast to estrogen-only therapy that pre-vented bone loss *(43)*. The oral estrogen–methyltestosterone combination not only sup-pressed several biochemical markers of bone reabsorption (as seen with estrogen alone) but was also associated with increases in the markers of bone formation *(45)*. Treatment of postmenopausal women with nandrolone decanoate has been shown to increase verte-bral BMD and has been used successfully for many years to treat osteoporosis *(46)*. Com-bined estradiol and testosterone replacement with subcutaneous implant pellets increases bone mass in postmenopausal women *(47,48)*, with the effects in the hip and spine being greater than with estradiol implants alone *(34)*. Thus, it appears that estradiol alone has an anti-reabsorptive effect on bone in postmenopausal women, whereas the addition of tes-tosterone, either orally or parenterally, results in increased bone formation.

Studies of men, either with a mutation of the gene encoding the aromatase enzyme *(49)* or a mutation of the estrogen receptor *(50)*, indicate that androgens may only exert a measurable direct anabolic effect on bone in women and men when there is sufficient circulating estrogen to facilitate skeletal maturation and epiphysial closure and prevent bone resorption.

These findings are encouraging; however, improving BMD is only clinically important if it is associated with enhanced mechanical strength and a reduced fracture rate. To date, no studies have addressed the impact of androgens on the incidence of fracture. However, the effects of androgens on the mechanical properties of bone have been studied in feral female cynomolgus monkeys *(51)*. Increases in intrinsic bone strength and resistance to mechanical stress were associated with increased BMD following testosterone therapy. Treatment also resulted in increased bone torsional rigidity and bending stiffness.

Androgen Replacement and Glucocorticosteroid-Related Bone Loss

Circulating DHEA and DHEA-S have been positively correlated with BMD in ageing women *(52–54)* and the progressive decline in DHEA with increasing age is believed to contribute to senile osteoporosis. It is not clear whether these adrenal preandrogens directly influence bone metabolism or whether their effects are mediated indirectly after conversion to estradiol, A, or testosterone. Older women treated with oral DHEA have restoration of circulating A, DHT, and testosterone to premenopausal levels, as well as increases in DHEA and DHEAS, with no changes in circulating levels of estrone or estradiol from baseline *(55)*. Furthermore, circulating DHEAS, but not estradiol, in postmenopausal women is positively correlated with BMD *(52)*. The therapeutic administration of glucocorticosteroids results in significant suppression of adrenal preandrogen secretion *(56)*, which, in turn, may be a major factor in the development of iatrogenic osteopenia and osteoporosis with long-term glucocorticosteroid use. Therefore, a possible role for androgen replacement could indeed be to prevent or treat glucocorticosteroid-induced bone loss in both pre- and postmenopausal women.

In summary, current data indicates that androgen replacement, in the form of testosterone, is potentially an effective alternative to the prevention of bone loss and the treatment of osteopenia and osteoporosis. However, as prospective data confirming a reduction in fracture rate with such therapy is lacking, it cannot presently be recommended for this sole indication. Further research into the biological actions of androgens in bone and clinical studies of testosterone replacement and fracture are therefore needed to define the appropriate clinical application of androgens in the prevention and treatment of bone loss.

Metabolic Effects of Androgen Therapy: Risks and Benefits

CARDIOVASCULAR DISEASE RISK

There are prevailing concerns regarding potential adverse metabolic effects of androgen replacement in women, particularly with respect to possible detrimental effects on body composition, lipid and lipoprotein metabolism, and vascular function. However, available clinical data are extremely reassuring in that androgen-replacement therapy in women does not appear to be associated with the undesirable metabolic consequences seen in women with androgen excess or with an increase in cardiovascular risk.

ANDROGENS AND BODY COMPOSITION

In postmenopausal women, neither measured nor estimated bioavailable testosterone are associated with waist-to-hip ratio measurements and there does not appear to be a causal relationship between androgens and visceral adiposity in this population *(18)*.

Testosterone replacement by implant is associated with a modest increase in lean body mass measured by dual-photon X-ray absorptiometry and a reduction in total body fat, with no variation in BMI *(34)*.

Testosterone levels are frequently low in human immunodeficiency virus (HIV)-positive premenopausal women *(57)* and testosterone replacement is associated with an increase in fat free mass and body cell mass in HIV-positive men *(58)*. Studies are underway to evaluate the effects of testosterone therapy on body composition parameters in HIV-positive premenopausal women, with the expectation that such therapy may result in an increase in lean body mass and partially reverse the wasting component of this disease. It is also conceivable that testosterone replacement may be of benefit to premenopausal women suffering other illnesses associated with loss of lean body mass, such as malignant disease with cachexia.

Contrary to popular myth, neither oral nor parenteral HRT results in increased body weight *(34,59)*. There is also no evidence that the addition of testosterone replacement leads to weight gain, although this treatment is associated with a reduction in total body fat and an increase in lean mass. With increasing age, women tend to lose muscle mass and replace this with increased fat mass, with an overall tendency for weight gain in most Western societies. The small increase in lean mass observed with testosterone replacement is probably of beneficial effect, which in the long term will contribute to preservation of muscle strength and skeletal stability. The only ethical issue provoked by androgen-replacement therapy in older women is whether treated women who participate in competitive sport have any advantage in terms of muscle strength over their untreated counterparts.

TESTOSTERONE REPLACEMENT AND LIPIDS AND LIPOPROTEINS

Menopause, both natural and surgically induced, is associated with the development of a more adverse lipoprotein profile; however, there appears to be no relationship between these observed lipid and lipoprotein changes and endogenous testosterone levels *(28)*. Postmenopausal estrogen-replacement therapy results in reductions in total and low-density lipoprotein (LDL) cholesterol and these favorable effects are not diminished with either oral or parenteral testosterone replacement *(45,46)*. Parenteral testosterone replacement does not affect high-density lipoprotein (HDL) cholesterol *(46)*, however, HDL-cholesterol and apolipoprotein A_1 decrease significantly when oral methyltestosterone is administered concurrently with oral estrogen *(45,60)*. Oral estrogen replacement is associated with increased triglyceride levels. In contrast concomitant administration of oral methyl testosterone has been associated with the reduction in triglycerides *(45)*. Tibolone, a synthetic steroid with estrogenic, progestogenic, and androgenic properties, does not only modify total cholesterol, apolipoprotein A and apolipoprotein B levels in postmenopausal women but also causes a reduction in circulating triglycerides and HDL *(60)*.

The measurement of circulating lipids is an accepted surrogate for lipid metabolism. However, more direct measurement of lipid metabolism are probably better indicators of the effects of exogenous steroid therapy on cardiovascular risk. Combined oral esterified estrogen and methyl testosterone therapy results in reduced arterial LDL degradation and cholesterol ester content in cynomolgus monkeys that does not differ from the effects observed when estrogen is given alone *(61)*. Combined estrogen and methyl testosterone therapy is also associated with reduced plasma concentrations of apoplipoprotein B, reduced LDL particle size, and increased total body LDL catabolism *(61)*. Small LDL particles are more susceptible to oxidation and are hence considered to be more atherogenic. However, because estrogens appear to increase oxidative modification of LDL in the arterial wall *(61)*, the reduction in LDL particle size observed with both oral estrogen and combined therapy may not be deleterious but may merely reflect selective removal of large LDL particles from the circulation.

ANDROGEN REPLACEMENT AND VASCULAR FUNCTION

The incidence of coronary heart disease in postmenopausal women is not associated with levels of circulating testosterone or DHEAS *(29,62)*. Intracoronary testosterone administration to anesthetized male and female dogs induces increases in coronary artery cross-sectional area peak flow velocity and calculated volumetric blood flow that is blocked by pretreatment with an inhibitor of nitric oxide synthesis *(63)*. The beneficial effects of estrogen replacement therapy on coronary artery reactivity in cynomolgus monkeys is not lost with the addition of oral methyl testosterone *(64)* and parenteral testosterone improves both endothelium-dependent and endothelium-independent vascular reactivity in estrogenized postmenopausal women *(65)*.

Cardiac myocytes and fibroblasts contain functional α and β estrogen receptors, and cardiac myocytes express cyp450 aromatase *(66)*. Incubation of cardiac myocytes with A or testosterone results in transactivation of an estrogen-receptor-specific reporter, with A resulting in a significantly higher induction than testosterone *(66)*. Furthermore, both A and testosterone upregulate inducible nitric oxide synthase in cardiac myocytes *(66)*. The capacity for cardiac myoctes to synthesize estrogen from androgenic precursors and activate downstream target genes is greater in cells from female than from male animals *(66)*.

Thus, the administration of testosterone to women does not appear to affect the key events in coronary artery lipid metabolism or coronary artery function. Parenteral testosterone replacement does not negate the favorable effects exerted by exogenous estrogen on lipid and lipoprotein levels, whereas oral methyltestosterone use not only opposes the HDL cholesterol elevating effects of oral estrogen but also reduces HDL cholesterol levels below baseline values. Whether this effect of oral methyltestosterone in the setting of concomitant lowering of total cholesterol, LDL cholesterol, and triglyceride levels is detrimental is not known. Certainly, a high cardiac risk profile, which includes a low HDL cholesterol level, should be considered a relative contraindication to oral testosterone replacement, but should not influence the use of parenteral testosterone replacement therapy.

ANDROGENS AND BREAST CANCER

Elevated endogenous androgen levels have been reported to be associated with breast cancer *(67,68)*. However, interpretation of the available data has been limited by multiple compounding factors in these published studies. In postmenopausal women with breast cancer, age-adjusted mean values of total and free testosterone have found to be higher than in controls *(69)* and intratumor concentrations of 5α-DHT and estradiol have been reported to be greater than circulating levels of these hormones *(70)*. Androgen receptors are found in more than 50% of breast tumors *(70)* and are associated with longer survival in women with operable breast cancer and a favorable response to hormone treatment in advanced disease *(71)*. As yet, it is not known whether there is any relationship between exogenous androgen therapy and the occurrence of breast cancer.

VIRILIZATION WITH EXOGENOUS ANDROGEN EXCESS

Cosmetic side effects of androgen replacement are rare if supra-physiological hormone levels are avoided (25,26,31–33,48), but the potential virilizing effects include development of acne, hirsutism, deepening of the voice, and excessive libido. Women troubled by existing hirsutism or acne should not be prescribed androgen therapy. Although enhance libido is mostly seen as a benefit of therapy, increases in sexual thoughts and fantasies may well be undesirable for some women, and this should be clearly borne in mind if androgen replacement is being considered for the prevention or management of bone loss.

Summary

Disorders of endogenous androgen excess are clearly associated with increased cardiovascular risk, perturbations in lipid and carbohydrate metabolism, a more android weight distribution, and cosmetic manifestations of virilization. All of these undesirable metabolic effects are extremely unlikely and uncommon with androgen-replacement therapy with the caveat that circulating androgen levels are maintained closed to, or within, the normal female reproductive range and that patients are closely clinically monitored. With respect to breast cancer risk, women who have endogenously high androgen levels do appear to be at increased risk. There is no evidence that this increase in risk can be extrapolated to so-called "physiological" exogenous androgen replacement therapy after menopause. However, until more data are available, physicians should be cognizant of the possibility that androgen replacement could influence breast cancer development and clinical vigilance must be maintained.

IDENTIFYING WOMEN MOST LIKELY TO BENEFIT FROM ANDROGEN REPLACEMENT

Although a list of potential indications for androgen therapy is provided, the decision to offer androgen replacement to a woman is totally based on clinical assessment, and the outcome of treatment is completely dependent upon the subjective self-assessment of response and reporting by the patient. Biochemical measurements are of limited value, but clearly may guide the clinician away from offering androgen replacement when the free androgen index or free testosterone level is in the high normal range.

The clinical settings in which administration of androgen replacement are most likely to enhance woman's health and well-being are listed in Table 1. Possible future indications may also include the use of androgens in wasting states, such as HIV-infected individuals and malignancy-related cachexia, and to prevent or treat bone loss, particularly iatrogenic bone loss from glucocorticosteriod therapy or premenopausal bone loss.

Some women actively seek clinical assistance for loss of libido and/or inadequate restoration of well-being despite adequate estrogen–progestogen replacement. Others may volunteer such problems while attending their physician for another reason, however many women suffer silently, believing that this is their "lot" or are unaware of any available therapeutic options. Many women will not raise the issue of diminished libido because they find the topic awkward. Sadly, a number of young women who suffer loss of libido following cancer therapy express difficulty discussing the issue with their oncologist, as they feel their problem will be seen as trivial relative their disease recovery or remission. In many women, following chemo- or radiotherapy the symptoms of the

Table 1
Clinical Settings in Which Androgen-Replacement Therapy May Be Beneficial

Premature ovarian failure, including Turner's syndrome
Premenopausal iatrogenic androgen deficiency states
Symptomatic androgen deficiency as a result of surgical menopause, chemotherapy, or irradiation
Symptomatic androgen deficiency following natural menopause

Potential indications
   Glucocorticosteroid-induced bone loss
   GNRH-analog treatment of endometriosis
   Management of wasting syndromes
   Premenopausal bone loss
   Premenopausal loss of libido with diminished serum free testosterone

iatrogenic menopause and androgen deficiency, including fatigue, loss of well-being, depression, and reduced libido, can be difficult to distinguish from the overall physical toll of their therapy, and, frequently, their premature menopause and associated androgen insufficiency goes undiagnosed and untreated. Therefore, all "at risk" women should be at least directly questioned about the symptoms of androgen deficiency and made aware of the therapeutic possibilities available.

Symptoms such as fatigue and loss of well-being are extremely difficult to quantitate and are similar to diminished libido; it can be very difficult for both the physician and the patient to absolutely ascertain the cause of these symptoms when the patient's circumstances are multifactorial. The keys to dissecting out whether testosterone deficiency is a major factor and whether replacement is likely to be successful are, in reality, very simple and include the following:

   Spending TIME talking to the patient,
   LISTENING CAREFULLY to what the woman says, and, most importantly,
   Asking the woman WHAT SHE BELIEVES to be the fundamental problem.

In general, women are very reliable assessors of their own health and well-being and, importantly, are reluctant to use any therapy unless they truly believe it will result in an improvement in their health. Obviously, in assessing a woman presenting with loss of libido, the physician needs to establish the individual's past sexual history, the changes that have occurred in her sexuality, the status of her current relationship, and the presence of any other extrinsic or intrinsic factors that may affect her libido, particularly stress and depression.

Premature Ovarian Failure, Including Turner's Syndrome

The management of young women with premature menopause, particularly Turner's syndrome, who have never been sexually active is more difficult and perhaps controversial. Androgen replacement should be considered for such women experiencing persistent fatigue, inadequate well-being, and lack of libido despite adequate estrogen and progestogen replacement. However, it is obviously difficult for a woman to identify herself as having inadequate libido when she has never experienced what may be "normal." Alternatively, young women who have not become sexually active should become fully informed about androgen replacement as a future option, or perhaps, in some instances, offered very low-dose androgen replacement as a component of their HRT regimen at an earlier stage. Whether young women with premature ovarian failure should be recommended to use androgen replacement to prevent bone loss, specifically from the neck of femur, is yet to be established.

Premenopausal Iatrogenic Androgen Deficiency States

Gonadotropin-releaseing hormone (GnRH) analogs are in common usage for the treatment of severe endometriosis. A clinical consequences of the use of this therapy include symptoms of estrogen deficiency, bone loss, and loss of libido. Low-dose testosterone replacement could possibly be used to prevent bone loss and diminish some of the symptoms that are side effects of this therapy, although this is not by any means an established clinical indication. The use of low-dose testosterone replacement to prevent or treat glucocorticosteroid-related osteopenia and osteoporosis also warrants further clinical research. The administration of androgen replacement in a setting of suppressed androgen levels with the use of the oral contraceptive pill is not currently an accepted practice. Ideally, women suffering such consequences of oral contraception would be best advised to consider other forms of contraception and experience restoration of their own endogenous androgen levels following resumption of their normal ovarian function.

Androgen Replacement Following Menopause

Androgen-replacement therapy has become an accepted component of HRT for the restoration of sexual and general well-being in women who have undergone a surgical menopause. Its use in naturally menopausal women, particularly in the perimenopausal years, remains controversial. This is because most studies published have focused on treating the surgically menopausal patient rather than the naturally menopausal woman. Most women, following natural menopause, do not experience any loss of libido. However, there is a significant subgroup of women who do experience clear decline in their sexuality in association with the menopause, which anecdotally appears to be more frequent in women experiencing an earlier menopause. Androgen replacement in women who have experienced a natural menopause continues to be a neglected component of HRT in the management of their postmenopausal symptoms. Not only are such women usually very responsive to androgen replacement in terms of restoration of their sexuality, but they also frequently describe an increased sense of well-being and overall energy related to their androgen-replacement therapy.

Whether premenopausal women who complain of loss of libido and who have low bioavailable testosterone levels should be offered androgen replacement is even more controversial. Certainly, such women do appear to be at greater risk of premenopausal bone loss and it is the author's experience that some symptomatic premenopausal women with low measurable testosterone levels clinically appear to benefit from androgen therapy. At present, this is a subgroup of women for whom clear recommendations cannot be made. However, their symptoms should not be dismissed or too quickly attributed to other psychosocial factors, as it is possible that relative testosterone deficiency is a major contributing factor. Currently, management of such women needs to be very open-minded and therapy completely individualized, but we must await the results of relevant clinical studies before specific therapeutic guidelines for the premenopausal woman can be made.

Table 2
Androgen Replacement Therapy Formulations Used for Women

	Route	Frequency	Dose range
Methyltestosterone[a] (in combination with esterified estrogen)	Oral	Daily	1.25–2.5 mg
Testosterone undecanoate	Oral	Daily or alternate days	40–80 mg
Testosterone implants	Subcutaneous	3–6 monthly	50 mg
Nandrolone decanoate	Intramuscular	6–12 weekly	25–50 mg
Testosterone matrix patch	Transdermal	Twice a week	150/300 µg

[a]Currently available in the United States.

Clearly, androgen replacement is a far more sensitive issue for the women than HRT in general. It is essential that a physician consulting in this area be sensitive to the enormous variations in women's's' knowledge, expectations, sexual practices, and needs and, in every case, tailor the therapy to the individual's circumstances.

HOW SHOULD ANDROGEN REPLACEMENT BE PRESCRIBED?

Although no form of androgen replacement is commercially available in the United States for the treatment of loss of libido in women, oral methyl testosterone can be prescribed for menopausal symptoms unresponsive to estrogen replacement alone, and testosterone implants have been approved for replacement therapy for women in the United Kingdom. The current global therapeutic options in terms of androgen replacement therapy are listed in Table 2.

To achieve a good therapeutic response, in terms of enhanced libido, with testosterone replacement, it appears that testosterone levels often need to be restored to at least the upper end of the normal physiological range for young ovulating women. The doses of androgen replacement required to achieve such an effect usually result in an initially postadministration peak testosterone level that is supraphysiological regardless of the mode of administration.

An oral estrogen–androgen preparation is currently available in the United States in two doses—esterified estrogen 0.625 mg plus methyl testosterone 1.25 mg, or esterified estrogen 1.25 mg plus methyl testosterone 2.5 mg. Methyltestosterone is not available in any other countries because liver damage has been reported with long-term high-dose therapy (72). A more recent study has not shown any short-term (12 mo) detrimental effects of these doses of methyl testosterone combined with estrogen on hepatic enzymes or blood pressure (73). Interestingly, women who use esterified estrogens combined with methyl testosterone report a lower instance of nausea compared with women receiving conjugated equine estrogen alone (72).

Testosterone undecanoate is an oral androgen mostly used for replacement therapy in hypogonadal men. Its clinical application in women has been little studied although in some countries, its use is quite widespread. It is believed to be absorbed via the lymphatic system, hence, for best effect, it is recommended that testosterone undecanoate be ingested with fat (e.g., with a glass of milk). The clinical role for testosterone undecanoate as a replacement therapy for women at present remains unclear and further research is required before its use can be recommended.

There has now been considerable clinical experience with the administration of testosterone implants in postmenopausal women, particularly in the Commonwealth countries. These implants are fused crystalline implants 4–5 mm in diameter containing testosterone BP (British Pharmacopoeia) as the active ingredient. Experience indicates that a dose of 50 mg in extremely effective and does not result in virilizing side effects *(34)*. This dose is obtained by bisecting a 100-mg implant under sterile conditions. The implant is inserted, under local anesthesia, subcutaneously, usually into the lower anterior abdominal wall using a trocar and cannular. This therapy provides a slow release of testosterone with an approximate duration of effect for a 50-mg implant of between 3 and 6 mo. As there is significant variation in the duration of the effect, women treated with testosterone implants must be carefully monitored and serum testosterone levels measured prior to the administration of each subsequent implant. It is recommended that additional testosterone implants should not be inserted unless total testosterone is in the normal range for young women. The use of testosterone implants greater than 100-mg would prudently be avoided.

The recent development of a transdermal testosterone matrix patch will provide yet another therapeutic option for women requiring androgen replacement. The patch, which is now undergoing clinical trial, delivers either 150 µg or 300 µg of testosterone per day. This patch will have some obvious advantages over both oral and implant therapy; however, many women will prefer to use a less apparent mode of replacement or may have difficulties with skin irritation or adhesion.

Nandrolone decanoate is approved in some countries for the treatment of postmenopausal osteoporosis. The dose, administered intramuscularly, should not exceed 50 mg and the frequency of the dose is best titrated against the patient's gross build. It is prudent that treatment is not given less than six weekly and patients should be very carefully monitored for hirsutism and voice deepening. In most women, treatment with nandrolone decanoate results in cessation of bone loss over time and, in some women, an increase in BMD.

A final potential alternative, which is not currently generally available, is a transdermal testosterone cream or gel. Although such preparations may be regionally available on specific prescription from compounding pharmacists, there is no pharmacokinetic data available or published clinical experience pertaining to their use.

The contraindications to and side effects of testosterone replacement are listed in Tables 3 and 4. Again it is emphasized that with judicious dosing and careful patient monitoring, side effects of testosterone replacement are rare. All postmenopausal women treated with testosterone replacement should be using concurrent estrogen-replacement therapy. There is no clinical data available regarding the use of testosterone replacement in postmenopausal women who are not on estrogen; however, one would predict that such use may well result in adverse metabolic and cosmetic side effects. The sole circumstance in which androgen therapy has been administered without concurrent estrogen use is the administration of the anabolic steroid nandrolone deconoate. Women treated with this steroid must be extremely carefully monitored for adverse effects, including voice change and hirsutism, which do occur in the setting of this compound being administered unopposed by estrogen.

Table 3
Contraindications to Testosterone Therapy

Pregnancy or lactation
Known or suspected androgen-dependent neoplasia
Severe acne
Moderate–severe hirsutism
Circumstances in which enhanced libido would be undesirable
Androgenic alopecia

Table 4
Side Effects from Excessive Dosage

Virilization: hirsutism, acne, temporal balding, voice deepening
Clitoromegaly
Fluid retention
Hepatocellular damage: has been associated with high dose 17α-alkylandrogens given orally
Lipids: oral androgens may adversely affect serum levels of lipids and lipoproteins.
Drug interactions: C-17-substituted derivatives of oral testosterone may decrease anticoagulant requirements. Androgens may elevate serum levels of oxyphenbutazone and in diabetic patients may rarely affect insulin requirements.

REFERENCES

1. Kirschner MAA, Bardin CW. Androgen production and metabolism in normal and virilized women. Metabolism 1972;21:667–688.
2. Judd HL, Yen SSC. Serum androstenedione and testosterone levels during the menstrual cycle. J Clin Endocr Metab 1973;36:475–481.
3. Vierhapper H, Nowotny P, Waldhausl W. Determination of testosterone production rates in men and women using stable isotope'dilution and mass spectrometry. J Clin Endocr Metab 1997;82:1492–1496.
4. Mushayandebvu T, Castracane DV, Gimpel T, Adel T, Santoro N. Evidence for diminished midcycle ovarian androgen production in older reproductive aged women. Fertil Steril 1996;65:721–723.
5. Dunn JF, Nisula BC, Rodboard D. Transport of steroid hormones. Binding of 21 endogenous steroids to both testosterone-binding globulin and cortico-steroid-binding globulin in human plasma. J Clin Endocr Metab 1981;53:58–68.
6. Longcope C, Franz C, Morello C, Baker K, Johnston Jr CC. Steroid and gonadotropin levels in women during the peri-menopausal years. Maturitas 1986;8:189–196.
7. Burger HG, Dudley EC, Hopper DL. The endocrinology of the menopausal transition: a cross-sectional study of a population-based sample. J Clin Endocr Metab 1995;80:3537–3545.
8. Zumoff B, Strain GW, Miller LK, Rosner W. Twenty-four hour mean plasma testosterone concentration declines with age in normal premenopausal women. J Clin Endocr Metab 1995;80:1429,1430.
9. Rannevik G, Jeppsson S, Johnell O. A longitudinal study of the perimenopausal transition: altered profiles of steroid and pituitary hormones, SHBG and bone mineral density. Matuitas 1986;8:189–196.
10. Zumoff B, Rosenfeld RS, Strain GW. Sex differences in the 24 hour mean plasma concentrations of dehydroisoandrosterone (DHA) and dehydroisoandrosterone sulfate (DHAS) and the DHA to DHAS ratio in normal adults. J Clin Endocrinol Metab 1980;51:330–334.
11. Meldrum Dr. Changes in circulating steroids with aging in post menopausal women. Obstet Gynecol 1997;57:624–628.
12. Bancroft J, Cawood EHH. Androgens and the menopause: a study of 40–60 year old women. Clin Endocrinol 1996;45:577–587.
13. Tazuke S, Khaw K-T, Chir MBB, Barrett-Connor E. Exogenous estrogen and endogenous sex hormones. Medicine 1992;71:44–51.

14. Mathur RS, Landgreve SC, Moody LO, Semmens JP, Williamson HO. The effect of estrogen treatment on plasma concentrations of steroid hormones, gonadotropins, prolactin and sex hormone-binding globulin in post-menopausal women. Maturitas 1985;7:129–133.

15. Krug R, Psych D, Pietrowsky R, Fehm HL, Born J. Selective influence of menstrual cycle on perception of stimuli with reproductive significance. Psychosom Med 1994;56:410–417.

16. Ushiroyama T, Sugimoto O. Endocrine function of the peri- and postmenopausal ovary. Horm Res 1995;44:64–68.

17. Castelo-Branco C, Martinez de Osaba MJ, Fortuny A, Iglesias X, Gonzalez-Merlo J. Circulating hormone levels in menopausal women receiving different hormone replacement therapy regimens. A comparison. J Reprod Med 1995;40:556–560.

18. Goodman-Gruen D, Barrett-Connor E. Total but not bioavailable testosterone is a predictor of central adiposity in postmenopausal women. Int J Obes 1995;19:293–298.

19. Hallstrom T. Sexuality in the climacteric. Clin Obstet Gynecol 1977;4:227–239.

20. McCoy NL, Davidson JM. A longitudinal study of the effects of menopause on sexuality. Maturitas 1985;7:203–210.

21. Frock J, Money J. Sexuality and the menopause. Psychother Psychosom 1992;57:29–33.

22. Bachmann GA, Leiblum SR. Sexuality in sexagenarian women. Maturitas 1991;13:45–50.

23. Utian WH. The true clinical features of postmenopausal oophorectomy and their response to estrogen replacement therapy. S Afr Med J 1972;46:732–737.

24. Campbell S, Whitehead M. Oestrogen therapy and the menopausal syndrome. Clin Obstet Gynecol. 1977;4:31–47.

25. Studd JWW, Chakravarti S, Oram D. The climacteric. Clin Obstet Gynecol. 1977;4:3–29.

26. Sherwin BN, Gelfand MM, Brender W. Androgen enhances sexual motivation in females: a prespective, crossover study of sex steroid administration in surgical menopause. Psychosom Med. 1997;47:339–351.

27. Bixo M, Backstrom T, Winblad B, Andersson A. Estradiol and testosterone in specific regions of the human female brain in different endocrine states. J Steroid Biochem Mol Biol 1995;55:297–303.

28. Wakatsuki A, Sagara Y. Lipoprotein metabolism in postmenopausal and oophorestomized women. Obstet.Gynecol 1995;85:523–528.

29. Barrett-Connor E, Goodman-Gruen D. Prospective study of endogenous sex hormones and fatal cardiovascular disease in postmenopausal women. Br Med J 1995;311:1193–1196.

30. Van Goozen SHM, Cohen-Kettenis PT, Gooren LIG, Frijda NH, Van de Poll NE. Gender differences in behaviour: activating effects of cross-sex hormones. Psychoneuroendocrinology 1995;20:343–363.

31. Studd JWW, Colins WP, Chakravarti S. Estradiol and testosterone implants in the treatment of psychosexual problems in postmenopausal women. Br J Obstet Gynaecol 1977;84:314,315.

32. Burger HG, Hailes J, Menelaus M, et al. The management of persistent symptoms with estradiol-testosterone implants: clinical, lipid and hormonal results. Maturitas 1984;6:351–358.

33. Burger HG, Hailes J, Nelson J, Menelaus M. Effect of combined implants of estradiol and testosterone on libido in postmenopausal women. Br Med J 1987;294:936,937.

34. Davis SR, McCloud PI, Strauss BJG, Burger HG. Testosterone enhances estradiol's effects on postmenopausal bone density and sexuality. Maturitas 1995;21:227–236.

35. Shifren JL, Braunstein G, Simon J, Casson P, Buster JE, Red Burki RE, Ginsburg ES, Rosen RC, Leiblum SR, Caramelli KE. Transdermal testosterone treatment in women with impaired sexual function after oophorectomy. N Eng J Med 2000;343(10):682–688.

36. Dow MGT, Hart DM, Forrest CA. Hormonal treatments of sexual unresponsiveness in postmenopausal women: a comparative study. Br J Obstet Gynaecol 1983;90:361–366.

37. Colvard DS, Eriksen EF, Keeting PE. Identification of androgen receptors in normal human osteoblast-like cells. Proc Natl Acad Sci USA 1989;86:854–857.

38. Kasperk CH, Wergedal JE, Farley JR, Llinkhart TA, Turner RT, Baylink DG. Androgens directly stimulate proliferation of bone cells in vitro. Endocrinology 1989;124:1576–1578.

39. Nilas L, Christiansen C. Bone mass and its relationship to age and the menopause. J Clin Endocrinol Metab 1987;65:697–699.

40. Slemenda C, Longcope C, Peacock M, Hui S, Johnston CC. Sex steroids, bone mass, and bone loss. A prospective study of pre-, peri- and postmenopausal women. J Clin Invest 1996;97:14–21.

41. Simberg N, Titinen A, Silfrast A, Viinikka L, Ylikorkala O. High bone density in hyperandrogenic women: effect of gonadotropin-releasing hormone agonist alone or in conjunction with estrogen-progestin replacement. J Clin Endocrinol Metab 1995;81:646–651.

42. Heiss CJ, Sanborn CF, Nichols DL. Associations of body fat distribution, circulating sex hormones and bone density in postmenopausal women. J Clin Endocrinol Metab 1995;80:1591–1596.

43. Jassal SK, Barrett-Connor E, Edelstein S. Low bioavailable testosterone levels predict future height loss in postmenopausal women. J Bone Min Res 1995;10(4):650–653.
44. Davidson BJ, Ross RK, Paganni Hill A, et al. Total free estrogens and androgens in post menopausal women with hip fractures. J Clin Endocrinol Metab 1982;54:115–120.
45. Raisz LG, Wiita B, Artis A, et al. Comparison of the effects of estrogen alone and estrogen plus androgen on biochemical markers of bone formation and resoprtion in postmenopausal women. J Clin Endocrinol Metab 1995;81:37–43.
46. Watts NB, Notelovitz M, Timmons MC. Comparison of oral estrogens and estrogens plus androgen on bone mineral density, menopausal symptoms and lipid-lipoprotein profiles in surgical menopause. Obstet Gynecol 1995;85:529–537.
47. Savvas M, Studd JWW, Fogelman I, Dooley M, Montgomery J, Murby B. Skeletal effects of oral estrogen compared with subcutaneous oestrogen and testosterone in postmenopausal women. Br Med J 1988;297:331–333.
48. Savvas M, Studd JWW, Norman S, Leather AT, Garnett TJ. Increase in bone mass after one year of percutaneous oestradiol and testosterone implants in post menopausal women who have previously received long-term oral oestrogens. Br J Obstet Gynaecol 1992;99:757–760.
49. Morishima A, Grumbach MM, Simpson ER. Aromatase deficiency in male and female siblings caused by a novel mutation and the physiological role of estrogens. J Clin Endocrinol Metab 1995;80:3689–3698.
50. Smith EP, Boyd J, Frank GR, et al. Estrogen resistance caused by a mutation in the oestrogen-receptor gene in a man. N Engl J Med 1994;331:1056–1061.
51. Kasra M, Grynpas MD. The effects of androgens on the mechanical properties of primate bone. Bone 1995;17:265–270.
52. Nawata H, Tariaka S. Aromatase in bone cell: association with osteoporosis in post menopausal women. J Steroid Biochem Mol Biol 1995;53:165–174.
53. Taelman P, Kayman JM, Janssens X, Vermeulen A. Persistence of increased bone resorption and possible role of dehydroepiandrosterone as a bone metabolism determinant in osteoporotic women in late menopause. Maturitas 1989;11:65–73.
54. Nordin BEC, Robertson A, Seamark RF, et al. The relation between calcium absorption serum DHEA and vertebral mineral density in postmenopausal women. J Clin Endocrinol Metab 1985;60:651–657.
55. Morales AJ, Nolan JJ, Nelson JC, Yen SSC. Effects of replacement dose of dehydroepiandrosterone in men and women of advancing age. J Clin Endocrinol Metab 1994;78:1360–1367.
56. Abraham GE. Ovarian and adrenal contribution to peripheral androgens during the menstrual cycle. J Clin Endocrinol Metab 1974;39:340–346.
57. Engelson ES, Goggin KJ, Rabkin JG, et al. Nutrition and testosterone status of HIV positive women. [Abstract] Proceedings of the XI Inter Conf on AIDS, Vancouver, 1996.
58. Engelson ES, Rabkin JG, Rabkin R, Kotler DP. Effects of testosterone upon body composition [Letter]. J Acquir Immune Defic Syndr Hum Retrovirol 1996;11:510,511.
59. Darling GM, Johns JA, McCloud PI, Davis SR. Estrogen and progestin compared with simvastatin for hypercholesterolemia postmenopausal women. N Engl J Med 1997;337(9):595–601.
60. Hickok LR, Toomey C, Speroff L. A comparison of esterified estrogens with and without methyltestosterone: Effects on endometrial histology and serum lipoproteins in postmenopausal women. Obstet Gynecol 1993;82:919–924.
61. Wagner JD, Zhang L, Williams JK, Register TC, Ackerman DM, Wiita B, Clarkson TB, Adams MR. Esterified estrogens with and without methyltestosterone decrease arterial LDL metabolism in Cynomolgus monkeys. Arteriosclerosis,Thrombosis Vascular Biol 1996;16:1473–1479.
62. Barrett-Connor E, Goodman-Gruen D. Dehydroepiandrosterone sulfate does not predict cardiovascular death in postmenopausal women. The Rancho Bernardo Study. Circulation 1995;91:1757–1760.
63. Chou TM, Sudhir K, Hutchison SJ, Ko E, Amidon TM, Collins P, Chatterjee K. Testosterone induces dilation of canine coronary conductance and resistance arteries in vivo. Circulation 1996;94:2614–2619.
64. Honore EK, Williams JK, Adams MR, Ackerman DM, Wagner JD. Methyltestosterone does not diminish the beneficial effects of estrogen replacement therapy on coronary artery reactivity in cynomolgus monkeys. Menopause: J N Am Menopause Soc 1996;3:20–26.
65. Worboys S, Kotsopoulos D, Teede H, McGrath BP, and Davis SR. Parental testosterone improves endothelium-dependent and independent vasodilation in postmenopausal women already receiving estrogen. J Clin Endocrinol Metab 2001;86(1):158–161.
66. Grohe C, Kahlert S, Lobbert K, Vetter H. Expression of oestrogen receptor alpha and beta in rat heart: role of local oestrogen synthesis. J Endocrinol 1998;156:R1–R7.

67. Secreto G, Toniolo P, Pisani P, et al. Androgens and breast cancer in premenopausal women. Cancer Res 1989;49:471–476.

68. Secreto G, Toniolo P, Berrino E, et al. Serum and urinary androgens and risk of breast cancer in postmenopausal women. Cancer Res 1991;51:2572–2576.

69. Berrino F, Muti P, Michelli A, Bolelli G, Krogh V, Sciajno R, Pisani P, Panico S, Secreto G. Serum sex hormone levels after menopause and subsequent breast cancer. J Natl Cancer Inst 1996;88:291–296.

70. Recchione C, Venturelli E, Manzari A, Cavalteri A, Martinetti A, Secreto G. Testosterone, dihydrotestosterone and oestradiol levels in postmenopausal breast cancer tissues. J Steroid Biochem Mol Biol 1995;52:541–546.

71. Wiren KM, Keenan EJ, Orwoll ES, Zhang X, Chang C. Transcriptional U-Regulation of the Human Androgen Receptor by Androgen in Bone Cells. Endocrinology 1997;138(6):2291–2300.

72. Barrett-Connor E, Timmons MC, Young R, Wiita B, Estratest Working Group. Interim safety analysis of a two-year study comparing oral estrogen-androgen and conjugated estrogens in surgically meno-pausal women. J Women's Health 1996;5:593–602.

73. Palacios S, Mendenez C, Jurado AR, Vargas JC. Effects of oestradiol administration via different routes on the lipid profile in women with bilateral oophorectomy. Maturitas 1994;(18):239–244.

27 Hormonal Therapy of the Infertile Woman

Shahar Kol, MD

CONTENTS

INTRODUCTION

Fertility requires anatomical and functional integrity of the sexual axis, starting at the level of the hypothalamus, going down to the pituitary, ending at the level of the ovaries, Fallopian tubes, and uterus. From the pharmacological point of view, the current arsenal allows for tight control and flexible manipulation of the sexual endocrine axis, offering a wide range of therapeutic interventions with the goal of achieving pregnancy. This chapter aims at presenting briefly the major therapeutic tools that are currently at our disposal.

ANOVULATION

Anovulation is the single most frequent reason for female infertility, affecting about 10% of the female population of reproductive years. The classification of anovulation into three groups by the World Health Organization (WHO) is used as a practical guideline to diagnosis and treatment.

Group I. Hypogonadotropic hypogonadal anovulation (hypothalamic amenorrhea): The patients are characterized by low serum gonadotropins and low estradiol. Because the endometrium is not primed with estradiol, progesterone withdrawal does not induce menstrual bleeding. Treatment is usually directed at inducing pituitary response by providing exogenous pulsatile gonadotropin-releasing hormone (GnRH) or by direct

From: *Endocrine Replacement Therapy in Clinical Practice*
Edited by: A. Wayne Meikle © Humana Press Inc., Totowa, NJ

stimulation of the ovaries with gonadotropins. If hyperprolactinemia is diagnosed, specific treatment is required.

Group II. Normogonadotropic normoestrogenic anovulation (hypothalamic–pituitary dysfunction): This is the largest group of anovulatory (or oligo-ovulatory) patients. These women have evidence of endogenous estrogen activity. Physical examination may reveal evidence of excess androgen production. Luteinizing hormone (LH) may be elevated or normal. Follicle-stimulating hormone (FSH) is usually normal. There is withdrawal bleeding in response to progesterone. Ultrasound examination of the ovaries typically shows multiple small follicles (polycystic ovary syndrome [PCOS]). Treatment is based on raising the FSH levels to initiate follicular growth and maturation, leading to ovulation.

Group III. Hypergonadotropic hypoestrogenic anovulation: Patients in this group are characterized by their elevated serum gonadotropins, signifying ovarian failure or premature menopause. Numerous therapeutic maneuvers have been suggested to produce viable pregnancies in this group, all yielding disappointing results. For this group of patients, oocyte donation is the only procedure that offers reasonable chances of achieving pregnancy.

Hyperprolactinemic Anovulation

Hyperprolactinemia is associated with galactorrhea, menstrual disturbances, infertility and osteoporosis. A single, moderately elevated serum prolactin level warrants repeated measurement, as prolactin is secreted episodically. Well-established elevated prolactin levels dictate (after physiologic and pharmacological etiologies have been ruled out) a radiological evaluation (computed tomography [CT] or preferably magnetic resonance imaging [MRI]) of the hypothalamic–pituitary region. Most patients with hyperprolactinemia can be treated medically. Neurosurgical evaluation is indicated in the uncommon cases of large mass or failed medical treatment. Hyperprolactinemia *per se* does not require treatment; however, infertility is clearly an indication for medical treatment. This consists of dopamine agonists, of which bromocriptine (introduced in 1971), has been the standard drug. Bromocriptine is usually begun at a low dose of 1.25 mg daily and increased gradually to 2.5–5.0 mg daily. Occasionally, higher doses are required. Although bromocriptine is effective in 80% of patients (shrinkage of the tumor and substantial reductions of serum prolactin concentrations) its bothersome side effects cause discontinuation of treatment by 5–10% of patients. The most common side effects are nausea, dizziness, and orthostatic hypotension. Efforts to minimize these side effects have led to the development of a number of compounds, of which cabergoline emerged as a leading product. Whereas bromocriptine is given once or twice daily, cabergoline is given once or twice weekly. A 459-patient double-blind study *(1)* of women with hyperprolactinemic amenorrhea compared the safety and efficacy of cabergoline with bromocriptine (the standard therapy). Patients were treated with either cabergoline (0.5–1.0 mg twice weekly) or bromocriptine (2.5–5.0 mg twice daily). Normoprolactinemia was achieved in 186 of the 223 (83%) women treated with cabergoline and 138 of the 236 (59%, $p < 0.001$) women treated with bromocriptine. Ovulation was documented in 72 and 52% of the women treated with cabergoline and bromocriptine, respectively ($p < 0.001$). Adverse effects were recorded in 68% of the women taking cabergoline and 78% of those taking bromocriptine ($p = 0.03$); 3% discontinued taking cabergoline, and 12% stopped taking bromocriptine ($p < 0.001$) because of drug intolerance. Gastrointestinal symptoms were significantly less frequent, less severe, and shorter-lived in the women treated with cabergoline. Taken together, these results suggest that cabergoline is more effective and better tolerated than bromocriptine.

Another large-scale (455 patients) retrospective, case-series study confirmed the high efficacy and tolerability of cabergoline *(2)*.

Quinagolide is a nonergot dopamine agonist used to treat hyperprolactinemia. This drug is administered once daily. It has similar efficacy to bromocriptine, but is probably less effective than cabergoline. It is better tolerated than twice-daily bromocriptine, but is probably inferior to cabergoline in this regard *(3)*. The superiority of cabergoline is also demonstrated in the treatment of patients with micro- and macroprolactinomas, who are resistant to bromocriptine and quinagolide. These patients respond favorably to cabergoline *(4)*.

Patient monitoring during treatment includes reassurance of compliance and repeat of prolactin levels at 3-mo intervals during the first year and yearly thereafter. If a mass effect is suspected, surgery consultation is warranted. If prolactin levels are stable for more than 2 yr, dosage can be reduced gradually, while monitoring prolactin levels, until complete cessation of medical treatment.

PULSATILE GnRH THERAPY

Indications

The identification and sequencing of GnRH in the early 1970s, opened the opportunity to significantly manipulate the reproductive axis at the hypothalamus–pituitary area. Significant efforts were invested in creating GnRH analog molecules that can induce agonistic or antagonistic effects. Currently, the fruits of these efforts are used routinely in fertility treatments (most notably in the field of in vitro fertilization [IVF]). Soon after its introduction, it became apparent that physiologic activity of GnRH requires pulsatile, or intermittent, administration, because sustained effect (by GnRH agonists) induces pituitary desensitization and gonadotropin suppression.

The ideal candidate for pulsatile GnRH therapy would be the rather rare patient with hypogonadotropic hypogonadism (HH). Exogenous pulsatile administration of the missing primary ingredient (GnRH) results in mimicking the natural ovulatory cycle. Given current significant efforts to minimize fertility-treatment-induced multiple pregnancy, a natural-like, monofollicular stimulation is highly attractive. Indeed, this mode of treatment is highly successful in HH patients.

Other candidates for pulsatile GnRH treatment would be PCOS patients. One of the suggested etiologies for this condition is persistently rapid GnRH pulse frequency, leading to excessive LH secretion and relatively low FSH *(5)*. Although the rational for pulsatile GnRH treatment in these patients is not readily understood, it offers the potential benefit of monofollicular stimulation.

Dosage

ROUTE

Pulsatile GnRH is usually given intravenously. This mode of delivery assures a rapid peak and prompt return to baseline of GnRH and LH that follows. Long-term intravenous administration is cumbersome and not complication–free (iv site infection), although using a sterile technique and proper maintenance seem to reduce the frequency of infection *(6)*. Pulsatile GnRH can also be given subcutaneously (sc), although this mode of delivery blunts the pulses. This notwithstanding, sc administration leads to ovulation in 75% of cycles in patients with HH and a conception rate of 30% *(7)*. The more physiologic iv administration is advantageous as the ovulation rate is higher (90%), although the conception rate is similar (27.6%) *(8)*.

FREQUENCY

Fixed-pulse frequencies of every 60–120 min have been used successfully *(9)*. An attempt to simulate the normal menstrual cycle *(10)* by changing the pulse frequency from every 60 min to every 4 h did not result in a significant improvement. A frequency of one pulse every 90 min has been advised by pharmaceutical companies, although a 60-min interval may result in further optimization *(11)*.

DOSE

A wide range of bolus dose (1–20 μg/bolus) has been used. When the sc route is used, higher dosage is needed. High dosage with the iv route is associated with a greater risk of multiple pregnancy. Most centers start stimulation with a low iv dose (2.5–5 μg/bolus), to be increased (to 10–20 μg/bolus) if needed (i.e., no response after 10–15 d of treatment).

LUTEAL SUPPORT

Once ovulation occurs, luteal support can be given by continuing GnRH pulses, although less expensive and simpler alternatives can be used, like human chorionic gonadotropin (hCG) (two to three injections of 1500–2500 U each in a 3-d interval), or exogenous progesterone.

Monitoring

During the follicular phase, vaginal ultrasound is used to assess follicular development. Appearance of a single growing follicle is taken to reflect a favorable response. Multiple follicular responses, although rare, may lead to cycle cancellation if multiple pregnancy is to be avoided. Estradiol measurements are not needed. Ovulation is detected by urinary LH kits, usually done at home, to allow timed intercourse or intrauterine insemination (IUI).

Outcomes

The best results are achieved with HH patients, as a primary pituitary disorder is rare and treatment often leads to normal gonadotropin secretion. An ovulation rate of 80–90% is usually reported *(12)* and a pregnancy rate of nearly 30% per ovulatory cycle. The multiple pregnancy rate is in the range of 5%, and the abortion rate is 20–25%.

Patients with PCOS do not respond as well as HH patients. The ovulation rate in these patients is 40–50%, with pregnancy in only 16% of the cycles *(11)*. Better results may be obtained by pretreatment with a GnRH analog for 6–8 wk to induce pituitary suppression.

Complications

A multiple pregnancy rate of 5–8%, which is significantly higher than the 1% rate observed in spontaneous pregnancies, should be regarded as a significant complication. A low starting pulse dose and accurate assessment of the number of growing follicles may lower this rate. Furthermore, if multiple pregnancy is likely, based on ovarian response, the patient should be informed in detail regarding possible consequences. A prudent professional advice in these cases would be to abort the cycle. A severe ovarian hyperstimulation syndrome (OHSS) has not been described with pulsatile GnRH treatment. The risk of iv catheter-related infections seems to be low *(13)*, as 2% of the patients had positive blood cultures at the time of catheter removal.

ANTIESTROGENS

Clomiphene

Clomiphene citrate (CC) was synthesized in 1956 and was first used in clinical trials 4 yr later. By now, it is the most widely used (and abused) ovulation promoter. The primary indication for CC is infertility associated with normoprolactinemic normogonadotropic normoestrogenic anovulation (WHO group II). Over the years, other indications were added, most notably controlled ovarian stimulation in unexplained infertility, and "mild male" factor in association with IUI. These indications have broadened the patient pool for CC considerably. Given its cost, route of administration (oral), and safety, CC has become a universal first-stage fertility drug. All too often we see patients who are given CC, before any fertility workup is done.

Monitoring During CC Therapy

In the typical anovulatory patient, CC may be initiated at any time. A starting point timed from uterine bleeding is hormonally meaningless in these patients. However, if bleeding occurs spontaneously or is induced (usually with a progestin), CC treatment is started on d 3–5 of the "cycle." The recommended starting dose is 50 mg daily for 5 d. If ovulation does not occur, the daily dose is increased by 50-mg increments. The maximal CC dose is 250 mg for 5 d. Lack of ovarian response to this dose is considered a CC failure. Treatment variations by extending CC intake duration to more than 7 d or more have been suggested. Theoretically, luteal support is not indicated, although one cannot rule out a compromised luteal function as a result of CC treatment.

Some practitioners believe that CC treatment monitoring can be limited to daily basal body temperature (BBT) measurement in order to document ovulation. This clearly represents a simple, low-cost monitoring plan. Indeed, a small randomized study concluded that "high-tech" monitoring (vaginal ultrasound and LH monitoring) offered no advantage over BBT alone *(14)*. However, detailed monitoring may be desirable if timed intercourse or IUI is planned, or for the purpose of documenting the number of responding follicles, or for the typical progesterone rise after ovulation. Objective monitoring is based on hormonal measurements and ultrasound. Because ovulation usually occurs 5–10 d after the last dose of CC, serum E_2 can be taken during this window of time followed by progesterone measurement in the projected mid-luteal phase to document ovulation. High-frequency transvaginal sonography (TVS) can be used as the only tool for follicular phase monitoring. Monitoring follicular response from the fifth day after the last CC dose onward by TVS is used to document the number of growing follicles. The purpose of the treatment is to achieve a single responding follicle that hopefully harbors a single fertilizable oocyte. Once the follicle reaches >20 mm in diameter, hCG (a single dose of 5000 IU) can be given if timed IUI is planned. If natural intercourse is preferred, hCG can also be given, although spontaneous ovulation may occur without any further intervention. However, in the case of a multi-follicular response, serious consideration should be given to aborting the cycle, if multiple pregnancy and ovarian hyperstimulation syndrome (OHSS) are to be avoided. In fact, these situations present a major contribution of TVS to treatment monitoring (i.e., allowing accurate estimation of the responding follicles). The risk of multiple pregnancy and OHSS is directly correlated with the number of responding follicles.

Other antiestrogens have been introduced as alternatives to CC, most notably tamoxifen, which presumably offers comparable ovulation and pregnancy rates *(15)*.

Another seemingly promising alternative is the use of an aromatase inhibitor for induction of ovulation. The preliminary reported experience with such a compound (letrozole) is favorable *(16)*. Not only was a high ovulation rate achieved but this approach also avoids the unfavorable effect on the endometrium that is associated with CC.

Outcomes

Of the anovulatory patient pool, about 80% can be expected to ovulate and consequently become pregnant unless other infertility factors exist. Once ovulation occurs conception becomes a matter of chance with somewhat lower pregnancy rates compared to those reported in the general population. Because CC is not given exclusively to the classical anovulatory patients, the conception rate for other groups of patients may be lower, although the ovulation rate is higher.

Complications

Hot flashes, probably secondary to antiestrogenic effect, are reported by 11% of patients. Visual symptoms (blurring, spots, and flashes) occur in 2% of patients and are reversible. More important is the antiestrogenic effect of CC at the level of the endometrium and cervical mucus. Although the direct effect on cervical glands is difficult to document and easy to bypass (by IUI), adverse changes in endometrial morphology were reported using TVS *(17)*. It appears that, in a subset of patients, endometrial growth during the proliferative phase is hampered by CC. This effect is documented by as a thin, poor endometrial lining, in spite of high estradiol levels. These effects prompted researchers to add estrogen to the treatment protocol, with apparent success *(18)*.

Use of Metformin and Insulin Sensitizers for Ovulation Induction

Polycystic ovary syndrome is commonly associated with obesity and insulin-resistance, leading to hyperinsulinemia. High insulin contributes to anovulation and hyperandrogenism, suggesting that an insulin sensitizer may decrease insulin secretion, followed by ovulation. Indeed, several studies have documented that agents like metformin *(19)* or troglitazone (this compound has been recalled by the manufacturer because of safety concerns) *(20)* increase the rate of ovulation with or without concomitant treatment with CC. A randomized, double-blind, placebo-controlled study of CC-resistant PCOS patients showed that treatment with metformin (1500 mg daily) significantly increased ovulation and pregnancy rates *(21)*. A similar study, with rather lean, Chinese PCOS patients, failed to show any improvement with metformin *(22)*, indicating that treatment individualization is always important and that body mass index (BMI) may correlate with the degree of response to metformin.

OVARIAN HYPERSTIMULATION SYNDROME

Ovarian hyperstimulation syndrome still remains the most important complication of controlled ovarian stimulation. In fact, it can be looked at as a situation in which the ovaries run "out of control," producing a typical syndrome during the luteal phase of the stimulated cycle. Being an iatrogenic complication associated with a purely elective medical procedure, all efforts must be made to prevent its occurrence. Mild stimulation, individualization of treatment protocol to suit each patient's needs and regarding patient safety as first priority may minimize OHSS occurrence.

Strategies for OHSS prevention include the following:

1. Cycle cancellation in a high-risk situation is a prudent approach. Ovarian stimulation is stopped and hCG is not given. It should be noted that spontaneous ovulation by an endogenous LH surge may still occur followed by OHSS. If pregnancy is achieved, the severity of OHSS often increases. Therefore, in addition to cycle abortion, the patient should be counseled about abstinence until menses. A spontaneous LH surge will not occur in GnRH-agonist-induced pituitary downregulated patients or if a GnRH antagonist is given to ascertain that ovulation is prevented.
2. Reducing the dose of hCG given for ovulation triggering is a popular approach, although it cannot guarantee total OHSS prevention.
3. Other modalities taken to lower the risk of OHSS include luteal phase support with a progesterone (instead of hCG), withholding fresh embryo transfer (and in that context averting "in vivo" ovarian stimulation to IVF), and use of a recombinant LH to trigger ovulation.
4. The single approach that combines efficient ovulation triggering and total OHSS prevention is the use of a singe bolus of a GnRH agonist *(23)*. This approach has been successfully used in both ovulation induction and IVF patients. The recent introduction of GnRH antagonists makes this protocol more applicable, especially in the IVF setting. A single dose (0.2 mg) of GnRH agonist reliably and effectively triggers ovulation. Oocyte retrieval (for IVF) or IUI is timed as if hCG were given. Luteal support with a progesterone is mandatory (estradiol may also be supplemented) because endogenous biosynthesis of sex steroids by the corpora lutea decreases sharply. In fact, a situation of complete luteolysis is attained, which is the key to OHSS prevention. Early luteolysis also assures that if pregnancy is achieved, the associated endogenous hCG will not "revive" the corpora lutea. If stimulation is performed for IUI (or natural intercourse, not for IVF) the subject of multiple pregnancy should be discussed with the patient. Although OHSS is completely prevented, there is no control over the number of embryos that may develop. Therefore, it is recommended to switch to IVF for the purpose of controlling the number of transferred embryos.
5. Numerous researchers have suggested that intravenous albumin at the time of oocyte retrieval in IVF may prevent or alleviate OHSS. There is no evidence to support this approach; therefore this treatment is not recommended *(24)*.

Treatment of OHSS is supportive in nature. In mild cases, bed rest and periodic observation is sufficient. Patients with severe OHSS should be hospitalized. Hemoconcentration and electrolyte imbalances are treated with intravenous fluid. Other therapeutic measures include plasma expanders, diuretics, paracentesis for tense ascites and finally, therapeutic abortion if all measures fail.

GONADOTROPIN THERAPY

In the late 1950s and early 1960s, exogenous gonadotropins were introduced as a novel therapeutic tool in infertility. In their early days, gonadotropins were produced from human pituitaries. It was only when urinary-derived products became available that this treatment gained popularity. The product, human menopausal gonadotropin (hMG), contains equal biological activity of FSH and LH (each 75 IU/ampoule) and has been used with impressive success for decades. In the mid-1990s, recombinant FSH products were introduced. The new recombinant products gradually replaced the urinary-derived ones for their advantages:

- High purity
- High specific activity
- Identical amino acid sequence compared to natural FSH
- No contamination with urinary proteins of undetermined origin
- No LH activity
- Reliable source for production, no need for cumbersome collection of urine

Recombinant FSH preparations also appear to be slightly superior to hMG based on the available evidence, although experience shows that ovarian stimulation in the face of no LH (endogenous or exogenously administered) is problematic. If GnRH agonist-induced pituitary downregulation results in very low LH levels, ovarian stimulation with recombinant FSH leads to very low estradiol levels and low pregnancy rates.

Recombinant LH is currently in its final stages of development; its marketing is anticipated in the near future.

Indications

The principal indication for gonadotropins is failure of PCOS patients to respond to antiestrogen therapy, mainly CC. In daily clinical practice, gonadotropins are also used in other situations:

1. Failure to achieve pregnancy with antiestrogens in PCOS patients, despite a favorable ovarian response leading to ovulation
2. Controlled ovarian stimulation before intrauterine insemination in "unexplained" or "mild male" infertility
3. Controlled ovarian stimulation for IVF
4. Treatment of male or female hypogonadotropic hypogonadism

Dose

The individualized treatment approach dictates tailoring the dose to the patient needs. The purpose of treatment in a PCOS patient is to reach ovulation of a single mature follicle (which hopefully contains a fertilizable oocyte). Consequently, a minimal starting dose is used (one ampoule, or even less), with dose increases as necessary. In contrast, the purpose of controlled ovarian stimulation in IVF is to obtain about 10 mature oocytes. In this situation, a higher starting dose is used (three ampoules). Recently, "soft" stimulation protocols have been advocated in IVF, aiming at achieving fewer oocytes, with transfer of only one or two embryos. This trend dictates a lower starting dose of only two ampoules.

Often, the starting dose is chosen based on previous performance of a given patient to gonadotropin treatment. A typical example is the high responder who needs only a minimal dose of gonadotropins for adequate response. Frequently, these patients are stimulated with a routine protocol to which they respond with a large number of growing follicles, and very high levels of E_2. A prudent approach in these situations is to abort the cycle, given a high risk of OHSS. A reduced starting dose in subsequent stimulation cycles may lead to adequate ovarian response. In contrast, a known "low responder" can be safely stimulated with four ampules a day. In other word, detailed history of previous exposure to gonadotropins is very helpful. "Fine-tuning" of the dose from cycle to cycle will maximize the chances for success.

Protocols

For the typical PCOS patient, the "chronic low-dose" protocol has gained popularity in recent years. Based on the follicular threshold concept, a low starting dose is used (50 IU daily) for up to 14 d of stimulation. If a dominant follicle is not observed, the daily dose is increased by 25–50 IU for an additional 7 d. If a follicle of ≥11 mm is observed, the dose is kept unchanged until hCG is given (when the dominant follicle is ≥17 mm).

Ovarian stimulation of cycling patients usually starts with two ampoules. The ovarian response is assessed after 4–5 d of stimulation, and dose adjustments are done. The aim of ovarian stimulation in these patients is to reach up to four follicles of adequate diameter for ovulation. A larger number of ovulating follicles may increase the risk of multiple pregnancy and OHSS. This consideration advocates "softer" stimulation with a lower starting dose, although this approach may result in a lower pregnancy rate,; however, the risk of multiple pregnancy is not eliminated *(25)*. Because the number of ovulatory follicles (≥17 mm) is not predictive of high-order multiple pregnancy, ultrasonography may not be a valuable tool in reducing the risk of this outcome. Whether peak serum E_2 concentrations can be used to reduce this risk is also questioned *(25)*. The conclusion is that in these cases, pregnancy is a statistical event; therefore, patients must be aware that complications (i.e., multiple pregnancy and OHSS) cannot be totally eliminated. A practical approach may be to prefer IVF to IUI *(25)*, because it offers a higher pregnancy rate and leaves the decision of how many embryos to transfer to the uterus in the hands of the couple and the treating physician.

Gonadotropins in IVF are usually given after pituitary downregulation is established with a GnRH agonist. The usual starting dose is three ampoules, although deviations based on patients characteristics are common. If a GnRH antagonist is used, ovarian stimulation is started on d 2 or 3 of the cycle, and the antagonist is added after 5 d of stimulation or when the leading follicle reaches a diameter of 14 mm.

Preparations

The use of gonadotropins in fertility treatment became widespread when large-scale industrial production from urine collected from postmenopausal women was established. The relative biological activity of LH and FSH (75 IU each) was not changed from those early days. The product is sold today by manufacturers under different trade names (Pergonal®, Humegon®, Menogon®, and others). Further chemical purification steps have resulted in the production of urinary-derived FSH, sold under the names Metrodin®, Metrodin HP® (highly purified), and others. Parallel to the global trend of using recombinant DNA technology to synthesize human peptides, recombinant human FSH became available in the mid-1990s. Preparations like Puregon® and Gonal-F® were extensively studied and found to be safe and effective *(26)*. Recombinant LH was also synthesized and used successfully in the experimental setting *(27)*; its marketing debut is expected soon.

Monitoring

Objective assessment of ovarian response to gonadotropins relies on blood hormonal levels and ultrasound. The purpose of monitoring is to achieve the degree of ovarian stimulation that suits the individual patient needs. This may range from a single growing follicle in a PCOS with patient up to 10 mature follicles in an IVF case. In most cases, E_2 measurement after the fourth gonadotropin dose is used. A transvaginal ultrasound scan with a high-frequency probe allows for detailed and accurate assessment of the ovarian response. In addition, ultrasound is used to document the endometrial response to ovarian stimulation. Gonadotropin dosage is changed based on those two parameters. hCG (5000–10,000IU) is frequently given to trigger ovulation when the leading follicle reaches a diameter of ≥18 mm. A spontaneous LH surge may occur (in cycles during which a GnRH agonist or antagonist are not used to neutralize the pituitary). Therefore, if accurate timing of ovulation is needed (to plan IUI), P and LH measurements are obtained as the patient approaches the presumed ovulation date. If an oocyte-retrieval procedure is planned (i.e., for IVF), hCG is given 35 h before the procedure.

It is the responsibility of the treating fertility expert to minimize the risk of OHSS based on the monitoring plan and his best clinical judgment. If in her or his best judgment the patient is at risk, the cycle should be aborted and a new one planned. In this case, intercourse should be avoided, because if pregnancy is achieved, OHSS is a threat even though hCG was not given.

In most cases, luteal phase support is not needed; therefore, scheduled monitoring is not indicated. In high-risk situations for OHSS, the patient is instructed to limit physical activity until the results of the cycle are known and to report any symptoms that may indicate the development of OHSS.

In failed cycles, menses occurs earlier than expected based on a 14-d luteal phase duration. To avoid redundant and meaningless pregnancy tests, a blood hCG level is taken if menses does not occur 14 d after IUI (or scheduled intercourse).

Outcomes

Most PCOS patients (up to 95%) will respond to gonadotropin treatment. Stimulation cycles in these patients will yield one or two ovulatory follicles if a gentle, patient approach is used. Once ovulation is achieved, about a 20% clinical pregnancy rate is expected per ovulatory cycle. This rate decreases with the patient's age. A 30% early (≤12 wk), pregnancy loss can be expected. If three or more leading follicles are observed serious consideration should be given to aborting the cycle because of the risks of OHSS and multiple pregnancy.

In other indications for gonadotropin treatment, multifollicular response is commonly achieved; the pregnancy rate depends on other variables (i.e., patient age, sperm quality, history of previous pregnancy, anatomical or mechanical pelvic anomalies). Generally speaking, a 15% pregnancy rate per cycle can be expected.

PREMATURE OVARIAN FAILURE

Premature ovarion failure (POF) is a major source of frustration for both the patient and the fertility expert. Although numerous etiologies are known for this condition (iatrogenic, infections, genetic, autoimmune), in most cases we are left with an idiopathic condition, facing a wide choice of treatments and protocols with a narrow chance for success.

Meaningful success rates in POF patients can only be obtained using donated oocytes. This sad truth should be conveyed honestly to the patient, before embarking on any stimulation protocol. Most patients may choose to "role the dice" for the slim chance of having their own genetic child. For those patients, a wide range of treatment protocols have been advocated, some of which were tested in controlled studies (28). The following therapeutic maneuvers try to enhance follicular recruitment and growth:

1. Suppression of pituitary FSH with estrogens and/or GnRH-a followed by ovarian stimulation (rebound phase)
2. Initiation of ovarian stimulation with GnRH-a followed by gonadotropins (the "flare" effect)
3. High doses of gonadotropins
4. Immune suppression with corticosteroids

The combined data of observational and controlled studies indicate that a POF patient has a 5–10% of conceiving after the diagnosis is made. Unfortunately, there is no evidence, at this stage, that any treatment can improve this pregnancy rate (28).

REFERENCES

1. Webster J, Piscitelli G, Polli A, et al. A Comparison of cabergoline and bromocriptine in the treatment of hyperprolactinemic amenorrhea. N Engl J Med 1994;331:904–909.
2. Verhelst J, Abs R, Maiter D, et al. Cabergoline in the treatment of hyperprolactinemia: a study in 455 patients. J Clin Endocrinol Metab 1999;84:2518–2522.
3. Webster J. A comparative review of the tolerability profiles of dopamine agonists in the treatment of hyperprolactinaemia and inhibition of lactation. Drug Saf 1996;14:342.
4. Colao A, Di Sarno A, Sarnacchiaro F, et al. Prolactinomas resistant to standard dopamine agonists respond to chronic cabergoline treatment. J Clin Endocrinol Metab 1997;82: 876–883.
5. Christian GM, Randolph JF, Kelch RP, Marshall JC. Reduction of GnRH pulse frequency is associated with subsequent selective FSH secretion in women with polycystic ovarian disease. J Clin Endocrinol Metab 1991;72:1278–1285.
6. Hopkins CC, Hall JE, Santoro NF, et al. Closed intravenous administration of gonadotropin releasing hormone (GnRH): safety of extended peripheral intravenous catheterization. Obstet Gynecol 1989;74:267–270.
7. Schriock ED, Jaffe RB. Induction of ovulation with gonadotropin-releasing hormone. Ob Gyn Sur 1986;41:414–423.
8. Martin K, Santoro N, Hall J, et al. Management of ovulatory disorders with pulsatile gonadotropin-releasing hormone. J Clin Endocrinol Metab 1990;71:1081A–1081G.
9. Crowley Jr. WF, McArthur JW. Stimulation of the normal menstrual cycle in Kallmann's syndrome by pulsatile administration of luteinizing hormone-releasing hormone (LHRH). J Clin Endocrinol Metab 1988;66:327.
10. Filicori M, Santoro N, Merriam GR and Crowley Jr. WF. Characterization of the physiologic pattern of episodic gonadotropin secretion throughout the human menstrual cycle. J Clin Endocrinol Metab 1986;62:1136–1144.
11. Filicori M, Flamigni C, Meriggiola MC, et al. Ovulation induction with pulsatile gonadotropin-releasing hormone: technical modalities and clinical perspectives. Fertil Steril 1991;56:1–12.
12. Filicori M, Flamigni C, Dellai P, et al. Treatment of anovulation with pulsatile gonadotropin-releasing hormone: prognostic factors and clinical results in 600 cycles. J Clin Endocrinol Metab 1994;79:1215–1220.
13. Hopkins CC, Hall JE, Santoro NF, at al. Closed intravenous administration of gonadotropin releasing hormone (GnRH): safety of extended peripheral intravenous catheterization. Obstet Gynecol 1989; 74:267–270.
14. Smith YR, Randolph JF Jr, Christman GM, et al. Comparison of low-technology and high technology monitoring of clomiphene citrate ovulation induction. Fertil Steril 1998;70:165–168.
15. Boostanfar R, jain JK, Mishell DR Jr, Paulson RJ. A prospective randomized trial comparing clomiphene citrate with tamoxifen citrate for ovulation induction. Fertil Steril 2001;75:1024–1026.

16. Mitwally MF, Casper RF. Use of aromatase inhibitor for induction of ovulation in patients with an inadequate response to clomiphene citrate. Fertil Steril 2001;75:305–309.
17. Randall JM, Templeton A. Transvaginal sonographic assessment of follicular and endometrial growth in spontaneous and clomiphene citrate cycles. Fertil Steril 1991;56:208–212.
18. Unfer V, Costabile L, Gerli S, et al. Low dose of ethinyl estradiol can reverse the antiestrogenic effects of clomiphene citrate on endometrium. Gynecol Obstet Invest 2001;51:120–123.
19. Nestler JE, Jakubowicz DJ, Evans WS, Pasquali R. Effects of metformin on spontaneous and clomiphene-induced ovulation in polycystic ovary syndrome. N Engl J Med 1998;338:1876–1880.
20. Mitwally MF, Kuscu NK, Yalcinkaya TM. High ovulatory rates with use of troglitazone in clomiphene-resistant women with polycystic ovary syndrome. Hum Reprod 1999;14:2700–2703.
21. Vendermolen DT, Ratts VS, Evans WS, et al. Metformin increases the ovulatory rate and pregnancy rate from clomiphene citrate in patients with polycystic ovary syndrome who are resistant to clomiphene citrate alone. Fertil Steril 2001;75:310–315.
22. Ng EHY, Wat NM, Ho PC. Effects of metformin on ovulation rate, hormonal and metabolic profiles in women with clomiphene-resistant polycystic ovaries: a randomized, double-blind placebo controlled trial. Hum Reprod 2001;16:1625–1631.
23. Lewit N, Kol S, Manor D, Itskovitz-Eldor J. Comparison of GnRH analogs and hCG for the induction of ovulation and prevention of ovarian hyperstimulation syndrome (OHSS): a case-control study. Hum Reprod 1996;11:1399–1402.
24. Ben-Chetrit A, Eldar-Geva T, Gal M, Huerta M, Mimon T, Algur N, Diamant YZ, Margalioth EJ. The questionable use of albumin for the prevention of ovarian hyperstimulation syndrome in an IVF programme: a randomized placebo-controlled trial. Hum Reprod 2001;16:1880–1884.
25. Gleicher N, Oleske DM, Tur-Kaspa, I, et al. Reducing the risk of high-order multiple pregnancy after ovarian stimulation with gonadotropins. N Engl J Med 2000;343:2–7.
26. Out HJ, Mannaerts BMJL, Driessen SGAJ, Coelingh Bennink HJT, for the European Puregon collaborative IVF study group. A prospective, randomized assessor-blind, multicenter study comparing recombinant and urinary follicle-stimulating hormone (Puregon vs. Metrodin) in in-vitro fertilization. Hum Reprod 1995;10:2534–2540.
27. The European Recombinant LH Study Group. Human recombinant luteinizing hormone is as effective as, but safer than, urinary human chorionic gonadotropin in inducing final follicular maturation and ovulation in in vitro fertilization procedures: results of a multicenter double-blind study. J Clin Endocrinol Metab 2001;86:2607–2618.
28. van Kasteren YM, Schoemaker J. Premature ovarian failure: a systematic review of therapeutic interventions to restore ovarian function and achieve pregnancy. Hum Reprod Update 1999;5:483–492.

INDEX

From: *Contemporary Endocrinology: Endocrine Replacement Therapy in Clinical Practice*
Edited by: A.W. Meikle © Humana Press, Totowa, NJ